Clinical Epigenetics

Clinical Epigenetics

Editor: Augustus Drew

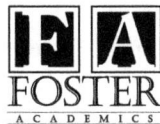

FA
FOSTER
ACADEMICS

www.fosteracademics.com

www.fosteracademics.com

FA
FOSTER
ACADEMICS

Cataloging-in-Publication Data

Clinical epigenetics / edited by Augustus Drew.
    p. cm.
Includes bibliographical references and index.
ISBN 978-1-63242-699-4
1. Epigenetics. 2. Medical genetics. 3. Human genetics. I. Drew, Augustus.
RB155 .C55 2019
616.042--dc23

Foster Academics,
118-35 Queens Blvd., Suite 400,
Forest Hills, NY 11375, USA

ISBN 978-1-63242-699-4 (Hardback)

Contents

Preface

The study of heritable phenotype changes which do not involve alterations in the DNA sequence is known as epigenetics. It involves the changes affecting gene activity and expression. Some common mechanisms which alter gene expression without altering the underlying DNA sequence include histone modification and DNA methylation. The action of repressor proteins which attach to silencer regions of the DNA, aids in controlling gene expression. The process of cellular differentiation is a common example of epigenetic change in the eukaryotes. Other epigenetic processes include position effect, gene silencing, paramutation, transvection, bookmarking, imprinting, X chromosome inactivation, the progress of carcinogenesis, etc. This book elucidates new techniques and their applications in a multidisciplinary manner. It elucidates the concepts and innovative models around prospective developments with respect to clinical epigenetics. As this field is emerging at a rapid pace, the contents of this book will help the readers understand the modern concepts and applications of the subject.

Various studies have approached the subject by analyzing it with a single perspective, but the present book provides diverse methodologies and techniques to address this field. This book contains theories and applications needed for understanding the subject from different perspectives. The aim is to keep the readers informed about the progresses in the field; therefore, the contributions were carefully examined to compile novel researches by specialists from across the globe.

Indeed, the job of the editor is the most crucial and challenging in compiling all chapters into a single book. In the end, I would extend my sincere thanks to the chapter authors for their profound work. I am also thankful for the support provided by my family and colleagues during the compilation of this book.

Editor

Epigenome-wide DNA methylation regulates cardinal pathological features of psoriasis

Aditi Chandra[1], Swapan Senapati[2], Sudipta Roy[3], Gobinda Chatterjee[4] and Raghunath Chatterjee[1*]

Abstract

Background: Psoriasis is a chronic inflammatory autoimmune skin disorder. Several studies suggested psoriasis to be a complex multifactorial disease, but the exact triggering factor is yet to be determined. Evidences suggest that in addition to genetic factors, epigenetic reprogramming is also involved in psoriasis development. Major histopathological features, like increased proliferation and abnormal differentiation of keratinocytes, and immune cell infiltrations are characteristic marks of psoriatic skin lesions. Following therapy, histopathological features as well as aberrant DNA methylation reversed to normal levels. To understand the role of DNA methylation in regulating these crucial histopathologic features, we investigated the genome-wide DNA methylation profile of psoriasis patients with different histopathological features.

Results: Genome-wide DNA methylation profiling of psoriatic and adjacent normal skin tissues identified several novel differentially methylated regions associated with psoriasis. Differentially methylated CpGs were significantly enriched in several psoriasis susceptibility (PSORS) regions and epigenetically regulated the expression of key pathogenic genes, even with low-CpG promoters. Top differentially methylated genes overlapped with PSORS regions including S100A9, SELENBP1, CARD14, KAZN and PTPN22 showed inverse correlation between methylation and gene expression. We identified differentially methylated genes associated with characteristic histopathological features in psoriasis. Psoriatic skin with Munro's microabscess, a distinctive feature in psoriasis including parakeratosis and neutrophil accumulation at the stratum corneum, was enriched with differentially methylated genes involved in neutrophil chemotaxis. Rete peg elongation and focal hypergranulosis were also associated with epigenetically regulated genes, supporting the reversible nature of these characteristic features during remission and relapse of the lesions.

Conclusion: Our study, for the first time, indicated the possible involvement of DNA methylation in regulating the cardinal pathophysiological features in psoriasis. Common genes involved in regulation of these pathologies may be used to develop drugs for better clinical management of psoriasis.

Keywords: Differentially methylated probes, Methylation-sensitive PCR, Bisulfite cloning and sequencing, Gene expression, Histopathology of psoriasis, Munro's microabscess, Rete peg elongation, Kogoj's abscess

Background

Psoriasis is a chronic inflammatory skin disease suggested to be mediated by complex interaction of genetic, epigenetic and environmental factors [1]. The disease prevalence is estimated to be between 0.2 and 11.8% across different population worldwide [2, 3]. It is characterised by hyper proliferation and abnormal differentiation of keratinocytes, manifested as distinct elevated dry red scaly plaques on skin surface. The epidermal changes are thought to be preceded by a faulty immune activation, mainly mediated by T cells [4]. Genome-wide association and linkage-based studies have identified several psoriasis susceptibility regions (PSORS) predisposing to the disease [1, 5–9]. However, many of them failed to be replicated in other populations, except HLA-Cw6 allele in patients with age of disease onset below 40 years [10–18].

Despite the different genetic backgrounds, basic phenotypic presentation of the disease remains essentially similar across different populations. Studies on

* Correspondence: rchatterjee@isical.ac.in
[1]Human Genetics Unit, Indian Statistical Institute, 203 B. T. Road, Kolkata, West Bengal 700108, India
Full list of author information is available at the end of the article

monozygotic twins showed that disease concordance is about 35–72% [19], thereby indicating the involvement of epigenetics in addition to the genetic susceptibility factors. Among all epigenetic mechanisms, DNA methylation has been reported to be one of the important factors for keratinocyte differentiation [20, 21]. It has been reported that the commonly used drug in psoriasis, e.g. methotrexate, can interfere with methyl transfer function of folate, thereby reverting to normal methylation state [22]. The reversible and relapsing nature of the disease again indicates involvement of epigenetic anomalies in psoriasis pathogenesis [1].

Histopathologic features including abnormal retention of nuclei in keratinocytes of stratum corneum (parakeratosis), aggregation of neutrophils in the parakeratotic stratum corneum (Munro's microabscess), unevenly thickened epidermis with elongated rete ridges, absence of granular layer (hypogranulosis) or locally thickened granular layer (focal hypergranulosis), occasional aggregation of neutrophils along with spongiosis in stratum spinosum (called spongiform pustules of Kogoj or Kogoj's abscess), dilated and tortuous blood vessels in the dermis and perivascular collection of immune cells are frequently observed in psoriasis.

Recent studies on skin tissues and peripheral blood mononuclear cells (PBMCs) of psoriasis patients established significant role of DNA methylation in disease pathogenesis [23–33]. Aberrant methylation and inversely correlated expression was shown for genes including demethylation of promoter2 of SHP-1 or protein tyrosine phosphatase non-receptor 6 (PTPN6) [23], hypermethylation of p16 [24] and secreted frizzled-related protein 4 (SFRP4) [25], hypomethylation of inhibitor of DNA binding 4 (ID4) [26] and 2′-5′-oligoadenylate synthetase 2 (OAS2) [27]. Overexpression of DNA methyltransferase 1 (DNMT1) and global hypermethylation was also reported in psoriatic tissues and PBMCs of psoriasis patients [28]. LINE-1 repeat elements were reported to be hypomethylated disrupting neighbouring gene expression in psoriatic tissue [29]. Genome-wide DNA methylation studies showed aberrant methylation in psoriatic skin tissue [30–33], which was reversed back to normal upon treatment [30, 33].

Several studies have reported reversal of aberrant DNA methylation [30, 33] as well as resolving of histopathological

features associated with psoriasis following therapy [34]. However, there had not been any report addressing if there is any association between the altered DNA methylation and crucial histopathological features observed in psoriasis. We have shown for the first time that DNA methylation regulates the expression of genes associated with key histopathologic features of psoriasis. We also report genome-wide DNA methylation alterations between psoriatic and adjacent normal skin tissue for the first time in Indian population. We report here that aberrant DNA methylation in psoriatic skins was significantly enriched in several PSORS regions and may affect the expression of key pathogenic genes. We further show that DNA methylation at the CpG-poor promoters can inversely regulate downstream gene expression.

Results

Characterisation of the differentially methylated probes (DMPs)

We conducted a genome-wide DNA methylation profiling of psoriatic and adjacent normal skin tissues from 24 patients belonging to Eastern Indian population (Table 1). Differentially methylated probes (DMPs) were identified using β values that were at least 15% differential ($|\Delta\beta| >$ 0.15) between disease and adjacent normal tissues with false discovery rate (FDR)-adjusted P value ≤ 0.05. In total, 4133 CpG sites were differentially methylated in disease compared to adjacent normal tissues (Additional file 1). Approximately 62% ($N = 2578$) of the DMPs were hypermethylated, while only 38% ($N = 1555$) were hypomethylated in disease tissues. Genomic distribution of the DMPs showed that they were mainly enriched in the introns, followed by promoters and intergenic regions (Fig. 1a,b). The distribution was similar for both hyper- and hypomethylated DMPs (Additional file 2: Figure S1a). Hypermethylation in all these regions is more prevalent than hypomethylation (Fig. 1b), as also observed previously [31], suggesting a trend towards global hypermethylation in psoriatic tissues. Unsupervised hierarchical clustering showed distinct classification of normal and disease samples (Fig. 1c). Highest enrichment of DMPs was observed in intronic regions (41%), followed by promoters (28%). Note that the 450k array design includes highest number of probes in the promoters, followed by intron and intergenic regions (Additional file 2: Figure S1b). Around 11%

Table 1 Demographic characteristics of discovery and validation cohort samples

Study subjects	Discovery cohort: 48 (24 paired) samples	Validation cohort: 30 (15 paired) samples
Mean age (in years)	37.94 (SD = 14.24) (range 12–74)	39.83 (SD = 10.77) (range 22–60)
Mean age of onset (in years)	33.17 (SD = 14.03) (range 10–73)	33.12 (SD = 11.21) (range 9–52)
Type I–type II	19–5	10–5
Type I–type II: age distribution	Mean age/onset 32.4/28.3	Mean age/onset 34.05/26.83
	Mean age/onset 54/51.5	Mean age/onset 51.4/45.7
Sex distribution	18 males, 6 females	10 males, 5 females

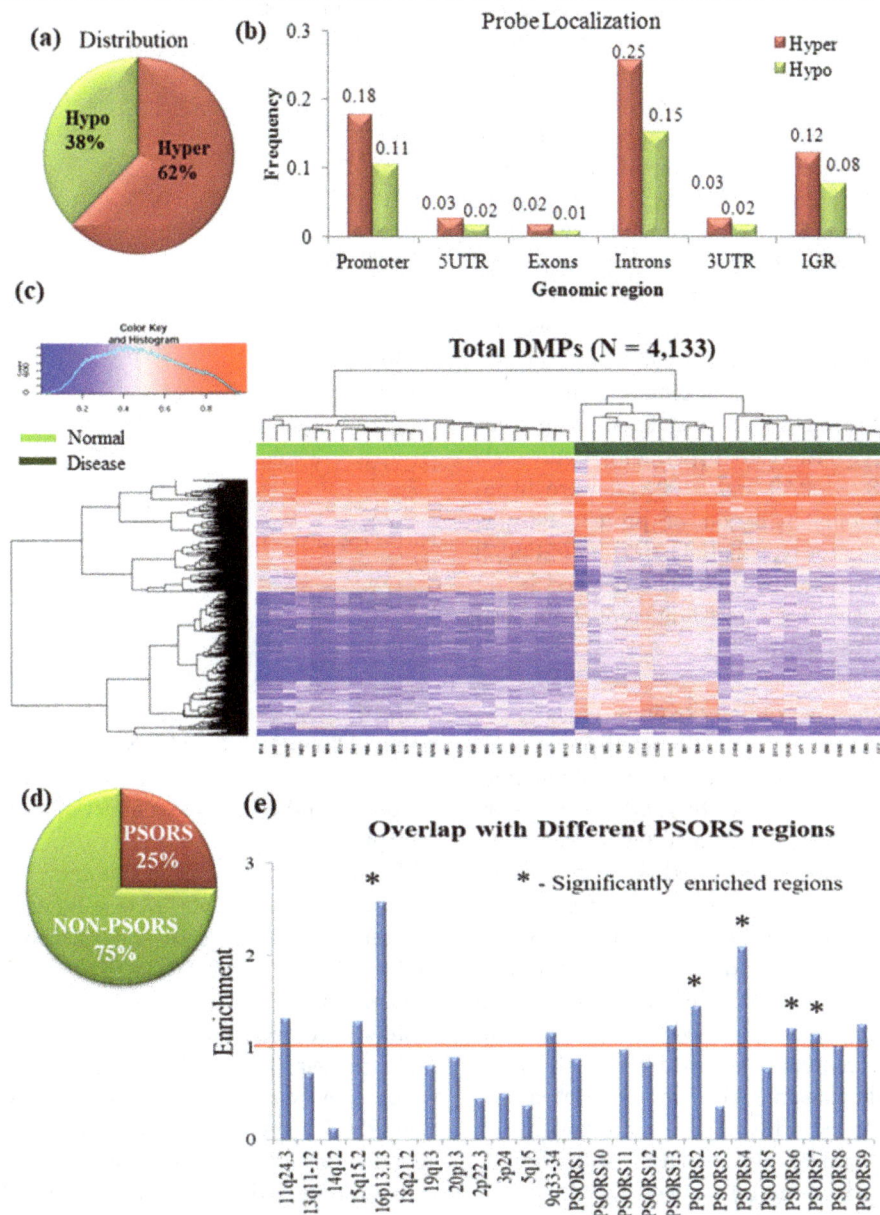

Fig. 1 Characterisation of differentially methylated probes (DMPs) (N = 4133). **a** Classification of the DMPs into hyper- and hypomethylated probes. **b** Distribution of the hyper- and hypomethylated probes across different genomic regions. **c** Hierarchical clustering with 4133 DMPs shows distinctly separate clusters for disease and adjacent normal samples. Normal samples are marked in light green, and disease samples are marked in dark green. **d** Overlap of DMPs with psoriasis susceptibility regions (PSORS) and non-PSORS. **e** Distribution of PSORS-overlapping DMPs across various known PSORS loci. Loci significantly enriched (P value ≤ 0.05) in hypergeometric test are marked (*)

of the DMPs were overlapped with repeat elements, and most of these DMPs were primarily enriched in the introns (45%) (Additional file 2: Figure S1c-d). Contrary to the overall distributions, DMPs overlapped with the repeat elements had higher frequency of hypomethylated CpGs than the hypermethylated CpGs (Additional file 2: Figure S1c). LINE elements contain largest proportion of hypomethylated sites (Additional file 2: Figure S1e).

Even though the majority of differential sites (58%) were in CpG-poor open sea regions, CpG islands (CGIs) and associated regions (CGI shores and shelves) showed higher degree of hypermethylation (47%) than hypomethylation (35%) (Additional file 2: Figure S2a-b). Unlike hypomethylated CGI shores, hypermethylated CGI shores were significantly differentially methylated, while shelves were not differential at all (Additional file 2: Figure S2c).

In order to identify the involvement of DNA methylation in regulating genes within psoriasis susceptibility regions, we determined DMPs that were overlapped with PSORS regions. A significant proportion (P value 5.1×10^{-3}) of DMPs ($N = 1040$) were overlapped with the PSORS loci (Fig. 1d). Significant enrichment was observed for PSORS2, PSORS4, PSORS6, PSORS7 and locus at 16p13.13 (Fig. 1e). On closer look at the differential sites, we observed that several of them were located at promoters of known psoriasis susceptibility genes. This include promoters of the shorter isoform of caspase recruitment domain family member 14 (CARD14) (in PSORS2) and several S100 calcium-binding genes (S100 A3, S100A5, S100A13) in epidermal differentiation complex (in PSORS4), which were hypermethylated, while others, e.g. S100A8, S100A9 and S100A12, were hypomethylated. The promoter region of protein tyrosine phosphatase non-receptor type 22 (PTPN22) (in PSORS7) showed significant hypomethylation. The detailed list of PSORS associated genes that showed differential methylation is presented in Additional file 3.

Differential methylation in promoter regions

We next identified the differentially methylated promoters and evaluated their downstream gene regulation. Approximately 29% ($N = 1168$) of the DMPs were overlapped with 764 promoters (Additional file 4). Hierarchical clustering using differentially methylated promoters classified normal and disease samples into two distinct clusters (Additional file 2: Figure S3a). Similar to the DMPs, 59% ($N = 451$) of the differentially methylated promoters were hypermethylated, while the remaining 41% ($N = 313$) were hypomethylated. Around 57% of hypermethylated promoters overlapped with CGI or associated regions, whereas only 33% hypomethylated promoters were overlapped with CGIs (Additional file 2: Figure S3b). Gene ontology (GO) analysis with the differentially methylated promoters showed enrichment of biological processes including regulation of immune system process, T cell activation, regulation of cell adhesion, regulation of leukocyte activation, inflammatory response, leukocyte and neutrophil migration among the top enriched processes (Table 2, Additional file 5: Table S1). Several genes reported to be involved in psoriasis pathogenesis including S100A9, S100A8, PTPN22, PTPN6, LAMA4, IL1B and IL12RA were involved in many of these enriched biological processes (Additional file 5: Table S1). On classification into hyper- and hypomethylated promoters, the hypermethylated promoters showed enrichment of biological processes including cellular development and differentiation, actin cytoskeletal organisation, cell adhesion and motility, while hypomethylated promoters showed enrichment of immune-activation processes including inflammation, T

Table 2 List of top enriched biological processes identified from gene ontology study with the differential promoters

GO term: biological process	Gene count (%)	Fold enrichment	P value (BH)
Regulation of immune system process	14.11	2.11	4.40×10^{-9}
T cell activation	6.31	2.91	4.90×10^{-7}
Regulation of cell adhesion	7.81	2.50	6.89×10^{-7}
Regulation of leukocyte activation	5.71	2.51	4.38×10^{-5}
Inflammatory response	7.66	2.48	1.11×10^{-6}
Cell migration	12.76	2.22	5.20×10^{-9}
Regulation of cell migration	7.21	2.17	7.15×10^{-5}
Leukocyte migration	5.40	2.96	2.77×10^{-6}
Neutrophil migration	2.40	5.26	2.86×10^{-5}
Positive regulation of MAPK cascade	5.56	2.36	1.85×10^{-4}
Extracellular matrix organisation	3.90	2.41	3.43×10^{-3}

cell activation, cytokine production and cellular proliferation (Additional file 6: Table S1).

Validation and downstream effect of promoter methylation

Differentially methylated promoters, obtained from the genome-wide array data, were validated in an independent set of paired disease and adjacent normal samples (Table 1). For the validation study, we included 10 promoters that had at least 3 DMPs. Among these, 8 promoters were overlapped with PSORS regions, while zinc finger protein (ZNF106) and signalling lymphocytic activation molecule family member 1 (SLAMF1) were outside PSORS regions. Cloning and sequencing of the bisulfite-converted products showed concordant results with genome-wide array data. Similar degree of hypermethylation for selenium-binding protein (SELENBP1), DENN domain containing 1C (DENND1C) and hypomethylation for S100A9, PTPN22 were observed (Fig. 2a). Differential methylation of these 10 promoters was also validated using bisulfite sequencing PCR (BSP) followed by qMSP. Around 80–100% of the samples showed similar differential methylation as observed in genome-wide data (Fig. 2b, Additional file 2: Figure S3c).

To determine the effect of differential promoter methylation, we checked the downstream gene expression of these selected promoters in paired disease and adjacent normal tissue samples. Significant downregulation for hypermethylated genes SELENBP1 and ZNF106 and significant upregulation for hypomethylated genes PTPN22 and S100A9 were observed in psoriatic tissues compared to adjacent normal (Fig. 2c, Additional file 2: Figure S3d).

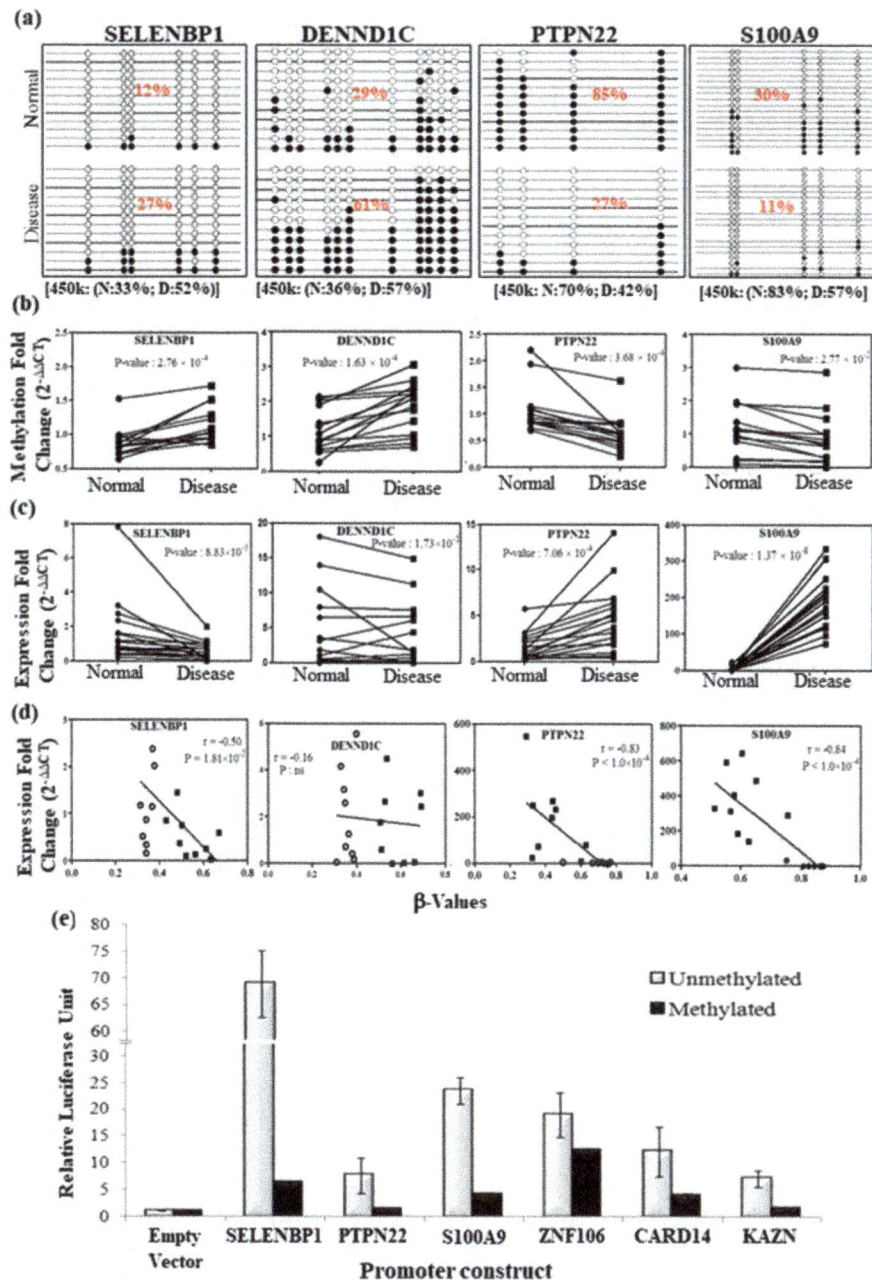

Fig. 2 Validation of differentially methylated promoters in an additional independent set of samples. **a** Graphical representation of cloning and sequencing of BSP products from adjacent normal and disease samples, for four selected promoter regions. The average promoter methylation (%) for the normal and disease samples are presented inside the figure. Average β values (%) for these selected promoters are presented at the bottom of the figure. **b** Validation of promoter methylation status in paired disease and adjacent normal samples through quantitative methylation-sensitive PCR (qMSP). **c** Gene expression fold change in disease and adjacent normal samples of corresponding genes. **d** Scatter plot showing inverse correlation between methylation level (β value) and gene expression fold change. **e** Relative luciferase expression of the unmethylated and methylated versions of the promoter constructs for selected genes. *P value ≤ 0.05

CARD14 and DENND1C also showed overall downregulation, but did not reach the level of significance at 0.05 (Fig. 2c, Additional file 2: Figure S3d). Note that there are other larger isoforms of these two genes which do not show differential promoter methylation. As the smaller isoforms had no unique exons, we could not exclusively check expression of those isoforms which harboured differentially methylated promoter. Average promoter methylation (β value) and corresponding gene expression (fold change) showed significant inverse correlation for SELENBP1 ($r = -0.5$), PTPN22 ($r = -0.83$) and S100A9 ($r = -0.84$), except for DENND1C ($r = -0.16$) (Fig. 2d).

Furthermore, in order to substantiate that the expression of these genes were actually controlled by the methylation states of their promoters, we cloned six CpG-poor promoters (SELENBP1, PTPN22, S100A9, ZNF106, CARD14, KAZN) into a CpG-less luciferase reporter vector (pCpGL) (Fig. 2e). The CpGs within the cloned promoter regions of pCpGL-promoter constructs were enzymatically methylated (Additional file 2: Figure S4), and both methylated and unmethylated plasmids were transiently transfected to the HEK293T cells. Unmethylated promoters were significantly overexpressed, while the methylated version abrogated the luciferase expression (Fig. 2e), suggesting that their aberrant expression in disease might be mediated by differential DNA methylation in psoriasis.

Epigenetic regulation of histopathological features of psoriasis

Next, we classified the patients based on the presence of key histopathologic features including Munro's microabscess, Kogoj's microabscess, elongation of rete pegs and focal hypogranulosis and determined the unique differentially methylated CpGs in the psoriatic skins associated with each of these features (Additional file 2: Figure S5, Table 3).

Significant DMPs were identified between psoriatic skin and adjacent normal tissues for the groups with and without Munro's microabscess (Table 3). We identified 831 and 48 DMPs that were uniquely differential in Munro's microabscess present and absent groups, respectively (Additional file 7). Around 1508 DMPs were commonly differential in both groups (Additional file 7). Principal component analysis (PCA) with top unique DMPs showed distinct clustering of the two groups (Fig. 3a, b). To determine the genes that might be regulated by these unique DMPs, GO analysis was performed with the promoters that were overlapped with these unique DMPs. Interestingly, the highest enrichment was observed for the neutrophil and leukocyte chemotaxis processes (Fig. 3c), indicating the epigenetic regulation of genes involved in Munro's microabscess. These processes include genes like histamine receptor H1 (HRH1), phosphodiesterase 4D (PDE4D), C-C motif chemokine ligand 25 (CCL25) and allograft inflammatory factor 1 (AIF1) (Fig. 3b). A disintegrin and metalloproteinase domain-containing

protein 10 (ADAM10), free fatty acid receptor 2 (FFAR2), interleukin 1 beta (IL1B) and triggering receptor expressed on myeloid cells 1 (TREM1), involved in neutrophil and leukocyte chemotaxis, were also differentially methylated in the psoriatic skin tissues of patients with Munro's microabscess (Additional file 5: Table S2).

Maximum length of the elongated rete pegs was measured from each patient. Correlation between maximum rete peg lengths and methylation status (β value) of the differential CpG sites were studied. We observed 391 CpG sites that showed significant correlation of methylation level with the rete peg length in the psoriatic skin (P value ≤ 0.05 and $\mid r \geq 0.4$) (Additional file 8); of these, 32 DMPs showed relatively high correlation ($\mid r \mid \geq 0.6$) (Fig. 4a). Nearest genes to these DMPs include CCAAT/enhancer binding protein alpha (CEBPA), laminin subunit alpha 4 (LAMA4) and gap junction protein gamma 2 (GJC2) (Fig. 4b; Additional file 2: Figure S6a, b; and Additional file 8).

Due to rapid proliferation and incomplete differentiation of psoriatic keratinocytes, the granular layer is absent in disease tissue. The granules appear prematurely in some samples leading to focal hypergranulosis. Analysing the samples with and without focal hypergranulosis identified 4450 unique DMPs in samples without focal hypergranulosis, while only 20 DMPs were unique in samples with focal hypergranulosis (Additional file 9). First two principal components of the PCA explained 79.3% of variations between these two groups (Fig. 4c). Genes with unique differentially hypomethylated promoters include G protein-coupled receptor 128 (GPR128) and human leukocyte antigen (HLA)-DMA, while hypermethylated promoters include macrophage stimulating 1 receptor (MST1R) and tenascin-XB (TNXB) in patients without focal hypergranulosis (Fig. 4d, Additional file 9).

Another characteristic feature, Kogoj's microabscess was detected in 9 samples, while remaining 15 samples did not show any sign of this histopathologic feature (Table 3, Additional file 2: Figure S5). On comparison of samples classified based on the presence of Kogoj's abscess, we identified 125 unique DMPs in samples containing this abscess, while only 25 DMPs were unique in the group without Kogoj's abscess (Additional file 10). These unique DMPs for the present and absent groups were mapped into 25 and 8 promoters, respectively. GO analysis identified regulation of transport and stress response processes for these genes. Nevertheless, the identified unique sites did not show separate clustering of the samples with and without Kogoj's microabscess (Fig. 5a).

Finally, we sought to identify if there are any common DMPs among the unique sets observed to be associated with different histopathological features. We identified 7 DMPs that were common between Munro's microabscess and rete peg elongation, 111 common between hypogranulosis and rete peg elongation, and 415 common between

Table 3 Histopathological characterisation of the discovery cohort samples

Histopathological parameter	Characteristics
Parakeratosis	Present: confluent- 19, focal- 3; NA: 3
Focal hypergranulosis	Present- 7, absent- 17
Munro's microabscess	Present- 11, absent- 10, NA- 3
Kogoj's microabscess	Present- 9, absent- 15
Elongation of rete pegs	Mild- 6, moderate- 14, severe- 4

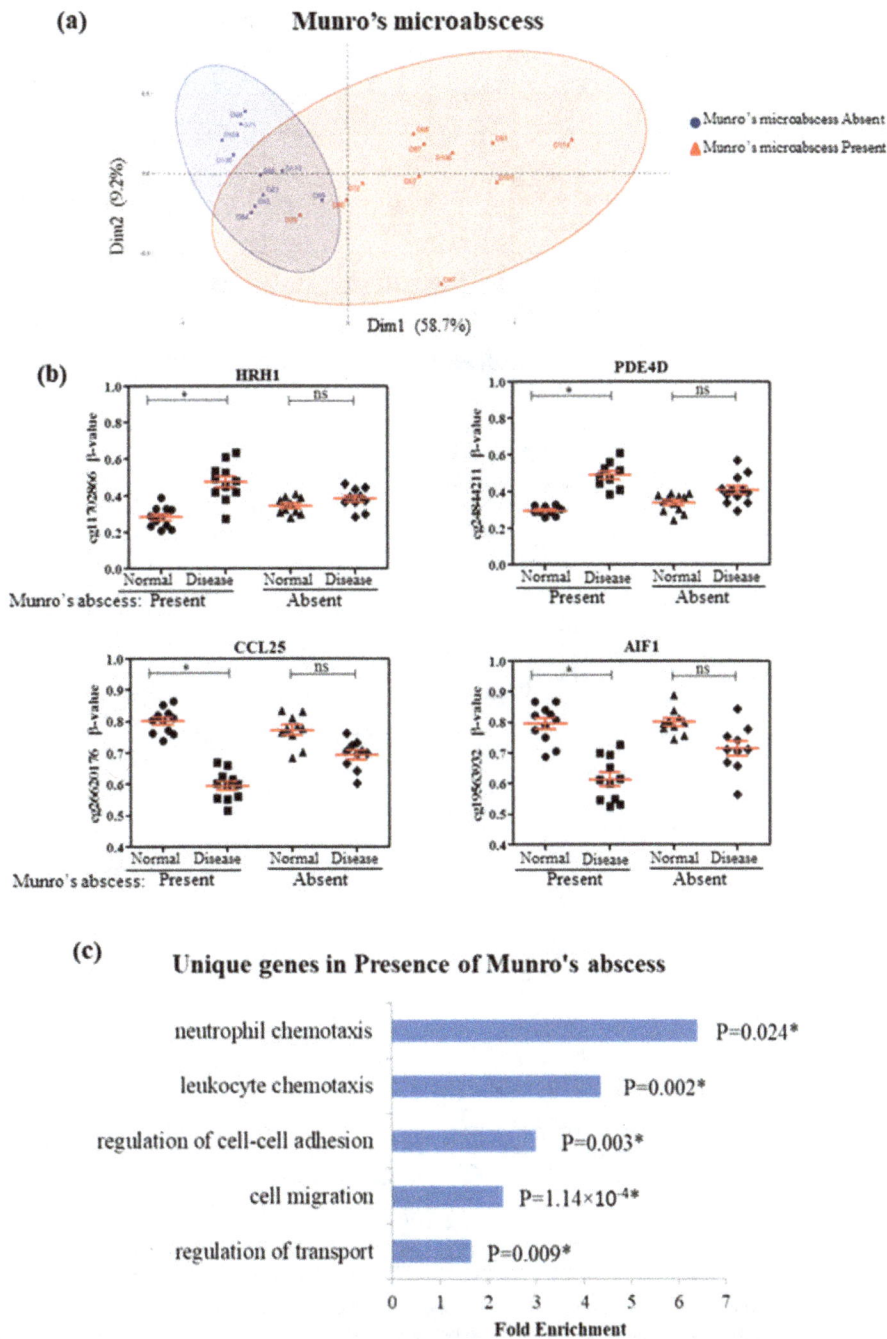

Fig. 3 DNA methylation in regulation of Munro's microabscess formation. **a** Principal component analysis (PCA) with top 100 differential CpG sites unique for Munro's abscess present samples shows distinct clusterings for samples with and without Munro's microabscess. **b** Candidate promoter-overlapping sites that are differential only in samples with Munro's microabscess but not in the other group. **c** Gene ontology study with gene promoters overlapping with unique DMPs. *P value ≤ 0.05

hypogranulosis and Munro's microabscess. However, only 6 hypermethylated probes were found to be common for all three characteristic histological features (Fig. 5b). Of these, 3 sites overlapped with promoters of synaptogyrin 1 (SYNGR1) (smaller isoform), NADH dehydrogenase 1 beta subcomplex 4 (NDUFB4) and testis-specific serine kinase 1B (TSSK1B), and two of the sites overlapped with PSORS loci.

Discussion

We have conducted a genome wide DNA methylation study among Indian psoriasis patients using Illumina Infinium Human Methylation 450k BeadChip. Twenty-four paired tissue samples were used as the discovery set. Using a cut-off of adjusted P value ≤ 0.05 and $|\Delta\beta| > 0.15$, we identified 4133 DMPs associated with psoriasis. Around

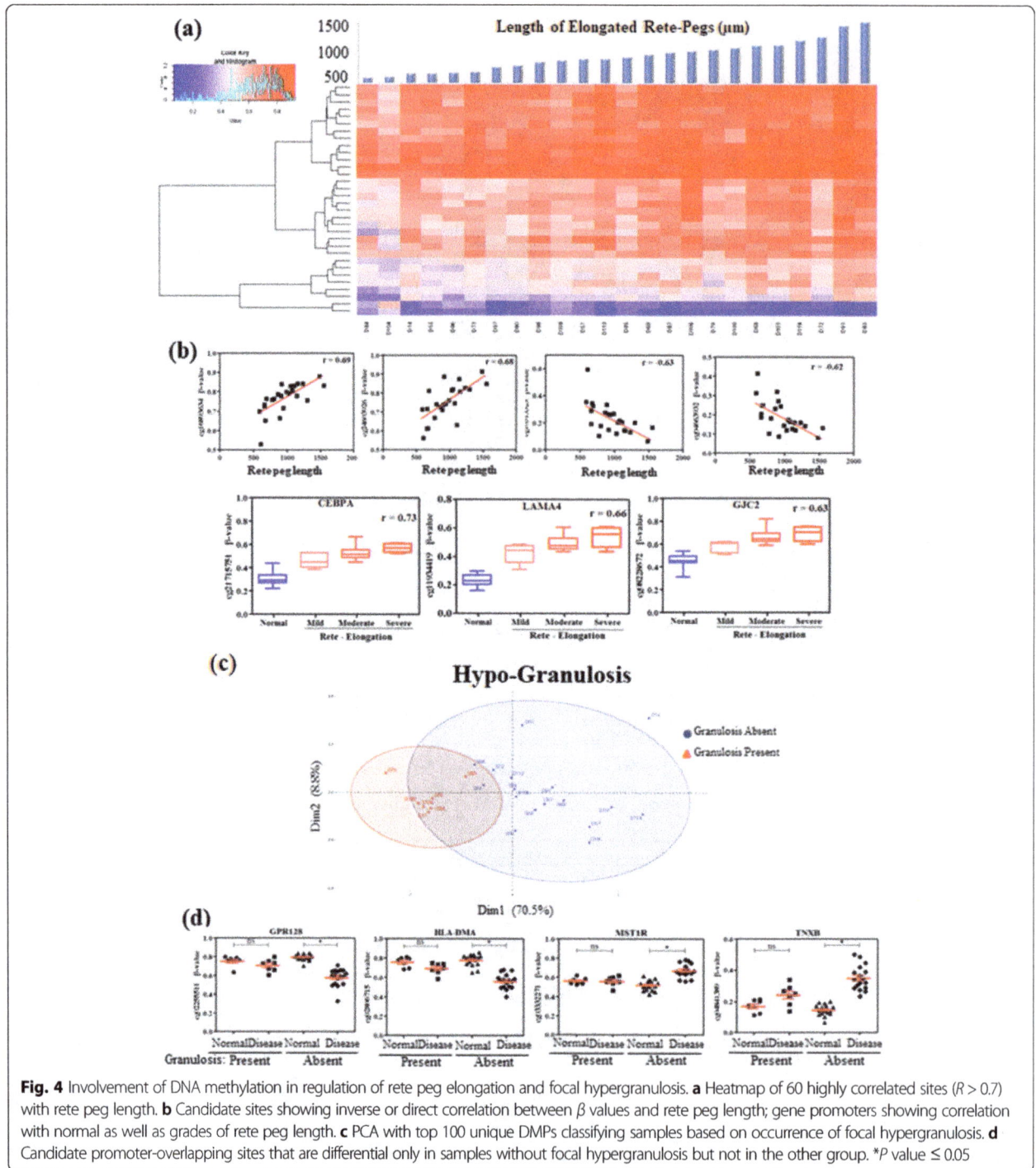

Fig. 4 Involvement of DNA methylation in regulation of rete peg elongation and focal hypergranulosis. **a** Heatmap of 60 highly correlated sites ($R > 0.7$) with rete peg length. **b** Candidate sites showing inverse or direct correlation between β values and rete peg length; gene promoters showing correlation with normal as well as grades of rete peg length. **c** PCA with top 100 unique DMPs classifying samples based on occurrence of focal hypergranulosis. **d** Candidate promoter-overlapping sites that are differential only in samples without focal hypergranulosis but not in the other group. *P value ≤ 0.05

40–50% DMPs, identified in previous studies [30, 32], which compared psoriatic and adjacent normal skin tissues, were also detected in our study. Precisely, 756 sites (including 440 hyper- and 316 hypomethylated DMPs) out of 1514 total differential sites, identified previously, were overlapped with DMPs identified in our study [32]. It is worth mentioning here that this study used 10% delta-beta cut-off ($|\Delta\beta| \geq 0.1$) and used Bonferroni correction to control for the multiple hypothesis tests [32]. Another study with Illumina Infinium Human Methylation 27k array, which used differential M values also showed ~44% (12 out 27 sites) overlap with our study [30]. Hierarchical clustering with the DMPs was able to accurately classify the normal and disease samples (Fig. 1c), again supporting the role of epigenetic alterations during psoriasis pathogenesis.

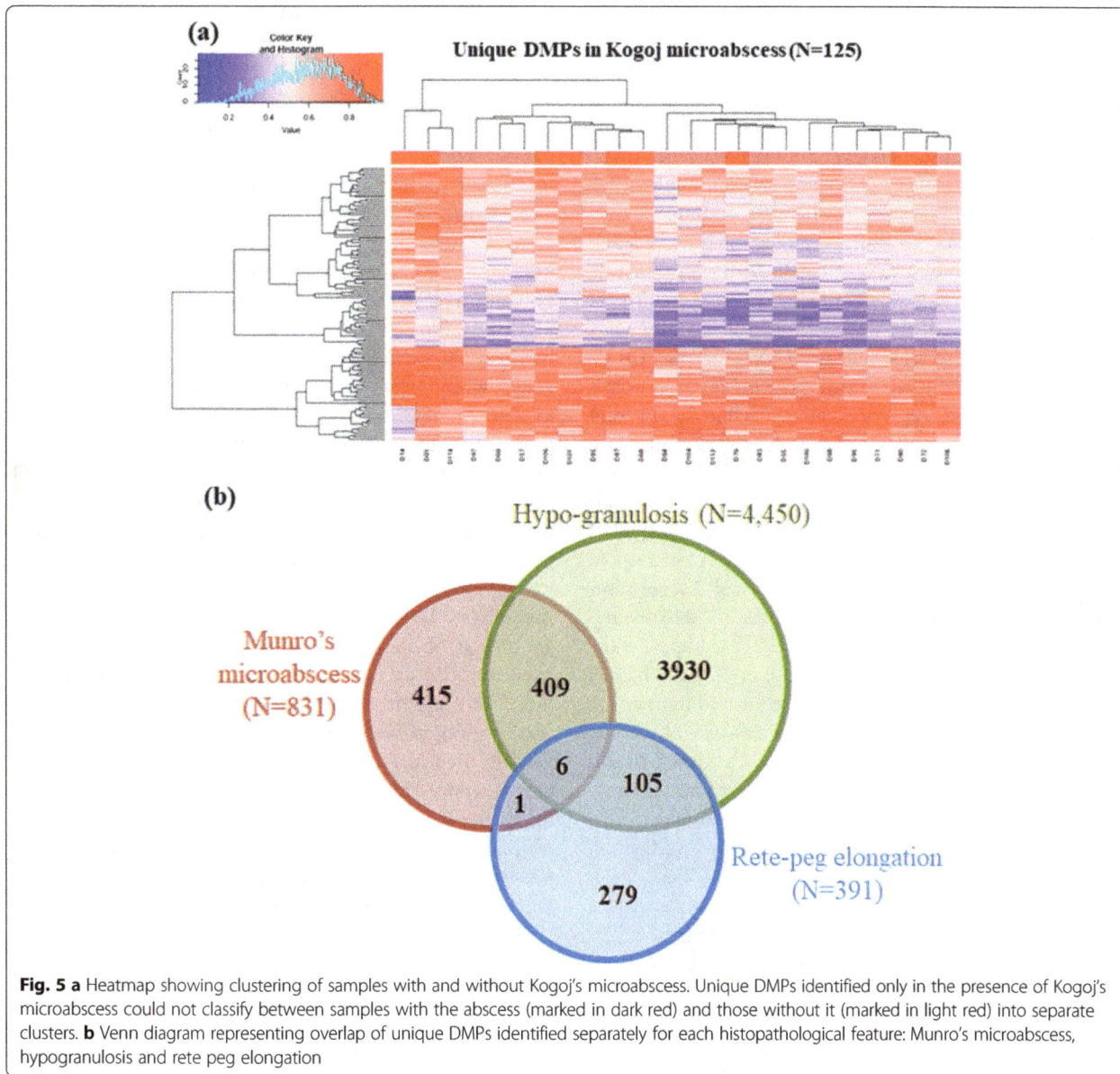

Fig. 5 a Heatmap showing clustering of samples with and without Kogoj's microabscess. Unique DMPs identified only in the presence of Kogoj's microabscess could not classify between samples with the abscess (marked in dark red) and those without it (marked in light red) into separate clusters. **b** Venn diagram representing overlap of unique DMPs identified separately for each histopathological feature: Munro's microabscess, hypogranulosis and rete peg elongation

Differential sites were mostly enriched in intronic regions, as also observed previously [31]. Introns are known to harbour different regulatory regions like enhancer elements, which might lead to an additional level of gene regulation associated with psoriasis; however, these remain mostly uncharacterised in context of psoriasis. Hypomethylation of LINE elements, observed in our study, is also supported by previous reports [29]. Higher proportion of hypermethylated probes was also commonly observed in previous studies [30, 31], while opposite result was obtained when the epidermal part was separately studied [33]. Since the epidermis is mostly enriched with keratinocytes, and LINE-1 hypomethylation was found to be restricted only to psoriatic keratinocytes [29], this can explain the opposite global

methylation pattern in the epidermis compartment. Global hypermethylation of psoriatic CD4+ T cells [35], dermal fibroblasts and contribution of other cell types, when total psoriatic skin tissues were considered, might have led to the global hypermethylation observed in our study as well as in previous studies [30, 31].

A subset of the genome-wide data was validated in an additional 15 pairs of samples using sodium bisulfite conversion followed by either sequencing of the cloned bisulfite converted product, or by quantitative methyl sensitive PCR (qMSP). Validation of some of these DMPs showed 80–100% concordance with the discovery set of samples. One may, in principle, argue to increase the $|\Delta\beta|$ cut-off to reduce the false positive rates, but simultaneously, it may also lead to missing out of the true positive signals. In the genome-wide data, when we considered $|\Delta\beta|$ cut-off > 0.3, we identified 60 DMPs, of which only 11 sites overlapped with promoters. With a $|\Delta\beta|$ cut-off > 0.2, we identified 861 DMPs (Additional file 1). In our validation study using cloning and sequencing of the bisulfite converted products, we considered 7 DMPs with $|\Delta\beta|$ between 0.15 and 0.2, 5 DMPs with $|\Delta\beta|$ between 0.2 and 0.3 and 3 DMPs with $|\Delta\beta|$ > 0.3. We observed a concordance of 80–100% for all these probes. qMSP validation in 15 additional samples comprising 38 DMPs, of which 35 had $|\Delta\beta|$ < 0.3, also showed similar results, thus confirming the reliability of DMPs obtained from the genome-wide data, and also added support to the $|\Delta\beta|$ cut-off of 0.15. We have considered total skin biopsy samples of psoriasis patients, which is a heterogeneous collection of different cell types. Number of cells of a particular cell type may also vary between normal and diseased tissues. However, due to different methylation levels of different cell types, actual differential methylation might be averaged out and missed at higher cut-offs. We have shown that these DMPs could generate distinct clusters for the normal and disease samples, thereby demonstrating the crucial role of DNA methylation in psoriasis pathogenesis (Fig. 1c). A subset of these sites showed intermediate methylation, at least in half of the samples, which might be the reflection of intermediate state of the disease or a distinct clinical sub-type of the disease. Furthermore, a high correlation of CpG methylation with the rete peg elongation is clearly evident from our analysis. Rete peg elongation increases with the state of this disease, which also indicates the possible involvement of CpG methylation with the disease progression.

For the first time, we have identified involvement of DNA methylation and key pathogenic genes that might regulate the characteristic histopathological features observed in psoriasis. Gene expression study showed inverse correlation with promoter methylation status for most of the genes, which was also evident from previous studies [19, 30, 31]. Additionally, cloning the CpG-poor promoters into CpG-less (pCpGL) luciferase vector further established the fact that only altering methylation levels of the promoter can significantly regulate the downstream gene expression (Fig. 2e). Our study showed the direct proof of silencing of gene expression through promoter methylation in case of psoriasis. Although previous studies used pGL3 vectors to demonstrate this phenomenon, but methylation of CpG sites in this vector backbone might have interfered with the results obtained [35].

Some studies have focused on psoriatic PBMCs [19, 28, 35], epidermis [33] or dermal compartments only [36], we, however, wanted to include both the epidermal and dermal compartments along with infiltrating immune cells, as all of these cell types contribute to the disease. Since DNA methylation levels can be influenced by environmental factors, we had not included unrelated healthy controls in our analysis,

whose different environmental exposure or unalike genetic background might add unnecessary differences thereby affecting data quality. In order to minimise influence of other factors, we thus compared methylation pattern of disease tissue with corresponding adjacent normal tissues from each patient. Both psoriatic and adjacent normal tissues were histopathologically analysed before considering for the genome-wide or validation studies.

Most interestingly, we observed overlapping of ~ 25% of the DMPs with PSORS loci (Fig. 1d), previously known psoriasis susceptibility regions conferring genetic predisposition to the disease. Prominent differential methylation was observed in promoter of several S100A genes within epidermal differentiation complex (EDC) located in PSORS4 (Additional file 6), complying with previous studies which also observed similar enrichment [30, 32]. Overexpression of S100A8-S100A9 has been reported in psoriatic tissue [37] and serum samples [38] as well, suggesting their prominent role in psoriasis pathogenesis. PTPN22, one of the top hypomethylated genes overlapping with PSORS7, showed inverse correlation of methylation with gene expression in our study. Although genetic association of this gene has been reported in psoriasis [39] as well as in other autoimmune diseases [40], there are no reports on its regulation by promoter methylation in psoriasis. Another top hypermethylated gene located in PSORS4, SELENBP1, has been identified in our study. This gene has not previously been reported in psoriasis. However, lower selenium levels observed in psoriasis patients [41] could be attributed to lowered expression of this gene. This suggests SELENBP1 as a potential candidate for studying the role of this gene and supplementation of this trace element in disease. Since both histopathological features and DNA methylation aberrations sometimes resolved on therapy, we wanted to study if DNA methylation could regulate these features. Due to the cell-type heterogeneity in different histopathological features, the results of differential methylation analysis are sometimes biased, which in turn increases the false positive results. Adjusting for the major cell-type compositions from the histopathological data may partially reduce the rate of false positives, however, that may substantially reduce the true positive predictions too. Here, to control the false positive rate, we have used a differential methylation threshold of $|\Delta\beta|$ > 0.15 between disease and adjacent normal tissue and a FDR-adjusted P value ≤ 0.05. Comparing the differences in methylation with respect to different histopathological features, a unique set of DMPs were observed from paired analysis of samples with Munro's microabscess, focal hypergranulosis and Kogoj microabscess. GO analysis with the unique differential promoters involved in Munro's abscess formation revealed neutrophil and leukocyte chemotaxis as the highest enriched biological processes which include genes like HRH1, PDE4D, CCL25, AIF1, ADAM10, FFAR2, IL1B and TREM1. HRH1 has been reported to promote keratinocyte proliferation, suppression of differentiation and wound healing in keratinocytes [42, 43]. IL1B has also been previously reported in proliferation and intra-epidermal microabscess in flaky skin mice [44]. Abnormal inflammation, infiltration and accumulation of neutrophils in stratum corneum, as observed in Munro's microabscess, thus, might be regulated by methylation, at least in part. This observation also adds support to our selected $\Delta\beta$ cut-off value, as differential methylation was not enriched on genes that are expressed by neutrophils, but with those that are involved in neutrophil chemotaxis, a feature that is actually observed in disease. A set of highly correlated ($|r| \geq 0.6$) methylated CpGs was identified with the rete peg elongation. Hypermethylated CpGs were observed in the promoter regions of C/EBPα, LAMA4, GJC2 and miR1178. C/EBPα has been reported to arrest cell proliferation through direct inhibition of CDK2 and CDK4 [45], while LAMA4 and GJC2 are involved in cell adhesion and differentiation. Increasing length of spinous layer with rete peg elongation thus can be attributed to the gradual hypermethylation and probable silencing of these genes.

Higher number of overlap of unique sites between Munro's microabscess and focal hypogranulosis suggests their common causal feature, i.e. both are caused due to abnormal differentiation of keratinocytes. Interestingly, the common sites observed between all three histopathological features can be important targets for disease therapeutics. Since Kogoj's abscess is a localised phenomenon, we could have easily missed particular sites containing this feature while selecting the site of biopsy. This might have limited the identification of actual genes that could regulate formation of Kogoj's microabscess and could be the possible reason for misclassification of groups with and without Kogoj's abscess. Studies from Indian population have also shown the inconsistent presence of this feature among psoriasis patients [46]. Regulation of histopathological features by DNA methylation is also established from the fact that after treatment, aberrant methylation levels revert back to normal and histopathological features resolve as well [30, 33, 34]. This observation further highlights the crucial role of DNA methylation in psoriasis pathogenesis.

Conclusions

In conclusion, our study demonstrates the significant involvement of DNA methylation in psoriasis development. It appears to control disease progression as well as involved in manifestation of characteristic histopathological features. Since DNA methylation is reversible, this also explains the dynamic nature of the disease during remission and relapse of the psoriatic plaques.

Identification of epigenetically regulated genes may be used to develop epigenetic drugs for disease management. Our study has identified a core set of DMPs and associated key molecules that are strongly involved in psoriasis pathogenesis, or presence of characteristic histopathologic features. Methylation status at these sites can be monitored and controlled to prevent disease occurrence or recurrence. These can thus be good targets for future clinical studies on psoriasis therapy. However, further validation and functional studies might be required to determine the precise clinically significant epigenetically regulated genes in psoriasis.

Methods
Study sample

Psoriasis patients ($N = 39$) were recruited from eastern region of India after obtaining written consent for participation in the study. Family history, comorbidities and other disease characteristics were recorded. Sample characteristics are summarised in Table 2. The disease was diagnosed by at least two dermatologists and confirmed by histopathological examination. Patients with generalised plaque type psoriasis were only included in the study to minimise clinical heterogeneity. Patients were kept without any systemic or topical therapy for at least 1 month prior to sample collection. Psoriatic and adjacent normal skin biopsies (4 mm) were obtained from each patient. A part of the sample was collected in formalin for histopathology; the remaining part was collected in RNA Later (Invitrogen) and stored at − 80 °C until further processing. The study was approved by the Institutional Ethics Committee for Human Research, Indian Statistical Institute, Kolkata, India and IPGMER, Kolkata, India, and conducted according to the Declaration of Helsinki Principles.

DNA methylation study and data analysis

DNA was isolated from blood and skin tissues with DNeasy Blood and Tissue kit (Qiagen, Germany) using manufacturer's instructions. Quality and concentration of each DNA sample was checked by Nanodrop Spectrophotometer (Nanodrop 2000). DNA isolated from 48 samples (24 psoriatic disease skin and 24 adjacent normal tissue) was subjected to Illumina Infinium Human Methylation 450k BeadChip, according to manufacturer's protocol. Raw data (.idat files) obtained was analysed using Chip Analysis of Methylation Pipeline (ChAMP) available as R-Bioconductor package [47, 48]. After initial pre-processing, data were normalised using beta mixture quantile (BMIQ) [49] method to correct for type 1 and type 2 probe bias. Batch effect removal was carried out using ComBat [50]. Illumina 450k bead array can profile 482,421 CpG sites, 3091 non-CpG sites and 65 random SNPs across the human genome [51, 52]. After removal of quality control probes, probes which failed to attain detection P value (cut-off ≤ 0.05), represented < 3 times in 5% samples, non-CpG probes, probes on sex chromosomes and those overlapping with polymorphic sites, we were left with 347,635 sites for downstream analysis. The batch-corrected β values were subjected to paired differential methylation analysis to identify differential probes. Differentially methylated probes (DMP) were identified using β values that were at least 15% differential ($|\Delta\beta| > 0.15$) between disease and adjacent normal tissues with FDR-adjusted P value ≤ 0.05. The co-ordinates of the PSORS regions were identified by previous studies and reviewed earlier [1]. The overlap between DMPs and PSORS loci were identified using bedtools, and significance of locus-wise enrichment was carried out using hypergeometric test in R. Heatmaps were generated using Euclidean distance and complete linkage method using heatmap.2 function available in gplots package in R.

Bisulfite sequencing PCR (BSP) and quantitative methylation-specific PCR (qMSP)

Promoters are defined in our study as 1500 bp regions, including 1000 bp upstream and 500 bp downstream from each transcription start site (TSS). We considered 10 promoters that had at least 3 DMPs for the validation. Among these, 8 promoters were overlapped with PSORS regions, while ZNF106 and SLAMF1 were outside PSORS regions. For validation of Illumina 450K methylation array data, 15 independent psoriatic and adjacent normal skin biopsy pairs were used (Table 1). Bisulfite treatment of the isolated DNA was carried out using EZ DNA Methylation Gold Kit (Zymo Research), according to manufacturer's protocol. Converted DNA samples were used for bisulfite sequencing PCR (BSP) to amplify the selected promoter regions. BSP products were cloned into TA-cloning vector pTZ57R/T (Thermo Scientific) and transformed into *E. coli* JM109 competent cells. Atleast 10 randomly selected white colonies were sequenced to determine the percentage of methylation status in normal and disease samples. Representative figure of the bisulfite converted followed by cloning and sequencing data for both disease and adjacent normal tissue DNA has been prepared using QUMA tool [53].

BSP products were also used as templates for qMSP to determine methylation fold change in disease compared to adjacent normal tissue. BSP and qMSP primers were designed using MethPrimer tool [54]. qMSP was carried out using SYBR green (iTaq Universal SYBR Green Supermix, Bio-Rad) on 7900HT Fast Real-Time PCR system (Applied Biosystems). Methylation fold change in disease tissue was calculated in comparison to normal as using $2^{-\Delta\Delta Ct}$ method as stated previously [55], with minor modifications. Instead of calculating the percent methylation from the $2^{-\Delta\Delta Ct}$, we used fold change.

Primers for BSP and qMSPs are provided in Additional file 6: Table S2.

Gene expression study

Seventeen paired samples were used to study the expression pattern of selected genes. Out of these, 9 samples overlapped with the samples used for Illumina 450k methylation array. Tissue samples were snap-frozen in liquid nitrogen and finely ground to powder. Total RNA was isolated using AllPrep DNA/RNA Mini Kit (Qiagen, Germany). RNA concentration and quality was checked with Nanodrop Spectrophotometer (Nanodrop Technologies, Wilmington, DE). One microgramme of total RNA was used for cDNA synthesis using Transcriptor First Strand cDNA synthesis kit (Roche). cDNA was diluted, and 10 ng was used in each reaction of qPCR analysis. Gene expression qPCR primers were obtained from whole transcriptome qPCR primer database available through UCSC browser [56] and were amplified using iTaq Universal SYBR Green Supermix (Bio-Rad) in 7900HT Fast Real-Time PCR system (Applied Biosystems). Gene expression was normalised to expression of RNaseP (RPP30). GAPDH was also used as endogenous control. However, since both the genes gave similar results, data for only RPP30 has been used here. Gene expression qPCR primer sequences are provided in Additional file 6: Table S3.

Cell culture

HEK293T cells were cultured in DMEM-F12 (Gluta-MAX) medium (ThermoFisher Scientific) with 10% fetal bovine serum (Gibco) and 1% antibiotic (Penicillin--Streptomycin, Gibco) and incubated in 5% CO_2 incubator at 37 °C. Cells were seeded on 24-well culture plates and grown until 80–90% confluency and changed to reduced serum media (Opti-MEM, Invitrogen), and then, transient transfection was done with the recombinant pCpGL luciferase constructs using Lipofectamine (Lipofectamine 2000, Thermo Scientific). Media were replaced with complete media after 6 h of transfection.

Luciferase reporter assay

Promoters with at least 3 differentially methylated sites were selected for luciferase reporter assay. Core promoter element (including the TSS) was cloned into the upstream MCS of CpG-less (pCpGL) luciferase vector (InvivoGen). Primers used for promoter cloning are presented in Additional file 6: Table S4. pCpGl vector does not contain any CpG sites within its backbone and includes Lucia luciferase gene. This is a synthetic form of secreted luciferase that utilises colenterazine as substrate. Promoter constructs (pCpGL-promoter) were transformed into *E. coli* GT115 (Invivogen) *pir* mutant strain that lacks Dcm methylase. Positive colonies selected with Zeocin resistance were cultured and verified by Sanger sequencing. One part of the amplified plasmid was completely methylated with CpG Methylase enzyme (M.SssI, NEB). Complete methylation was checked by digestion with methylation-sensitive restriction enzymes HpaII, AciI and HinP1I (all purchased from NEB) (Additional file 2: Figure S4). Around 200 ng of methylated and unmethylated versions of each construct and an empty vector were transfected into HEK293T cells in triplicate. Minimal promoter-pGL4.24 (Promega), which utilises luciferin substrate, was used as transfection control. Twenty-four hours after transfection, luciferase activity was measured on Glomax 20/20 luminometer (Promega). Lucia luciferase value was normalised to that of firefly luciferase, and promoter activity of the constructs was calculated as fold change over the activity of M.SssI treated and untreated empty vector.

Histological analysis

Formalin-fixed samples were cut into 2-mm thickness, and the slices were embedded in paraffin. Thin slices of 4-μm thickness were made from formalin-fixed paraffin embedded (FFPE) blocks using a microtome. After being mounted on poly-L-lysine-coated slides, and air dried, each slide was stained for haematoxylin and eosin (H&E) and covered with a cover slip using DPX mounting media and left to dry before image capture. The H&E-stained slides were used to assess overall abnormality of histopathology, including rete peg elongation, the presence of Munro's microabscesses, Kogoj's microabscesses and focal hypergranulosis (Additional file 2: Figure S5). A part of the normal tissues were also analysed histopathologically, and only histopathologically normal tissues were included in the study.

Among the 24 psoriasis samples studied in discovery set, all had characteristic histopathological features but varied only in terms of degree of rete peg elongation, the presence of Munro's microabscesses, Kogoj's microabscesses and focal hypergranulosis. In case of Munro's microabscess, 11 samples were positive, 10 samples did not show the feature, while 3 samples could not be studied due to loss of stratum corneum during histopathological processing. The presence of granular layer along with focal hypergranulosis was observed in 7 samples, while others lacked this feature (Table 3). As in most of the cases, there are comparable numbers of patients with and without a specific histopathological feature; in the combined analysis, some of the feature-associated DMPs might have averaged out. So a separate paired differential methylation analysis was conducted between present and absent groups, for each histopathological feature. Unique sites were defined as those which were atleast 15% differential in either present or absent group, but not significantly different in the counterpart.

Pearson's correlation coefficient between the methylation status (β values) of 4133 DMPs and maximum rete peg length was carried out using cor.test function in R. Probes with correlation P value ≤ 0.05 were considered for further analysis.

GO enrichment

To functionally characterise the genes that were differentially methylated, we tested for enrichment of GO terms with DAVID GO (https://david.ncifcrf.gov/). Gene ontology was done using genes that had overlapped with the differentially methylated probes (DMPs) at their promoters (from 1000 bp upstream to the + 500 bp downstream with respect to the TSS) [57, 58]. A term was identified as significant if the adjusted P value was ≤ 0.05. For the unique DMPs in Munro's microabscess, we presented the unique GO terms with a cut-off enrichment score ≥ 1.5 and P value ≤ 0.05.

Statistical analysis

Statistical tests were performed in R, unless otherwise mentioned. Spearman rank correlation coefficient was determined for the gene expression fold change and methylation (β values). The Fisher exact test was conducted for comparisons with small sample size. All P values were adjusted using Benjamini-Hochberg multiple hypothesis testing correction, and adjusted P value ≤ 0.05 was considered to be significant.

Additional files

Additional file 1: List of total 4133 DMPs identified in the study. (XLSX 706 kb)

Additional file 2: Figure S1. Characterisation of DMPs. (a) Distribution of DMPs across different genomic regions; separate study of localization of hyper- and hypomethylated DMPs. (b) Figure showing comparison of frequency of DMPs and total probes in 450 k array across different genomic regions. *Indicates significantly enriched regions according to hypergeometric test. (c) Overlap of DMPs across regions containing repeat elements, (d) their distribution over genomic regions and (e) sub-classification into different types of repeat elements. **Figure S2.** Characterisation of differential CGI. (a) Hierarchical clustering of differential CGI. Normal samples are marked in light green and disease samples are marked with dark green. (b) Distribution of DMPs over CGI and associated regions (shores and shelves) and non-CGI regions (Open Sea); separate classification of hyper- and hypomethylated DMPs across CGI and associated regions. (c) Extent of hyper- and hypomethylation over CGI and associated shores and shelves. **Figure S3.** Characterisation of differential promoters. (a) Heatmap of differentially methylated promoters. Normal samples are marked in light green and disease samples are marked with dark green. (b) Classification of differential promoters into hyper- and hypomethylation; overlap of hyper- and hypomethylayed promoters with CGI and associated regions and non-CGI regions. (c) Validation of candidate promoter methylation in additional samples by qMSP. (d) Gene expression analysis of corresponding genes between disease and adjacent normal samples. **Figure S4.** Verification of complete methylation of promoter-pCpGL constructs. Unmethylated and methylated promoter constructs were digested with methylation sensitive restriction enzymes (HinP1I, AciI, HpaII) and run on 1% agarose gel. Lane1: 100 bp ladder; 2: SELENBP1 unmethylated uncut construct; 3: SELENBP1 unmethylated cut; 4:

SELENBP1 methylated cut; Lane5: 100 bp ladder; 6: S100A9 unmethylated uncut construct; 7: S100A9 unmethylated cut; 8: S100A9 methylated cut. **Figure S5.** Description of Histopathological features studied :(a) ×10 magnification images of histopathological sections of adjacent normal and psoriatic disease tissue samples, (b) ×40 magnification image of stratum corneum in samples with and without Munro's microabscess. (c) ×40 magnification image of stratum corneum and stratum spinosum junction showing Kogoj's microabscess and focal hypergranulosis. **Figure S6.** Correlation of methylation status of sites with $R > 0.6$ with rete peg length. (a) Heatmap of sites correlated ($r > 0.6$) with rete peg elongation. (b) PCA with highly correlated ($R > 0.7$) sites. (PDF 1185 kb)

Additional file 3: List of differentially methylated promoters that overlap with PSORS loci. Significantly (hypergeometric test) enriched PSORS loci are presented in bold. (XLSX 29 kb)

Additional file 4: Total list of differentially methylated promoters. Hypo- and hypermethylated promoters are presented in two sheets. (XLSX 86 kb)

Additional file 5: List of top enriched biological processes (including the list of genes involved in each process) identified from gene ontology analysis of differentially methylated promoters (Table S1) and unique differentially methylated promoters in Munro's microabscess (Table S2). (XLSX 13 kb)

Additional file 6 Table S1. List of biological processes enriched in gene ontology study for the hypermethylated and hypomethylated promoters. Table S2. List of primers used for BSP and qMSP validation. Table S3. List of primers used for gene expression study. Table S4. List of primers used for cloning promoter regions. (DOCX 21 kb)

Additional file 7: List of unique and common differential probes obtained on classification of samples with and without Munro's microabscess. (XLSX 544 kb)

Additional file 8: List of probes correlated with rete peg length. (XLSX 44 kb)

Additional file 9 List of unique and common differential probes obtained on classification of samples with and without focal hypergranulosis. (XLSX 972 kb)

Additional file 10: List of unique and common differential probes obtained on classification of samples with and without Kogoj's microabscess. (XLSX 672 kb)

Abbreviations

ADAM10: A disintegrin and metalloproteinase domain-containing protein 10; AIF1: Allograft inflammatory factor 1; BMIQ: Beta-mixture quantile; BSP: Bisulfite sequencing PCR; CARD14: Caspase recruitment domain family member 14; CCL25: C-C motif chemokine ligand 25; CEBPA: CCAAT/enhancer binding protein alpha; CGI: CpG island; ChAMP: Chip Analysis of Methylation Pipeline; DENND1C: DENN domain containing 1C; DMPs: Differentially methylated probes; DNMT1: DNA methyltransferase 1; FDR: False discovery rate; FFAR2: Free fatty acid receptor 2; FFPE: Formalin-fixed paraffin embedded; GJC2: Gap junction protein gamma 2; GO: Gene ontology; GPR128: G protein-coupled receptor 128; H&E: Haematoxylin and eosin; HLA-DMA: Human leukocyte antigen-DMA; HRH1: Histamine receptor H1; ID4: Inhibitor of DNA binding 4; IL1B: Interleukin 1 beta; KAZN: Kazrin; LAMA4: Laminin subunit alpha 4; LINE-1: Long interspersed nuclear elements 1; MST1R: Macrophage stimulating 1 receptor; NDUFB4: NADH dehydrogenase 1 beta subcomplex 4; OAS2: 2'-5'-Oligoadenylate synthetase 2; PCA: Principal component analysis; pCpGL: CpG-less luciferase reporter vector; PDE4D: Phosphodiesterase 4D; PSORS: Psoriasis susceptibility; PTPN22: Protein tyrosine phosphatase non-receptor type 22; PTPN6: Protein tyrosine phosphatase non-receptor 6; qMSP: Quantitative methylation-specific PCR; RPP30: RNase P; S100A3, S100A5, S100A13, S100A8, S100A9, S100A12: S100 calcium-binding genes; SELENBP1: Selenium-binding protein; SFRP4: Secreted frizzled-related protein 4; SYNGR1: Synaptogyrin 1; TNXB: Tenascin-XB; TREM1: Triggering receptor expressed on myeloid cells 1; TSS: Transcription start site; TSSK1B: Testis-specific serine kinase 1B; ZNF106: Zinc finger protein 106

Acknowledgements

AC is working as a CSIR-NET SRF and is thankful to CSIR for providing the fellowship. The authors would like to acknowledge all volunteers who participated in the study.

Funding

This work is funded by the Science & Engineering Research Board (SERB), DST, Govt. of India (EMR/2015/002436) and intramural research funding of Indian Statistical Institute to RC.

Authors' contributions

RC conceived and supervised the project. AC performed the experiments and data analysis with some help from RC. GC and SS examined and recruited the patients. SR performed the histopathological analysis. AC and RC wrote the manuscript with input from the other authors. All authors read and approved the final manuscript.

Competing interests

The authors declare that they have no competing interests.

Author details

[1]Human Genetics Unit, Indian Statistical Institute, 203 B. T. Road, Kolkata, West Bengal 700108, India. [2]Uttarpara, Hooghly, West Bengal 712258, India. [3]MDDC, Lansdowne Place, Kolkata, West Bengal, India. [4]Department of Dermatology, IPGMER/SSKM Hospital, Kolkata, West Bengal, India.

References

1. Chandra A, Ray A, Senapati S, Chatterjee R. Genetic and epigenetic basis of psoriasis pathogenesis. Mol Immunol. 2015;64:313–23.
2. Chandran V, Raychaudhuri SP. Geoepidemiology and environmental factors of psoriasis and psoriatic arthritis. J Autoimmun. 2010;34:J314–21.
3. Dogra S, Yadav S. Psoriasis in India: prevalence and pattern. Indian J Dermatol Venereol Leprol. 2010;76:595–601.
4. Lowes MA, Suarez-Farinas M, Krueger JG. Immunology of psoriasis. Annu Rev Immunol. 2014;32:227–55.
5. Nair RP, Duffin KC, Helms C, Ding J, Stuart PE, Goldgar D, Gudjonsson JE, Li Y, Tejasvi T, Feng BJ, et al. Genome-wide scan reveals association of psoriasis with IL-23 and NF-kappaB pathways. Nat Genet. 2009;41:199–204.
6. Strange A, Capon F, Spencer CC, Knight J, Weale ME, Allen MH, Barton A, Band G, Bellenguez C, Bergboer JG, et al. A genome-wide association study identifies new psoriasis susceptibility loci and an interaction between HLA-C and ERAP1. Nat Genet. 2010;42:985–90.
7. Zhang XJ, He PP, Wang ZX, Zhang J, Li YB, Wang HY, Wei SC, Chen SY, Xu SJ, Jin L, et al. Evidence for a major psoriasis susceptibility locus at 6p21(PSORS1) and a novel candidate region at 4q31 by genome-wide scan in Chinese hans. J Invest Dermatol. 2002;119:1361–6.
8. Zhang XJ, Huang W, Yang S, Sun LD, Zhang FY, Zhu QX, Zhang FR, Zhang C, Du WH, Pu XM, et al. Psoriasis genome-wide association study identifies susceptibility variants within LCE gene cluster at 1q21. Nat Genet. 2009;41: 205–10.
9. Tang H, Jin X, Li Y, Jiang H, Tang X, Yang X, Cheng H, Qiu Y, Chen G, Mei J, et al. A large-scale screen for coding variants predisposing to psoriasis. Nat Genet. 2014;46:45–50.
10. Das A, Chandra A, Lahiri A, Datta S, Senapati S, Chatterjee R. Genetics of psoriasis. In: eLS; 2016. p. 1–9.
11. Chandra A, Lahiri A, Senapati S, Basu B, Ghosh S, Mukhopadhyay I, Behra A, Sarkar S, Chatterjee G, Chatterjee R. Increased risk of psoriasis due to combined effect of HLA-Cw6 and LCE3 risk alleles in Indian population. Sci Rep. 2016;6:24059.
12. Chandra A, Senapati S, Ghosh S, Chatterjee G, Chatterjee R. Association of IL12B risk haplotype and lack of interaction with HLA-Cw6 among the psoriasis patients in India. J Hum Genet. 2017;62:389–95.

13. Ammar M, Bouchlaka-Souissi C, Soumaya K, Bouhaha R, Ines Z, Bouazizi F, Doss N, Dhaoui R, Ben Osman A, Ben Ammar-El Gaaied A, et al. Failure to find evidence for deletion of LCE3C and LCE3B genes at PSORS4 contributing to psoriasis susceptibility in Tunisian families. Pathol Biol (Paris). 2014;62:34–7.

14. Borgiani P, Vallo L, D'Apice MR, Giardina E, Pucci S, Capon F, Nistico S, Chimenti S, Pallone F, Novelli G. Exclusion of CARD15/NOD2 as a candidate susceptibility gene to psoriasis in the Italian population. Eur J Dermatol. 2002;12:540–2.

15. Litjens NH, van der Plas MJ, Ravensbergen B, Numan-Ruberg SC, van Assen Y, Thio HB, van Dissel JT, van de Vosse E, Nibbering PH. Psoriasis is not associated with IL-12p70/IL-12p40 production and IL12B promoter polymorphism. J Invest Dermatol. 2004;122:923–6.

16. Nair RP, Stuart P, Ogura Y, Inohara N, Chia NV, Young L, Henseler T, Jenisch S, Christophers E, Voorhees JJ, et al. Lack of association between NOD2 3020insC frameshift mutation and psoriasis. J Invest Dermatol. 2001;117:1671–2.

17. Riveira-Munoz E, He SM, Escaramis G, Stuart PE, Huffmeier U, Lee C, Kirby B, Oka A, Giardina E, Liao W, et al. Meta-analysis confirms the LCE3C_LCE3B deletion as a risk factor for psoriasis in several ethnic groups and finds interaction with HLA-Cw6. J Invest Dermatol. 2011;131:1105–9.

18. Sandoval-Talamantes AK, Brito-Luna MJ, Fafutis-Morris M, Villanueva-Quintero DG, Graciano-Machuca O, Ramirez-Duenas MG, Alvarado-Navarro A. The 3′UTR 1188A/C polymorphism of IL-12p40 is not associated with susceptibility for developing plaque psoriasis in Mestizo population from western Mexico. Immunol Lett. 2015;163:221–6.

19. Gervin K, Vigeland MD, Mattingsdal M, Hammero M, Nygard H, Olsen AO, Brandt I, Harris JR, Undlien DE, Lyle R. DNA methylation and gene expression changes in monozygotic twins discordant for psoriasis: identification of epigenetically dysregulated genes. PLoS Genet. 2012;8: e1002454.

20. Chatterjee R, Vinson C. CpG methylation recruits sequence specific transcription factors essential for tissue specific gene expression. Biochim Biophys Acta. 1819;2012:763–70.

21. Rishi V, Bhattacharya P, Chatterjee R, Rozenberg J, Zhao J, Glass K, Fitzgerald P, Vinson C. CpG methylation of half-CRE sequences creates C/EBPalpha binding sites that activate some tissue-specific genes. Proc Natl Acad Sci U S A. 2010;107:20311–6.

22. Kim YI, Logan JW, Mason JB, Roubenoff R. DNA hypomethylation in inflammatory arthritis: reversal with methotrexate. J Lab Clin Med. 1996;128:165–72.

23. Ruchusatsawat K, Wongpiyabovorn J, Shuangshoti S, Hirankarn N, Mutirangura A. SHP-1 promoter 2 methylation in normal epithelial tissues and demethylation in psoriasis. J Mol Med (Berl). 2006;84:175–82.

24. Chen M, Chen ZQ, Cui PG, Yao X, Li YM, Li AS, Gong JQ, Cao YH. The methylation pattern of p16INK4a gene promoter in psoriatic epidermis and its clinical significance. Br J Dermatol. 2008;158:987–93.

25. Bai J, Liu Z, Xu Z, Ke F, Zhang L, Zhu H, Lou F, Wang H, Fei Y, Shi YL, Wang H. Epigenetic downregulation of SFRP4 contributes to epidermal hyperplasia in psoriasis. J Immunol. 2015;194:4185–98.

26. Ruchusatsawat K, Wongpiyabovorn J, Protjaroen P, Chaipipat M, Shuangshoti S, Thorner PS, Mutirangura A. Parakeratosis in skin is associated with loss of inhibitor of differentiation 4 via promoter methylation. Hum Pathol. 2011;42:1878–87.

27. Gu X, Boldrup L, Coates PJ, Fahraeus R, Nylander E, Loizou C, Olofsson K, Norberg-Spaak L, Garskog O, Nylander K. Epigenetic regulation of OAS2 shows disease-specific DNA methylation profiles at individual CpG sites. Sci Rep. 2016;6:32579.

28. Zhang P, Su Y, Chen H, Zhao M, Lu Q. Abnormal DNA methylation in skin lesions and PBMCs of patients with psoriasis vulgaris. J Dermatol Sci. 2010; 60:40–2.

29. Yooyongsatit S, Ruchusatsawat K, Noppakun N, Hirankarn N, Mutirangura A, Wongpiyabovorn J. Patterns and functional roles of LINE-1 and Alu methylation in the keratinocyte from patients with psoriasis vulgaris. J Hum Genet. 2015;60:349–55.

30. Roberson ED, Liu Y, Ryan C, Joyce CE, Duan S, Cao L, Martin A, Liao W, Menter A, Bowcock AM. A subset of methylated CpG sites differentiate psoriatic from normal skin. J Invest Dermatol. 2012;132:583–92.

31. Zhang P, Zhao M, Liang G, Yin G, Huang D, Su F, Zhai H, Wang L, Su Y, Lu Q. Whole-genome DNA methylation in skin lesions from patients with psoriasis vulgaris. J Autoimmun. 2013;41:17–24.

32. Zhou F, Wang W, Shen C, Li H, Zuo X, Zheng X, Yue M, Zhang C, Yu L, Chen M, et al. Epigenome-wide association analysis identified nine skin DNA methylation loci for psoriasis. J Invest Dermatol. 2016;136:779–87.

33. Gu X, Nylander E, Coates PJ, Fahraeus R, Nylander K. Correlation between reversal of DNA methylation and clinical symptoms in psoriatic epidermis following narrow-band UVB phototherapy. J Invest Dermatol. 2015;135: 2077–83.

34. Ozkanli S, Zemheri E, Karadag AS, Akbulak O, Zenginkinet T, Zindanci I, Bilgili SG, Akdeniz N. A comparative study of histopathological findings in skin biopsies from patients with psoriasis before and after treatment with acitretin, methotrexate and phototherapy. Cutan Ocul Toxicol. 2015;34:276–81.

35. Park GT, Han J, Park SG, Kim S, Kim TY. DNA methylation analysis of CD4+ T cells in patients with psoriasis. Arch Dermatol Res. 2014;306:259–68.

36. Hou R, Yin G, An P, Wang C, Liu R, Yang Y, Yan X, Li J, Li X, Zhang K. DNA methylation of dermal MSCs in psoriasis: identification of epigenetically dysregulated genes. J Dermatol Sci. 2013;72:103–9.

37. Gudjonsson JE, Ding J, Johnston A, Tejasvi T, Guzman AM, Nair RP, Voorhees JJ, Abecasis GR, Elder JT. Assessment of the psoriatic transcriptome in a large sample: additional regulated genes and comparisons with in vitro models. J Invest Dermatol. 2010;130:1829–40.

38. Benoit S, Toksoy A, Ahlmann M, Schmidt M, Sunderkotter C, Foell D, Pasparakis M, Roth J, Goebeler M. Elevated serum levels of calcium-binding S100 proteins A8 and A9 reflect disease activity and abnormal differentiation of keratinocytes in psoriasis. Br J Dermatol. 2006;155:62–6.

39. Smith RL, Warren RB, Eyre S, Ke X, Young HS, Allen M, Strachan D, McArdle W, Gittins MP, Barker JN, et al. Polymorphisms in the PTPN22 region are associated with psoriasis of early onset. Br J Dermatol. 2008;158:962–8.

40. Zheng J, Ibrahim S, Petersen F, Yu X. Meta-analysis reveals an association of PTPN22 C1858T with autoimmune diseases, which depends on the localization of the affected tissue. Genes Immun. 2012;13:641–52.

41. Naziroglu M, Yildiz K, Tamturk B, Erturan I, Flores-Arce M. Selenium and psoriasis. Biol Trace Elem Res. 2012;150:3–9.

42. Gutowska-Owsiak D, Salimi M, Selvakumar TA, Wang X, Taylor S, Ogg GS. Histamine exerts multiple effects on expression of genes associated with epidermal barrier function. J Investig Allergol Clin Immunol. 2014;24:231–9.

43. Gutowska-Owsiak D, Selvakumar TA, Salimi M, Taylor S, Ogg GS. Histamine enhances keratinocyte-mediated resolution of inflammation by promoting wound healing and response to infection. Clin Exp Dermatol. 2014;39:187–95.

44. Schon M, Behmenburg C, Denzer D, Schon MP. Pathogenic function of IL-1 beta in psoriasiform skin lesions of flaky skin (fsn/fsn) mice. Clin Exp Immunol. 2001;123:505–10.

45. Wang H, Iakova P, Wilde M, Welm A, Goode T, Roesler WJ, Timchenko NA. C/EBPalpha arrests cell proliferation through direct inhibition of Cdk2 and Cdk4. Mol Cell. 2001;8:817–28.

46. Mehta S, Singal A, Singh N, Bhattacharya SN. A study of clinicohistopathological correlation in patients of psoriasis and psoriasiform dermatitis. Indian J Dermatol Venereol Leprol. 2009;75:100.

47. Morris TJ, Butcher LM, Feber A, Teschendorff AE, Chakravarthy AR, Wojdacz TK, Beck S. ChAMP: 450k chip analysis methylation pipeline. Bioinformatics. 2014;30:428–30.

48. Tian Y, Morris TJ, Webster AP, Yang Z, Beck S, Feber A, Teschendorff AE. ChAMP: updated methylation analysis pipeline for Illumina BeadChips. Bioinformatics. 2017;33:3982–4.

49. Teschendorff AE, Marabita F, Lechner M, Bartlett T, Tegner J, Gomez-Cabrero D, Beck S. A beta-mixture quantile normalization method for correcting probe design bias in Illumina Infinium 450 k DNA methylation data. Bioinformatics. 2013;29:189–96.

50. Johnson WE, Li C, Rabinovic A. Adjusting batch effects in microarray expression data using empirical Bayes methods. Biostatistics. 2007;8:118–27.

51. Bibikova M, Barnes B, Tsan C, Ho V, Klotzle B, Le JM, Delano D, Zhang L, Schroth GP, Gunderson KL, et al. High density DNA methylation array with single CpG site resolution. Genomics. 2011;98:288–95.

52. Sandoval J, Heyn H, Moran S, Serra-Musach J, Pujana MA, Bibikova M, Esteller M. Validation of a DNA methylation microarray for 450,000 CpG sites in the human genome. Epigenetics. 2011;6:692–702.

53. Kumaki Y, Oda M, Okano M. QUMA: quantification tool for methylation analysis. Nucleic Acids Res. 2008;36:W170–5.

54. Li LC, Dahiya R. MethPrimer: designing primers for methylation PCRs. Bioinformatics. 2002;18:1427–31.

55. Lu L, Katsaros D, de la Longrais IA, Sochirca O, Yu H. Hypermethylation of let-7a-3 in epithelial ovarian cancer is associated with low insulin-like growth factor-II expression and favorable prognosis. Cancer Res. 2007;67: 10117–22.

56. Zeisel A, Yitzhaky A, Bossel Ben-Moshe N, Domany E. An accessible database for mouse and human whole transcriptome qPCR primers. Bioinformatics. 2013;29:1355–6.

57. Huang DW, Sherman BT, Tan Q, Collins JR, Alvord WG, Roayaei J, Stephens R, Baseler MW, Lane HC, Lempicki RA. The DAVID gene functional classification tool: a novel biological module-centric algorithm to functionally analyze large gene lists. Genome Biol. 2007;8:R183.

58. Huang DW, Sherman BT, Tan Q, Kir J, Liu D, Bryant D, Guo Y, Stephens R, Baseler MW, Lane HC, Lempicki RA. DAVID bioinformatics resources: expanded annotation database and novel algorithms to better extract biology from large gene lists. Nucleic Acids Res. 2007;35:W169–75.

2

Loss of maternal EED results in postnatal overgrowth

Lexie Prokopuk[1], Jessica M. Stringer[1,2], Craig R. White[3], Rolf H. A. M. Vossen[4], Stefan J. White[4], Ana S. A. Cohen[5], William T. Gibson[5] and Patrick S. Western[1*] ⓘ

Abstract

Background: Investigating how epigenetic information is transmitted through the mammalian germline is the key to understanding how this information impacts on health and disease susceptibility in offspring. EED is essential for regulating the repressive histone modification, histone 3 lysine 27 tri-methylation (H3K27me3) at many developmental genes.

Results: In this study, we used oocyte-specific Zp3-Cre recombinase (Zp3Cre) to delete Eed specifically in mouse growing oocytes, permitting the study of EED function in oocytes and the impact of depleting EED in oocytes on outcomes in offspring. As EED deletion occurred only in growing oocytes and females were mated to normal wild type males, this model allowed the study of oocyte programming without confounding factors such as altered in utero environment. Loss of EED from growing oocytes resulted in a significant overgrowth phenotype that persisted into adult life. Significantly, this involved increased adiposity (total fat) and bone mineral density in offspring. Similar overgrowth occurs in humans with Cohen-Gibson (OMIM 617561) and Weaver (OMIM 277590) syndromes, that result from de novo germline mutations in EED or its co-factor EZH2, respectively. Consistent with a role for EZH2 in human oocytes, we demonstrate that de novo germline mutations in EZH2 occurred in the maternal germline in some cases of Weaver syndrome. However, deletion of Ezh2 in mouse oocytes resulted in a distinct phenotype compared to that resulting from oocyte-specific deletion of Eed.

Conclusions: This study provides novel evidence that altering EED-dependent oocyte programming leads to compromised offspring growth and development in the next generation.

Keywords: Epigenetic inheritance, Germ, Oocyte, Polycomb, Histone, Weaver, EED, EZH2, Overgrowth, H3K27me3

Background

Factors regulating oocyte (egg) and sperm programming and early embryonic development have been associated with the fetal origins of disease, including reduced cognitive ability and increased chronic diseases, such as type-2 diabetes, obesity, heart disease and behavioural anomalies [1–5]. The causes of these defects are poorly understood, but are likely to be in part due to altered epigenetic programming of oocytes or sperm that significantly impact on embryonic development and underlie the fetal origin of some of these disorders [1, 2, 4].

Defining how inherited epigenetic information regulates fetal development and postnatal phenotypic outcomes is therefore important for understanding how inherited epigenetic information impacts on human health and disease. While the establishment of aberrant epigenetic states has been associated with disease, functional analyses of epigenetic inheritance that isolate in vivo effects generated in the germline are not possible in humans. Here, we have used genetic mouse models to mediate oocyte-specific deletion of Eed and Ezh2 to understand how changes in epigenetic information established in the oocyte can impact on phenotypic outcomes in offspring.

H3K27me3 is a critical epigenetic modification that is catalysed by polycomb repressive complex 2 (PRC2), a highly conserved epigenetic modifying complex. PRC2 is comprised of three core protein subunits: Embryonic

* Correspondence: patrick.western@hudson.org.au
[1]Centre for Reproductive Health, Hudson Institute of Medical Research and Department of Molecular and Translational Science, Monash University, Clayton, Victoria 3168, Australia
Full list of author information is available at the end of the article

Ectoderm Development (EED), Enhancer of Zeste 1/2 (EZH1/2) and Suppressor of Zeste 12 (SUZ12). Global loss of function to any one of these components results in drastically compromised enzymatic activity of PRC2, substantial loss of H3K27me3 and embryonic lethality in mice [6–8]. Recent studies of germ cells have demonstrated enrichment of H3K27me3 at key developmental genes in male and female germ cells [9–11] and the maintenance of some H3K27me3 marked histones in mature sperm [12–14]. Furthermore, oocyte-specific deletion of *Ezh2* results in loss of H3K27me3 in the zygote and ~ 40% growth restriction in maternal offspring [15]. In humans, de novo germline mutations in *EED* or *EZH2* lead to Cohen-Gibson (OMIM 617561) or Weaver (OMIM 28229590) syndromes, which are characterised by overgrowth, skeletal defects and advanced bone age [16–23], indicating that PRC2 activity may be required in the human germline for regulating outcomes in offspring. Together, these studies raise the possibility that PRC2 and H3K27me3 may underpin epigenetic inheritance effects on offspring development and postnatal outcomes.

During female fetal development, germ cells commit to oogenesis and enter meiotic prophase [24]. Folliculogenesis occurs in early postnatal life and results in establishment of a finite pool of quiescent primordial follicles that underpin the female reproductive lifespan. Subsequently, primordial follicles are continuously released in reproductively mature females, initiating a prolonged period of oocyte growth and maturation that takes around 21 days in mice and up to 12 months in humans [25]. While most of this period involves oocyte growth while in a diploid state, it is completed by rapid maturation of each oocyte through meiosis I and meiosis II, ultimately producing a haploid oocyte at fertilisation [26]. Before completion of the first meiotic division, the diploid oocyte enters the germinal vesicle (GV) stage, characterised by decondensed chromatin and a period of high transcription that includes the production of maternal factors (proteins and RNAs) that are required for directing preimplantation development in the offspring [27]. In addition to maternal factors, the mature oocyte carries specific epigenetic information required for offspring development, but the nature, extent and effects of this information on offspring development are not yet fully understood [28, 29].

Germ cell-specific knockout mouse models have been valuable for analysing the function of maternal factors in the absence of confounding effects such as in utero environment and nutritional influences derived from the mother [15, 28, 30]. *Zp3Cre*, is a well-established model for generating oocyte-specific gene deletion mediated by transcription of *Cre recombinase* under control of the *Zona Pellucida 3* (*Zp3*) promoter [31]. This model allows the production of offspring from oocytes that lack specific genes only during their maturation and can be effectively used for functional analyses of maternal inheritance [15, 31–33].

Although deletion of the PRC2 component, *Ezh2*, in the growing oocyte leads to restricted growth in offspring [15], little is known about the role of *Eed* in the female germline. However, the PRC1 components, *Ring finger protein 2* (*Rnf2*) and *Ring finger protein 1* (*Ring1*), are regulated throughout oogenesis and absence of maternal RNF2 and RING1 proteins leads to developmental arrest at the two-cell stage of embryogenesis [30]. Moreover, injection of the H3K27me3-specific demethylase, *Kdm6b*, into zygotes resulted in ectopic maternal expression of specific genes that are normally expressed only from the paternal allele, demonstrating that maternal H3K27me3 regulates DNA methylation-independent imprinting [34]. These data suggest oocyte-specific roles for polycomb group proteins in the establishment of maternal factors and/or epigenetic modifications that are required for correct development of offspring.

In this study, we used *Zp3Cre* to delete *Eed* specifically from growing oocytes. The resulting oocytes lacked H3K27me3 and produced offspring with significant overgrowth that involved increased adiposity (percentage fat) and increased bone mineral density. These data demonstrate that EED is required in the oocyte for programming developmental outcomes that affect life-long outcomes in offspring. This contrasted with growth restriction that resulted from deletion of *Ezh2* in growing oocytes, indicating that while EED mediates epigenetic inheritance through the maternal germline, the function of EZH2 is more complex.

Results

Immunofluorescent studies of oocyte development demonstrated that H3K27me3 is increasingly enriched in the nucleus of oocytes during follicle growth [35]. In this study, we used a *Zp3Cre* transgene to mediate oocyte-specific deletion of *Eed*, in order to determine the effect loss of maternal PRC2 function had on offspring (Fig. 1a). The *Eed*$^{fl/fl}$ model was originally developed by Orkin and colleagues, and results in deletion of exons 3–6 of *Eed* and loss of the ability for PRC2 to catalyse H3K27 methylation [36]. Genotyping of progeny from *Eed* floxed females carrying *Zp3Cre* mated to wild type males demonstrated that *Eed* deletion was 100% efficient in oocytes (Additional file 1: Figure S1; *Chi-square test, nsd*). Mouse oocyte growth encompasses 22–24 days, after which they complete meiosis during maturation within a single day, ultimately producing haploid ova [37, 38]. Deletion using *Zp3Cre* occurs early during oocyte growth, resulting in loss of the target gene during the majority of the diploid (4C) oocyte growth

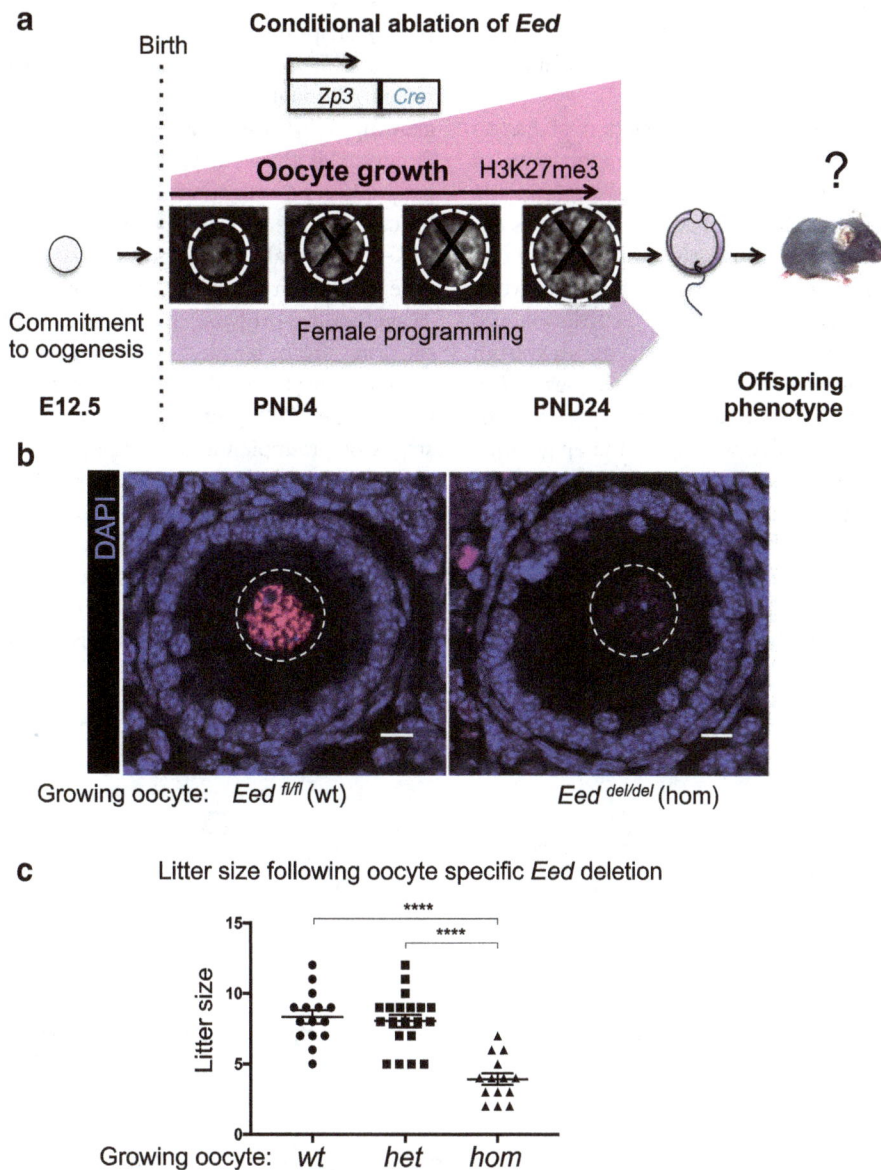

Fig. 1 Deletion of *Eed* significantly reduced H3K27me3 in growing oocytes: **a** Schematic of the study aims—germ cells commit to female development after E12.5 and new epigenetic information is established in growing oocytes after birth. H3K27me3 is enriched as oocytes grow, with strong enrichment in the maturing oocyte. Using an *Eedfl-Zp3*Cre mouse model, we investigated the impacts of deleting *Eed* in the growing oocyte on offspring weight and growth. As EED deletion occurs only in growing oocytes, this model allows the study of EED-dependent maternal programming without contributions from confounding factors such as in utero environment. **b** Representative confocal images of immunofluorescence in ovary sections from adult *Eed*$^{fl/fl}$ and *Eed*$^{fl/fl}$.*Zp3*-Cre female mice producing *Eed*$^{fl/fl}$ (wild type; *wt*) and *Eed*$^{del/del}$ (homozygous; *hom*) oocytes, respectively. Merged channels: H3K27me3 (red) and DAPI (DNA; blue). *Eed*$^{fl/fl}$ (*wt*) and *Eed*$^{del/del}$(*hom*) oocytes are shown within the white dashed line. Images are representative of four biological replicates. 10-μm scale bars. **c** Average litter sizes from mothers producing *Eed*$^{fl/fl}$ (*wt*), *Eed*$^{wt/del}$ (heterozygous; *het*) and *Eed*$^{del/del}$ (*hom*) growing oocytes: $n = 15, 20$ and 13 litters per genotype, respectively, and 7 different mothers per genotype group. ****$P < 0.0001$. One-way ANOVA plus post hoc Tukey's multiple comparisons test. Error bars ± SEM

phase [31]. Critically, immunofluorescence demonstrated that *Eed*$^{del/del}$ oocytes contained markedly reduced nuclear H3K27me3, consistent with substantial loss of PRC2 function in these cells (Fig. 1b). Initially, we determined whether deleting *Eed* in oocytes affected average litter size produced from *Eed*$^{wt/wt}$ *Eed*$^{wt/del}$ and *Eed*$^{del/del}$ growing oocytes. Despite severe depletion of H3K27me3, *Eed*$^{del/del}$ oocytes produced live born pups in normal sex ratios. However, the average litter size produced by females producing *Eed*$^{del/del}$ oocytes was significantly reduced compared to females producing *Eed*$^{wt/wt}$ or *Eed*$^{wt/del}$ oocytes, although the causes for the litter size reduction remain unknown (Fig. 1c, $n = 13–20$ litters per genotype). This model therefore provides an opportunity to study offspring derived from oocytes that lack EED and H3K27me3, specifically during oocyte growth, maturation and preimplantation development, prior to activation of the paternal *Eed* allele.

Mating females with oocyte-specific deletion of *Eed* to wild type C57BL/6 males provided the opportunity to compare isogenic offspring in the absence of confounding maternal in utero effects (Fig. 2). Importantly, oocytes developing in *Eed*$^{wt/fl}$;*Zp3-Cre* transgenic mothers have one intact copy of *Eed* during the oocyte growth period, when epigenetic modifications including DNA methylation and H3K27me3 are established. In contrast, oocytes from *Eed*$^{fl/fl}$;*Zp3-Cre* transgenic females lack both copies of *Eed* (*Eed*$^{del/del}$) and have no EED function in their growing oocytes. Therefore, in this model, we expect the epigenome of *Eed*^{del} haploid oocytes produced by *Eed*$^{fl/wt}$;*Zp3-Cre* females to be relatively normal as they developed in the presence of reduced, yet sufficient, EED function during their growth and maturation. However, *Eed*^{del} haploid oocytes produced by *Eed*$^{fl/fl}$;*Zp3-Cre* females lacked EED protein during oocyte growth and maturation (Fig. 2).

This model allowed the production of heterozygous (HET) offspring from females producing *Eed*$^{del/del}$ (hom) or *Eed*$^{wt/del}$ (het) growing oocytes mated to wild type males. Although HET offspring from *Eed*$^{del/del}$ or *Eed*$^{wt/del}$ growing oocytes were isogenic, they have two critical differences. Firstly, we expect these offspring to be epigenetically different, reflecting the presence or absence of EED function in the growing oocyte. Secondly, these offspring lacked maternal EED during the zygotic to paternal genome activation phase of preimplantation development. Therefore, we proposed that differences between the HET offspring from females producing *Eed*$^{del/del}$ or *Eed*$^{wt/del}$ growing oocytes could be attributed to altered programming in *Eed*$^{del/del}$ growing oocytes and during the earliest stages of preimplantation development. Similar comparisons were made between wild type (WT) offspring from *Eed*$^{wt/fl}$;*Zp3-Cre* and *Eed*$^{wt/wt}$ females, which respectively produced *Eed*$^{wt/del}$ and *Eed*$^{wt/wt}$ growing oocytes (Fig. 2).

To identify postnatal differences in offspring due to compromised EED-dependent programming in the oocyte and early development, we initially weighed postnatal day

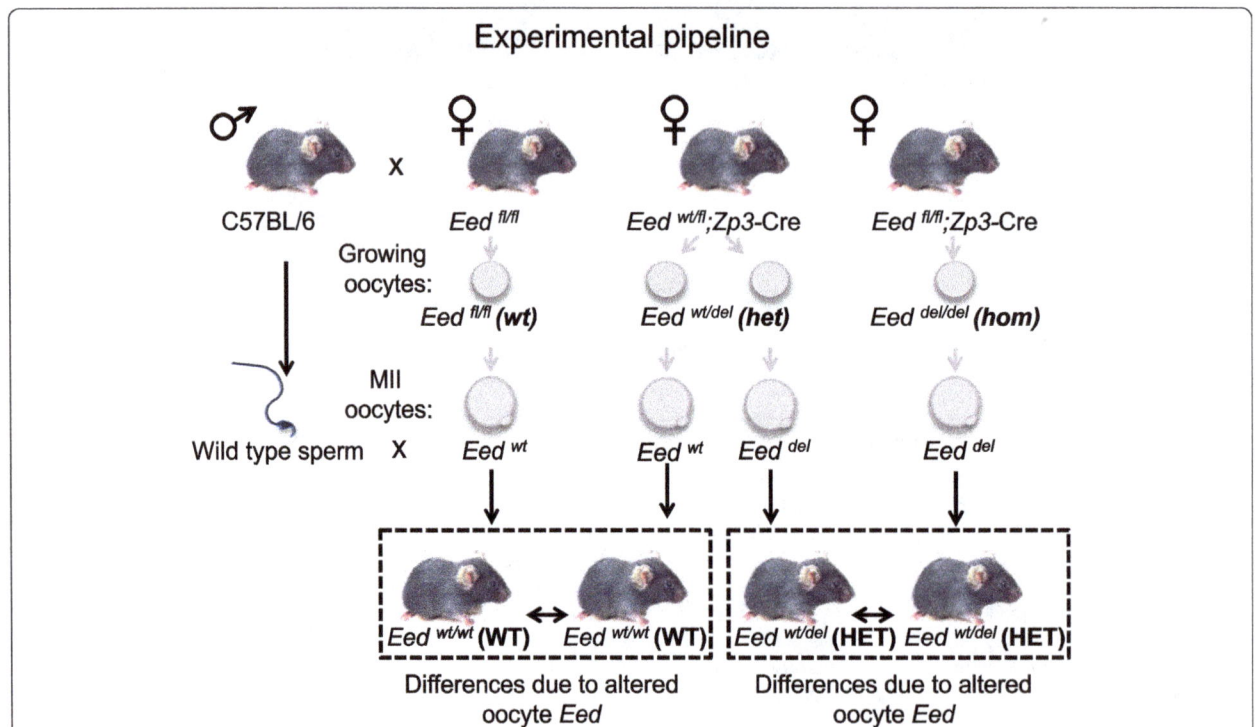

Fig. 2 Schematic of experimental breeding to determine epigenetic differences in isogenic offspring from *Eed* floxed females: Wild type males were mated with *Eed*$^{fl/fl}$, *Eed*$^{fl/del}$;*Zp3-Cre* and *Eed*$^{fl/del}$;*Zp3Cre* female mice that produce *Eed*^{del} or *Eed*^{wt} haploid oocytes derived from *Eed*$^{fl/fl}$ (wild type; wt), *Eed*$^{wt/del}$(heterozygous; het) or *Eed*$^{del/del}$ (homozygous; hom) growing oocytes. *Het* oocytes grow and mature in the presence of functional EED, while *hom* oocytes grow and mature in the absence of EED function. Production of offspring by mating *Eed*$^{fl/del}$;*Zp3-Cre* and *Eed*$^{fl/del}$;*Zp3Cre* female mice with isogenic wild type males allowed the comparison of isogenic HET offspring from *het* and *hom* oocytes. As the resulting HET offspring were isogenic and carry identical heterozygous *Eed* deletion, differences detected could be ascribed to loss of epigenetic regulation by EED in the oocyte and before cavitation of paternal *Eed* in the preimplantation embryo. Similar comparisons were made between WT offspring produced from *Eed*$^{fl/fl}$ and *Eed*$^{fl/del}$;*Zp3-Cre* females. Comparison of WT and HET offspring produced by *Eed*$^{fl/fl}$ and *Eed*$^{fl/del}$;*Zp3-Cre* females provides an internal control identifying the contribution of *Eed* heterozygosity to the phenotype. Genetically identical offspring are shown in purple dashed box

(PND) 2 pups generated from $Eed^{del/del}$, $Eed^{wt/del}$ and $Eed^{wt/wt}$ growing oocytes and isogenic wild type sperm (Figs. 2 and 3a). Remarkably, complete loss of EED specifically in the growing oocyte resulted in a 29% increase in weight of PND2 HET offspring from $Eed^{del/del}$ growing oocytes (average weight 2.19 g, $n = 51$) compared to PND2 HET offspring from $Eed^{wt/del}$ growing oocytes (average weight 1.69 g, $n = 52$) (Fig. 3a $P < 0.0001$, one-way ANOVA). In addition, HET offspring from $Eed^{del/del}$ growing oocytes had increased nose to rump length, compared to isogenic age-matched HET offspring from $Eed^{wt/del}$ growing oocytes (Fig. 3b–d). Similarly, HET offspring from $Eed^{del/del}$ growing oocytes were significantly longer and heavier than WT offspring from $Eed^{wt/del}$ growing oocytes, but there was no difference in length or weight between HET and WT offspring generated from $Eed^{wt/del}$ or

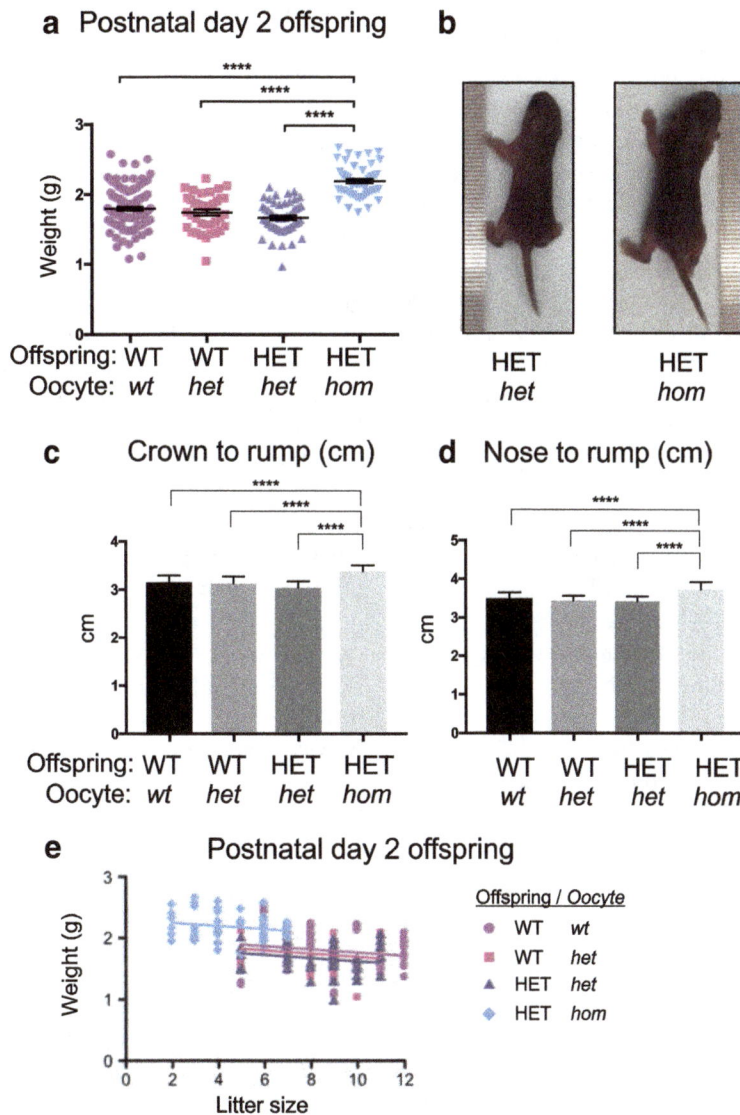

Fig. 3 Offspring from $Eed^{del/del}$ oocytes have increased weight and length that is independent of litter size. **a** Postnatal day (PND) 2 weights of WT and HET offspring produced from $Eed^{fl/fl}$ (wt), $Eed^{wt/del}$ (het) and $Eed^{del/del}$(hom) oocytes and wild type sperm (WT offspring from *wt* oocytes $n = 118$; WT offspring from *het* oocytes $n = 37$; HET offspring from *het* oocytes $n = 52$; HET offspring from *hom* oocytes $n = 51$). **b** Representative images showing two isogenic PND2 male pups. Left: HET offspring from a *het* growing oocyte; Right: HET offspring from a *hom* growing oocyte. **c** Crown to rump measurements of PND2 male and female pups. **d** Nose to rump measurements of PND2 male and female pups. **c–d** WT offspring from *wt* oocytes $n = 29$; WT offspring from *het* oocytes $n = 10$; HET offspring from *het* oocytes $n = 10$; HET offspring from *hom* oocytes $n = 23$) ****$P < 0.0001$. One-way ANOVA plus post hoc Tukey's multiple comparisons test. Data represents mean ± SEM. **e** Relationship between PND2 weight and litter size: Litter size vs offspring weight ($t_{33.5} = -1.32$, $P = 0.20$; variance components: litter ID = 0.0398, residual = 0.0345). Accounting for litter size vs offspring weight: HET pups from $Eed^{del/del}$ oocytes were heavier than HET pups produced from $Eed^{wt/del}$ oocytes ($t_{34.8} = 3.44$, $P = 0.002$), WT pups from either $Eed^{wt/del}$ ($t_{36.3} = 2.81$, $P = 0.008$) and $Eed^{wt/wt}$ ($t_{33.1} = 2.29$, $P = 0.03$) oocytes

$Eed^{wt/wt}$ growing oocytes (Fig. 3d). There was no bias in this PND2 overgrowth phenotype between the sexes (Additional file 1: Figure S2).

One possible explanation for the increased pup weight at PND2 was the reduced average litter size observed for females producing $Eed^{del/del}$ growing oocytes (Fig. 1c). To account for this, we analysed the weight data using linear mixed models to statistically evaluate the litter size dependent, and litter size independent contributions to offspring weight. To account for non-independence of pups from individual litters, we included litter identification as a random effect in the analysis. Initially, we ensured that there were no differences in offspring weight due to litter size differences that were attributable individual oocyte genotypes. This revealed that the relationship between litter size and offspring weight among WT and HET pups produced from $Eed^{wt/wt}$, $Eed^{wt/del}$ and $Eed^{del/del}$ oocytes was consistent (litter size by offspring group interaction: $F_{3,48.4} = 0.048$, $P = 0.99$; variance components: litter ID = 0.0423, residual = 0.0346). Next, we determined the relationship between litter size and offspring weight for all genotypes. This revealed that as litter size decreased, there was a minor increase in offspring weight ($t_{33.5} = -1.32$, $P = 0.20$; variance components: litter ID = 0.0398, residual = 0.0345; Fig. 3e). However, this effect was not significant and was insufficient to account for the substantial increase in the weight of HET offspring generated from $Eed^{del/del}$ growing oocytes compared to HET or WT offspring generated from $Eed^{wt/del}$ or $Eed^{wt/wt}$ oocytes. In contrast, after removing the weight change attributable to litter size, there remained a highly significant increase in weight of HET pups produced from $Eed^{del/del}$ growing oocytes compared to HET pups produced from $Eed^{wt/del}$ oocytes ($t_{34.8} = 3.44$, $P = 0.002$) and WT pups produced from either $Eed^{wt/del}$ ($t_{36.3} = 2.81$, $P = 0.008$) or $Eed^{wt/wt}$ ($t_{33.1} = 2.29$, $P = 0.03$) growing oocytes (Fig. 3e). Given that this increase in offspring weight only occurred in the HET pups generated from $Eed^{del/del}$ growing oocytes and was not accounted for by litter size differences, we concluded that loss of EED in the oocyte and early embryo resulted in substantial, postnatal overgrowth.

As the Eed HET pups produced were isogenic, the simplest explanation for this difference is that loss of maternal EED in the mouse oocyte and zygote led to a significant early developmental programming effect that impacted on postnatal weight in offspring from $Eed^{del/del}$ compared to $Eed^{wt/del}$ growing oocytes. As EED is known only to regulate epigenetic outcomes, this postnatal effect is likely to result from altered epigenetic programming in the oocyte and early embryo.

Recent studies in humans have demonstrated that de novo germline mutations in EED lead to Cohen-Gibson (OMIM 617561) syndrome, which is characterised by overgrowth, skeletal defects and advanced bone age [16–20]. DEXA scanning of the PND2 mouse offspring produced in this study revealed increased bone mineral density (BMD) in HET offspring from $Eed^{del/del}$ growing oocytes compared to HET controls generated from $Eed^{wt/del}$ growing oocytes ($Eed^{wt/wt}$ $n = 28$, $Eed^{wt/del}$ $n = 14$, $Eed^{del/del}$ $n = 19$; $P < 0.05$, one-way ANOVA; Fig. 4a). Moreover, fat content was also significantly increased in PND2 HET offspring from $Eed^{del/del}$ oocytes compared to HET offspring from $Eed^{wt/del}$ growing oocytes, and WT offspring from $Eed^{wt/del}$ and $Eed^{wt/wt}$ oocytes (Fig. 4b, $P < 0.01$, one-way ANOVA). Lean muscle content was significantly reduced in HET offspring from $Eed^{del/del}$ growing oocytes, compared to WT offspring from $Eed^{wt/wt}$ oocytes (Fig. 4c, $P < 0.05$, one-way ANOVA), but there was no significant difference between HET offspring from $Eed^{wt/del}$ and $Eed^{del/del}$ oocytes. The ponderal index (weight/crown-length^3) of WT and HET offspring from $Eed^{wt/wt}$ and $Eed^{wt/del}$ growing oocytes, respectively, was not significantly different indicating that there was no substantial effect on corpulence in these offspring. However, while there was an unexpected marginal decrease in ponderal index in WT pups from $Eed^{wt/del}$ growing oocytes compared to all other treatment groups, the significance of this change remains unknown (Fig. 4d, $*P < 0.05$, $**P < 0.01$ one-way ANOVA).

To determine the weight phenotype observed in PND2 offspring persisted through adult life, female and male offspring from $Eed^{wt/wt}$, $Eed^{wt/del}$ and $Eed^{del/del}$ growing oocytes were weighed at PND30, PND49 and PND130 (Fig. 5a–b, Additional file 1: Figure S2). HET offspring from $Eed^{del/del}$ growing oocytes remained significantly heavier than age-matched WT offspring from $Eed^{wt/wt}$ oocytes at PND30 (females), PND49 and PND130 (Additional file 1: Figure S2). However, there was no statistical difference in male weights at PND30, a growth period encompassing the transition of adolescence to adulthood in mice. Although the reason for this discrepancy remains unknown, individual variation in growth and maturation at this time point may explain the greater individual variability evident in the data. Notwithstanding this limitation, our findings are consistent with Cohen-Gibson patients [16], as the weight differences between animals were partially ameliorated through time and between sexes such that there was no longer a consistent statistically significant difference between HET offspring from $Eed^{wt/del}$ and $Eed^{del/del}$ growing oocytes at PND30 and at older ages (Fig. 5a–b, Additional file 1: Figure S2). Calculation of the change in average sex-specific weights in each group at PND30 and PND49 relative to PND2, detected no difference in the growth rates of WT and HET offspring produced from $Eed^{wt/wt}$ and $Eed^{del/del}$ growing oocytes (Fig. 5c–d).

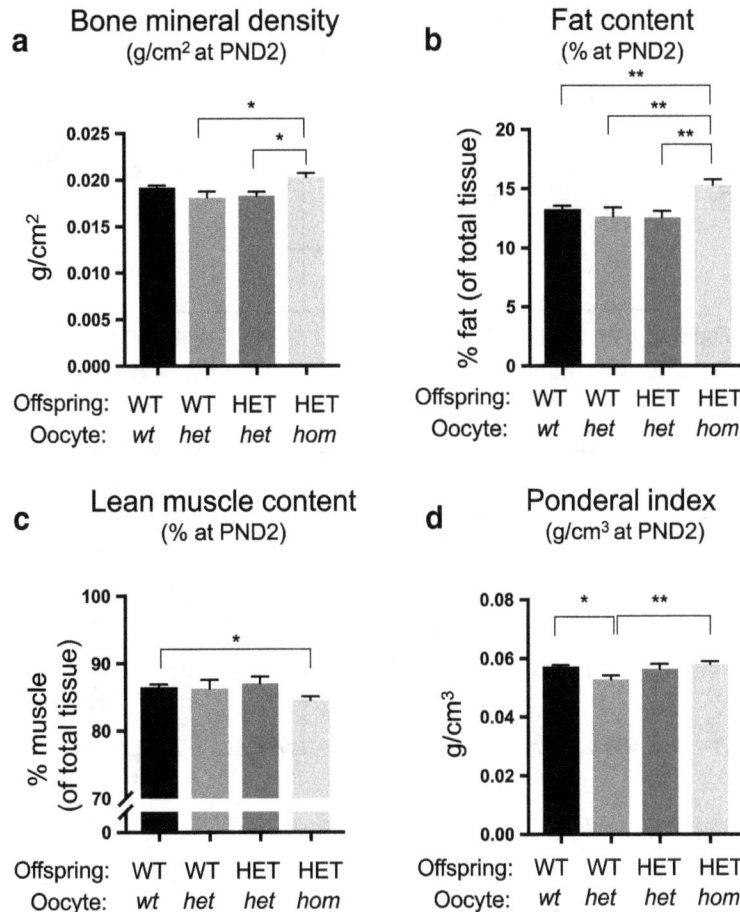

Fig. 4 Offspring from *Eed*^{del/del} oocytes have increased bone mineral density and fat content, but reduced lean muscle. **a–d** Postnatal day (PND) 2: bone mineral density (**a**), lean muscle content (**b**), fat content (**c**), ponderal index (**d**) in WT and HET offspring produced from *Eed*^{fl/fl} (*wt*), *Eed*^{wt/del} (*het*) and *Eed*^{del/del}(*hom*) oocytes and wild type sperm (**a–d**: WT offspring from *wt* oocytes n = 28; WT offspring from *het* oocytes n = 6; HET offspring from *het* oocytes n = 8; HET offspring from *hom* oocytes n = 19). *$P < 0.05$, **$P < 0.01$, one-way ANOVA plus post hoc Tukey's multiple comparisons test. Error bars ± SEM

In humans, de novo germline mutations in *EZH2* lead to Weaver Syndrome (OMIM 28229590) and de novo germline mutations in *EED* lead to Cohen-Gibson syndrome, both of which are characterised by overgrowth [16–18, 21–23]. To determine the germline origin of the EZH2/EED de novo mutation, comparative SNPs were analysed in the *EZH2* and *EED* genomic regions in DNA samples from Weaver syndrome patients and their parents (Fig. 6a). Long range, targeted sequencing revealed that the causative EZH2 mutations in human patients occurred either in the maternal or paternal germlines (Fig. 6b). Although patient numbers are quite restricted in this study, parent-of-origin appeared to have no effect on birth weight in human patients. Unfortunately, analysis of two patients carrying EED mutations were uninformative, one patient lacked informative SNPs in the sequenced region and data from the other patient was inconclusive as amplification of the template failed for this individual.

An earlier study in mice found that deletion of *Ezh2* in growing oocytes resulted in reduced birth weight in maternal offspring [15]. As the offspring produced after deletion of *Eed* in growing oocytes resulted in overgrown offspring, we independently generated offspring from *Ezh*^{fl/fl} (*Zp3-Cre* negative), *Ezh2*^{wt/fl};*Zp3*-Cre and *Ezh2*^{fl/fl};*Zp3*-Cre mothers. Consistent with deletion of *Eed* in growing oocytes, deletion of *Ezh2* using the same *Zp3Cre* strategy was highly efficient (Additional file 1: Figure S3) and resulted in substantially reduced H3K27me3 in growing oocytes. The degree to which H3K27me3 was lost in *Ezh2*^{del/del} and *Eed*^{del/del} oocytes was comparable, indicating that loss of EZH2 is unlikely to be compensated for by the related protein EZH1. In contrast to *Eed*, oocyte-specific deletion of *Ezh2* resulted in significantly reduced PND2 weight in HET offspring from *Ezh2*^{del/del} growing oocytes compared to WT pups from *Ezh2*^{wt/del} and *Ezh2*^{wt/wt} growing oocytes. However, there was no difference in PND2 weight between HET

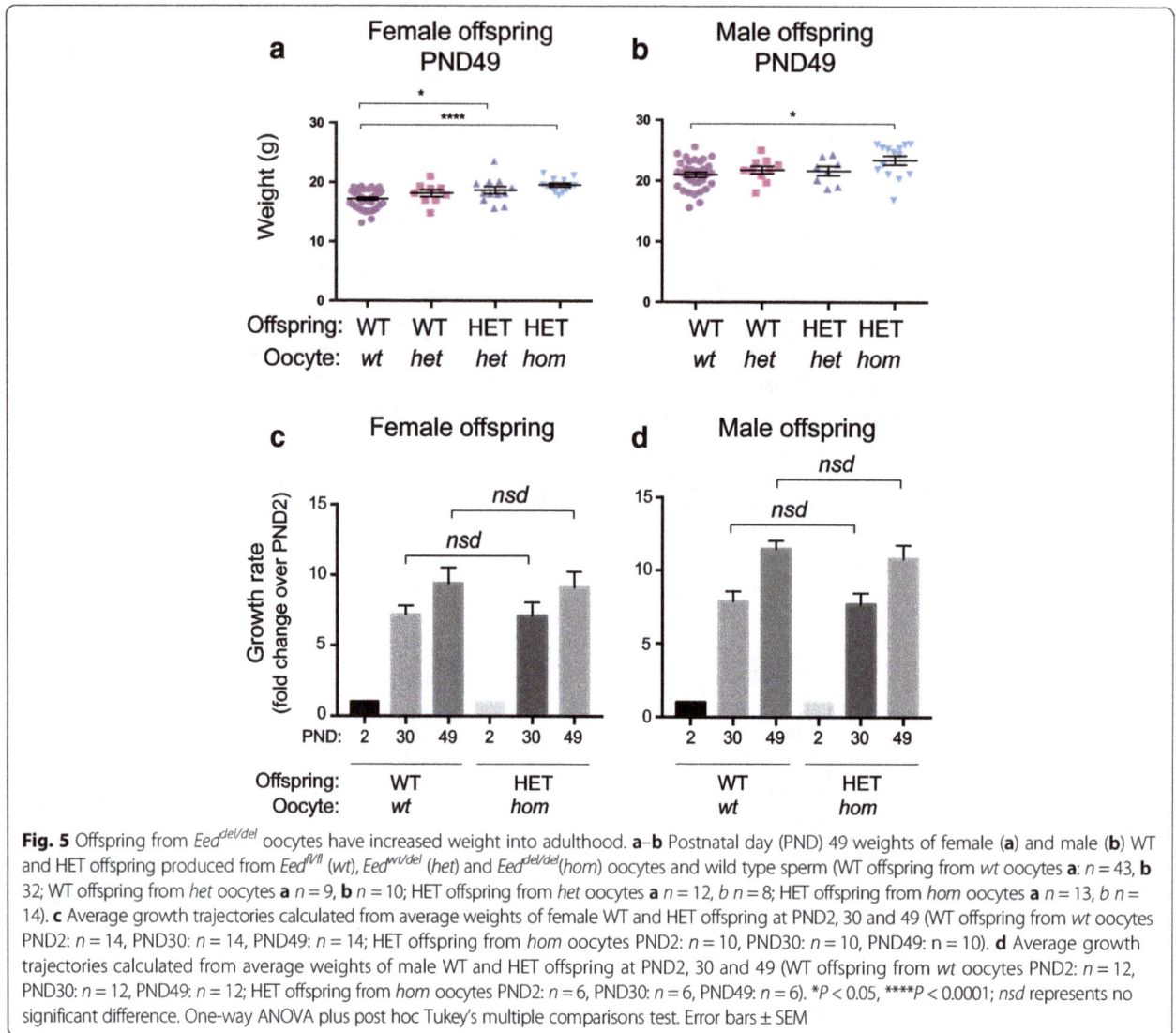

Fig. 5 Offspring from *Eed*$^{del/del}$ oocytes have increased weight into adulthood. **a–b** Postnatal day (PND) 49 weights of female (**a**) and male (**b**) WT and HET offspring produced from *Eed*$^{fl/fl}$ (*wt*), *Eed*$^{wt/del}$ (*het*) and *Eed*$^{del/del}$(*hom*) oocytes and wild type sperm (WT offspring from *wt* oocytes **a**: $n = 43$, **b** 32; WT offspring from *het* oocytes **a** $n = 9$, **b** $n = 10$; HET offspring from *het* oocytes **a** $n = 12$, *b n* = 8; HET offspring from *hom* oocytes **a** $n = 13$, b $n =$ 14). **c** Average growth trajectories calculated from average weights of female WT and HET offspring at PND2, 30 and 49 (WT offspring from *wt* oocytes PND2: $n = 14$, PND30: $n = 14$, PND49: $n = 14$; HET offspring from *hom* oocytes PND2: $n = 10$, PND30: $n = 10$, PND49: n = 10). **d** Average growth trajectories calculated from average weights of male WT and HET offspring at PND2, 30 and 49 (WT offspring from *wt* oocytes PND2: $n = 12$, PND30: $n = 12$, PND49: $n = 12$; HET offspring from *hom* oocytes PND2: $n = 6$, PND30: $n = 6$, PND49: $n = 6$). *$P < 0.05$, ****$P < 0.0001$; *nsd* represents no significant difference. One-way ANOVA plus post hoc Tukey's multiple comparisons test. Error bars ± SEM

offspring from *Ezh2*$^{del/del}$ and *Ezh2*$^{wt/del}$ growing oocytes (Fig. 7). Significantly, this indicated that deletion of *Ezh2* in growing oocytes resulted in a genetically defined, heterozygous vs wild type reduction in offspring weight, rather than the epigenetically defined, heterozygous vs heterozygous difference in offspring weight observed for deletion of *Eed* in growing oocytes. A caveat to this is that *Ezh2* HET offspring from *Ezh2*$^{wt/del}$ growing oocytes were not significantly different in weight to WT offspring from *Ezh2*$^{wt/del}$ or *Ezh2*$^{wt/wt}$ growing oocytes. Therefore, it is likely that this phenotype results from a combination of genetic and epigenetic effects mediated through the maternal germline.

Discussion

We have established a model in which oocyte-specific deletion of *Eed* results in overgrowth in postnatal offspring. Heterozygous offspring from *Eed*$^{del/del}$ growing oocytes had increased body weight, length, fat content and bone mineral density compared to isogenic heterozygous control offspring from *Eed*$^{wt/del}$ growing oocytes. Our findings are reminiscent of weight gains observed in offspring in other epigenetic models, including mice with disrupted maternal imprinting of H19 [39]. This is an interesting parallel considering recent evidence has demonstrated a role for H3K27me3 in DNA methylation-independent maternal imprinting [34].

Growth trajectories were similar between offspring from all *Eed* oocyte genotypes and mice from *Eed*$^{del/del}$ growing oocytes remained moderately larger throughout adulthood (18 weeks of age), although this overgrowth phenotype was ameliorated through time. These phenotypic effects demonstrate the importance of maternal PRC2 for establishing fetal growth patterns and provide evidence that maternal EED regulates offspring growth and postnatal outcomes. Linear regression analysis indicated that litter size did not strongly correlate with weight at PND2. Therefore, while litter size may make a

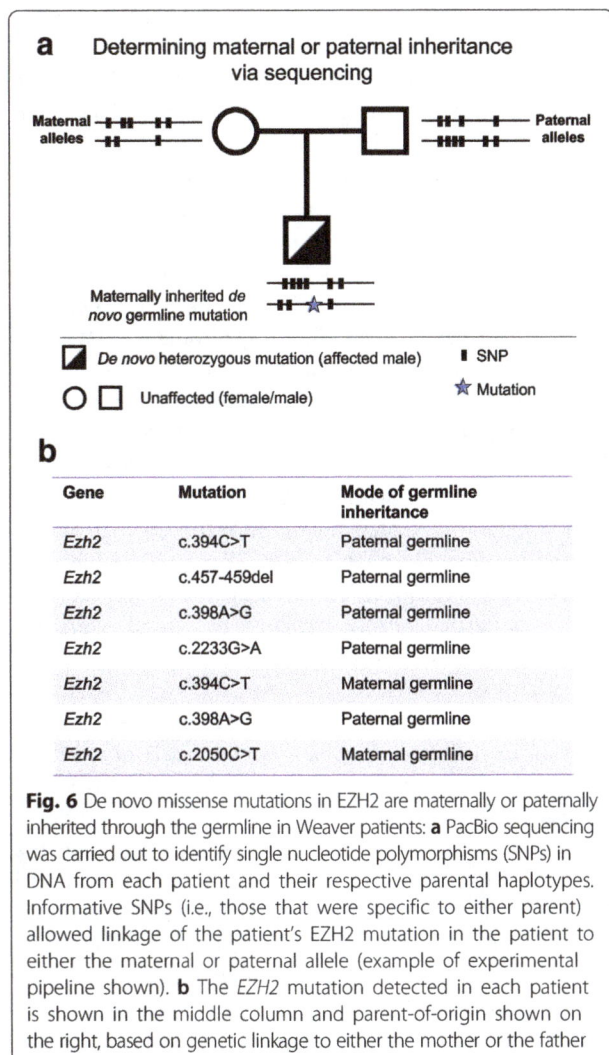

Fig. 6 De novo missense mutations in EZH2 are maternally or paternally inherited through the germline in Weaver patients: **a** PacBio sequencing was carried out to identify single nucleotide polymorphisms (SNPs) in DNA from each patient and their respective parental haplotypes. Informative SNPs (i.e., those that were specific to either parent) allowed linkage of the patient's EZH2 mutation in the patient to either the maternal or paternal allele (example of experimental pipeline shown). **b** The *EZH2* mutation detected in each patient is shown in the middle column and parent-of-origin shown on the right, based on genetic linkage to either the mother or the father

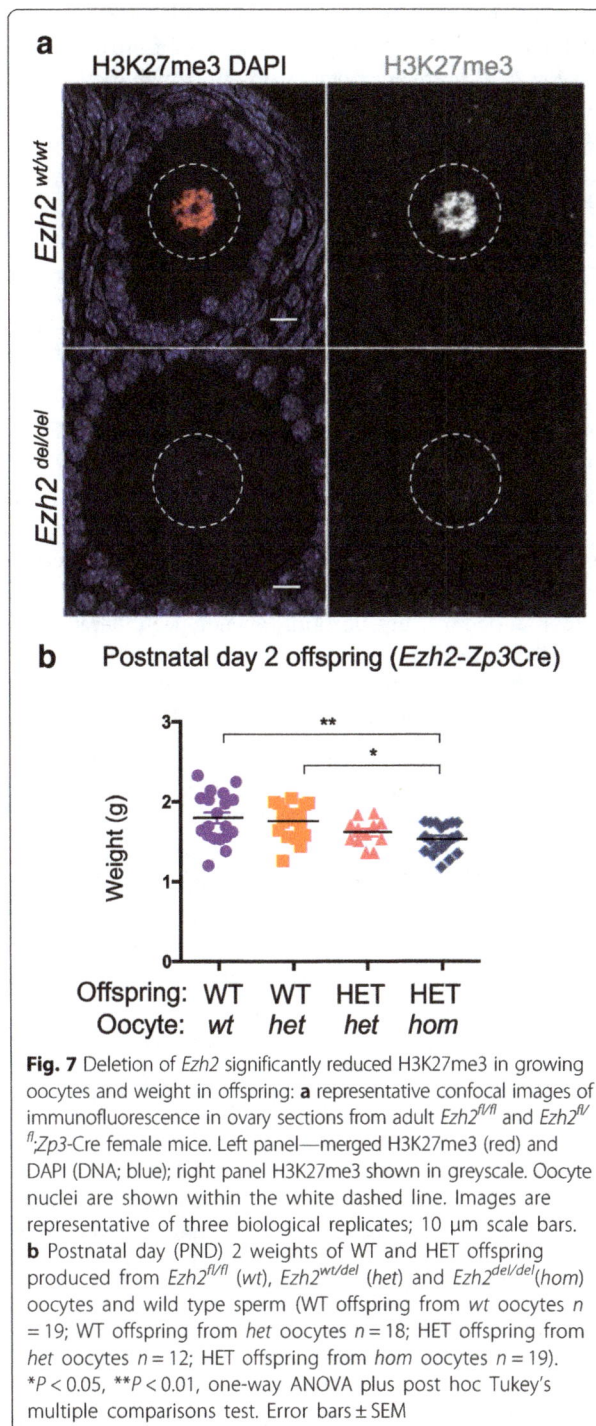

Fig. 7 Deletion of *Ezh2* significantly reduced H3K27me3 in growing oocytes and weight in offspring: **a** representative confocal images of immunofluorescence in ovary sections from adult $Ezh2^{fl/fl}$ and $Ezh2^{fl/fl}$;Zp3-Cre female mice. Left panel—merged H3K27me3 (red) and DAPI (DNA; blue); right panel H3K27me3 shown in greyscale. Oocyte nuclei are shown within the white dashed line. Images are representative of three biological replicates; 10 μm scale bars. **b** Postnatal day (PND) 2 weights of WT and HET offspring produced from $Ezh2^{fl/fl}$ (wt), $Ezh2^{wt/del}$ (het) and $Ezh2^{del/del}$(hom) oocytes and wild type sperm (WT offspring from *wt* oocytes n = 19; WT offspring from *het* oocytes n = 18; HET offspring from *het* oocytes n = 12; HET offspring from *hom* oocytes n = 19). *$P < 0.05$, **$P < 0.01$, one-way ANOVA plus post hoc Tukey's multiple comparisons test. Error bars ± SEM

minor confounding contribution to PND2 offspring size, the majority of the overgrowth phenotype was attributable to differences in EED-dependent regulation in the oocyte.

In contrast to the offspring overgrowth observed for loss of EED in the oocyte, we found that oocytes lacking EZH2 resulted in reduced offspring birth weight. The observed EZH2-dependent growth restriction was consistent with a previous study [15]. However, the pattern of inheritance for EED-mediated effects to offspring was not consistent with *Ezh2* regulating a clear epigenetic inheritance effect from the oocyte as HET offspring generated from $Ezh2$ $^{wt/del}$ and $Ezh2$ $^{del/del}$ oocytes were equivalent, but WT and HET offspring differed in birth weight. In contrast, loss of *Eed* in oocytes resulted in postnatal overgrowth in HET offspring generated from Eed $^{del/del}$ oocytes compared to HET offspring from Eed $^{wt/del}$ oocytes. As these offspring were isogenic and derived from oocytes that lacked EED during oocyte growth and preimplantation development, it appears

that these effects are mediated by altered epigenetic patterning in the oocyte and early life. Furthermore, this *Eed*-mediated, inherited phenotype persisted into the later stages of life (> 18 weeks old). Moreover, while in the previous study, the EZH2-mediated growth restriction was resolved by 4 weeks of age [15], the increased offspring size initiated by lack of EED in the oocyte was more persistent and affected animals through adulthood.

Despite the dependence of PRC2 on EZH2 and EED for catalysing H3K27me3, offspring generated from $Eed^{del/del}$ and $Ezh2^{del/del}$ growing oocytes produced remarkably different overgrowth and growth restriction phenotypes in offspring. Growth restricted offspring were produced from $Ezh2^{del/del}$ oocytes, but there was no difference in weight between HET and HET offspring from $Ezh2^{del/wt}$ and $Ezh2^{del/del}$ oocytes, or between WT and WT offspring from $Ezh2^{del/wt}$ and $Ezh2^{wt/wt}$ oocytes. However, there was a significant difference in weight between genetically different HET and WT offspring. These observations indicate that the growth restriction observed in $Ezh2$ HET vs WT offspring is dependent on $Ezh2$ heterozygosity rather than on epigenetic or maternal factor differences identified for EED. One possible explanation is that haploinsufficiency of PRC2 occurs due to compensation for the loss of EZH2 by EZH1 in $Ezh2^{del/del}$ growing oocytes, whereas PRC2 function is entirely lost in $Eed^{del/del}$ oocytes. However, this scenario seems unlikely as H3K27me3 levels were similar in $Eed^{del/del}$ and $Ezh2^{del/del}$ oocytes, but offspring phenotypes differed substantially for these two models. Moreover, although growth restriction was related to $Ezh2$ heterozygosity in offspring, Eed heterozygosity did not result in a growth phenotype.

An alternative explanation is that the functions of EZH2 and EED differ in these models. EED is known to function only in PRC2 and is essential for PRC2 function [40]. However, EZH2 can methylate non-histone protein targets [41–43] and result in phenotypic change that is PRC2 independent. For example, EZH2 methylates PLZF in T cells, leading to the ubiquitination of PLZF and its subsequent degradation [43]. Furthermore, T cell-specific deletion of $Ezh2$ did not affect H3K27me3 levels and induced rapid expansion of natural killer T (NKT) cells. In contrast, conditional deletion of $Suz12$ or Eed halted NKT cell development due to PRC2 destabilisation [43]. Furthermore, PLZF exerts growth-suppressive activities [44] and regulates limb-axial skeletal patterning in mice [45]. Interestingly, skeletal development is compromised when $Ezh2$ is deleted from mesenchymal stem cells in mice, resulting in reduced skeletal size and reduced body weight [46]. Therefore, although further analyses are required to determine the role of $Ezh2$ in this system, it remains possible that the growth restriction observed in $Ezh2$ heterozygotes derived from $Ezh2^{del/del}$ oocytes may result from PRC2 independent EZH2 effects in the embryo rather than reduced H3K27me3 in the oocyte.

Significantly, de novo germline mutations in EED or $EZH2$ in humans lead to Cohen-Gibson and Weaver syndromes, characterised by overgrowth, skeletal defects and learning/cognitive disabilities [16–18, 21, 22]. As deletion of Eed in the maternal germline also resulted in offspring overgrowth, it appears likely that this mouse model, at least in part, reflects the developmental defects typified in Cohen-Gibson syndrome patients. In mice, this appears to be either an epigenetically inherited phenomenon, or to result from loss of a maternal factor activity of EED, for which the only known activity is to regulate epigenetic state through H3K27 methylation. De novo germline mutations in human EED lead to Cohen-Gibson, also characterised by fetal overgrowth. Moreover, EED is very highly conserved between mice and humans and loss of EED in the oocyte results in similar offspring phenotypes in both species. Therefore, the $EedZP3Cre$ mouse model appears highly relevant for both the study of maternal epigenetic inheritance and Cohen-Gibson syndrome in humans.

An apparent anomaly in the mouse and human models is that murine offspring produced from oocytes lacking $Ezh2$ were born with growth restriction, but patients with de novo missense mutations in either $EZH2$ or EED were born with overgrowth [16–18]. The sequencing data presented here demonstrated that in two affected families, de novo p.Pro132Ser (c.394 C>T) and p.Arg684Cys (c.2050 C>T) changes in $EZH2$ were maternally inherited. Both patients presented with increased length at birth (94th and 95th percentiles) and the patient with the p.Arg684Cys (c.2050 C>T) mutation was in the 95th percentile for weight and was delivered preterm. Consistent with the mouse model, which lacks the EZH2 SET domain and is catalytically inactive [47], the maternally derived $EZH2$ mutations in both patients reduced histone methyltransferase activity, although the impact of Pro132Ser was less severe than that mediated by Arg684Cys [23]. The reasons for the differing phenotypes in mouse and human (i.e., growth restriction in mouse and overgrowth in Weaver patients) are not clear. However, mesenchymal stem cell-specific $Ezh2$ deletion in mice resulted in large offspring with increased size and weight in heterozygous animals, but reduced size and weight in homozygous animals, demonstrating that partial loss of $Ezh2$ activity (via heterozygosity of a loss-of-function mutation) and complete loss of $Ezh2$ (via deletion) have differing impacts on skeletal size and birth weight [46]. Whether similar effects of EZH2 dosage in human patients result in variable skeletal development remains to be determined. However, human data in DECIPHER associates copy number variations in either EZH2 or EED suggesting that both over- and under-growth can be related to alterations of PRC2 dosage [48].

Epigenetic modifications are established and removed through the activity of specific chromatin modifying complexes, which can be altered by mutations, dysregulated transcription, drugs or other environmental influences. The most prominent examples of epigenetic dysregulation have been found in cancer, with mutations in human tumours commonly detected in genes that regulate chromatin organisation [49]. For example, gain-of-function mutations in $EZH2$, EED or $SUZ12$ occur in multiple cancer types, and both EZH2 and EED are current targets for cancer therapy [49]. A prominent example is provided by Tazemetostat (Epizyme, Inc.), an EZH1/2 inhibitor in stage I/II clinical trials for treatment of refractory malignant mesothelioma, lymphomas and a number of other tumours [50]. Significantly, as observed in *Eed* and *Ezh2* deleted oocytes, H3K27me3 is substantially and rapidly reduced in growing oocytes of mice treated with pre-clinical doses of Tazemetostat for just 10 days [51]. While the impacts of maternal Tazemetostat treatment on offspring outcomes remain unknown, our study demonstrates that loss of H3K27me3 in growing oocytes substantially affects life-long offspring outcomes.

Importantly, a range of cancers affect men and women of reproductive age, including tumours carrying gain-of-function mutations in *EZH2*. Our mouse model provides evidence that loss of maternal PRC2 function in the germline of adult females disrupts H3K27me3 and results in defects in offspring growth. Based on these findings, it is likely that drugs targeting PRC2 will alter the epigenome in the oocytes of patients undergoing cancer therapy, raising the possibility that these drugs will affect health outcomes in offspring should the patient conceive during or soon after treatment [52]. Indeed, since the oocyte pool in all women is finite, and oocyte growth and maturation spans 12 months in humans, these drugs may have effects in patients' oocytes long after the termination of treatment. Further evaluation of the impacts of drugs that target PRC2 and other epigenetic modifier enzymes on oocytes and sperm is essential to assess the risks of these drugs in reproductive biology. Such studies would reveal the potential risks of drugs that target epigenetic modifier complexes and would facilitate development of more informed clinical approaches for patients of reproductive age [52], potentially including germline preservation or avoidance of pregnancy after treatment has been completed.

Conclusions

Using a genetic approach that deleted *Eed* specifically in the growing oocyte, we have demonstrated that this conserved and developmentally important epigenetic modifier mediates programming effects in the oocyte and in the earliest stages of development that are important for life-long outcomes in mice. Further understanding of this and other similar models is essential for determining how epigenetic modifiers regulate early life and long-term developmental outcomes in human health and the developmental origins of disease.

Methods
Mouse strains, animal housing, breeding and ethics
Mice were housed at Monash Medical Centre Animal Facility using a 12-h light-dark cycle. Food and water were available ad libitum and room temperature was

21–23 °C with controlled humidity. With the exception of breeding pairs and newborn mice (up to 3 weeks old), males and females were weaned at 21 days and kept in cages of up to five individuals. All animal work was undertaken in accordance with Monash University Animal Ethics Committee (AEC) approvals. *Zp3Cre* mice (C57BL/6-Tg 93knw/J; Jackson Labs line 003651) were constructed by Professor Barbara Knowles and obtained from The Jackson Laboratory. *Eed* floxed mice (*Eed^{fl/fl}*) (B6; 129S1-*Eed^{tm1Sho}*/J; Jackson Labs line 0022727) were constructed by Stuart Orkin and colleagues [36] and obtained from the Jackson Laboratory. *Ezh2* floxed mice (*Ezh2^{fl/fl}*) were constructed by Alexander Tarakhovsky and colleagues [47]. The *Eed* and *Ezh2* lines were backcrossed to a pure C57BL6/J and shared with us by Rhys Allen and Marnie Blewitt, Walter and Eliza Hall Institute for Medical Research, Melbourne.

Genotyping
Colony maintenance animals were genotyped via tail collection at PND2 or ear punch at weaning by Transnetyx (Cordova, TN) using real-time PCR assays designed for each gene (details available on request). Assays were designed based on the genomic structure of *Eed* and *Ezh2* in relation to the conditional genetic modifications established in [36] and [47], respectively.

Tissue fixation and embedding
Ovaries were fixed in 4% paraformaldehyde (PFA) in PBS overnight at 4 °C. Samples were then washed in PBS and left in a 30% sucrose solution overnight at 4 °C. Samples were then placed in disposable cryostat moulds (Sakura Finetek, #4565) filled with OCT (Sakura Finetek, #4583) and frozen in dry ice. Blocks were stored at − 80 °C.

Immunofluorescence
Eight micron sections were cut from OCT embedded ovaries fixed in 4% PFA, mounted on Superfrost Plus slides and dried for 5 min before immersing in 1 × PBS. Sections were then permeabilised by incubation in 1% Triton × 100 (Sigma, #T8787) in PBS for 10 min at room temperature (RT). Slides were washed in PBS. Sections were blocked in PBS containing 5% BSA (Sigma, #A9647) and 10% donkey serum (Sigma, #D9663) and incubated for 45 min at RT. Blocking solution was replaced by PBS containing 1% BSA and appropriately diluted H3K27me3 antibody (1:400, rabbit anti-H3K27me3 Cell Signaling Technologies #C36B11) and incubated for 1 h at RT. Slides were washed three times for 5 min in PBS and secondary antibodies diluted in 1% BSA in 1 × PBS according to antibody dilutions (1:300, donkey anti-rabbit 594, Alexa Fluor Life Technologies #A21207. Secondary antibody incubation was carried out in a dark box for 1 h at RT. Slides were washed three times in

PBS (5 min each wash) and mounted in ProLong Gold® containing DAPI (Life Technologies, #P36931) and left in a dark box overnight to dry. For control slides, only a secondary antibody was applied. Confocal images were taken as single optical sections using a Nikon® C1 inverted Confocal microscope. All pictures were taken at × 80, using a × 40 oil immersion lens.

Phenotypic analysis of offspring

Offspring were weighed at PND2 and/or 30, 49 and 130. At PND30, 49 and 130, female and male mice were analysed separately to account for age-related sex-specific differences. Crown to rump (rump defined by base of tail) and nose to rump measurements were taken by one individual to minimise variances in method. Maternal genotypes were concealed to ensure no bias during collection of data.

Lunar PIXImus DEXA (bone mineral density, lean muscle, fat content)

PND2 offspring were measured, euthanised and stored at − 20 °C. Lunar PIXImus for small animals was used to measure bone and tissue composition using dual-energy X-ray absorptiometry (DEXA). Quality control is ensured by calibrating Lunar PIXImus to a QC phantom upon each run. Animal is place inside the region of interest (ROI), and scan is completed, $n = 61$. All data was collected using Lunar Piximus 2.0 software.

Long-range PCR and sequencing of patient and parental DNA samples

Regions spanning the defined mutations in the EZH2 gene of patients were amplified using long-range PCR in patient and parental DNA samples and processed for single molecule real-time (SMRT) sequencing (Pacific Bioscience) by the Leiden Genome Technology Centre, Department of Human Genetics, Leiden University Medical Center, the Netherlands. All samples were obtained by Professor William Gibson under University of British Columbia and British Columbia Children's Hospital Human Ethics approval numbers H08-00784, H09-01228 and H10-03215, University of British Columbia, Vancouver, Canada. Sample preparation and workflow was carried out as previously described [53]. Primer sequences are included in Additional file 1.

Statistical analysis

One-way ANOVA plus Tukey's post hoc test was used to statistically analyse all quantitative data. Pearson r correlation test used to analyse weight vs. litter size. PRISM software v6.0e; GraphPad Prism 7 was used to analyse and graph data sets. Where data are presented graphically, statistically significant ($P < 0.05$) post hoc outcomes are represented by an asterisk.

A linear mixed model with litter ID as a random effect was used to test for differences among offspring groups while accounting for the relationship between offspring weight and litter size. Tests of significance for fixed effects were undertaken using Satterthwaite approximation for degrees of freedom and type III sums of squares for ANOVA. Linear mixed models were implemented in R v3.3.2 (R Core [54]) using lme4 v1.1-13 and lmerTest v2.0-33 [55, 56].

Abbreviations

E: Embryonic day; EED: Embryonic Ectoderm Development; eGFP: Enhanced GFP; EZH1: Enhancer of Zeste 1; EZH2: Enhancer of Zeste 2; H3K27me3: Trimethylated lysine 27 on histone 3; MVH: Mouse vasa homologue (also known as DDX4); *Nsd*: No significant difference; PRC2: Polycomb repressive complex 2; SUZ12: Supressor of Zeste 12; Zp3-Cre: Zona pellucida 3 Cre recombinase

Acknowledgements

We thank Monash Animal Research Platform staff for assistance with mouse care; MMC Histology Platform and MMI Micro Imaging Facility for technical advice. We thank Stuart Orkin, Barbara Knowles and Alexander Tarakhovsky for respectively sharing the *Eed^fl/fl*, *Ezh2^fl/fl*, and *ZP3Cre* lines and Marnie Blewitt, Rhys Allen, John Carroll and Eileen McLaughlin for sharing mice. We also thank the patients and families involved in the study.

Funding

This work was supported by the National Health and Medical Research Grants 1144966 and 1144887 awarded to PW, funding from the Monash University Faculty of Medicine, Nursing and Health Sciences funding granted to PW and the Victorian Government's Operational Infrastructure Support Program. LP was supported by an Australian Postgraduate Award.

Authors' contributions

PW conceived and designed the study, obtained financial support, collected and analysed data. LP and JS collected and processed the samples. LP optimised and performed experiments and analysed data. CW performed the linear mixed model analysis and analysed data. RV, SW, AC and WG designed assays and performed patient sequencing and data analysis. LP, PW and JS drafted the manuscript, with contributions and review from all authors. All authors read and approved the final manuscript.

Authors' information

LP is now located at the Stem Cells and Cancer Division of the Walter and Eliza Hall Institute of Medical Research, Parkville, Victoria, Australia.

Author details

[1]Centre for Reproductive Health, Hudson Institute of Medical Research and Department of Molecular and Translational Science, Monash University, Clayton, Victoria 3168, Australia. [2]Monash Biomedicine Discovery Institute, Monash University, Clayton, Victoria 3800, Australia. [3]Centre for Geometric Biology, School of Biological Sciences, Monash University, Clayton, Victoria 3800, Australia. [4]Leiden Genome Technology Centre, Department of Human Genetics, Leiden University Medical Center, Leiden, the Netherlands. [5]Department of Medical Genetics, University of British Columbia and British Columbia Children's Hospital Research Institute, Vancouver, BC, Canada.

References

1. Stegemann R, Buchner DA. Transgenerational inheritance of metabolic disease. Semin Cell DevBiol. 2015;43:131–40.

2. Fernandez-Twinn DS, Constancia M, Ozanne SE. Intergenerational epigenetic inheritance in models of developmental programming of adult disease. Semin Cell DevBiol. 2015;43:85–95.

3. Gapp K, Woldemichael BT, Bohacek J, Mansuy IM. Epigenetic regulation in neurodevelopment and neurodegenerative diseases. Neuroscience. 2014; 264:99–111.

4. Keverne EB. Significance of epigenetics for understanding brain development, brain evolution and behaviour. Neuroscience. 2014;264:207–17.

5. Barker DJ. The origins of the developmental origins theory. J Intern Med. 2007;261(5):412–7.

6. Pasini D, Bracken AP, Jensen MR, Denchi EL, Helin K. Suz12 is essential for mouse development and for EZH2 histone methyltransferase activity. EMBO J. 2004;23(20):4061–71.

7. Faust C, Schumacher A, Holdener B, Magnuson T. The Eed mutation disrupts anterior mesoderm production in mice. Development. 1995;121(2): 273–85.

8. O'Carroll D, Erhardt S, Pagani M, Barton SC, Surani MA, Jenuwein T. The polycomb-group gene Ezh2 is required for early mouse development. Mol Cell Biol. 2001;21(13):4330–6.

9. Lesch BJ, Dokshin GA, Young RA, McCarrey JR, Page DC. A set of genes critical to development is epigenetically poised in mouse germ cells from fetal stages through completion of meiosis. Proc Natl Acad Sci U S A. 2013; 110(40):16061–6.

10. Sachs M, Onodera C, Blaschke K, Ebata KT, Song JS, Ramalho-Santos M. Bivalent chromatin marks developmental regulatory genes in the mouse embryonic germline in vivo. Cell Rep. 2013;3(6):1777–84.

11. Ng JH, Kumar V, Muratani M, Kraus P, Yeo JC, Yaw LP, Xue K, Lufkin T, Prabhakar S, Ng HH. In vivo epigenomic profiling of germ cells reveals germ cell molecular signatures. Dev Cell. 2013;24(3):324–33.

12. Erkek S, Hisano M, Liang CY, Gill M, Murr R, Dieker J, Schubeler D, van der Vlag J, Stadler MB, Peters AH. Molecular determinants of nucleosome retention at CpG-rich sequences in mouse spermatozoa. Nat Struct Mol Biol. 2013;20(7):868–75.

13. Brykczynska U, Hisano M, Erkek S, Ramos L, Oakeley EJ, Roloff TC, Beisel C, Schubeler D, Stadler MB, Peters AH. Repressive and active histone methylation mark distinct promoters in human and mouse spermatozoa. Nat Struct Mol Biol. 2010;17(6):679–87.

14. Hammoud SS, Nix DA, Zhang H, Purwar J, Carrell DT, Cairns BR. Distinctive chromatin in human sperm packages genes for embryo development. Nature. 2009;460(7254):473–8.

15. Erhardt S, Su IH, Schneider R, Barton S, Bannister AJ, Perez-Burgos L, Jenuwein T, Kouzarides T, Tarakhovsky A, Surani MA. Consequences of the depletion of zygotic and embryonic enhancer of zeste 2 during preimplantation mouse development. Development. 2003;130(18):4235–48.

16. Cohen ASA, Tuysuz B, Shen YQ, Bhalla SK, Jones SJM, Gibson WT. A novel mutation in EED associated with overgrowth. J Hum Genet. 2015;60(6):339–42.

17. Cohen ASA, Gibson WT. EED-associated overgrowth in a second male patient. J Hum Genet. 2016;61(9):831–4.

18. Cooney E, Bi WM, Schlesinger AE, Vinson S, Potocki L. Novel EED mutation in patient with Weaver syndrome. Am J Med Genet A. 2017;173(2):541–5.

19. Imagawa E, Higashimoto K, Sakai Y, Numakura C, Okamoto N, Matsunaga S, Ryo A, Sato Y, Sanefuji M, Ihara K, et al. Mutations in genes encoding polycomb repressive complex 2 subunits cause Weaver syndrome. Hum Mutat. 2017;38(6):637–48.

20. Tatton-Brown K, Loveday C, Yost S, Clarke M, Ramsay E, Zachariou A, Elliott A, Wylie H, Ardissone A, Rittinger O, et al. Mutations in epigenetic regulation genes are a major cause of overgrowth with intellectual disability. Am J Hum Genet. 2017;100(5):725–36.

21. Gibson WT, Hood RL, Zhan SH, Bulman DE, Fejes AP, Moore R, Mungall AJ, Eydoux P, Babul-Hirji R, An JH, et al. Mutations in EZH2 cause Weaver syndrome. Am J Hum Genet. 2012;90(1):110–8.

22. Tatton-Brown K, Hanks S, Ruark E, Zachariou A, Duarte SD, Ramsay E, Snape K, Murray A, Perdeaux ER, Seal S, et al. Germline mutations in the oncogene EZH2 cause Weaver syndrome and increased human height. Oncotarget. 2011;2(12):1127–33.

23. Cohen AS, Yap DB, Lewis ME, Chijiwa C, Ramos-Arroyo MA, Tkachenko N, Milano V, Fradin M, McKinnon ML, Townsend KN, et al. Weaver syndrome-associated EZH2 protein variants show impaired histone methyltransferase function in vitro. Hum Mutat. 2016;37(3):301–7.

24. Smith P, Wilhelm D, Rodgers RJ. Development of mammalian ovary. J Endocrinol. 2014;221(3):R145–61.

25. Eppig JJ. Oocyte control of ovarian follicular development and function in mammals. Reproduction. 2001;122(6):829–38.

26. Petronczki M, Siomos MF, Nasmyth K. Un menage a quatre: the molecular biology of chromosome segregation in meiosis. Cell. 2003;112(4):423–40.

27. Kim K-H, Lee K-A. Maternal effect genes: findings and effects on mouse embryo development. Clin ExpReprodMed. 2014;41(2):47–61.

28. Prokopuk L, Western PS, Stringer JM. Transgenerational epigenetic inheritance: adaptation through the germline epigenome? Epigenomics. 2015;7(5):829–46.

29. Hogg K, Western PS. Refurbishing the germline epigenome: out with the old, in with the new. Semin Cell DevBiol. 2015;45:104–13.

30. Posfai E, Kunzmann R, Brochard V, Salvaing J, Cabuy E, Roloff TC, Liu ZC, Tardat M, van Lohuizen M, Vidal M, et al. Polycomb function during oogenesis is required for mouse embryonic development. Genes Dev. 2012; 26(9):920–32.

31. Lewandoski M, Wassarman KM, Martin GR. Zp3-cre, a transgenic mouse line for the activation or inactivation of loxP-flanked target genes specifically in the female germ line. Curr Biol. 1997;7(2):148–51.

32. Bao S, Tang F, Li X, Hayashi K, Gillich A, Lao K, Surani MA. Epigenetic reversion of post-implantation epiblast to pluripotent embryonic stem cells. Nature. 2009;461(7268):1292–5.

33. Kemler R, Hierholzer A, Kanzler B, Kuppig S, Hansen K, Taketo MM, de Vries WN, Knowles BB, Solter D. Stabilization of beta-catenin in the mouse zygote leads to premature epithelial-mesenchymal transition in the epiblast. Development. 2004;131(23):5817–24.

34. Inoue A, Jiang L, Lu F, Suzuki T, Zhang Y. Maternal H3K27me3 controls DNA methylation-independent imprinting. Nature. 2017;547(7664):419–24.

35. Prokopuk L, Stringer JM, Hogg K, Elgass KD, Western PS. PRC2 is required for extensive reorganization of H3K27me3 during epigenetic reprogramming in mouse fetal germ cells. Epigenetics Chromatin. 2017;10:1–20.

36. Xie H, Xu J, Hsu JH, Nguyen M, Fujiwara Y, Peng C, Orkin SH. Polycomb repressive complex 2 regulates normal hematopoietic stem cell function in a developmental-stage-specific manner. Cell Stem Cell. 2014;14(1):68–80.

37. Racki WJ, Richter JD. CPEB controls oocyte growth and follicle development in the mouse. Development. 2006;133(22):4527–37.

38. Li R, Albertini DF. The road to maturation: somatic cell interaction and self-organization of the mammalian oocyte. Nat Rev Mol Cell Biol. 2013;14(3):141–52.

39. Leighton PA, Ingram RS, Eggenschwiler J, Efstratiadis A, Tilghman SM. Disruption of imprinting caused by deletion of the H19 gene region in mice. Nature. 1995;375(6526):34–9.

40. Cao Q, Wang X, Zhao M, Yang R, Malik R, Qiao Y, Poliakov A, Yocum AK, Li Y, Chen W, et al. The central role of EED in the orchestration of polycomb group complexes. Nat Commun. 2014;5:3127.

41. Yan JL, Ng SB, Tay JLS, Lin BH, Koh TL, Tan J, Selvarajan V, Liu SC, Bi CL, Wang S, et al. EZH2 overexpression in natural killer/T-cell lymphoma confers growth advantage independently of histone methyltransferase activity. Blood. 2013;121(22):4512–20.

42. Bracken AP, Pasini D, Capra M, Prosperini E, Colli E, Helin K. EZH2 is downstream of the pRB-E2F pathway, essential for proliferation and amplified in cancer. EMBO J. 2003;22(20):5323–35.

43. Vasanthakumar A, Xu DK, Lun ATL, Kueh AJ, van Gisbergen KPJM, Iannarella N, Li XF, Yu L, Wang D, Williams BRG, et al. A non-canonical function of Ezh2 preserves immune homeostasis. EMBO Rep. 2017;18(4):619–31.

44. Shaknovich R, Yeyati PL, Ivins S, Melnick A, Lempert C, Waxman S, Zelent A, Licht JD. The promyelocytic leukemia zinc finger protein affects myeloid cell growth, differentiation, and apoptosis. Mol Cell Biol. 1998;18(9):5533–45.

45. Barna M, Hawe N, Niswander L, Pandolfi PP. Plzf regulates limb and axial skeletal patterning. Nat Genet. 2000;25(2):166–72.

46. Hemming S, Cakouros D, Codrington J, Vandyke K, Arthur A, Zannettino A, Gronthos S. EZH2 deletion in early mesenchyme compromises postnatal bone micro architecture and structural integrity and accelerates remodeling. FASEB J. 2017;31(3):1011.

47. Su IH, Basavaraj A, Krutchinsky AN, Hobert O, Ullrich A, Chait BT, Tarakhovsky A. Ezh2 controls B cell development through histone H3 methylation and Igh rearrangement. Nat Immunol. 2003;4(2):124–31.

48. Firth HV, Richards SM, Bevan AP, Clayton S, Corpas M, Rajan D, Van Vooren S, Moreau Y, Pettett RM, Carter NP. DECIPHER: database of chromosomal imbalance and phenotype in humans using Ensembl resources. Am J Hum Genet. 2009;84(4):524–33.

49. Jones PA, Issa JPJ, Baylin S. Targeting the cancer epigenome for therapy. Nat Rev Genet. 2016;17(10):630–41.
50. Knutson SK, Kawano S, Minoshima Y, Warholic NM, Huang KC, Xiao YH, Kadowaki T, Uesugi M, Kuznetsov G, Kumar N, et al. Selective inhibition of EZH2 by EPZ-6438 leads to potent antitumor activity in EZH2-mutant non-Hodgkin lymphoma. Mol Cancer Ther. 2014;13(4):842–54.
51. Prokopuk L, Hogg K, Western PS. Pharmacological inhibition of EZH2 disrupts the female germline epigenome. Clin Epigenetics. 2018; In press
52. Western PS. Epigenomic drugs and the germline: collateral damage in the home of heritability? Mol Cell Endocrinol. 2018; In press
53. Buermans HPJ, Vossen RHAM, Anvar SY, Allard WG, Guchelaar HJ, White SJ, den Dunnen JT, Swen JJ, van der Straaten T. Flexible and scalable full-length CYP2D6 long amplicon PacBio sequencing. Hum Mutat. 2017;38(3):310–6.
54. Team RC. R: a language and environment for statistical computing [computer software], v3.3.2 edn. Vienna: R Foundation for Statistical Computing; 2016.
55. Bates D, Mächler M, Bolker B, Walker S. Fitting linear mixed-effects models using lme4. J Stat Softw. 2015;67(1):1–48.
56. Kuznetsova A, Brockhoff PB, Christensen RHB. lmerTest package: tests in linear mixed effects models. J Stat Softw. 2017;82(13):1–26.

3

Circulating microRNAs as potential cancer biomarkers: the advantage and disadvantage

Hao Wang[1], Ran Peng[2], Junjie Wang[2], Zelian Qin[1*] and Lixiang Xue[1,2*]

Abstract

MicroRNAs are endogenous single-stranded non-coding small RNA molecules that can be secreted into the circulation and exist stably. They usually exhibit aberrant expression under different physiological and pathological conditions. Recently, differentially expressed circulating microRNAs were focused on as potential biomarkers for cancer screening. We herein review the role of circulating microRNAs for cancer diagnosis, tumor subtype classification, chemo- or radio-resistance monitoring, and outcome prognosis. Moreover, circulating microRNAs still have several issues hindering their reliability for the practical clinical application. Future studies need to elucidate further potential application of circulating microRNAs as specific and sensitive markers for clinical diagnosis or prognosis in cancers.

Keywords: Cancer, Circulating microRNA, Biomarker, Diagnosis, Prognosis

Background

Cancer is one of the leading causes of death worldwide. In recent years, some significant improvements have been made in tumor diagnosis and treatment. However, early detection is still critical for improving outcomes and reducing recurrence and mortality of cancer patients. The absence of obvious symptoms and insufficiently sensitive biomarkers in early stages of carcinoma limits early diagnosis. Biopsy and imaging examination as golden standards greatly improve the detection rate, but their applications are limited by their own invasive or radiation-related characteristics, respectively. In addition, traditional tumor diagnostic markers like carcinoembryonic antigen (CEA) and CA199 usually exhibit low sensitivity. Therefore, it is urgent to identify novel, more sensitive, and easy-to-detect biomarkers which can be used in diagnosis and prognosis of cancers.

Novel methods are currently under development for cancer detection, including those based on the detection of microRNAs (miRNAs). MicroRNAs are endogenous, single-stranded, non-coding small RNA with length of ~ 22 nucleotide (nt). The first miRNA was discovered in 1993 in *Caenorhabditis elegans* which participated in

embryo development [1]. In the next two decades, miRNAs were found in plants, animals, protists, and viruses but not in bacteria. These small RNA molecules function as antisense RNA to negatively regulate their target genes at the post-transcription level. Most miRNAs have only modest effects on the translation of their target genes, but they constitute highly complex networks with their targets and downstream effectors [2]. A single gene is simultaneously targeted by multiple miRNAs, while each miRNA is able to target numerous genes via similar seed sequence. It was reported that miRNAs regulated more than 30% of the human genome and are involved in almost all fundamental cell processes [3, 4]. A group of target genes may function through a common signaling pathway and accordingly facilitate similar cell behaviors, such as proliferation, apoptosis, differentiation, migration, invasion, metabolism, and stress response.

The expression patterns of miRNAs are usually altered in different development stages and various pathology conditions like senescence, cardiovascular diseases, and cancers [2, 5, 6]. Dysregulations of miRNAs were often observed in different kinds of cancers due to dysfunction of the miRNA biogenesis process, transcription of miRNA-encoding genes, and regulator of mature miRNAs like circular-RNA [2]. Some of these altered miRNAs were significantly overexpressed and regarded as

* Correspondence: qinzl@bjmu.edu.cn; lixiangxue@hsc.pku.edu.cn
[1]Medical Research Center, Peking University Third Hospital, Beijing, China
Full list of author information is available at the end of the article

oncogenes or "oncomiRs" which accelerate tumor occurrence, development, and metastasis. Meanwhile, those that decreased in cancer patients were considered tumor suppressors [2, 6]. The differential expression of miRNAs can be detected by polymerase chain reaction (PCR), Northern blotting, microarray, and deep sequencing and have potential for clinical applications [7, 8].

miRNAs in different cell types can be secreted into the extracellular space and then transported to the circulating body fluid like peripheral blood. It was reported that 10% of the known human miRNAs could be detected in plasma. About 30% of them were mirtrons, rare miRNAs originated from short-chain, hairpin-structured introns of mRNA and through a special biogenesis pathway [9–11]. These miRNAs are detectable in plasma or serum in a remarkably stable form, encapsulated into the extracellular vesicles or bound with special lipid proteins, thus being resistant to RNase digestions [12–15]. Therefore, these small molecules are capable to be ideal candidates to serve as biomarkers for cancer detection by liquid biopsies. Besides peripheral blood, various body fluids, including saliva, cerebrospinal fluid, ascites, urine, breast milk, and semen, allow for miRNA detection [16].

This review mainly discussed the potential application of circulating miRNAs as clinical cancer biomarkers. We herein are more focused on those cancers with higher incidence rates and mortalities, more difficult detection in early stages, and heavier burdens on people and society, like cancers of the lung, liver, colorectal, stomach, and breast.

Potential clinical application of circulating miRNAs

The differential expression of circulating miRNAs exhibited promising potential for cancer screening without additional injury for patients. The abnormal levels of distinct miRNAs could be observed at an early stage, during progression, and after metastasis of cancers. Thus, these small RNA molecules may function as favorable clinical biomarkers for distinguishing tumors, treatment strategy selection, and outcomes. In non-small cell lung cancers (NSCLC) patients, for example, a large group of miRNAs have been identified to be differentially expressed in different stages of disease and to contribute to the diagnosis, treatment determination, and prognosis (Fig. 1).

Circulating miRNAs as biomarkers for early diagnosis

A growing number of circulating miRNAs was reported to be dysregulated in the early stage of cancers. The altered expression may be observed before the obvious clinical symptoms or clear biopsy and image examination evidence. Plasma miR-21-5p, miR-20a-5p, miR-141-3p, miR-145-5p, miR-155-5p, and miR-223-3p significantly increased for NSCLC patients at stages I and II [17–19]. Serum miR-126-3p, miR-182-5p, miR-183-5p, and miR-210-3p were also found to possess early detective value for NSCLC patients, exhibiting similar sensitivity and specificity with traditional tumor marker CEA [20]. Two miRNA precursors, pri-miR-944 and pri-miR-3662, were also capable of distinguishing NSCLC at stages I–IIIA [21]. Significantly decreased levels of miR-125a-3p were observed in plasma exosomes of colon cancer patients [22], as well as increased levels of miR-23a-3p, miR-27a-3p, miR-142-5p, and miR-376c-3p in serum [23]. A group of miRNA, including miR-642b-3p, miR-1202-5p, miR-1207-5p, miR-1225-5p, miR-4270-5p, and miR-4281-3p, was upregulated in plasma of breast cancer patients with stage I [24]. Serum miR-1825-3p was specifically downregulated in glioma at early stage, and its level was correlated with tumor progression and poor prognosis [25]. These evidences suggest that the

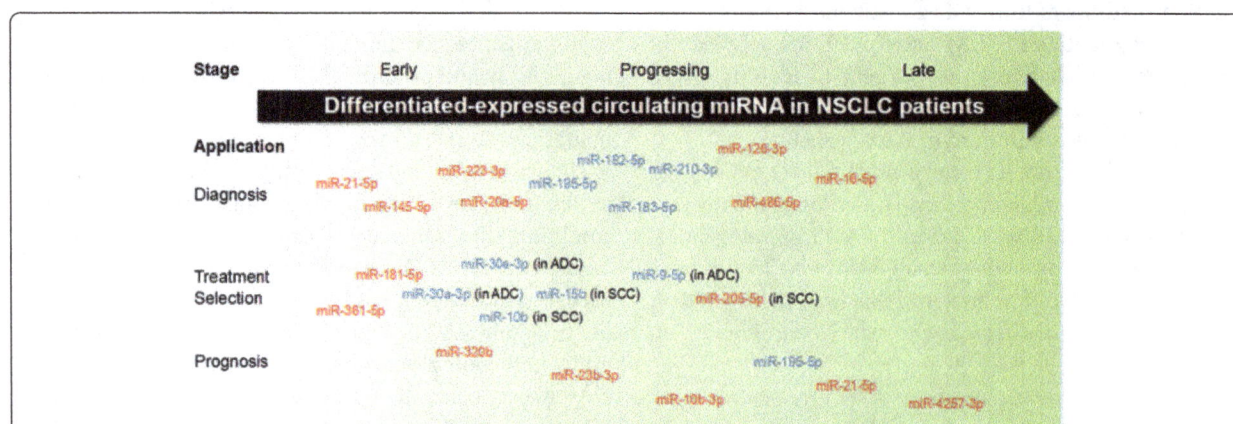

Fig. 1 The potential clinical applications of circulating miRNAs as tumor biomarkers for NSCLC. Diverse circulating miRNAs functioned at various aspects of clinical screening. In NSCLC patient for example, some differentially expressed miRNAs facilitated cancer diagnosis and prognosis while others contributed to treatment strategy selection by distinguishing tumor subtypes, monitoring tumor progression, or predicting the drug resistance. The expression levels of these cell-free miRNAs could be significantly differentiated at early stage, during the tumor progression, or until the late stage. Red color indicated increased expressed miRNAs in peripheral blood of NSCLC patients, while blue color indicated decreased ones

circulating miRNA detection might be introduced for early-stage cancer screening.

Circulating miRNAs as diagnosis biomarkers to distinguish different subtypes of cancer

Cancers can be divided into different subtypes by tissue origination or pathological mechanisms. For example, NSCLCs include two major pathologic subtypes, adenocarcinoma (ADC) and squamous cell carcinoma (SCC) [26]. Breast cancers are well known as heterogeneous diseases, which can be sub-classified by the presence of estrogen receptor (ER), progesterone receptor (PR), and HER2/neu receptor [27, 28]. The sub-classification of specific tumors is valuable for determining tumor mechanisms and making therapeutic decisions. Of note, certain differentially expressed miRNAs in parallel with the different subtypes draw more and more attention recently. They could be optimal to determine tumor subtype and pathology, contributing to the selection for a more efficient therapeutic approach.

Taking NSCLC as an example, the accurate sub-classification into ADC and SCC is important for deciding treatment methods. Expression patterns of several miRNAs were different not only between the plasma of NSCLC patients and healthy individuals, but also between ADC and SCC patients. Levels of miR-16-5p and miR-486-5p were elevated in ADC and SCC cases compared to those of healthy ones. miR-9-5p expression was stable between overall NSCLC patients and healthy controls, but exhibited significant declination in ADC patients instead of SCC ones. Another plasma miRNA, miR-205-5p, was upregulated only in SCC patients [29]. Additionally, Jin et al. found several ADC- and SCC-specific differentially expressed miRNAs by RNA sequencing [30]. miR-181-5p, miR-361-5p, and miR-320b were significantly elevated in plasma exosomes of NSCLC patients. The levels of miR-181-5p and miR-361-5p were increased by more than 10 times in ADC patients than SCC patients, and miR-320b in SCC samples increased by over 10 times than in ADC ones. miR-30a-3p and miR-30e-3p were specifically downregulated in ADC patients, while miR-10b-5p and miR-15b-5p were decreased in SCC patients. Therefore, investigators suggest that these miRNA panels may be not only applicable in NSCLC diagnosis, but also helpful to subtype discrimination. Interestingly, cell-free miRNA precursors were also found to have diagnostic potential. Pri-miR-944 was suggested to distinguish SCC from ADC, while pri-miR-3662 distinguished ADC from SCC [21]. In addition, the mature forms of these two miRNAs were also revealed to have the potential in indicating the diagnostic accuracy for operable SCC and ADC, respectively [31].

The subtyping of heterogeneous breast cancer is also of great importance for clinical therapy. The positively expressed ER, PR, or HER2/neu in tumors could be directed as therapeutic targets. On the contrary, patients bearing triple-negative breast cancer (TNBC), which expressed none of these receptors, were usually treated with traditional chemotherapy or radiotherapy [27]. TNBC was associated with higher stage at diagnosis and poorer prognosis. Therefore, biomarkers of specific breast cancer subtypes have also been focused on, especially for TNBC from the miRNA point of view. Shin et al. [32] observed the declined levels of miR-16-5p, miR-21-5p, and miR-199a-5p in plasma and tumor tissues of TNBC patients compared with both non-TNBC and healthy individuals, as well as the elevated levels of miR-92a-3p and miR-342-3p. Among them, miR-199a-5p exhibited the highest value to distinguished TNBC from non-TNBC. This small molecule was validated to be downregulated since the stage I of tumor and to decrease with tumor progression [32]. Meanwhile, exosomal levels of miR-373-3p were increased in TNBC but not luminal carcinomas and higher in ER/PR-negative tumors than receptor-positive tumors [33]. Interestingly, serum levels of miR-373-3p showed no significant difference between TNBC and luminal carcinomas.

In other cancers, different tumor subtypes may also be distinguished by circulating miRNAs. Exosomal levels of miR-101-3p and miR-483-5p in plasma of adrenocortical cancer were significantly higher than those of adrenocortical adenomas, which could be adopted to preoperative diagnosis of adrenocortical malignancy [34]. On the other hand, papillary and follicular thyroid cancer might be distinguished by the expression of exosomal miR-21-5p, miR-31-5p, and miR-181a-5p in combination [35].

Circulating miRNAs contribute to monitor tumor metastasis

The occurrence of tumor metastasis leads to a significant impairment of curative effect, resulting to the poor survival rate and high risk of recurrence. There are currently no reliable biomarkers for predicting metastatic spread to different sites. According to the characteristics of relative tissue specificity of miRNAs, the candidates for this purpose become favorable since more and more circulating miRNAs were found to be associated with clinical tumor stage and/or metastasis. In osteosarcoma patients, miR-497-5p was significantly downregulated in primary tumor tissues, metastatic tissues, and serum compared to healthy controls [36–41]. This small molecule targeted multiple genes like IGF-1R [38], VEGFA [39], AMOT [40], and P21 [42] to inhibit osteosarcoma cell proliferation, migration, and invasion and enhance apoptosis. Furthermore, the declined miR-497-5p expression was associated with clinical stage, distant metastasis, and promoted cisplatin resistance [36, 39].

Elevated levels of miR-205-5p in plasma were correlated with tumor stage and pathological grade in patients with bladder cancer [43]. miR-148a-3p expression was reduced in plasma of ovarian cancer patients and correlated with histopathologic grade and lymph node metastasis [44]. Plasma levels of miR-520g were higher in breast cancer patients with low differentiation degree grade, mammary gland invasion, and lymph node metastasis [45]. Additionally, both miR-106a-5p and miR-196a/b-3p were upregulated in gastric cancer patients, and their levels were associated with TNM stage and metastatic potential [46, 47]. In the future, further clarifying the miRNAs from the original tumor sites or the targeted metastatic tissue/organ might be helpful to predict the upcoming metastasis event.

Circulating miRNAs predicted the sensitivity of tumor to clinical treatment

Chemotherapy and radiotherapy are important approaches for tumor treatment, which are often in combination with surgical operation. However, some types of tumor cells may gain resistance after long-time treatment due to the heterogeneity of tumors. As a result, parts of patients would have worse outcomes upon a certain treatment. Investigators expect to find accurate biomarkers to detect or predict the resistance of different cancers, in order to select superior treatment strategies.

In pancreatic ductal adenocarcinoma (PDAC), a main subtype of pancreatic cancer, miR-155-5p was upregulated in tumor tissues and plasma, and the expressions in tissues were associated with tumor stage and poor prognosis [48–50]. Besides, long-term administration of gemcitabine in tumor cells further overexpressed miR-155-5p which was released into exosomes to induce gemcitabine resistance via anti-apoptotic activity. Therefore, higher miR-155-5p expression showed chemoresistance and poor prognosis for PDAC patients receiving gemcitabine treatment [51]. Levels of miR-1914-3p and miR-1915-3p in plasma from chemo-resistant colorectal cancer (CRC) patients were decreased compared to those from responders. These two miRNAs were demonstrated to facilitate cell resistance to 5-Fu and oxaliplatin by NFIX in vitro [52]. Aberrant reduction of miR-497-5p in plasma of osteosarcoma patients implied the poor response to chemotherapy [36]. Furthermore, lower miR-146-5p levels in serum exosomes were associated with the cisplatin resistance and shorter progression-free survival (PFS) for NSCLC patients [53]. These putative resistant miRNAs may be favorable for monitoring the resistant and tolerance of treatment and for selection of clinical therapeutic approach. In line with these findings, targeting those miRNAs and their downstream targets might become the novel strategy to rescue the resistance against chemotherapy or radiotherapy.

Circulating miRNAs as prognostic biomarkers of cancers

Accumulating evidences suggested that circulating levels of miRNAs may be associated with the outcomes. The expressions of miR-222-3p in serum exosomes were associated with poor outcomes of NSCLC patients [54]. After internalized via caveolin- and lipid raft-mediated endocytosis, miR-222-3p promoted the proliferation, chemoresistance, migration, and invasion of recipient cells. Elevated levels of miR-23b-3p, miR-10b-3p, and miR-21-5p in exosomes were associated with poor overall survival (OS) of NSCLC patients [55]. Additionally, higher levels of miR-21-5p and miR-4257-3p existed in exosomes of recurrent NSCLC patients compared with those without recurrent and the healthy controls [56]. The level of these two exosomal miRNAs was associated with disease-free survival (DFS), while miR-4257-3p alone was also associated with node metastasis and TNM stage. On the other hand, miR-21-5p was also upregulated in the circulating exosomes, primary tumor tissues, and liver metastasis tissues [57]. Exosomal level of miR-21-5p was associated with liver metastasis, TNM stage, and poor prognosis, including shorter OS and DFS.

Besides the tumor type mentioned above, circulating miRNAs also showed tight correlation with prognosis in other types of tumors. The levels of let-7b and miR-18a-5p were significantly associated with DFS and OS in multiple myeloma patients [58]. miR-4772-3p levels were negatively associated with the risk of recurrence and death in serum exosomes derived from stage II and stage III colon cancer patients [59]. Higher levels of plasma miR-148a were associated with longer OS in ovarian cancer patients [44, 60]. Lower plasma levels of miR-185-5p were correlated with poor survival in glioma patients [61]. These findings above suggest the promise of applying circulating miRNAs as biomarkers for early prediction upon certain treatment and improvement of the outcomes in most types of cancer.

The advantage of circulating miRNAs as diagnosis and prognosis biomarkers

Traditional cancer markers are mainly produced by tumor tissues or normal embryo tissues, while absence or in tiny amount in tissue and blood of healthy adults. The most validated traditional cancer markers include alpha-fetoprotein (AFP), carcinoembryonic antigen (CEA), and carbohydrate antigen (CA) [62, 63]. They are generally broad-spectrum biomarkers for diagnosis of various types of cancers. CEA, CA199, and CA125 were generally accepted to be validated to have positive predictive value as circulating biomarkers for different cancers. Other screening strategies include mammography for breast cancer [64, 65], colonoscopy for CRC [66], and prostate-specific antigen (PSA) for prostate cancer [67]. However, still missing are more effective, accurate, specific, and sensitive screening biomarkers to fulfill the detective and predictive functions in the care of cancer patients. Circulating miRNAs have the particular advantage as a potential clinical application.

Circulating miRNAs are non-invasive biomarkers

Circulating miRNAs are easy to obtain without severe damage. Besides, a great number of potential effective miRNA biomarkers are stable in healthy people. Their expression levels may not be obviously affected by age, gender, body mass index (BMI), smoking status, or other basic characteristics when evaluating pathogenic potential. Hence, the altered expression pattern might be introduced to routine examination for monitoring and early diagnosis of cancers.

Although cell-free miRNAs from plasma and serum are the most common circulating miRNA biomarkers, other body fluid samples like urine and saliva are also applicable as the resource of circulating miRNAs. miR-186-5p was overexpressed in not only tumor tissues and blood, but also urine from bladder cancer patients [68]. Several miRNAs including miR-210-3p were upregulated in urine from transitional cell carcinoma patients and capable to facilitate cancer diagnosis [69]. All members of let-7 families were significantly elevated in urine from clear-cell renal cell cancer (ccRCC) patients [70], while a combination of urinary exosomal miR-34b-5p, miR-126-3p, and miR-449a-3p could be favorable for ccRCC diagnosis [71]. A panel of four breast cancer-related miRNAs (miR-21-5p, miR-125b-5p, miR-155-5p, and miR-451-5p) was also differentially expressed in urine samples of breast cancer patients and exhibited their diagnostic value [72]. Elevated levels of miR-143-3p and miR-30e-5p in urine samples of PDAC patients shown their potential as diagnostic biomarkers in the early stage [73]. Therefore, these easily accessible cell-free small molecules have been widely applied for clinical use.

Circulating miRNAs may be used for screening tumors with higher sensitivity

Up to now, polymerase chain reaction (PCR) is still the major examination technology for circulating miRNA. Amplification is a critical step and characteristic of all kinds of PCR, which magnifies the initial difference between samples, even if the difference is quite small. Therefore, the current detection method makes circulating miRNAs more sensitive biomarkers. Monitoring of the aberrant expression can be easier and earlier compared with biopsy and/or image examination which reflects the actual size without amplification, although the latter are regarded as the golden standard so far.

The dynamic expression pattern of circulating miRNAs may be associated with the progression of tumors

The generation of miRNAs is dynamic and prompt upon the internal or external stimuli. This feature endows miRNAs the ability to observe the whole time course changes in real time and dynamic manner from tumorigenesis throughout the following progression. miR-195-5p was reported to inhibit the proliferation, migration, and invasion of NSCLC cells via multiple targets [74–77], and the lower miR-195-5p levels in plasma were showed to be associated with lymph node metastasis and advanced clinical stage [78]. Serum miR-373-3p was downregulated in pancreatic cancer patients, and miR-373-3p level was negatively correlated with TNM stage, lymph node metastasis, and distant metastasis [79]. In periampullary carcinoma, miR-192-5p levels were increased and correlated with tumor stage and aggressiveness [80]. A panel of miRNAs including miR-34a-5p, miR-34b-5p, and miR-34c-5p was significantly downregulated in TNBC patients. Among these miRNAs, miR-34a-5p expression was positively correlated with lymph node metastasis together with miR-34b-5p and correlated with tumor grade and distant metastasis together with miR-34c-5p [81]. These observations revealed the possibility of circulating miRNAs for evaluating the stage and progression of tumors. The whole dynamic expression pattern of miRNAs could depict the development landscape of cancer during the entire progression.

The disadvantage and limitation of circulating miRNAs as diagnosis and prognosis biomarkers

The diversified origin of circulating miRNAs influences the effectiveness partially

Most of potential miRNA biomarkers ubiquitously exist in both healthy individuals and cancer patients. The differences in their expression levels between healthy people and patients are usually quite tiny. So the way of sampling cannot be ignored to distinguish cancers from healthy state or other benign injury accurately.

Currently circulating miRNAs are obtained from venous plasma or serum. miRNA profiles in venous and arterial plasma were largely similar, so the levels of most miRNAs have no significant difference between vein and artery. Five elevated miRNAs (miR-20b-3p, miR-28-3p, miR-192-5p, miR-223-3p, and miR-296-5p) were identified from serum of esophageal squamous cell carcinoma (ESCC) patients [82]. The investigators compared their content in venous and arterial serum and found no statistic difference. However, the use of venous miRNAs for cancer detection was still challenged in some cases. Ten arterial highly expressed miRNAs and fourteen venous highly expressed miRNAs were identified in plasma samples of healthy male rats [83]. The miRNA profiles in arterial plasma showed higher correlation with that in tissue. Studies with human samples had similar observations. Levels of upregulated miRNAs (miR-10-3p, miR-21-5p, miR-409-3p, and miR-425-5p) were even higher in arterial plasma compared with venous plasma from lung adenocarcinoma patients [84]. Levels of let-7g-5p, miR-15b-5p, miR-155-5p, and miR-328-5p were found to be significantly higher in mesenteric vein than in peripheral vein and tumor tissue from colon cancer patients, suggesting that tumor drain vein contained more complete biomarkers origin from tumor tissues than peripheral vein [85]. Thus, the blood sampling methods should be carefully considered for some specific miRNA biomarkers.

Exosomal miRNAs in peripheral blood have also drawn more and more attention in the aspect of biomarkers. It is known that most of the miRNAs in blood were packaged in extracellular vesicles like microvesicles and exosomes. Several miRNAs were reported to differently express in plasma, serum, and peripheral blood exosomes. For example, miR-181b-5p and miR-21-5p were enriched in the exosomes of lung cancer patients instead of healthy individuals [86]. Plasma levels of miR-19b-3p, miR-21-5p, miR-221-3p, miR-409-3p, miR-425-5p, and miR-584-5p were elevated in lung adenocarcinoma patients, but only miR-19-3p, miR-21-5p, and miR-221-3p were found to be upregulated in plasma exosomes [84]. Similarly, a panel of five serum miRNAs overexpressed in ESCC patients, including miR-20b-5p, miR-28-3p, miR-192-5p, miR-223-3p, and miR-296-5p. Only miR-296-5p was found to be upregulated in ESCC serum exosomes [82]. Likewise, miR-132-3p and miR-185-5p were overexpressed in gastric cancer patients' serum instead of exosomes [87]. miR-101-3p was elevated both in serum and exosomes from breast cancer patient, but expression levels of miR-372-3p and miR-373-3p increased in exosome and serum, respectively [33]. These observations implied the importance of selecting a proper sampling method for certain circulating miRNAs.

Single miRNA molecule has limitations in both sensitivity and specificity

High sensitivity and specification are the fundamental demands and the most important evaluation criteria for circulating miRNAs as diagnostic or prognostic biomarkers for clinical application. Single miRNA molecules could hardly meet the criteria for many candidate miRNA biomarkers because their levels in patients and healthy controls were overlapped. This observation suggested that the level of an applicable miRNA biomarker should possess high individual difference, which increased the possibility of false negative or positive diagnosis.

On the other hand, many cell-free miRNAs showed altered expression patterns in various types of cancers instead of a certain cancer type. miR-21-5p, miR-155-5p, and miR-210-3p are good examples, as all of them are involved in cancers like NSCLC [17–20, 88], breast cancer [89–92], and colorectal cancer [57, 93, 94].

Additionally, there was similar expression between benign injury and malign tumor. miR-21-5p levels in plasma significantly increased in CRC patients, but this candidate biomarker could not distinguish the carcinoma and benign polyps [95]. Therefore, there should be a strict process of screening from bench to bedside.

Therefore, a larger sample size was essential to obtain the basal line of candidate of interest and decide whether it could clearly separate the health and disease status. Only those who have high sensitivity and specificity in people with different characteristics have the potential for clinical application (Fig. 2). In addition, more advanced technologies like digital PCR were developed in last years. These advanced methods could be further appropriate to overcome these difficulties.

Contribution of miRNAs in different cancers is complicated. A certain miRNA can be oncomiR in this kind of tumor and suppressor in another. Circulating miR-21-5p was reported to be upregulated in patients of NSCLC [17–19, 55, 56, 72], liver cancer [57], and gastric cancer [96, 97], but downregulated in patients suffered from breast cancer [32, 72]. The levels of miR-195 in peripheral blood were lower in patients with hepatocellular carcinoma [98] and cervical cancer [99]. On the contrary, its increased plasma levels were observed in osteosarcoma patients [100] and associated with poor prognosis of head and neck cancer patients [101]. It was of great importance for careful assessment when discussing the clinical application value for the certain miRNA molecules in a certain tumor.

Recently, more and more investigators turned to incorporate several miRNAs to improve the diagnostic

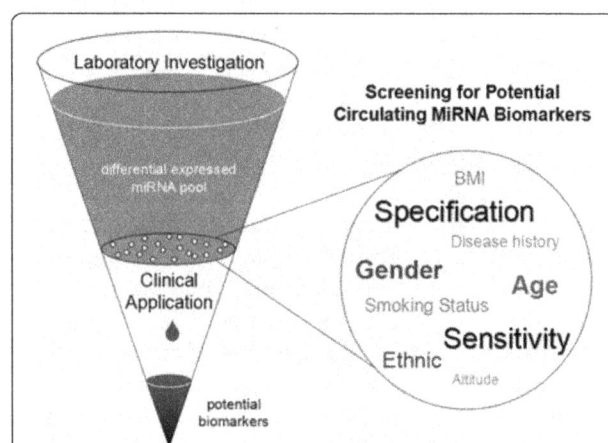

Fig. 2 Screening for potential circulating miRNA biomarkers for clinical applications. A great number of differentially expressed miRNAs were identified in laboratory investigations to constitute the candidate pool. In the further screening, candidates which had no correlation with individual characteristics were retained, as well as those with high specificity and sensitivity in order to distinguish cancer patients from healthy people accurately. They were considered as potential clinical biomarkers for large-scale validation

effect or combine miRNAs with traditional biomarkers like CEA. Several panels of miRNAs were already introduced to ESCC detection [102]. Plasma levels of miRNA pair miR-19b-3b and miR-297-5p were found to be diagnostically significant for prostate cancer [103]. A combination of exosomal miR-126-3p, miR-449a-5p, and miR-34b-5p was adopted to the diagnosis of ccRCC, and combination of miR-126-3p and miR-34b-5p could identify carcinoma and benign injury [71]. It appears that the combination of different miRNAs or miRNAs with other clinical indicators will be the tendency for precise cancer detection in the future.

Perspective

A growing number of circulating miRNAs were found to have potential to act as diagnostic or prognostic biomarkers for various types of cancer patients, especially for long-term, slow progress solid tumors which are hard to detect at early stage. However, the difference between criteria of scientific research and clinical application is quite obvious. This gap makes it important to carefully examine for any potential miRNA biomarkers. An appropriate applicable biomarker for specific cancer should not only be significantly differentially expressed, but also be capable of defining the correlation with the outcome of patients.

The limited sample size was another unavoidable obstacle. In practical clinical application, the level of circulating biomarkers would be under the influence of multiple individual classifications, including age, gender, ethnic, lifestyle, history of diseases, and so on. Although many investigators validated that the miRNAs they focused were not affected by individual characteristics, the proportion may be limited, and larger sample size cohort studies were still needed for further assessment. Detection results could also be affected by measurement principle, method, instrument, and the operation of technicians. So expanding the sample size could be a critical process to ensure the accuracy for cancer diagnosis. In addition, the absolute quantitative detection method may be promising as well as a basic level of the circulating biomarker in healthy controls.

Differentially expressed circulating miRNAs may also play other roles for patients suffering from different cancers except for functioning as biomarkers. Some of them may be just results or by-products of diseases, and the others participated in the occurrence and development of tumors directly or indirectly. There are few studies to reveal the association between the levels of aberrant expressions of miRNAs and therapeutic options so far. However, those miRNAs that participated in tumor pathology may reflect and in turn change the cellular transcriptome via complex regulatory network. Exogenous overexpression or inhibition of those functional miRNAs would probably rescue the pathological development and do favor to the treatment and improvement. Therefore, the circulating miRNA biomarkers could further serve as valuable research targets and candidate small molecule drugs for clinical treatment.

So far, multiple independent validation studies are still demanded for clinical application. The combination of miRNAs with other biomarkers and precise selection of their origin could contribute to further researches. Obtaining the comprehensive view of miRNAs, identified and unidentified, as well as the lncRNAs, circularRNAs, and other ncRNAs is still on the way. With clearer regulatory guidance, a more precise approach could be expected to provide a promising detection to improve treatment outcomes.

Conclusion

In conclusion, circulating miRNAs exhibited promising potential to serve as effective non-invasive cancer biomarkers for clinical application. They may be valuable in various aspects including cancer screening in the early stage, subtype classification and drug sensitivity prediction for treatment strategy selection, and screening the chemo- or radio-resistance of tumors to prognosis the outcomes and recurrences. Larger scale studies are expected to further promote the sensitivity, specificity, and applicability of potential circulating miRNA biomarkers in the future.

Abbreviations
ADC: Adenocarcinoma; AFP: Alpha-fetoprotein; BMI: Body mass index; CA: Carbohydrate antigen; ccRCC: Clear-cell renal cell cancer; CEA: Carcinoembryonic antigen; CRC: Colorectal cancer; DFS: Disease-free survival; ER: Estrogen receptor; ESCC: Esophageal squamous cell carcinoma; miRNA: MicroRNA; NSCLC: Non-small cell lung cancers; OS: Overall survival; PCR: Polymerase chain reaction; PDAC: Pancreatic ductal adenocarcinoma; PR: Progesterone receptor; PSA: Prostate-specific antigen; SCC: Squamous cell carcinoma; TNBC: Triple-negative breast cancers

Acknowledgements
We appreciate the valuable comments from Prof. Qinghua Cui in Peking University Health Science Center and the kindly linguistic assistance from Qiaochu Zhang from Dep. Bioengineering and Biomedical engineering in Rice University, Houston, Texas.

Funding
This work was supported by grants from the National Natural Science Foundation of China (NSFC No.91749107, No.81672091) and Beijing Natural Science Foundation (BJNSF No. 7172232).

Authors' contributions
HW, RP, and JW acquired the materials and wrote the manuscript draft. ZQ and LX designed the drafting and reviewed and edited the manuscript. All authors read and approved the manuscript.

Competing interests
The authors declare that they have no competing interests.

Author details
[1]Medical Research Center, Peking University Third Hospital, Beijing, China.
[2]Department of Radiation Oncology, Peking University Third Hospital, Beijing, China.

References

1. Lee RC, Feinbaum RL, Ambros V. The C. elegans heterochronic gene lin-4 encodes small RNAs with antisense complementarity to lin-14. Cell. 1993;75:843–54.
2. Bracken CP, Scott HS, Goodall GJ. A network-biology perspective of microRNA function and dysfunction in cancer. Nat Rev Genet. 2016;17:719–32.
3. Baek D, Villen J, Shin C, Camargo FD, Gygi SP, Bartel DP. The impact of microRNAs on protein output. Nature. 2008;455:64–71.
4. Bushati N, Cohen SM. microRNA functions. Annu Rev Cell Dev Biol. 2007;23: 175–205.
5. Zhu Y, Xiong K, Shi J, Cui Q, Xue L. A potential role of microRNAs in protein accumulation in cellular senescence analyzed by bioinformatics. PLoS One. 2017;12:e0179034.
6. Lin S, Gregory RI. MicroRNA biogenesis pathways in cancer. Nat Rev Cancer. 2015;15:321–33.
7. Calin GA, Croce CM. MicroRNA signatures in human cancers. Nat Rev Cancer. 2006;6:857–66.
8. Rosenfeld N, Aharonov R, Meiri E, Rosenwald S, Spector Y, Zepeniuk M, et al. MicroRNAs accurately identify cancer tissue origin. Nat Biotechnol. 2008;26:462–9.
9. Berezikov E, Chung WJ, Willis J, Cuppen E, Lai EC. Mammalian mirtron genes. Mol Cell. 2007;28:328–36.
10. Flynt AS, Greimann JC, Chung WJ, Lima CD, Lai EC. MicroRNA biogenesis via splicing and exosome-mediated trimming in Drosophila. Mol Cell. 2010;38: 900–7.
11. Westholm JO, Lai EC. Mirtrons: microRNA biogenesis via splicing. Biochimie. 2011;93:1897–904.
12. Valadi H, Ekström K, Bossios A, Sjöstrand M, Lee JJ, Lötvall JO. Exosome-mediated transfer of mRNAs and microRNAs is a novel mechanism of genetic exchange between cells. Nat Cell Biol. 2007;9:654–9.
13. Mitchell PS, Parkin RK, Kroh EM, Fritz BR, Wyman SK, Pogosova-Agadjanyan EL, et al. Circulating microRNAs as stable blood-based markers for cancer detection. Proc Natl Acad Sci U S A. 2008;105:10513–8.
14. Shen J, Stass SA, Jiang F. MicroRNAs as potential biomarkers in human solid tumors. Cancer Lett. 2013;329:125–36.
15. Lindner K, Haier J, Wang Z, Watson DI, Hussey DJ, Hummel R. Circulating microRNAs: emerging biomarkers for diagnosis and prognosis in patients with gastrointestinal cancers. Clin Sci (Lond). 2015;128:1–15.
16. Vanni I, Alama A, Grossi F, Dal Bello MG, Coco S. Exosomes: a new horizon in lung cancer. Drug Discov Today. 2017;22:927–36.
17. Zhang H, Mao F, Shen T, Luo Q, Ding Z, Qian L, Huang J. Plasma miR-145, miR-20a, miR-21 and miR-223 as novel biomarkers for screening early-stage non-small cell lung cancer. Oncol Lett. 2017;13:669–76.
18. Geng Q, Fan T, Zhang B, Wang W, Xu Y, Hu H. Five microRNAs in plasma as novel biomarkers for screening of early-stage non-small cell lung cancer. Respir Res. 2014;15:149.
19. Arab A, Karimipoor M, Irani S, Kiani A, Zeinali S, Tafsiri E, Sheikhy K. Potential circulating miRNA signature for early detection of NSCLC. Cancer Genet. 2017;216-217:150–8.
20. Zhu W, Zhou K, Zha Y, Chen D, He J, Ma H, et al. Diagnostic value of serum miR-182, miR-183, miR-210, and miR-126 levels in patients with early-stage non-small cell lung cancer. PLoS One. 2016;11:4.
21. Powrózek T, Kuźnar-Kamińska B, Dziedzic M, Mlak R, Batura-Gabryel H, Sagan D, et al. The diagnostic role of plasma circulating precursors of miRNA-944 and miRNA-3662 for non-small cell lung cancer detection. Pathol Res Pract. 2017;213:1384–7.
22. Wang J, Yan F, Zhao Q, Zhan F, Wang R, Wang L, et al. Circulating exosomal miR-125a-3p as a novel biomarker for early-stage colon cancer. Sci Rep. 2017;7:1.
23. Vychytilova-Faltejskova P, Radova L, Sachlova M, Kosarova Z, Slaba K, Fabian P, et al. Serum-based microRNA signatures in early diagnosis and prognosis prediction of colon cancer. Carcinogenesis. 2016;37:941–50.
24. Hamam R, Ali AM, Alsaleh KA, Kassem M, Alfayez M, Aldahmash A, Alajez NM. microRNA expression profiling on individual breast cancer patients identifies novel panel of circulating microRNA for early detection. Sci Rep. 2016;6:25997.
25. Xing W, Zeng F. A novel serum microRNA-based identification and classification biomarker of human glioma. Tumour Biol. 2017;39:5.
26. Blandin Knight S, Grosbie PA, Balata H, Chudziak J, Hussell T, Dive C. Progress and prospects in early detection in lung cancer. Open Biol. 2017;7:9.
27. Hon JD, Singh B, Sahin A, Du G, Wang J, Wang VY, et al. Breast cancer molecular subtypes: from TNBC to QNBC. Am J Cancer Res. 2016;6:1864–72.
28. Rahim B, O'Regan R. AR signaling in breast cancer. Cancers (Basel). 2017;9:3.
29. Sromek M, Glogowski M, Chechlinska M, Kulinczak M, Szafron L, Zakrzewska K, et al. Changes in plasma miR-9, miR-16, miR-205 and miR-486 levels after non-small cell lung cancer resection. Cell Oncol (Dordr). 2017;40:529–36.
30. Jin X, Chen Y, Chen H, Fei S, Chen D, Cai X, et al. Evaluation of tumor-derived exosomal miRNA as potential diagnostic biomarkers for early-stage non-small cell lung cancer using next-generation sequencing. Clin Cancer Res. 2017;23:5311–9.
31. Powrózek T, Krawczyk P, Kowalski DM, Winiarczyk K, Olszyna-Serementa M, Milanowski J. Plasma circulating microRNA-944 and microRNA-3662 as potential histologic type-specific early lung cancer biomarkers. Transl Res. 2015;166:315–23.
32. Shin VY, Siu JM, Cheuk I, Ng EK, Kwong A. Circulating cell-free miRNAs as biomarker for triple-negative breast cancer. Br J Cancer. 2015;112:1751–9.
33. Eichelser C, Stückrath I, Müller V, Milde-Langosch K, Wikman H, Pantel K, Schwarzenbach H. Increased serum levels of circulating exosomal microRNA-373 in receptor-negative breast cancer patients. Oncotarget. 2017;5:9650–63.
34. Perge P, Butz H, Pezzani R, Bancos I, Nagy Z, Paloczi K, et al. Evaluation and diagnostic potential of circulating extracellular vesicle-associated microRNAs in adrenocortical tumors. Sci Rep. 2017;7:1.
35. Samsonov R, Burdakov V, Shtam T, Radzhabova Z, Vasilyev D, Tsyrlina E, et al. Plasma exosomal miR-21 and miR-181a differentiates follicular from papillary thyroid cancer. Tumour Biol. 2016;37:12011–21.
36. Pang PC, Shi XY, Huang WL, Sun K. miR-497 as a potential serum biomarker for the diagnosis and prognosis of osteosarcoma. Eur Rev Med Pharmacol Sci. 2016;20:3765–9.
37. Wang C, Li Q, Liu F, Chen X, Nesa EU, Guan S, et al. Downregulation of microRNA-497 is associated with upregulation of synuclein gamma in patients with osteosarcoma. Exp Ther Med. 2016;12:3761–6.
38. Liu Q, Wang H, Singh A, Shou F. Expression and function of microRNA-497 in human osteosarcoma. Mol Med Rep. 2016;14:439–45.
39. Shao XJ, Miao MH, Xue J, Xue J, Ji XQ, Zhu H. The down-regulation of microRNA-497 contributes to cell growth and cisplatin resistance through PI3K/Akt pathway in osteosarcoma. Cell Physiol Biochem. 2015;36:2051–62.
40. Ruan WD, Wang P, Feng S, Xue Y, Zhang B. MicroRNA-497 inhibits cell proliferation, migration, and invasion by targeting AMOT in human osteosarcoma cells. Onco Targets Ther. 2016;9:303–13.
41. Ge L, Zheng B, Li M, Niu L, Li Z. MicroRNA-497 suppresses osteosarcoma tumor growth in vitro and in vivo. Oncol Lett. 2016;11:2207–12.
42. Gui ZL. MicroRNA-497 suppress osteosarcoma by targeting MAPK/Erk pathway. Bratisl Lek Listy. 2017;118:449–52.
43. Fang Z. Circulating miR-205: a promising biomarker for the detection and prognosis evaluation of bladder cancer. Tumour Biol. 2016;37:8075–82.
44. Gong ZL, Wu TL, Zhao GC, Lin ZX, Xu HG. Decreased expression of microRNA-148a predicts poor prognosis in ovarian cancer and associates with tumor growth and metastasis. Biomed Pharmacother. 2016;83:58–63.
45. Ren GB, Wang L, Zhang FH, Meng XR, Mao ZP. Study on the relationship between miR-520g and the development of breast cancer. Eur Rev Med Pharmacol Sci. 2016;20:657–63.
46. Yuan R, Wang G, Xu Z, Zhao H, Chen H, Han Y, et al. Up-regulated circulating miR-106a by DNA methylation promised a potential diagnostic and prognostic marker for gastric cancer. Anti Cancer Agents Med Chem. 2016;16:1093–100.
47. Tsai MM, Wang CS, Tsai CY, Huang CG, Lee KF, Huang HW, et al. Circulating microRNA-196a/b are novel biomarkers associated with metastatic gastric cancer. Eur J Cancer. 2016;64:137–48.

48. Papaconstantinou IG, Manta A, Gazouli M, Lyberopoulou A, Lykoudis PM, Polymeneas G, Voros D. Expression of microRNAs in patients with pancreatic cancer and its prognostic significance. Pancreas. 2013;42:67–71.

49. Greither T, Grochola LF, Udelnow A, Lautenschlager C, Wurl P, Taubert H. Elevated expression of microRNAs 155, 203, 210 and 222 in pancreatic tumors is associated with poorer survival. Int J Cancer. 2010;126:73–80.

50. Wang J, Chen J, Chang P, LeBlanc A, Li D, Abbruzzesse JL, et al. MicroRNAs in plasma of pancreatic ductal adenocarcinoma patients as novel blood-based biomarkers of disease. Cancer Prev Res (Phila). 2009; 2:807–13.

51. Mikamori M, Yamada D, Eguchi H, Hasegawa S, Kishimoto T, Tomimaru Y, et al. MicroRNA-155 controls exosome synthesis and promotes gemcitabine resistance in pancreatic ductal adenocarcinoma. Sci Rep. 2017;7:42339.

52. Hu J, Cai G, Xu Y, Cai S. The plasma microRNA miR-1914* and -1915 suppresses chemoresistant in colorectal cancer patients by down-regulating NFIX. Curr Mol Med. 2016;16:70–82.

53. Yuwen DL, Sheng BB, Liu J, Wenyu W, Shu YQ. MiR-146a-5p level in serum exosomes predicts therapeutic effect of cisplatin in non-small cell lung cancer. Eur Rev Med Pharmacol Sci. 2017;21:2650–8.

54. Wei F, Ma C, Zhou T, Dong X, Luo Q, Geng L, et al. Exosomes derived from gemcitabine-resistant cells transfer malignant phenotypic traits via delivery of miRNA-222-3p. Mol Cancer. 2017;16:1.

55. Liu Q, Yu Z, Yuan S, Xie W, Li C, Hu Z, et al. Circulating exosomal microRNAs as prognostic biomarkers for non-small-cell lung cancer. Oncotarget. 2017;8: 13048–58.

56. Dejima H, Iinuma H, Kanaoka R, Matsutani N, Kawamura M. Exosomal microRNA in plasma as a non-invasive biomarker for the recurrence of non-small cell lung cancer. Oncol Lett. 2017;13:1256–63.

57. Tsukamoto M, Iinuma H, Yagi T, Matsuda K, Hashiguchi Y. Circulating exosomal microRNA-21 as a biomarker in each tumor stage of colorectal cancer. Oncology. 2017;92:360–70.

58. Manier S, Liu CJ, Avet-Loiseau H, Park J, Shi J, Campigotto F, et al. Prognostic role of circulating exosomal miRNAs in multiple myeloma. Blood. 2017;129:2429–36.

59. Liu C, Eng C, Shen J, Lu Y, Takata Y, Mehdizadeh A, et al. Serum exosomal miR-4772-3p is a predictor of tumor recurrence in stage II and III colon cancer. Oncotarget. 2016;7:76250–60.

60. Gu Y, Zhang M, Peng F, Fang L, Zhang Y, Liang H, et al. The BRCA1/2-directed miRNA signature predicts a good prognosis in ovarian cancer patients with wild-type BRCA1/2. Oncotarget. 2015;6:2397–406.

61. Tang H, Liu Q, Liu X, Ye F, Xie X, Xie X, Wu M. Plasma miR-185 as a predictive biomarker for prognosis of malignant glioma. J Cancer Res Ther. 2015;11:630–4.

62. Ugrinska A, Bombardieri E, Stokkel MP, Crippa F, Pauwels EK. Circulating tumor markers and nuclear medicine imaging modalities: breast, prostate and ovarian cancer. Q J Nucl Med. 2002;46:88–104.

63. Wang Y, Yan J, Wang L. The diagnostic value of serum carcino-embryonic antigen, alpha fetoprotein and carbohydrate antigen 19-9 for colorectal cancer. J Cancer Res Ther. 2014;10(Suppl):307–9.

64. Baltzer PAT, Kapetas P, Marino MA, Clauser P. New diagnostic tools for breast cancer. Memo. 2017;10:175–80.

65. Modiri A, Goudreau S, Rahimi A, Kiasaleh K. Review of breast screening: toward clinical realization of microwave imaging. Med Phys. 2017;44:e446–58.

66. Issa IA, Noureddine M. Colorectal cancer screening: an updated review of the available options. World J Gastroenterol. 2017;23:5086–96.

67. Sadi MV. PSA screening for prostate cancer. Rev Assoc Med Bras (1992). 2017;63:722–5.

68. He X, Ping J, Wen D. MicroRNA-186 regulates the invasion and metastasis of bladder cancer via vascular endothelial growth factor C. Exp Ther Med. 2017;14:3253–8.

69. Geva GA, Gielchinsky I, Aviv N, Max KEA, Gofrit ON, Gur-Wahnon D, Ben-Dov IZ. Urine cell-free microRNA as biomarkers for transitional cell carcinoma. BMC Res Notes. 2017;10:1.

70. Fedorko M, Juracek J, Stanik M, Svoboda M, Poprach A, Buchler T, et al. Detection of let-7 miRNAs in urine supernatant as potential diagnostic approach in non-metastatic clear-cell renal cell carcinoma. Biochem Med (Zagreb). 2017;27:411–7.

71. Butz H, Nofech-Mozes R, Ding Q, Khella HWZ, Szabó PM, Jewett M, et al. Exosomal microRNAs are diagnostic biomarkers and can mediate cell-cell communication in renal cell carcinoma. Eur Urol Focus. 2016;2:210–8.

72. Erbes T, Hirschfeld M, Rucker G, Jaeger M, Boas J, Iborra S, et al. Feasibility of urinary microRNA detection in breast cancer patients and its potential as an innovative non-invasive biomarker. BMC Cancer. 2015;15:193.

73. Debernardi S, Massat NJ, Radon TP, Sangaralingam A, Banissi A, Ennis DP, et al. Noninvasive urinary miRNA biomarkers for early detection of pancreatic adenocarcinoma. Am J Cancer Res. 2015;5:3455–66.

74. Zhou Y, Tian L, Wang X, Ye L, Zhao G, Yu M, et al. MicroRNA-195 inhibits non-small cell lung cancer cell proliferation, migration and invasion by targeting MYB. Cancer Lett 2014; 347: 65–74.

75. Wang X. MiR-195 inhibits the growth and metastasis of NSCLC cells by targeting IGF1R. Tumour Biol. 2014;35:8765–70.

76. Guo H, Li W, Zheng T, Liu Z. MiR-195 targets HDGF to inhibit proliferation and invasion of NSCLC cells. Tumour Biol. 2014;35:8861–6.

77. Liu B, Qu J, Xu F, Guo Y, Wang Y, Yu H, Qian B. MiR-195 suppresses non-small cell lung cancer by targeting CHEK1. Oncotarget. 2015;6: 9445–56.

78. Su K, Zhang T, Wang Y, Hao G. Diagnostic and prognostic value of plasma microRNA-195 in patients with non-small cell lung cancer. World J Surg Oncol. 2016;14:1.

79. Hua Y, Chen H, Wang L, Wang F, Wang P, Ning Z, et al. Low serum miR-373 predicts poor prognosis in patients with pancreatic cancer. Cancer Biomark. 2017;20:95–100.

80. Murali Manohar K, Sasikala M, Kvsrr Y, Sunil V, Talukdar R, Murthy H, et al. Plasma microRNA192 in combination with serum CA19-9 as non-invasive prognostic biomarker in periampullary carcinoma. Tumour Biol. 2017;39:3.

81. Zeng Z, Chen X, Zhu D, Luo Z, Yang M. Low expression of circulating microRNA-34c is associated with poor prognosis in triple-negative breast cancer. Yonsei Med J. 2017;58:697–702.

82. Huang Z, Zhang L, Zhu D, Shan X, Zhou X, Qi LW, et al. A novel serum microRNA signature to screen esophageal squamous cell carcinoma. Cancer Med. 2017;6:109–10.

83. Xu W, Zhou Y, Xu G, Geng B, Cui Q. Transcriptome analysis reveals non-identical microRNA profiles between arterial and venous plasma. Oncotarget. 2017;8:28471–80.

84. Zhou X, Wen W, Shan X, Zhu W, Xu J, Guo R, et al. A six-microRNA panel in plasma was identified as a potential biomarker for lung adenocarcinoma diagnosis. Oncotarget. 2017;8:6513–25.

85. Monzo M, Santasusagna S, Moreno I, Martinez F, Hernández R, Muñoz C, et al. Exosomal microRNAs isolated from plasma of mesenteric veins linked to liver metastases in resected patients with colon cancer. Oncotarget. 2017;8: 30859–69.

86. Tian F, Shen Y, Chen Z, Li R, Ge Q. No significant difference between plasma miRNAs and plasma-derived exosomal miRNAs from healthy people. Biomed Res Int. 2017;2017:1304816.

87. Huang Z, Zhu D, Wu L, He M, Zhou X, Zhang L, et al. Six serum-based miRNAs as potential diagnostic biomarkers for gastric cancer. Cancer Epidemiol Biomark Prev. 2017;26:188–96.

88. Heegaard NH, Schetter AJ, Welsh JA, Yoneda M, Bowman ED, Harris CC. Circulating micro-RNA expression profiles in early stage nonsmall cell lung cancer. Int J Cancer. 2012;130:1378–86.

89. Chen H, Liu H, Zou H, Chen R, Dou Y, Sheng S, et al. Evaluation of plasma miR-21 and miR-152 as diagnostic biomarkers for common types of human cancers. J Cancer. 2016;7:490–9.

90. Eichelser C, Flesch-Janys D, Chang-Claude J, Pantel K, Schwarzenbach H. Deregulated serum concentrations of circulating cell-free microRNAs miR-17, miR-34a, miR-155, and miR-373 in human breast cancer development and progression. Clin Chem. 2013;59:1489–96.

91. Sochor M, Basova P, Pesta M, Dusilkova N, Bartos J, Burda P, et al. Oncogenic microRNAs: miR-155, miR-19a, miR-181b, and miR-24 enable monitoring of early breast cancer in serum. BMC Cancer. 2014;14:448.

92. Madhavan D, Peng C, Wallwiener M, Zucknick M, Nees J, Schott S, et al. Circulating miRNAs with prognostic value in metastatic breast cancer and for early detection of metastasis. Carcinogenesis. 2016;37:461–70.

93. Wang W, Qu A, Liu W, Liu Y, Zheng G, Du L, et al. Circulating miR-210 as a diagnostic and prognostic biomarker for colorectal cancer. Eur J Cancer Care (Engl). 2017;26:e12448

94. Ulivi P, Canale M, Passardi A, Marisi G, Valgiusti M, Frassineti GL, et al. Circulating plasma levels of miR-20b, miR-29b and miR-155 as predictors of bevacizumab efficacy in patients with metastatic colorectal cancer. Int J Mol Sci. 2018;19:307

95. Montagnana M, Benati M, Danese E, Minicozzi AM, Paviati E, Gusella M, et al. Plasma expression levels of circulating miR-21 are not useful for diagnosing and monitoring colorectal cancer. Clin Lab. 2016;62:967–70.

96. Sierzega M, Kaczor M, Kolodziejczyk P, Kulig J, Sanak M, Richter P. Evaluation of serum microRNA biomarkers for gastric cancer based on blood and tissue pools profiling: the importance of miR-21 and miR-331. Br J Cancer. 2017;117:266–73.

97. Zheng Y, Cui L, Sun W, Zhou H, Yuan X, Huo M, et al. MicroRNA-21 is a new marker of circulating tumor cells in gastric cancer patients. Cancer Biomark. 2011-2012;10:71–7.

98. Sohn W, Kim J, Kang SH, Yang SR, Cho JY, Cho HC, Shim SG, Paik YH. Serum exosomal microRNAs as novel biomarkers for hepatocellular carcinoma. Exp Mol Med. 2015;47:e184.

99. Zhang Y, Zhang D, Wang F, Xu D, Guo Y, Cui W. Serum miRNAs panel (miR-16-2*, miR-195, miR-2861, miR-497) as novel non-invasive biomarkers for detection of cervical cancer. Sci Rep. 2015;5:17942.

100. Lian F, Cui Y, Zhou C, Gao K, Wu L. Identification of a plasma four-microRNA panel as potential noninvasive biomarker for osteosarcoma. PLoS One. 2015;10:e0121499.

101. Summerer I, Unger K, Braselmann H, Schuettrumpf L, Maihoefer C, Baumeister P, et al. Circulating microRNAs as prognostic therapy biomarkers in head and neck cancer patients. Br J Cancer. 2015;113:76–82.

102. Zhou X, Wen W, Zhu J, Huang Z, Zhang L, Zhang H, et al. A six-microRNA signature in plasma was identified as a potential biomarker in diagnosis of esophageal squamous cell carcinoma. Oncotarget. 2017;8:34468–80.

103. Osip'yants AI, Knyazev EN, Galatenko AV, Nyushko KM, Galatenko VV, Shkurnikov MY, Alekseev BY. Changes in the level of circulating hsa-miR-297 and hsa-miR-19b-3p miRNA are associated with generalization of prostate cancer. Bull Exp Biol Med. 2017;162:379–82.

4

Circulating tumour DNA for monitoring colorectal cancer—a prospective cohort study to assess relationship to tissue methylation, cancer characteristics and surgical resection

Erin L. Symonds[1,2*], Susanne K. Pedersen[3], David H. Murray[3], Maher Jedi[1^], Susan E. Byrne[1], Philippa Rabbitt[4], Rohan T. Baker[3], Dawn Bastin[1] and Graeme P. Young[1]

Abstract

Background: Cell-free circulating tumour-derived DNA (ctDNA) can be detected by testing for methylated *BCAT1* and *IKZF1* DNA, which has proven sensitivity for colorectal cancer (CRC). A prospective correlative biomarker study between presence of methylated *BCAT1* and *IKZF1* in tissue and blood was conducted in cases with CRC to explore how detection of such ctDNA biomarkers relates to cancer characteristics, methylation in tissue and surgical resection of the primary cancer.

Methods: Enrolled patients with invasive CRC had blood collected at diagnosis, prior to any treatment or surgery (peri-diagnostic sample). A subgroup of patients also had cancer and adjacent non-neoplastic tissue collected at surgical resection, as well as a second blood sample collected within 12 months of surgery (post-surgery sample). DNA was extracted from all samples and assayed for methylated *BCAT1* and *IKZF1* to determine the degree of methylation in tissue and the presence of ctDNA in blood.

Results: Of 187 cases providing peri-diagnostic blood samples, tissue was available in 91, and 93 provided at least one post-surgery blood sample for marker analysis. Significant methylation of either *BCAT1* or *IKZF1* was seen in 86/91 (94.5%) cancer tissues, with levels independent of stage and higher than that observed in adjacent non-neoplastic specimens ($P < 0.001$). ctDNA methylated in *BCAT1* or *IKZF1* was detected in 116 (62.0%) cases at diagnosis and was significantly more likely to be detected with later stage ($P < 0.001$) and distal tumour location ($P = 0.004$). Of the 91 patients who provided pre-and post-surgery blood samples, 47 patients were ctDNA-positive at diagnosis and 35 (74.5%) became negative after tumour resection.

(Continued on next page)

* Correspondence: erin.symonds@sa.gov.au
^Deceased
[1]Flinders Centre for Innovation in Cancer, College of Medicine and Public Health, Flinders University of South Australia, Bedford Park, South Australia 5042, Australia
[2]Bowel Health Service, Flinders Medical Centre, Bedford Park, South Australia, Australia
Full list of author information is available at the end of the article

(Continued from previous page)

Conclusion: This study has shown that *BCAT1* and *IKZF1* methylation are common events in CRC with almost all cancer tissues showing significant levels of methylation in the two genes. The presence of ctDNA in blood is stage-related and show rapid reversion to negative following surgical resection. Monitoring methylated *BCAT1* and *IKZF1* levels could therefore inform adequacy of surgical resection.

Keywords: Colorectal cancer, *BCAT1*, *IKZF1*, Methylation, Circulating tumour DNA, Surgical resection, Residual disease

Background

Colorectal cancer (CRC) is the second leading cause of death from cancer in the developed world [1]. Even though most CRC patients achieve remission with initial treatment, more than 25% will suffer recurrence [2]. Therefore, to achieve early detection of recurrence, patients are usually entered into a follow-up regimen including regular blood testing, radiology and colonoscopy. The current blood biomarker used, carcinoembryonic antigen (CEA), has limited sensitivity and specificity for recurrence [3, 4]. Better blood markers for adequacy of initial therapy should aid identification of subjects at risk of recurrence or in need of extended initial therapy such as addition of or prolongation of chemotherapy. These markers should be present in all colorectal tumours regardless of the genetic alterations and should be absent from the blood following complete surgical resection of the tumour.

Somatic and epigenetic alterations of DNA are associated with CRC development, and a number of studies show that tumour-derived DNA can be detected in the cell-free fraction of blood (circulating tumour DNA, ctDNA) [5–8]. Detecting ctDNA by assaying for somatic mutations [9, 10] has the potential to inform response to therapy, existence of minimal residual disease and development of metastases [11, 12]. However, none of the common somatic mutations linked to CRC development occurs universally, and all appear with a low frequency [5, 13]. Furthermore, the mutation profile becomes more heterogeneous as the cancer evolves over time, whereas epigenetic markers are more stable during oncogenesis [5]. Thus, aberrant DNA methylation, which occurs frequently in CRC [5, 6] might more reliably inform response to therapy and presence of residual disease.

A panel of methylated DNA biomarkers shown to have good sensitivity and specificity for CRC is *BCAT1* (branched chain amino acid transaminase 1) and *IKZF1* (IKAROS family zinc finger 1) [14–16]. Deregulation of *IKZF1* and *BCAT1* is involved in tumour growth and invasiveness in several cancers, including CRC [6, 17]. There is a biological plausibility that methylated *BCAT1* and *IKZF1* may be more significant in oncogenesis than simply epiphenomena resulting from disturbances in gene methylation processes as both play an important

functional role in maintaining a healthy state in normal tissue [18–20]. BCAT1 controls the metabolism of branched chain amino acids which are essential nutrients for growth, and it has been demonstrated that when *BCAT1* expression is blocked, the lifespan increases nearly 25% in nematodes [21]. The *BCAT1* gene locus is aberrantly methylated in several pathologies, including CRC [20, 22] where abnormal expression has been reported to be a predictor of distant metastases [17]. *IKZF1* encodes a DNA-binding protein, which during normal development restricts the G1-S transitioning of the cell cycle by regulating a small set of cell cycle regulator genes [23, 24]. *IKZF1* mutations and deletions leading to generation of isoforms lacking DNA binding capability are common in hematologic neoplasia, e.g. lymphoblastic leukemia where such mutations/deletions abolish cell cycle control and leads to hyperproliferation. In CRC, *IKZF1* promoter methylation has been linked to loss of proper regulation of proliferation and differentiation [24].

If detection of methylated *BCAT1*/*IKZF1* ctDNA is to be useful in patient management, it is important to better understand the principles underlying the presence of these epigenetic markers in blood and how this relates to tissue expression and to tumour debulking. The aim of this study was therefore to assess the relationship between tissue levels and detection in blood and to examine the effects of surgical resection on presence of ctDNA.

Methods

Study overview

This was a prospective observational study of cases with invasive CRC that examined the relationship of ctDNA status with clinicopathological measures and with levels of methylated *BCAT1* and *IKZF1* DNA in surgically resected tissues. In addition, the effect of surgical resection on ctDNA status was assessed. A methylation-specific validated real-time PCR-based method was used to assess the presence of methylated *BCAT1* and *IKZF1* in bisulphite-converted DNA isolated from plasma [25]. The degree of methylation of *BCAT1* and *IKZF1* DNA were also measured in tissue (tumour and adjacent non-neoplastic epithelium).

The study was approved by the Southern Adelaide Clinical Human Research Ethics Committee (reference number 134.045). Written informed consent was obtained from all participants. The study is registered at Australian and New Zealand Clinical Trials Registry (#12611000318987).

Population

Any adults (18 years of age or older) who were recently diagnosed with invasive colorectal adenocarcinoma (AJCC stages I–IV) at Flinders Medical Centre (Bedford Park, SA, Australia) or Repatriation General Hospital (Daw Park, SA) were approached about volunteering for the study during 2011–2016. Following consent, patients were enrolled in the study provided that they met diagnostic criteria for invasive colorectal adenocarcinoma, were adequately staged, and were provided a blood sample prior to any treatment (the peri-diagnostic sample). Diagnosis and extent of disease were determined on the basis of colonoscopy and other clinicopathological findings. CRC were staged (following AJCC and TNM) [26], and distal tumours were classed as those distal to the transverse colon.

Clinical procedures

Venous blood for ctDNA testing was collected into two 9 mL K3EDTA Vacuette tubes (Greiner Bio-One, Frickenhausen, Germany) prior to any treatment including primary surgery from 187 participants ("peri-diagnostic plasma sample") and when feasible at subsequent clinical review within 12 months after surgery from 93 participants ("post-surgery plasma sample"). Blood collection tubes were kept on ice prior to plasma processing (no more than 4 h from blood collection). Plasma was prepared by centrifugation at 1500g for 10 min at 4 °C (deceleration at lowest setting), followed by retrieval of the plasma fraction and a repeat centrifugation. The resulting plasma was stored at − 80 °C. Frozen plasma samples were shipped on dry ice to Clinical Genomics (North Ryde, NSW, Australia) and stored at − 80 °C until testing.

Resected tissue samples were also available for a subgroup of patients who had received no neoadjuvant therapy ($n = 91$). Samples collected were fresh (non-fixed) non-necrotic cancer tissue and adjacent non-neoplastic tissue (greater than 10 mm from the tumour, median 75 mm) which were obtained by a supervising pathologist. Samples were stored in RNAlater (Thermo Fisher Scientific Australia) for at least 48 h at 4 °C before stored at − 80 °C until further analysis.

No study-wide control of radiological imaging, pathology procedures, or quality was undertaken as the study aimed to assess marker performance relative to outcomes determined in usual clinical practice. All procedures were performed by hospital-accredited specialists and so met site-specific standards for venipuncture, monitoring, imaging and equipment.

Methylation testing

For ctDNA testing, cell-free circulating DNA was extracted from 4.5 mL plasma using the QIASymphony Circulating Nucleic Acid Kit (Qiagen, Hilden, Germany) and bisulphite-converted using the EpiTect Fast Bisulphite Conversion kit (Qiagen) as previously described [16]. The resulting bisulphite-converted DNA was simultaneously analyzed in triplicate using a real-time multiplex PCR assay simultaneously detecting a methylated region in BCAT1 and IKZF1 as well as a region in ACTB (proxy measure of the total amount of DNA) using a Light-Cycler 480 II instrument (Roche Diagnostics, IN, USA) [16, 25, 27]. We have previously shown this assay to be sensitive for the detection of low copy numbers of the methylated genes [25]. A blood sample was deemed ctDNA positive for clinical purposes if at least one PCR replicate was positive for methylated BCAT1 and/or IKZF1 [16, 27].

For tissue DNA analysis, DNA was extracted from 10 to 20 mg tissue according to the manufacturer's instructions (DNAeasy® Blood & Tissue kit, Qiagen), except for using 40 µL Proteinase K and a lysis time of 3 h at 56 °C. DNA (500 ng) was bisulphite-converted using an EpiTect Fast 96 Bisulphite Conversion kit (Qiagen) as previously described [16] with the exception of omitting carrier RNA and a 30 µL elution.

When consideration was given to percentage of methylated ctDNA, the level was expressed as the ratio of total mass of BCAT1 and IKZF1 measured in total amount of DNA volume. A sample was deemed positive when the %methylation was above the 75th percentile value of BCAT1 and IKZF1 of the non-neoplastic tissue (9.7% for BCAT1 and 0.5% for IKZF1).

Statistical analyses

Hypothesis testing included Mann-Whitney, Kruskal-Wallis, chi-square and Fisher's exact tests. Analyses were performed using two-sided tests, and a significance level of less than 5% was considered statistically significant. The binomial distribution was assumed for calculations of exact 95% confidence intervals (95%CI). All analyses were performed using Stata, version 13.1.

Once the data was collected, a power analysis was performed for a logistic regression analysis to compare the blood positivity across different cancer characteristics. The analysis was performed using a z test with a binomial distribution, an alpha of 5%, plasma positivity of 62% and a proportion comparison of 0.5 to 0.7. A power of 0.78 was estimated.

Logistic regression was used for multivariate analysis. Variables that were included were those where the relationship with the outcome was significant at $P \leq 0.1$ in the univariate analysis or had been shown in previous studies to be clinically significant. Age, tumour size, lymphatic invasion, perineural invasion, extramural vascular invasion, intramural vascular invasion and differentiation were included in the multivariate analysis. The final model was prepared using a backward selection method, and the goodness of fit was assessed using the Pearson chi-square test.

Results

Study population

Figure 1 shows the disposition of 442 patients approached. The characteristics of cases according to clinical information and specimen availability are summarized in Additional file 1: Table S1. The stage distribution differed between all cases and just those cases providing a post-surgical blood sample as not all stage IV cases proceeded to surgery.

Peri-diagnostic ctDNA status

Peri-diagnostic blood samples were available for 187 cases, and 116 (62.0%, 95%CI 54.7–69.0) tested positive for methylated BCAT1 and/or IKZF1. When methylation changes were assessed for different clinicopathological features, similar results were seen for BCAT1 and IKZF1 except for location where BCAT1 had a higher positivity rate with distally located tumours (Table 1). Overall ctDNA positivity varied by AJCC and TNM staging, size, location and lymphatic invasion by univariate analysis (Table 1). CRC stages II, III and IV were strong predictors for ctDNA positivity compared to stage I. After multivariate modeling, only stage and location remained as significant predictors; patients with tumours located in the distal colon or rectum were 3.0 times more likely to be ctDNA positive than those with proximal tumours (95% CI 1.4–6.2) (Table 2).

Methylation in colonic tissue

Tumour tissue was available in 91 cases, with matched non-neoplastic tissue in 87. Cancer tissues exhibited significantly greater methylation than adjacent non-neoplastic tissues ($P < 0.001$ for each marker; Fig. 2). Detectable methylation in one or both genes was present in 98.9% (90/91) of cancer tissue, with methylated BCAT1 present in 89/91 (97.8%) and methylated IKZF1 present in 79/91 (86.8%). The one tumour that was negative for both BCAT1 and IKZF1 methylation had a single somatic mutation in MSH2 and MSH6. Using the upper IQR values measured in non-neoplastic tissues as positivity thresholds, hypermethylation of BCAT1 and IKZF1 was observed in 82/91 (90.1%) and 75/91 (82.4%) of cancers,

respectively, with 86/91 (94.5%) having elevated levels for either marker. The only variables having any effect on methylation levels in cancers were age older than 65 years and tumour location for BCAT1 (Table 3). These differences were not seen in non-neoplastic tissue ($P > 0.05$, data not shown).

Comparison of tumour tissue methylation and peri-diagnostic ctDNA status

For the subgroup of patients who had surgical tissue assayed, there was no difference in methylation in tumour tissue between the 56 ctDNA-positive and 35 ctDNA-negative cases at peri-diagnosis (median (IQR): BCAT1, 43.4% (27.1–59.2) and 52.6% (26.1–68.2), respectively, $P = 0.533$; IKZF1, 59.3% (20.5–84.4) and 59.0% (16.6–100.3), respectively, $P = 0.430$). Detection of ctDNA was not concordant with tissue levels; levels of tissue methylation were not dependent on stage, whereas detection in blood was (Fig. 3). Most tumour tissues displayed elevated methylation of both BCAT1 and IKZF1 ($n = 78$, 85.7%), while ctDNA methylated in both genes was only detected in 30 patients (33.0%) (Additional file 1: Table S2).

Post-surgery ctDNA status

Plasma was available in 93 cases for detection of methylated ctDNA within 12 months of surgery (median (IQR) 1.9 months (1.6–4.0 months), Additional file 1: Figure S1). Thirty-five (74.5%) of the 47 cases who were ctDNA positive prior to surgery became negative after resection as shown in Fig. 4; plasma was collected in 26 of these within 3 months of surgery, indicating that reversion to a negative ctDNA status occurred rapidly. In the 12 cases who failed to revert to negative, eight had not received their full cancer treatment (i.e. adjuvant chemotherapy or resection of distant metastases) at the time of the blood collection.

Discussion

This study explored how the methylated BCAT1 and IKZF1 DNA biomarkers for ctDNA related to cancer characteristics, aberrant methylation in CRC tissue and surgical resection as understanding these relationships might aid management of patients diagnosed with CRC by informing completeness of surgical resection.

For a ctDNA marker to be useful, the measured molecular features (e.g. mutation or methylation) should be present in the majority of cancer tissues and ideally should be independent of location, stage and molecular pathogenesis. Percentage methylation of either marker was much higher in cancer than non-neoplastic tissue, indicating that this was not a field effect. Our observations showed that all but one tumour had detectable methylation, with tumour tissue levels being independent of stage. The variables that related to degree of

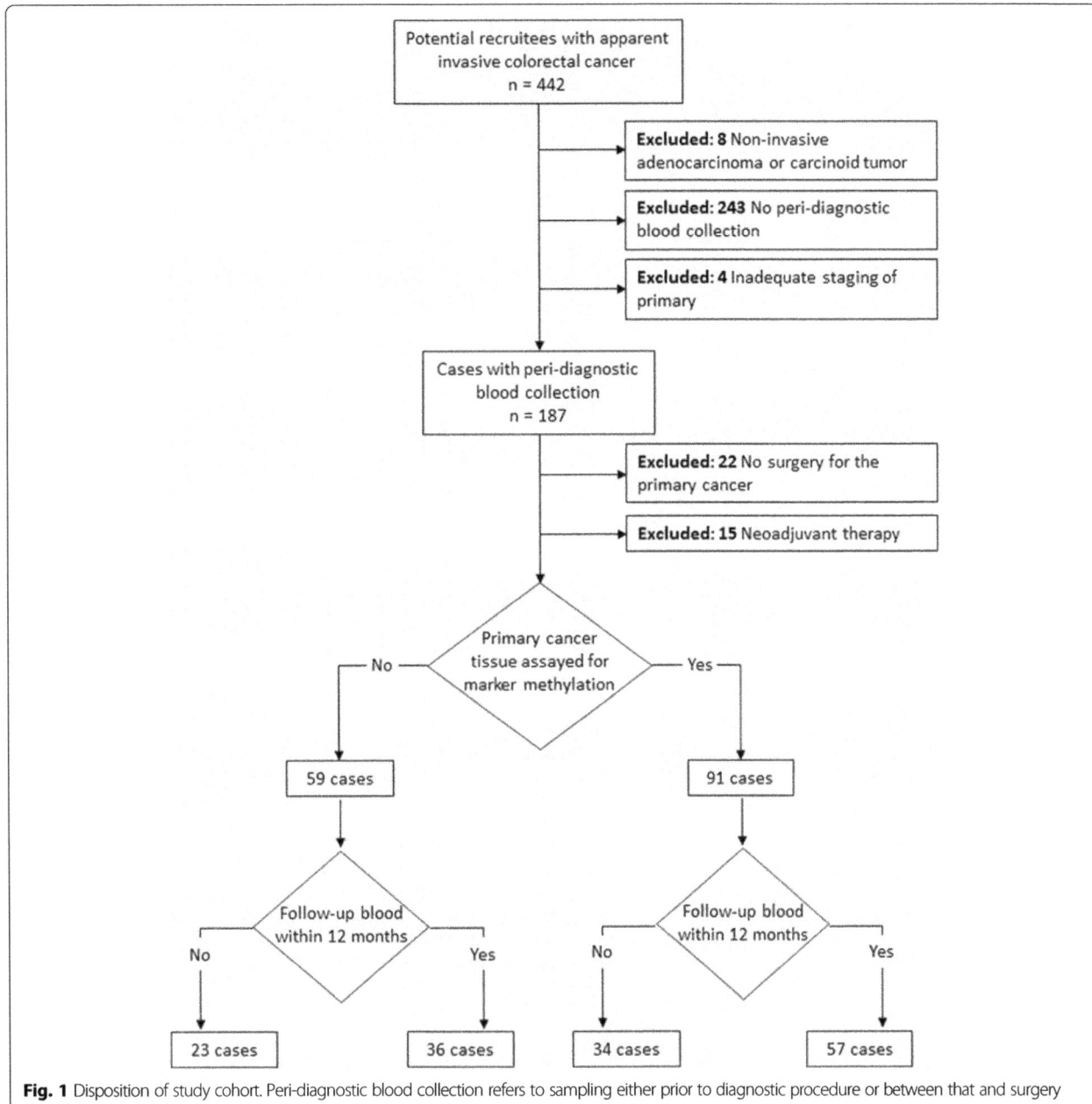

Fig. 1 Disposition of study cohort. Peri-diagnostic blood collection refers to sampling either prior to diagnostic procedure or between that and surgery

methylation in tissue was cancer compared to non-cancer tissue (either marker), age (lower methylation in younger people in cancer tissue, *BCAT1* only) and tumour location (higher methylation in proximal locations, *BCAT1* only). *IKZF1* also had slightly higher methylation levels in proximal cancers, but this did not reach statistical significance. Genome-wide hypermethylation has previously been reported to be more pronounced in proximal tumours than distal tumours [28]. Despite these differences in quantitative levels, there were no differences in the proportion of cancers considered positive for each methylated biomarker (i.e. with %methylation above the 75th percentile of non-neoplastic tissue). In

addition, these differences were not reflected in the blood results, with distal tumours more likely to be ctDNA positive, which is likely to be related to morphological differences. Thus, *BCAT1* or *IKZF1* hypermethylation of tissue is common at all stages of CRC and appears to be more frequent than the somatic mutation frequency reported for known hot-spot genes such as *KRAS*, *TP53* and *APC* [5, 13].

ctDNA blood tests (regardless of whether the marker is genetic or epigenetic) appear to be limited in their capacity to detect stage I cases compared to all other stages [12, 29, 30]. There was only one patient who was negative for both methylated *BCAT1* and *IKZF1* in the

Table 1 Plasma *BCAT1*, *IKZK1* and overall ctDNA positivity for different clinicopathological findings of patients with invasive colorectal cancer (n = 187)

Factor	Category	N	Methylated *BCAT1* DNA			Methylated *IKZF1* DNA			ctDNA positivity (combined *BCAT1/IKZF1*)		
			No. positive	% positive (95% CI[1])	P[2]	No. positive	% positive (95% CI[1])	P[2]	No. positive	% positive (95% CI[1])	P[2]
Age	< 65 years	67	29	43.3 (31.2–56.0)	0.154	28	41.8 (29.8–54.5)	0.332	39	58.2 (45.5–70.2)	0.421
	≥ 65 years	120	65	54.2 (44.8–63.3)		59	49.2 (39.9–58.4)		77	64.2 (54.9–72.7)	
Gender	Female	75	34	45.3 (33.8–57.3)	0.270	31	41.3 (30.1–53.3)	0.244	42	56.0 (44.1–67.5)	0.164
	Male	112	60	53.6 (43.9–63.0)		56	50.0 (40.4–59.6)		74	66.1 (56.5–74.7)	
Stage	I	40	4	10.0 (2.8–23.7)	< 0.001	2	5.0 (0.6–16.9)	< 0.001	6	15.0 (5.7–29.8)	< 0.001
	II	54	29	53.7 (39.6–67.4)		25	46.3 (32.6–60.4)		35	64.8 (50.6–77.3)	
	III	63	37	58.7 (45.6–71.0)		36	57.1 (44.0–69.5)		47	74.6 (62.1–84.7)	
	IV	30	24	80.0 (61.4–92.3)		24	80.0 (61.4–92.3)		28	93.3 (77.9–99.2)	
T stage	T1	26	2	7.7 (0.9–22.1)	< 0.001	1	3.8 (0.1–19.6)	< 0.001	2	7.7 (0.9–25.1)	< 0.001
	T2	23	6	26.1 (10.2–48.4)		3	13.0 (2.8–33.6)		8	34.8 (16.4–57.3)	
	T3	96	55	57.3 (46.8–67.3)		56	58.3 (47.8–68.3)		69	71.9 (61.8–80.6)	
	T4	34	24	70.6 (52.5–84.9)		21	61.8 (43.6–77.8)		29	85.3 (68.9–95.0)	
	Unknown	8	7	87.5 (47.3–99.7)		6	75.0 (34.9–96.8)		8	100.0 (63.1–100.0)	
N stage	N0	100	41	41.0 (31.3–51.3)	0.024	36	36.0 (26.6–46.2)	0.007	50	50.0 (39.8–60.2)	0.001
	N1/N2	73	44	60.3 (48.1–71.5)		44	60.3 (48.1–71.5)		56	76.7 (65.4–85.8)	
	Unknown	14	9	64.3 (35.1–87.2)		7	50.0 (23.0–77.0)		10	71.4 (41.9–91.6)	
M stage	M0	147	66	44.9 (36.7–53.3)	0.002	58	39.5 (31.5–47.8)	< 0.001	82	55.8 (47.4–64.0)	0.001
	M1	30	24	80.0 (61.4–92.3)		24	80.0 (61.4–92.3)		28	93.3 (77.9–99.2)	
	Unknown	10	4	40.0 (12.2–73.8)		5	50.0 (18.7–81.3)		6	60.0 (26.2–87.8)	
Size (mm)	< 20 mm	14	2	14.3 (1.8–42.8)	< 0.001	2	14.3 (1.8–42.8)	< 0.001	3	21.4 (4.7–50.8)	< 0.001
	20–50 mm	100	44	44.0 (34.1–54.3)		37	37.0 (27.6–47.2)		56	56.0 (45.7–65.9)	
	> 50 mm	65	44	67.7 (54.9–78.8)		45	69.2 (56.6–80.1)		52	80.0 (68.2–88.9)	
	Unknown	8	4	50.0 (15.7–84.3)		3	37.5 (8.5–75.5)		5	62.5 (24.5–91.5)	
Location	Proximal	75	28	37.3 (26.4–49.3)	0.011	31	41.3 (30.1–53.3)	0.306	37	49.3 (37.6–61.1)	0.011
	Distal	111	65	58.6 (48.8–67.8)		56	50.5 (40.8–60.1)		78	70.3 (60.9–78.6)	
	Unknown	1	1	100.0 (2.5–100.0)		0	0.0 (0.0–97.5)		1		
Lymphatic invasion	Yes	38	24	63.2 (46.0–78.2)	0.014	25	65.8 (48.6–80.4)	0.001	30	78.9 (62.7–90.4)	0.002
	No	121	49	40.5 (31.7–49.8)		44	36.4 (27.8–45.6)		61	50.4 (41.2–59.6)	
Perinueural invasion	Yes	20	9	45.0 (23.1–68.5)	0.860	10	50.0 (27.2–72.8)	0.541	15	75.0 (50.9–91.3)	0.104
	No	138	65	47.1 (38.6–55.8)		59	42.8 (34.4–51.4)		77	55.8 (47.1–64.2)	
Extramural vascular invasion	Yes	9	6	66.7 (29.9–92.5)	0.313	7	77.8 (40.0–97.2)	0.054	8	88.9 (51.8–99.7)	0.089
	No	178	88	49.4 (41.9–57.0)		80	44.9 (37.5–52.6)		108	60.7 (53.1–67.9)	
Intramural vascular invasion	Yes	3	2	66.7 (9.4–99.2)	0.567	2	66.7 (9.4–99.2)	0.481	2	66.7 (9.4–99.2)	0.868
	No	184	92	50.0 (42.6–57.4)		85	46.2 (38.8–53.7)		114	62.0 (54.5–69.0)	
Differentiation	Poor	34	21	61.8 (43.6–77.8)	0.241	20	58.8 (40.7–75.4)	0.124	25	73.5 (55.6–87.1)	0.160
	Moderate	118	54	45.8 (36.6–55.2)		48	40.7 (31.7–50.1)		67	56.8 (47.3–65.9)	
	Well	14	6	42.9 (17.7–71.1)		6	42.9 (17.7–71.1)		7	50.0 (23.0–77.0)	
	Unknown	21	13	61.9 (38.4–81.9)		13	61.9 (38.4–81.9)		17	81.0 (58.1–94.6)	

[1] Confidence interval
[2] *P* value, Pearson's chi-square test

tissue and who also returned a negative blood result. We report sensitivity for CRC of 62% across all stages, and the test was significantly more likely to be positive with more advanced clinical stage of cancer, which is consistent with our earlier findings [15, 16] and other commonly used CRC screening tests. In brief, we previously reported that at a matching specificity, the *BCAT1/IKZF1* blood test had equal sensitivity to a commonly used faecal

Table 2 Association between tumour characteristics and ctDNA positivity

Factor	Odds ratio (95% CI)	P value
Stage		< 0.001
I	1 (reference)	
II	12.5 (4.3–36.6)	
III	16.6 (5.7–48)	
IV	92.1 (16.5–513.8)	
Location		0.004
Proximal colon	1 (reference)	
Distal colon and rectum	3.0 (1.4–6.2)	

immunochemical test (62 versus 64%, respectively) [16]. There are two commercially available molecular tests for CRC screening, ColoGuard (multi-target stool DNA test, including two methylation markers) and ProColon (methylated *SEPT9*). The multi-target stool DNA test has a reported sensitivity of 92% [31] but a lower specificity (87%) than what we report for the *BCAT1/IKZF1* blood test (92%) [16]. The estimated sensitivity and specificity for the ProColon blood test is 48 and 92%, respectively [30].

Our results show clearly that absence of *BCAT1* or *IKZF1* in blood at diagnosis does not reflect an absence of marker methylation in the tissue. Consequently, infrequent aberrant methylation is not likely to be a limiting factor for the *BCAT1/IKZF1* blood test. It is not clear if the usefulness of ctDNA testing for primary diagnosis is somehow biologically limited in early cancer and dependent on tissue vascularity, invasion or cellular turnover (e.g. apoptosis or necrosis). It is also uncertain if ctDNA biomarker assays are technologically limited in assay sensitivity, or if they will vary in usefulness between specific markers. However, it is likely that complex panels will be needed for ctDNA tests assaying for the less frequent somatic mutations, whereas ctDNA tests assaying for just a few methylation markers, such as those reported here, are sufficient. The literature is sparse on direct paired comparison studies (tissue versus blood), especially for methylation biomarkers. Using other molecular markers of cancer (microRNA, mRNA), Wang et al. reported the circulating levels of miR-601 and miR-760 to be significantly lower in CRC patients compared to that of healthy subjects, yet they found no differences in the expression levels of these miRNA markers between cancer and non-cancer tissues [32]. Conversely, good concordances have been reported for colorectal neoplastic tissue and plasma detection for CRC biomarkers such as *TYMS* and *LISCH7* mRNAs, [33, 34] *KRAS* mutation and *SEPT9* methylation, [35] albeit the levels in plasma were much lower than that found in tissue. For *Sept9*, methylation rates were 64.5% in tissue and 14.5% in plasma, while *KRAS* mutation was found in 33.6% of tissues and 2.9% of plasma samples [35].

There is considerable interest in understanding the association between ctDNA and detection of minimal residual disease and likelihood of overall recurrence and survival [9, 36]. In this respect, the epigenetic markers we applied showed that three quarters of patients who were ctDNA positive at diagnosis became negative after

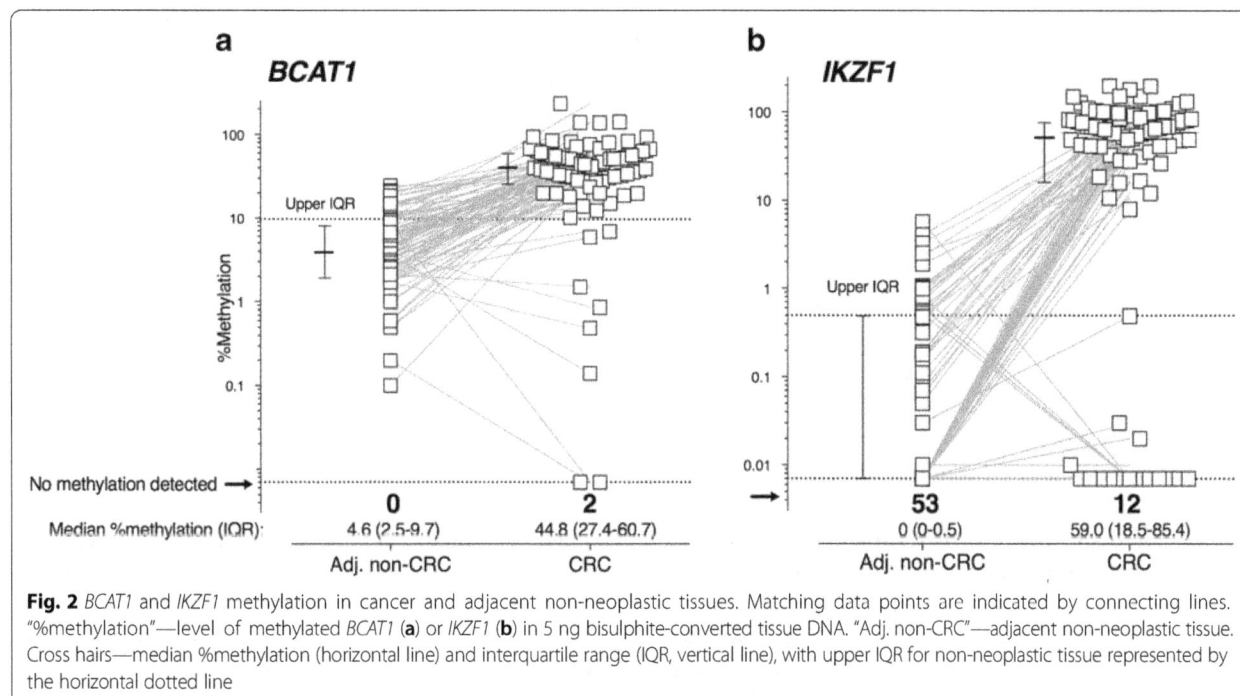

Fig. 2 *BCAT1* and *IKZF1* methylation in cancer and adjacent non-neoplastic tissues. Matching data points are indicated by connecting lines. "%methylation"—level of methylated *BCAT1* (**a**) or *IKZF1* (**b**) in 5 ng bisulphite-converted tissue DNA. "Adj. non-CRC"—adjacent non-neoplastic tissue. Cross hairs—median %methylation (horizontal line) and interquartile range (IQR, vertical line), with upper IQR for non-neoplastic tissue represented by the horizontal dotted line

Table 3 *BCAT1* and *IKZF1* methylation in 91 cancer tissue samples according to case demographics and tumour characteristics

Variable factor	Category	N	%Methylation, median (IQR)			
			BCAT1	P	IKZF1	P
Age	< 65	32	35.8 (14–57.5)	0.039[1]	52.5 (11.4–69.7)	0.143[1]
	≥ 65	59	50.1 (31.4–67.8)		64.8 (31.3–96.3)	
Gender	Female	45	46.9 (31.0–60.7)	0.444[1]	59 (41.6–96.3)	0.359[1]
	Male	46	42.2 (26.9–63.1)		59.3 (10.7–83.3)	
Stage	I	19	50.1 (19.8–81.3)	0.581[2]	56.9 (9.1–115.6)	0.659[2]
	II	34	44.6 (20.2–58.9)		48.7 (0.5–82)	
	III	29	43.3 (32.9–51.9)		61.1 (42.6–84.7)	
	IV	9	57.7 (36.1–71.4)		54.3 (41.4–98.7)	
T stage	T1	8	68.6 (54.4–93.0)	0.066[2]	88.7 (34.4–132.4)	0.362[2]
	T2	13	27.5 (18.8–51.4)		32.1 (9.1–100.3)	
	T3	48	50.5 (32.7–60.0)		65.1 (31.8–84.0)	
	T4	22	32.6 (23.6–52.9)		42.1 (10.7–69.0)	
N stage	N0	57	50.9 (26.9–63.3)	0.680[2]	63.4 (15.8–97.8)	0.538[2]
	N1/N2	33	43.3 (30.3–59.4)		59 (41.4–76.1)	
	Nx	1	26.9 (26.9–26.9)		9.1 (9.1–9.1)	
M stage	M0	79	44.8 (26.9–63.1)	0.282[2]	60.8 (18.5–91)	0.785[2]
	M1	9	57.7 (36.1–71.4)		54.3 (41.4–98.7)	
	Mx	3	31.7 (18.8–35.4)		50.3 (0.0–85.5)	
Size (mm)	< 20 mm	4	59.6 (34.9–103.7)	0.551[2]	68.5 (14.3–152.9)	0.856[2]
	20–50 mm	52	41.5 (27.9–57)		57 (16.2–88.3)	
	> 50 mm	34	47.8 (23.6–67.8)		62.1 (28–84.7)	
	Unknown	1	81.3 (81.3–81.3)		68.8 (68.8–68.8)	
Location	Proximal	50	51.6 (31.0–67.3)	0.029[1]	68.9 (41.6–98.7)	0.055[1]
	Distal	41	37.9 (19.8–51.9)		41.4 (16.6–68.8)	
Lymphatic invasion	Yes	25	42.2 (33.9–63.1)	0.650[1]	63.4 (40.8–85.5)	0.827[1]
	No	66	48.3 (26.9–58.9)		57 (18.5–91)	
Perineural invasion	Yes	13	37.9 (19.9–56.4)	0.626[1]	41.4 (10.7–84.7)	0.708[1]
	No	78	48.3 (27.4–63.1)		59.9 (28.5–96.1)	
Extramural vascular invasion	Yes	4	42.0 (32.2–67.2)	0.816[1]	56.8 (24.6–102.3)	0.816[1]
	No	87	44.8 (26.9–63.1)		59.0 (18.5–91.0)	
Intramural vascular invasion	Yes	1	28.3 (28.3–28.3)	0.446[1]	41.2 (41.2–41.2)	0.594[1]
	No	90	45.8 (26.9–63.1)		59.9 (18.5–91.0)	
Differentiation	Poor	26	47.4 (30.3–67.8)	0.320[2]	59.9 (32.6–96.3)	0.691[2]
	Moderate	53	44.8 (26.9–58.9)		57.1 (12.0–83.3)	
	Well	7	36.1 (19.8–39)		48.7 (18.5–70.6)	
	Unknown	5	56.2 (51.4–63.3)		81.2 (76.3–84.7)	

[1]Mann-Whitney test on medians (two-tailed)
[2]Kruskal-Wallis test on medians (two-tailed)

surgical resection. Many of the patients who remained positive had not completed their cancer treatment. The effect of surgical resection on detectable biomarker in blood adds credibility to the premise that these markers could be useful for monitoring of patients in that they are responsive to debulking. This observational study

has been conducted in a usual-care moderate-sized clinical service where follow-up protocols are subject to variance according to practitioner protocols and risk for recurrence, rather than in the context of a formal highly structured prospective clinical trial where blood would be collected at set intervals following surgery and other

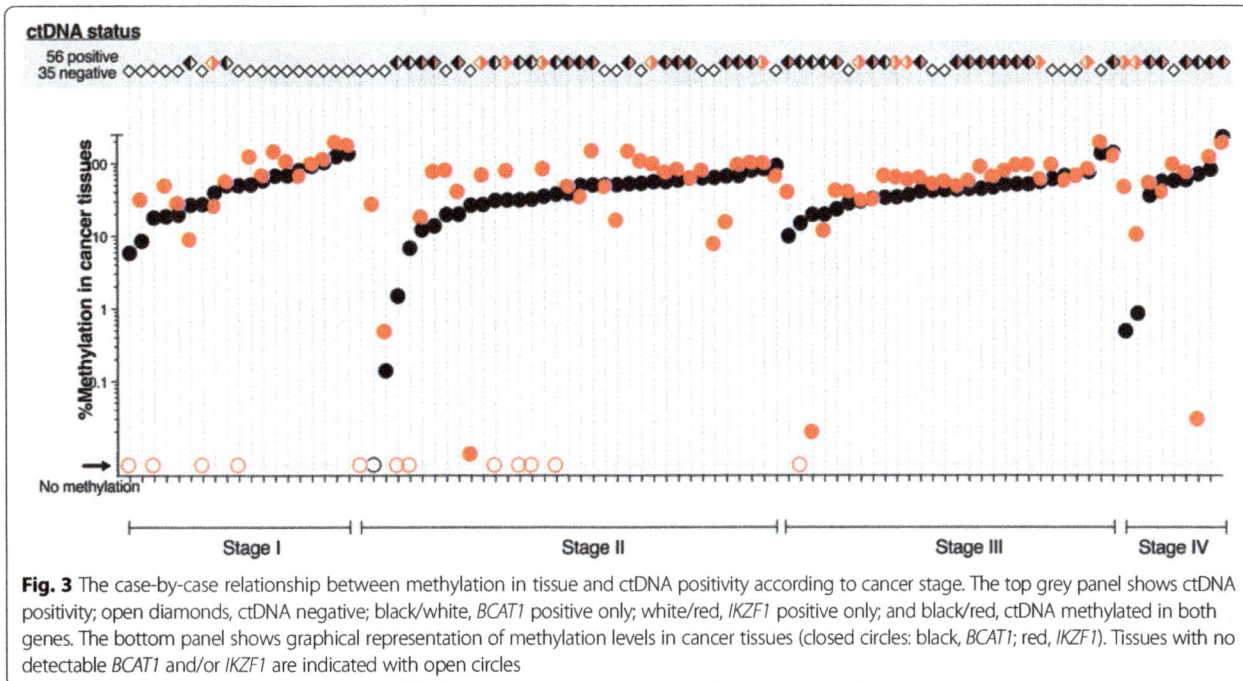

Fig. 3 The case-by-case relationship between methylation in tissue and ctDNA positivity according to cancer stage. The top grey panel shows ctDNA positivity; open diamonds, ctDNA negative; black/white, *BCAT1* positive only; white/red, *IKZF1* positive only; and black/red, ctDNA methylated in both genes. The bottom panel shows graphical representation of methylation levels in cancer tissues (closed circles: black, *BCAT1*; red, *IKZF1*). Tissues with no detectable *BCAT1* and/or *IKZF1* are indicated with open circles

therapies. Future prospective studies with tightly controlled and more frequent venipuncture would clarify the best time to draw blood after surgery, but it seems possible that it could be within 3 months, as most of the cases became negative within this time frame. A small study investigating the effect of surgery on mutation markers of ctDNA reported that cases became negative within 3 to 5 days [37]. All these observations are consistent with the estimated short half-life of circulating DNA [38] and indicate that these markers are highly and quite rapidly responsive to surgical debulking and thus adds credibility to the premise that these methylation

markers are applicable for dynamic monitoring of residual disease [29]. As this study focused on the effects of surgery on ctDNA clearance, the length of follow-up was consequently not long enough to show what our findings mean for clinical outcomes such as risk for recurrence and death.

Conclusions

Non-invasive analysis of ctDNA for post-treatment surveillance has the potential to become a practice-changing tool as it may create a window of opportunity for intervention at time points where curative modalities

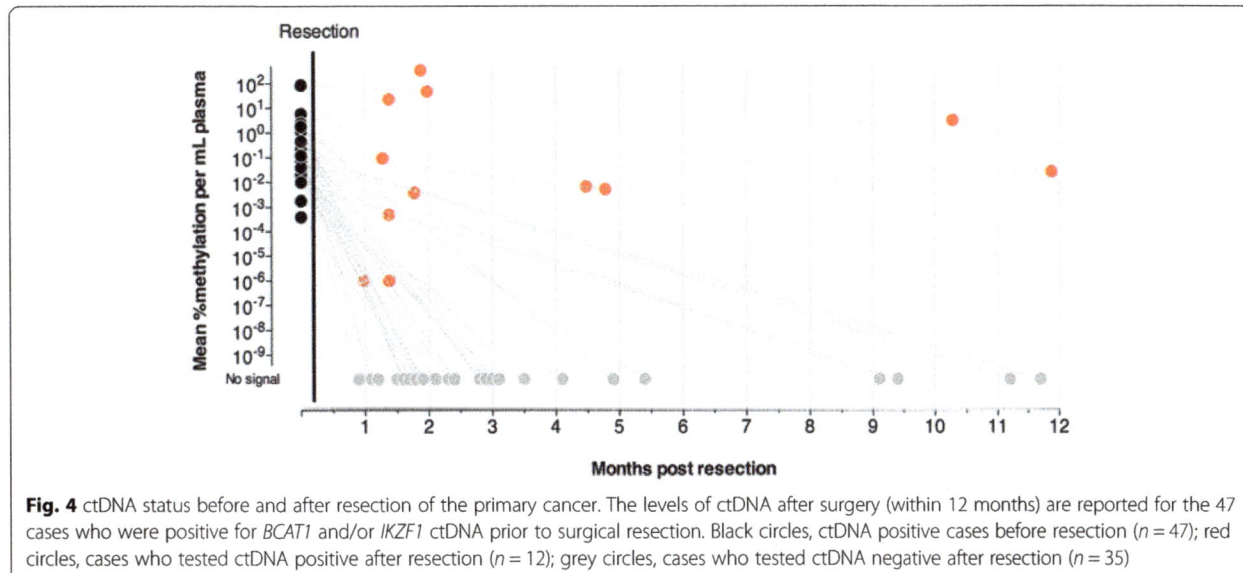

Fig. 4 ctDNA status before and after resection of the primary cancer. The levels of ctDNA after surgery (within 12 months) are reported for the 47 cases who were positive for *BCAT1* and/or *IKZF1* ctDNA prior to surgical resection. Black circles, ctDNA positive cases before resection (*n* = 47); red circles, cases who tested ctDNA positive after resection (*n* = 12); grey circles, cases who tested ctDNA negative after resection (*n* = 35)

are still an option. Our findings demonstrate that detection of ctDNA using this noninvasive test for methylated *BCAT1/IKZF1* is informative with respect to completeness of surgical resection. Hypermethylation in the two investigated genes are near ubiquitous in CRC tissue, and their appearance in the blood as markers of ctDNA is related to cancer behavior (stage) and is not limited by lack of tissue expression. Testing for ctDNA by measuring for appearance of methylated *BCAT1/IKZF1* could aid patient management through selection of cases for intensified surveillance for recurrence and might allow identification of patients who would benefit from adjustments in adjuvant therapies.

Abbreviations
BCAT1: Branched chain amino acid transaminase 1; CEA: Carcinoembryonic antigen; CRC: Colorectal cancer; ctDNA: Circulating tumour-derived DNA; *IKZF1*: IKAROS family zinc finger 1

Acknowledgements
Tissue specimens used in this research were kindly provided by the Flinders Tumour Bank.

Funding
This study was funded in part by the National Health and Medical Research Council (APP1006242, APP1017083) and Clinical Genomics Pty Ltd.

Authors' contributions
GPY and ES coordinated the study. MJ, SEB and DB were responsible for the data collection. PR and ES were responsible for the auditing of data. DHM, RTB, GPY, SKP and ES were responsible for the data analysis and interpretation of results. GPY, SKP and ES drafted the manuscript. All authors read and approved the final manuscript to be published.

Competing interests
GPY is a paid consultant to Clinical Genomics. SKP, DHM and RTB are paid employees of Clinical Genomics. The other authors declare that they have no competing interests.

Author details
[1]Flinders Centre for Innovation in Cancer, College of Medicine and Public Health, Flinders University of South Australia, Bedford Park, South Australia 5042, Australia. [2]Bowel Health Service, Flinders Medical Centre, Bedford Park, South Australia, Australia. [3]Clinical Genomics Pty Ltd, North Ryde, New South Wales, Australia. [4]Colorectal Surgery, Division of Surgery and Perioperative Medicine, Flinders Medical Centre, Bedford Park, South Australia, Australia.

References
1. Siegel RL, Miller KD, Fedewa SA, Ahnen DJ, Meester RGS, Barzi A, Jemal A. Colorectal cancer statistics, 2017. CA Cancer J Clin. 2017;67:177–93.
2. Sargent D, Sobrero A, Grothey A, O'Connell MJ, Buyse M, Andre T, Zheng Y, Green E, Labianca R, O'Callaghan C, et al. Evidence for cure by adjuvant therapy in colon cancer: observations based on individual patient data from 20,898 patients on 18 randomized trials. Journal of clinical oncology : official journal of the American Society of Clinical Oncology. 2009;27:872–7.
3. Chao M, Gibbs P. Caution is required before recommending routine carcinoembryonic antigen and imaging follow-up for patients with early-stage colon cancer. Journal of clinical oncology : official journal of the American Society of Clinical Oncology. 2009;27:e279–80. author reply e281
4. Meyerhardt JA, Mangu PB, Flynn PJ, Korde L, Loprinzi CL, Minsky BD, Petrelli NJ, Ryan K, Schrag DH, Wong SL, et al. Follow-up care, surveillance protocol, and secondary prevention measures for survivors of colorectal cancer: American Society of Clinical Oncology clinical practice guideline endorsement. Journal of clinical oncology : official journal of the American Society of Clinical Oncology. 2013;31:4465–70.
5. Vogelstein B, Papadopoulos N, Velculescu VE, Zhou S, Diaz LA Jr, Kinzler KW. Cancer genome landscapes. Science. 2013;339:1546–58.
6. Kibriya MG, Raza M, Jasmine F, Roy S, Paul-Brutus R, Rahaman R, Dodsworth C, Rakibuz-Zaman M, Kamal M, Ahsan H. A genome-wide DNA methylation study in colorectal carcinoma. BMC Med Genet. 2011;4:50.
7. Diehl F, Li M, Dressman D, He Y, Shen D, Szabo S, Diaz LA Jr, Goodman SN, David KA, Juhl H, et al. Detection and quantification of mutations in the plasma of patients with colorectal tumors. Proc Natl Acad Sci U S A. 2005; 102:16368–73.
8. Tie J, Kinde I, Wang Y, Wong HL, Roebert J, Christie M, Tacey M, Wong R, Singh M, Karapetis CS, et al. Circulating tumor DNA as an early marker of therapeutic response in patients with metastatic colorectal cancer. Annals of oncology : official journal of the European Society for Medical Oncology / ESMO. 2015;26:1715–22.
9. Tie J, Wang Y, Tomasetti C, Li L, Springer S, Kinde I, Silliman N, Tacey M, Wong HL, Christie M, et al. Circulating tumor DNA analysis detects minimal residual disease and predicts recurrence in patients with stage II colon cancer. Sci Transl Med. 2016;8:346ra392.
10. Wood LD, Parsons DW, Jones S, Lin J, Sjoblom T, Leary RJ, Shen D, Boca SM, Barber T, Ptak J, et al. The genomic landscapes of human breast and colorectal cancers. Science. 2007;318:1108–13.
11. Diaz LA Jr, Williams RT, Wu J, Kinde I, Hecht JR, Berlin J, Allen B, Bozic I, Reiter JG, Nowak MA, et al. The molecular evolution of acquired resistance to targeted EGFR blockade in colorectal cancers. Nature. 2012;486:537–40.
12. Bettegowda C, Sausen M, Leary RJ, Kinde I, Wang Y, Agrawal N, Bartlett BR, Wang H, Luber B, Alani RM, et al. Detection of circulating tumor DNA in early- and late-stage human malignancies. Sci Transl Med. 2014;6:224ra224.
13. Markowitz SD, Bertagnolli MM. Molecular origins of cancer: molecular basis of colorectal cancer. N Engl J Med. 2009;361:2449–60.
14. Pedersen SK, Baker RT, McEvoy A, Murray DH, Thomas M, Molloy PL, Mitchell S, Lockett T, Young GP, LaPointe L. A two-gene blood test for methylated DNA sensitive for colorectal cancer. PLoS One. 2015;10:e0125041.
15. Pedersen SK, Symonds EL, Baker RT, Murray DH, McEvoy A, Van Doorn SC, Mundt MW, Cole SR, Gopalsamy G, Mangira D, et al. Evaluation of an assay for methylated BCAT1 and IKZF1 in plasma for detection of colorectal neoplasia. BMC Cancer. 2015;15:654.
16. Symonds EL, Pedersen SK, Baker RT, Murray DH, Gaur S, Cole SR, Gopalsamy G, Mangira D, LaPointe LC, Young GP. A blood test for methylated BCAT1 and IKZF1 vs. a fecal immunochemical test for detection of colorectal neoplasia. Clin Transl Gastroenterol. 2016;7:e137.
17. Yoshikawa R, Yanagi H, Shen CS, Fujiwara Y, Noda M, Yagyu T, Gega M, Oshima T, Yamamura T, Okamura H, et al. ECA39 is a novel distant metastasis-related biomarker in colorectal cancer. World journal of gastroenterology : WJG. 2006;12:5884–9.
18. Schjerven H, McLaughlin J, Arenzana TL, Frietze S, Cheng D, Wadsworth SE, Lawson GW, Bensinger SJ, Farnham PJ, Witte ON, et al. Selective regulation of lymphopoiesis and leukemogenesis by individual zinc fingers of Ikaros. Nat Immunol. 2013;14:1073–83.
19. Tonjes M, Barbus S, Park YJ, Wang W, Schlotter M, Lindroth AM, Pleier SV, Bai AH, Karra D, Piro RM, et al. BCAT1 promotes cell proliferation through amino acid catabolism in gliomas carrying wild-type IDH1. Nat Med. 2013; 19:901–8.
20. Vincent A, Omura N, Hong SM, Jaffe A, Eshleman J, Goggins M. Genome-wide analysis of promoter methylation associated with gene expression profile in pancreatic adenocarcinoma. Clinical cancer research : an official journal of the American Association for Cancer Research. 2011;17:4341–54.
21. Mansfeld J, Urban N, Priebe S, Groth M, Frahm C, Hartmann N, Gebauer J, Ravichandran M, Dommaschk A, Schmeisser S, et al. Branched-chain amino acid catabolism is a conserved regulator of physiological ageing. Nat Commun. 2015;6:10043.
22. Oster B, Thorsen K, Lamy P, Wojdacz TK, Hansen LL, Birkenkamp-Demtroder K, Sorensen KD, Laurberg S, Orntoft TF, Andersen CL. Identification and validation of highly frequent CpG island hypermethylation in colorectal adenomas and carcinomas. International journal of cancer Journal international du cancer. 2011;129:2855–66.

23. Malinge S, Thiollier C, Chlon TM, Dore LC, Diebold L, Bluteau O, Mabialah V, Vainchenker W, Dessen P, Winandy S, et al. Ikaros inhibits megakaryopoiesis through functional interaction with GATA-1 and NOTCH signaling. Blood. 2013;121:2440–51.

24. Javierre BM, Rodriguez-Ubreva J, Al-Shahrour F, Corominas M, Grana O, Ciudad L, Agirre X, Pisano DG, Valencia A, Roman-Gomez J, et al. Long-range epigenetic silencing associates with deregulation of Ikaros targets in colorectal cancer cells. Molecular cancer research : MCR. 2011;9:1139–51.

25. Murray D, Baker R, Gaur S, Young G, Pedersen S. Validation of a circulating tumor-derived DNA blood test for detection of methylated BCAT1 and IKZF1 DNA. The Journal of Applied Laboratory Medicine. 2017;2:165–75.

26. Edge S, Byrd D, Compton C, Fritz A, Greene F, Trotti A. AJCC Cancer Staging Manual, 7th edition. New York: Springer; 2011.

27. Young GP, Pedersen SK, Mansfield S, Murray DH, Baker RT, Rabbitt P, Byrne S, Bambacas L, Hollington P, Symonds EL. A cross-sectional study comparing a blood test for methylated BCAT1 and IKZF1 tumor-derived DNA with CEA for detection of recurrent colorectal cancer. Cancer Med. 2016;5:2763–72.

28. Lee MS, Menter DG, Kopetz S. Right versus left colon cancer biology: integrating the consensus molecular subtypes. J Natl Compr Cancer Netw. 2017;15:411–9.

29. Garrigou S, Perkins G, Garlan F, Normand C, Didelot A, Le Corre D, Peyvandi S, Mulot C, Niarra R, Aucouturier P, et al. A study of hypermethylated circulating tumor DNA as a universal colorectal cancer biomarker. Clin Chem. 2016;62: 1129–39.

30. Church TR, Wandell M, Lofton-Day C, Mongin SJ, Burger M, Payne SR, Castanos-Velez E, Blumenstein BA, Rosch T, Osborn N, et al. Prospective evaluation of methylated SEPT9 in plasma for detection of asymptomatic colorectal cancer. Gut. 2014;63:317–25.

31. Imperiale TF, Ransohoff DF, Itzkowitz SH, Levin TR, Lavin P, Lidgard GP, Ahlquist DA, Berger BM. Multitarget stool DNA testing for colorectal-cancer screening. N Engl J Med. 2014;370:1287–97.

32. Wang Q, Huang Z, Ni S, Xiao X, Xu Q, Wang L, Huang D, Tan C, Sheng W, Du X. Plasma miR-601 and miR-760 are novel biomarkers for the early detection of colorectal cancer. PLoS One. 2012;7:e44398.

33. Garcia V, Garcia JM, Pena C, Silva J, Dominguez G, Hurtado A, Alonso I, Rodriguez R, Provencio M, Bonilla F. Thymidylate synthase messenger RNA expression in plasma from patients with colon cancer: prognostic potential. Clinical cancer research : an official journal of the American Association for Cancer Research. 2006;12:2095–100.

34. Garcia JM, Pena C, Garcia V, Dominguez G, Munoz C, Silva J, Millan I, Diaz R, Lorenzo Y, Rodriguez R, et al. Prognostic value of LISCH7 mRNA in plasma and tumor of colon cancer patients. Clinical cancer research : an official journal of the American Association for Cancer Research. 2007;13:6351–8.

35. Danese E, Minicozzi AM, Benati M, Montagnana M, Paviati E, Salvagno GL, Lima-Oliveira G, Gusella M, Pasini F, Lippi G, et al. Comparison of genetic and epigenetic alterations of primary tumors and matched plasma samples in patients with colorectal cancer. PLoS One. 2015;10:e0126417.

36. Thierry AR, Mouliere F, El Messaoudi S, Mollevi C, Lopez-Crapez E, Rolet F, Gillet B, Gongora C, Dechelotte P, Robert B, et al. Clinical validation of the detection of KRAS and BRAF mutations from circulating tumor DNA. Nat Med. 2014;20:430–5.

37. Ng SB, Chua C, Ng M, Gan A, Poon PS, Teo M, Fu C, Leow WQ, Lim KH, Chung A, et al. Individualised multiplexed circulating tumour DNA assays for monitoring of tumour presence in patients after colorectal cancer surgery. Sci Rep. 2017;7:40737.

38. Diehl F, Schmidt K, Choti MA, Romans K, Goodman S, Li M, Thornton K, Agrawal N, Sokoll L, Szabo SA, et al. Circulating mutant DNA to assess tumor dynamics. Nat Med. 2008;14:985–90.

5

Multifactorial analysis of the stochastic epigenetic variability in cord blood confirmed an impact of common behavioral and environmental factors but not of in vitro conception

D. Gentilini[1,5], E. Somigliana[2], L. Pagliardini[3], E. Rabellotti[3], P. Garagnani[4], L. Bernardinelli[5], E. Papaleo[3], M. Candiani[6], A. M. Di Blasio[1] and P. Viganò[3*]

Abstract

Background: An increased incidence of imprint-associated disorders has been reported in babies born from assisted reproductive technology (ART). However, previous studies supporting an association between ART and an altered DNA methylation status of the conceived babies have been often conducted on a limited number of methylation sites and without correction for critical potential confounders. Moreover, all the previous studies focused on the identification of methylation changes shared among subjects while an evaluation of stochastic differences has never been conducted. This study aims to evaluate the effect of ART and other common behavioral or environmental factors associated with pregnancy on stochastic epigenetic variability using a multivariate approach.

Results: DNA methylation levels of cord blood from 23 in vitro and 41 naturally conceived children were analyzed using the Infinium HumanMethylation450 BeadChips. After multiple testing correction, no statistically significant difference emerged in the number of cord blood stochastic epigenetic variations or in the methylation levels between in vitro- and in vivo-conceived babies. Conversely, four multiple factor analysis dimensions summarizing common phenotypic, behavioral, or environmental factors (cord blood cell composition, pre or post conception supplementation of folates, birth percentiles, gestational age, cesarean section, pre-gestational mother's weight, parents' BMI and obesity status, presence of adverse pregnancy outcomes, mother's smoking status, and season of birth) were significantly associated with stochastic epigenetic variability. The stochastic epigenetic variation analysis allowed the identification of a rare imprinting defect in the locus GNAS in one of the babies belonging to the control population, which would not have emerged using a classical case-control association analysis.

Conclusions: We confirmed the effect of several common behavioral or environmental factors on the epigenome of newborns and described for the first time an epigenetic effect related to season of birth. Children born after ART did not appear to have an increased risk of genome-wide changes in DNA methylation either at specific loci or randomly scattered throughout the genome. The inability to identify differences between cases and controls suggests that the number of stochastic epigenetic variations potentially induced by ART was not greater than that naturally produced in response to maternal behavior or other common environmental factors.

Keywords: Epigenome-wide analysis, Assisted reproduction technology, DNA methylation, Imprinted genes, Multiple factor analysis, Stochastic epigenetic variations

* Correspondence: vigano.paola@hsr.it
[3]Reproductive Sciences Laboratory, Division of Genetics and Cell Biology, IRCCS Ospedale San Raffaele, Via Olgettina 58, 20132 Milan, Italy
Full list of author information is available at the end of the article

Background

Currently, there is still poor consensus on the possibility that assisted reproduction technology (ART) could affect the epigenome of in vitro-conceived babies [1–3].

Most of the studies addressing the DNA methylation status of children conceived through in vitro fertilization (IVF) with or without intracytoplasmic sperm injection (ICSI) have specifically evaluated alterations in imprinted regions [1, 2]. This on the basis of a suggested link between ART and imprinting disorders. A recent meta-analysis including the results of all the studies regardless of the type of the imprinting disorder, showed a significant association between imprinting diseases and ART (odds ratio = 3.67; 95% confidence interval = 1.39–9.74) [2]. Beckwith-Wiedemann syndrome, as an example, has an estimated worldwide frequency of 1 in 13,700 naturally conceived babies and a weighted relative risk of 5.2 in children conceived by ART [2, 4]. Therefore, there is evidence to suggest an adverse effect of ART procedures, as well as of the underlying subfertility, on imprinting status. The biological rationale behind this idea is that because of the dynamic epigenetic reprogramming occurring during oocyte growth and preimplantation development, environmental perturbations during this time period may affect imprinting establishment and maintenance. Proper allelic expression of imprinted genes are known to play an important role in embryonic and neonatal growth, placental function, and postnatal behavior [1, 2, 4–7].

On the other hand, no evidence of generalized changes in DNA methylation of the imprinted genes KvDMR/KCNQIOTI, PEGI/MESR, IGF2, PEG3, and H19 in association with ART was found [2]. For instance, results of a meta-analysis of four studies comparing percentage methylation of IGF2 locus between ART and spontaneously conceived babies did not show any significant difference [2]. Although imprinting syndromes are usually associated with profound methylation changes, even the smaller scale changes that could be caused by ART methodologies could potentially predispose to epigenetic alterations at the key loci associated with the syndromes. However, it is unlikely that these hypothetical changes in the methylation status of newborns will be located in genomic regions shared among subjects. Considering that the reprogramming mechanism is driven by a relatively small number of "players" [8], it is difficult to figure out a mechanism where a potential interference related to IVF techniques will result in a small localized damage instead of a stochastic and more widespread effect. Indeed, the stochastic nature of these events has been previously suggested based on data both in humans and animal models [9, 10]. In addition to a potential damage, a stochastic effect could also be related to a rescue mechanism similar to the one observed in the germinal cells of the progeny of Dnmt3L2/2 female mice, where a hierarchy of factors involved in the establishment and maintenance of maternal germline imprints has been found, the loss of one possibly rescued in a stochastic fashion by the activity of the others [11].

Given the supposed small and stochastic effects associated with ART, the analysis of mean methylation levels may not be ideal in exploring differences between in vivo- and in vitro-conceived children. This analysis may be useful in identifying epigenetic alterations shared by a group of subjects and potentially associated with their phenotype but would not reflect differences in individual variation or other features of the methylation spectrum. Rare stochastic epigenetic variations that are not shared among subjects fail to be identified by a classic Epigenome Wide Association Study (EWAS) based on mean methylation values comparison [12]. To overcome this problem, we have conducted an analysis of stochasticity based on the previously introduced concept of stochastic epigenetic variations (SEVs) [12]. SEV is defined as a single CpG with a methylation level detected as an outlier when compared to the methylation level found for the same CpG in a control population. This allows to obtain both a measure of stochasticity at a whole-genome level (total number of SEVs) and a topographic information on genomic regions with an enriched number of SEVs. A previous application of this method permitted to obtain an estimation of the number of epigenetic alterations produced by aging, revealing an exponential association between age and number of SEVs [12]. Only four studies have previously evaluated DNA methylation at a genome-wide level in cord blood of human offspring from ART procedures, and this was done based on the comparison of the mean methylation levels [10, 13–15]. Importantly, correction for phenotypic parental or fetal traits was limited to none or very few confounders although parental BMI, mode of delivery, birth weight, smoke, and intrauterine growth restriction have been previously linked to changes in methylation levels of several genes [16–19].

In this report, we present different analytical approaches in evaluating global DNA methylation of umbilical cord blood from in vitro and naturally conceived newborns mostly with the aim to measure random epigenetic variations and the impact of potential confounders on their number.

Results

Dimensionality reduction of all phenotypic traits using multiple factor analysis

Differences at phenotypic level between naturally conceived ($n = 41$) and in vitro-conceived babies ($n = 23$) were evaluated. The phenotypic traits considered were birth weight, birthweight centiles, mother's age, parity status, gestational age, cesarean section, sex of the baby, presence of adverse pregnancy outcomes (diabetes, pre-eclampsia and placenta praevia), pre-gestational mother weight, parents' BMI and obesity, gestational weight increase, maternal smoking status, pre-post conception folate supplementation, blood cell composition [CD8 T Cells (CD8T), CD4 T Cells (CD4T), natural killer (NK) cells, B cells, monocytes, granulocytes], and season of birth. The correlogram in Additional file 1: Figure S1 shows all the phenotypes analyzed and the presence of a consistent degree of correlation among traits. The number of dimensions to use in the analysis was reduced using the multiple factor analysis of mixed data. Considering the first two obtained dimensions (Dims), the overlap of cases and controls shown in Fig. 1a suggested a phenotypic similarity between the two groups. Taken together, the first 10 dimensions collected 72% of the total variability among the subjects analyzed. Correlations between dimensions and phenotypic traits were evaluated and are shown in Fig. 1b. The logistic regression analysis indicated that the Dim 1 and Dim 3 were significantly associated with case-control status ($p = 0.03$ and $p = 0.01$, respectively) and were subsequently used as covariates in the case-control differential methylation analysis.

Phenotypic traits that were mainly captured by Dim1 and Dim 3 were highlighted by elevated correlation levels (Fig. 1b).

Visual inspection of DNA methylation level using principal component analysis (PCA)

The genome-wide DNA methylation analysis of cord blood was performed using the Infinium HumanMethylation450 BeadChip. Dimensional reduction was used to visually inspect the dataset for strong signals in the methylation values. The PCA was performed considering methylation signals from single CpG sites and also considering four sets of genomic regions: genes, promoters, CpG islands, and tiling (not overlapping regions of 5 kb length). Results reported in Fig. 2 show that there was no strong difference in the methylation level between naturally conceived and in vitro-conceived babies considering both sites and genomic regions.

Differential methylation analysis

Differential methylation analysis was computed both for site (single CpG) and region level. Dimensions obtained from the multifactorial analysis, which were significantly

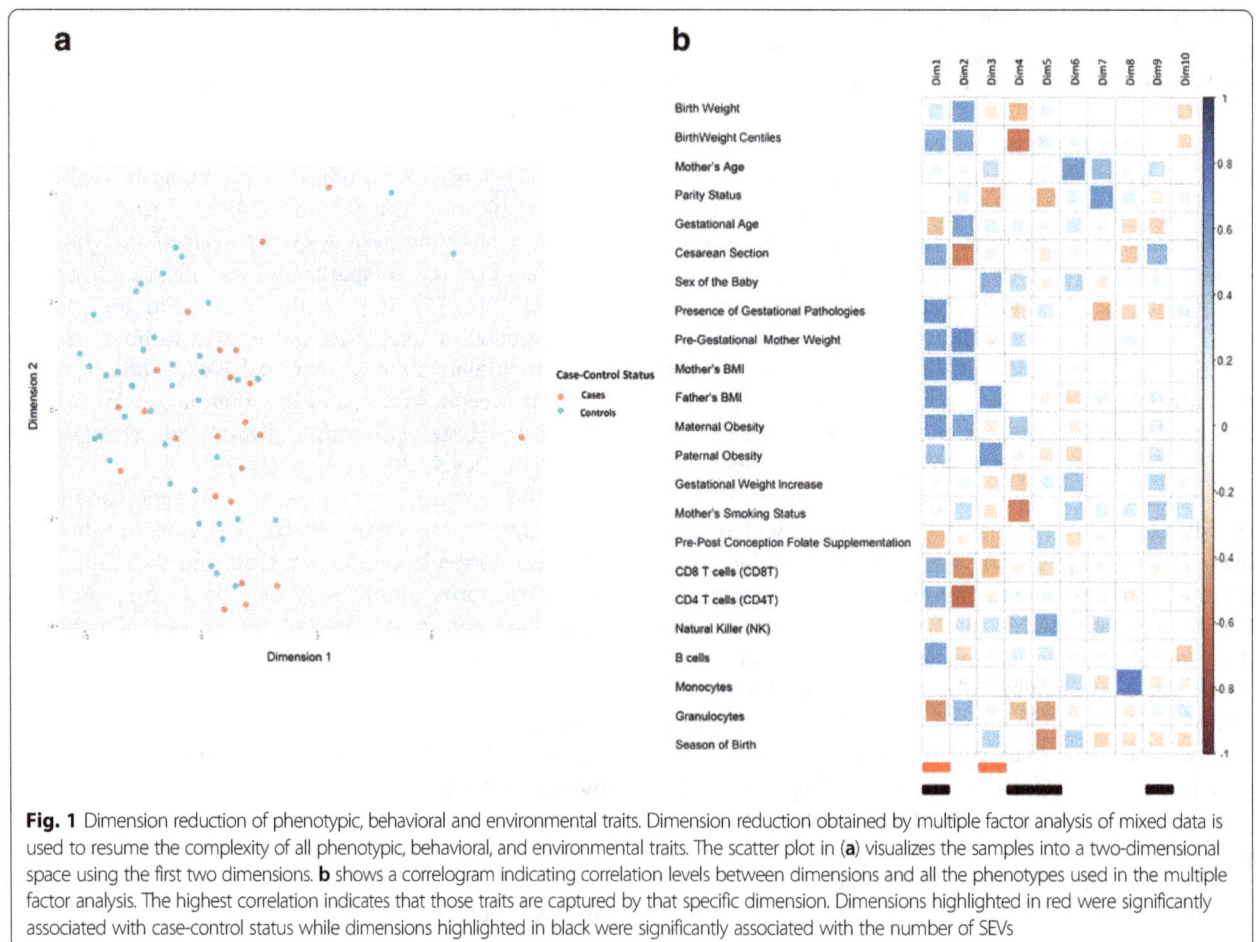

Fig. 1 Dimension reduction of phenotypic, behavioral and environmental traits. Dimension reduction obtained by multiple factor analysis of mixed data is used to resume the complexity of all phenotypic, behavioral, and environmental traits. The scatter plot in (**a**) visualizes the samples into a two-dimensional space using the first two dimensions. **b** shows a correlogram indicating correlation levels between dimensions and all the phenotypes used in the multiple factor analysis. The highest correlation indicates that those traits are captured by that specific dimension. Dimensions highlighted in red were significantly associated with case-control status while dimensions highlighted in black were significantly associated with the number of SEVs

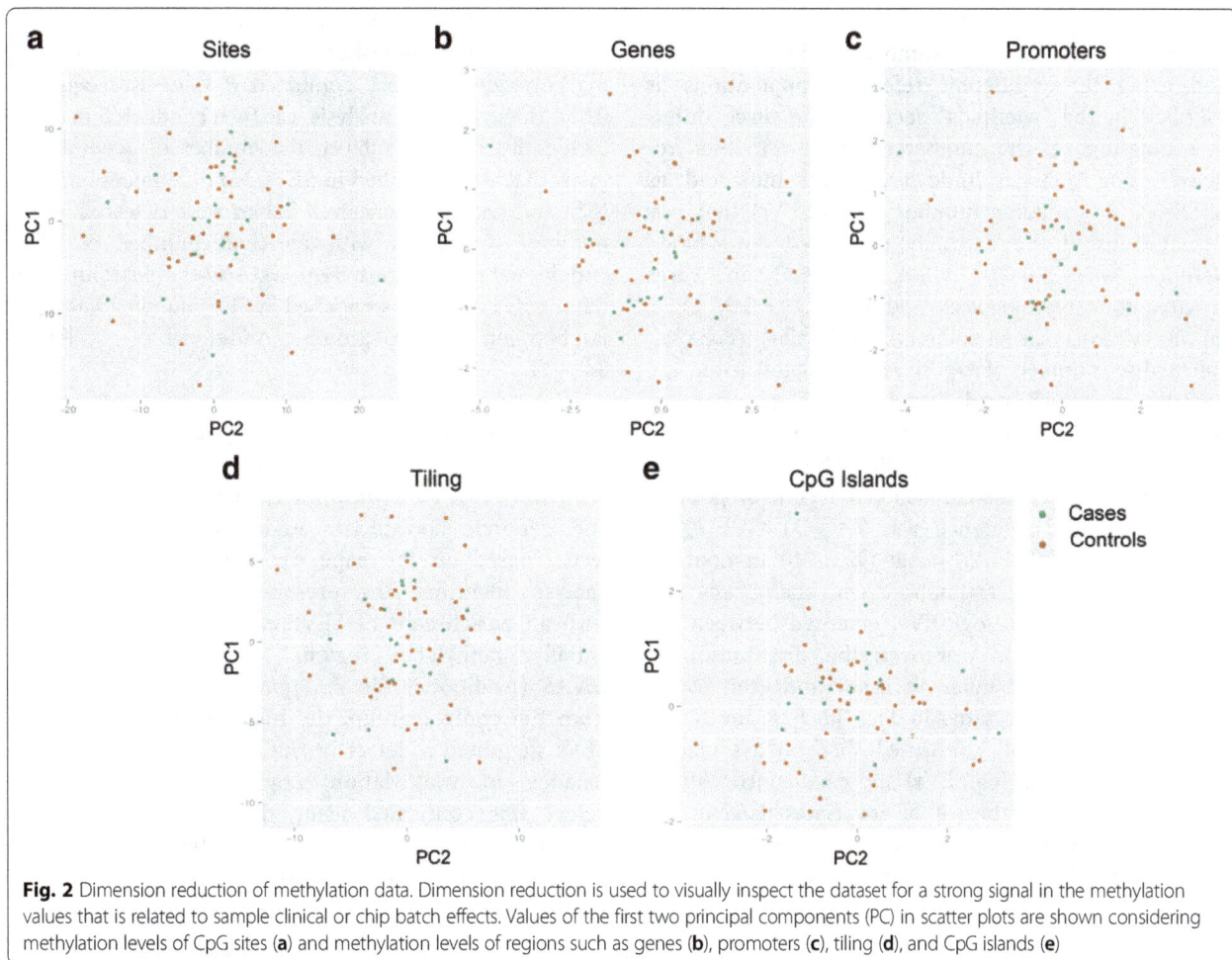

Fig. 2 Dimension reduction of methylation data. Dimension reduction is used to visually inspect the dataset for a strong signal in the methylation values that is related to sample clinical or chip batch effects. Values of the first two principal components (PC) in scatter plots are shown considering methylation levels of CpG sites (**a**) and methylation levels of regions such as genes (**b**), promoters (**c**), tiling (**d**), and CpG islands (**e**)

associated with the case-control status, and the chip batch were used as covariates to adjust the differential methylation analysis. Moreover, surrogate variables analysis (SVA) was applied in order to correct for potential unmeasured or unmodeled confounders. At site level, no statistical differences in methylation between cases and controls with a genome-wide approach ($p < 10^{-7}$) emerged. A list of the top 50 ranked probes as differently methylated is reported in Additional file 2: Table S1. Differential methylation analysis performed at regional level was conducted considering the CpG islands, promoters, genes, and tiling. After multiple testing correction, no statistical differences in region methylation levels emerged between cases and controls. QQ plots showing the level of inflation factor for adjusted and not adjusted analyses are reported in Additional file 3: Figure S2.

Comparative analysis of differences in methylation status with previous EWAS

The differential methylation analysis is based on the assumption that differences in methylation status are shared among subjects. We have thus evaluated the consensus among previous EWAS reporting differentially methylated genes in the cord blood between in vivo- and in vitro-conceived babies. The results presented with the Venn diagram in Additional file 4: Figure S3 showed a lack of consistency among the studies, with only 6 out of 214 genes found to be differentially methylated in at least two different studies (*NAP1L5*, *L3MBTL*, *GNAS*, *PEG10*, *PRCP*, and *RUNX3*). Importantly, none of these genes were differentially methylated between cases and controls in the present study, despite considering both adjusted and unadjusted p values in the regional analysis conducted for genes and promoters. Considering all the 214 genes reported in the literature, only *RNF185* [10] was found in our study to include one of the top 50 ranked probes reported in Additional file 2: Table S1. However, no enrichment of differentially methylated probes was observed for the gene *RNF185* in our population, with only a single probe out of eight associated with the gene resulting to be nominally significant. Additionally, no differences were detected in the regional analysis for genes and promoters (unadjusted p values: 0.09 and 0.19 for gene and promoter, respectively).

Stochastic epigenetic variations analysis

For each subject, the total number of SEVs was calculated using three different reference populations as described in the "Methods" section. The three different estimations of the number of SEVs were then reported using a logarithmic scale and indicated as log(SEVs). The median number of log(SEVs) that was calculated using the naturally conceived cord blood reference was 5.9 (Q1 = 5.8; Q2 = 6.6) in cases (in vitro-conceived babies) and 6.0 (Q1 = 5.9; Q2 = 6.3) in controls (in vivo-conceived babies) (Fig. 3a). The median number of log(SEVs) calculated using the naturally conceived cord blood GEO data reference was 7.5 (Q1 = 7.3; Q2 = 7.7) in cases and 7.4 (Q1 = 7.2; Q2 = 7.6) in controls (Fig. 3b). The median number of log(SEVs) calculated using the general population whole blood reference was 7.4 (Q1 = 7.2; Q2 = 7.6) in cases and 7.4 (Q1 = 7.2; Q2 = 7.6) in controls (Fig. 3c). For all the estimations, no statistically significant differences in log(SEVs) emerged between the two groups analyzed. Moreover, the distribution of log(SEVs) was very similar in cases and controls as shown in the densitograms in Fig. 3d–f. A multivariate logistic regression confirmed that no association was present between log(SEVs) and case-control status after adjustment for the set of covariates used in the differential methylation analysis. Three different regression models were performed according to the three estimations of SEVs, and the results were finally combined using the Fisher's method. After multiple testing correction, Fisher's combined P value was equal to 0.38. An enrichment analysis was then conducted in order to identify, in each subject, the number of genomic regions that were enriched in SEVs. No differences between ICSI and naturally conceived babies were detected in the number of regions with enriched number of SEVs (Additional file 5: Figure S4A–C). Also the distribution of the number of regions enriched in SEVs number was similar between the two groups. (Additional file 5: Figure S4D–F).

Stochastic epigenetic variations and imprinting defects

We have also checked for the presence of regions enriched in SEVs in imprinted loci. The list of genes and genomic coordinates under imprinting was selected based on the paper by Court et al. [20]. The analysis identified the presence of a single subject with an enrichment of SEVs located at several differentially methylated regions (DMRs) in the locus *GNAS* (Additional file 6: Figure S5). In this subject from the control group, the high number of reported SEVs suggested a defect in the establishment or maintenance of methylation imprints. The epigenetic defect was confirmed using the methylation-specific multiplex ligation-dependent probe amplification (MS-MLPA) (data not shown).

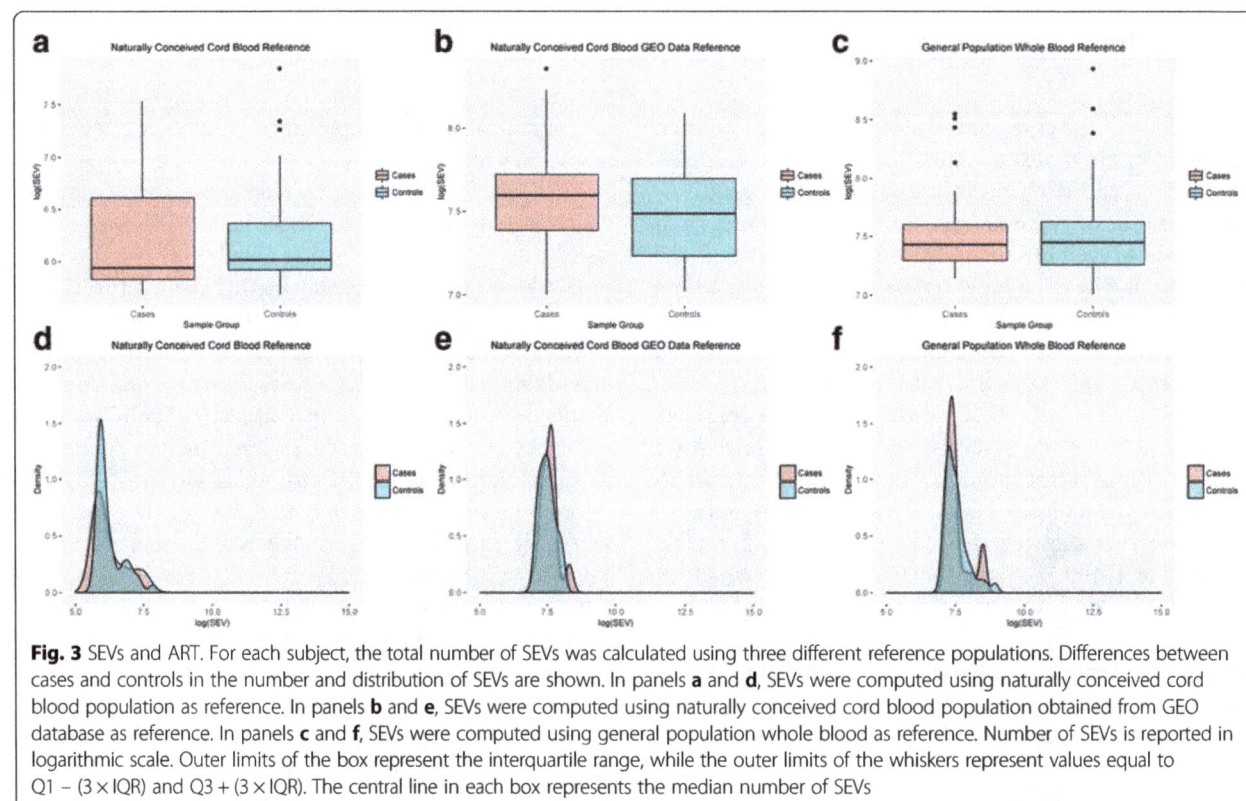

Fig. 3 SEVs and ART. For each subject, the total number of SEVs was calculated using three different reference populations. Differences between cases and controls in the number and distribution of SEVs are shown. In panels **a** and **d**, SEVs were computed using naturally conceived cord blood population as reference. In panels **b** and **e**, SEVs were computed using naturally conceived cord blood population obtained from GEO database as reference. In panels **c** and **f**, SEVs were computed using general population whole blood as reference. Number of SEVs is reported in logarithmic scale. Outer limits of the box represent the interquartile range, while the outer limits of the whiskers represent values equal to Q1 − (3 × IQR) and Q3 + (3 × IQR). The central line in each box represents the median number of SEVs

Stochastic epigenetic variations association analysis with phenotypic, behavioral, and environmental traits

A multivariate regression analysis was performed in order to identify phenotypic traits potentially associated with SEVs. Three different regression models were performed according to the three estimations of SEVs and the results were finally combined using Fisher's method. Each multivariate regression model was created considering the logarithmic number of SEVs as dependent variable and the first 10 dimensions obtained from the phenotypic multiple factor analysis as independent variables. Results were adjusted considering the chip batch effect. The multivariate regression showed that the Dim 1, Dim 4, Dim 5, and Dim 9 were strongly associated with the number of SEVs. After multiple testing correction, Fisher's combined p values were $p = 4.0 \times 10^{-4}$, $p = 4.0 \times 10^{-4}$, $p = 1.3 \times 10^{-3}$, and $p = 5.0 \times 10^{-4}$, respectively. The phenotypic traits captured by those dimensions are shown in the correlogram in Fig. 1b. Birthweight centiles, gestational age, cesarean section, presence of adverse pregnancy outcomes, pre-gestational mother's weight, parents' BMI and obesity, and cord blood cells composition (CD8T, CD4T, and B Cells) were significantly correlated to Dim 1 ($p < 0.01$, $\rho > | 0.5 |$). Birthweight centiles, mother's smoking status were significantly correlated to Dim 4 ($p < 0.01$, $\rho > | 0.5 |$), cord blood cells composition (NK cells) and season of birth were significantly correlated to Dim 5 ($p < 0.01$, $\rho > | 0.5 |$) while Dim 9 captured mainly cesarean section and pre- or post-conception folates supplementation ($p < 0.01$, $\rho > | 0.4 |$). The four most significant traits observed to be correlated with SEVs (pre or post conception folates supplementation, cesarean section, mother's obesity status and season of birth) are shown in Additional file 7: Figure S6. The number of SEVs reported has been obtained using the naturally conceived cord blood reference.

Discussion

We report the most comprehensive multifactorial analysis of cord blood DNA methylation of in vitro conceived babies and the first analysis of the stochastic variations potentially induced by ART techniques. Although the use of ART has allowed millions of otherwise infertile couples to conceive children, some concern still remains about the safety of these procedures [2, 21]. An increase in imprinting disorders has been found in children conceived through IVF and ICSI, but no evidence of generalized changes in DNA methylation could be appreciated [2]. Our results are in line with this observation based on two different approaches: (i) a conventional epigenome-wide association analysis. At both site and region levels, no differences in methylation status between naturally and in vitro conceived emerged

as statistically significant; (ii) a previously published method aimed at investigating the number and the localization of stochastic epigenetic variations [12, 22].

Although several studies have tried to investigate the methylation status of ART-conceived babies, only four EWAS were previously conducted on this topic. Melamed et al. have evaluated 27,578 CpG sites in cord blood from 10 children conceived in vitro and 8 conceived in vivo [10]. Castillo-Fernandez et al. investigated the links between IVF and DNA methylation patterns in 47 IVF and 60 non-IVF newborn twins (from 54 twin pairs) in whole cord blood cells and cord blood mononuclear cells using genome-wide methylated DNA immunoprecipitation coupled with deep sequencing [13]. Estill et al. reported the methylation profiles of neonatal blood spots of 137 babies conceived naturally or with four different ART techniques [14]. Finally, El Hajj N et al. evaluated the methylome of 48 babies conceived with ICSI [15]. Both Estill et al. and El Hajj N et al. used the Infinium HumanMethylation450 BeadChips to analyze the methylation levels [14, 15]. Notwithstanding the lack of an adequate correction for crucial confounding factors, only a small number of CpG sites was differentially methylated at a genome-wide level and the magnitude of differences identified was also extremely small [10, 13–15]. Furthermore, when considering all the studies together, we observed a substantial inconsistence among their results. Only six genes have been confirmed in at least two studies (*NAP1L5, L3MBTL, GNAS, PEG10, PRCP,* and *RUNX3*).

Interestingly, a review of literature concerning those genes revealed that they are already known to be epigenetically associated with other pregnancy conditions. *NAP1L5*, for example, has been previously identified to be differently methylated in cord blood samples characterized by intrauterine exposure to gestational diabetes mellitus [23]. *L3MBTL* has been reported to be differently methylated in cord blood of babies exposed to smoking during pregnancy [24] and is epigenetically associated with gestational age [25]. Increased methylation at differentially methylated regions of *GNAS* has been described in infants born in conditions of gestational diabetes [26]. An increase in DNA methylation at the *SGCE/PEG10* DMR has been previously positively associated with paternal BMI [27], maternal stress [28], and also with maternal prenatal physical activity [29]. Methylation of *PRCP* gene in newborns [30] as well as *RUNX3* [24] was found to be significantly associated with maternal smoking status. Hypermethylation of *RUNX3* CpG sites has been also associated with decreased gestational age [24]. Taken together, this evidence hints at the presence of confounding factors in previously reported results on epigenetics of ART. This observation seems to be supported by analysis of the

QQ-plot obtained from unadjusted analysis presented herein. The elevated genomic inflation factor (lambda = 1.7; Additional file 3: Figure S2) observed in unadjusted analysis sheds light on the excess of false positive rate potentially produced under inadequate correction. The influence of confounding factors on epigenome of cord blood has been extensively described. Soubry et al., for example, demonstrated a significant association between parental BMI and DNA methylation of imprinted genes [29]. This finding should be considered as relevant since a significant effect of ART has been reported to affect imprinted loci [15].

An increased variability of DNA methylation in IVF conceived babies was previously underlined, hinting at the presence of epigenetic changes not shared among subjects [10] and thus supporting the idea that the effect of ART might be more likely to be stochastic rather than confined to some genetic regions. Our novel analytical approach addressing the number of stochastic epigenetic variations [12, 22] showed no differences in cord blood from in vitro and in vivo conceived babies.

The analysis of SEVs proposed in the present study proved to be a powerful approach to study the epigenetic variability and allowed to study the impact of several conditions on the newborn epigenome. Interestingly, four dimensions obtained from the dimensional reduction of phenotypic traits were significantly associated with the number of SEVs. Cord blood cell composition, pre or post conception supplementation of folates, birth percentiles, gestational age, cesarean section, pre-gestational mother's weight, parental BMI and obesity, presence of adverse pregnancy outcomes, mother's smoking status, and season of birth were the traits mainly captured by these dimensions. Some of these factors such as parental BMI, gestational age, birth weight, and smoking are already known for playing a role on the newborn epigenome [20, 25, 27–29, 31]. Of note, we observed and reported for the first time the existence of an epigenetic signature associated with season of birth. The number of stochastic epigenetic variations was lower in subjects born in autumn. This observation should be considered important for at least two reasons: (i) seasonality of birth has already been reported to be associated with an increased incidence of several pathological conditions such as type I diabetes [32, 33], cardiovascular disease [34], skin cancer [35], and autoimmune diseases [36]. Moreover, seasonality of birth has been also studied in the field of aging and is associated with life expectancy [37–40]; (ii) the magnitude of the effect of seasonality, a natural event, on epigenome of newborns appeared to be greater compared to the one induced by ART.

We have also evaluated the presence of SEVs in imprinted loci failing to find significant differences between cases and controls. A single epigenetic alteration

in the locus GNAS was found in a control subject. It is important to note that the new method applied in this study allowed not only to evaluate the number of SEVs located across the whole genome, but also succeeded in the identification of a single epigenetic alteration subsequently confirmed using MS-MLPA and not shared among subjects. A standard case-control analysis would have failed to identify this particular defect. To our knowledge, this is the first study addressing a genome-wide analysis of imprinted loci taking into account the probable random effect of ART and applying a test that does not require the possible epigenetic variation to be present in more than one subject. In any case, we realize that these phenomena do represent rare events, and we probably need a greater sample size to completely exclude a direct effect at the level of specific imprinting genes.

The present work has clarified that the number of stochastic epigenetic variations potentially induced by ART technology was, at worst, comparable to that naturally produced in response to maternal behavior or other common environmental factors, thus debunking the idea of a severe impact of ART in the epigenome of the newborns and implying a reconsideration of the epigenetic safety of these techniques.

Another crucial aspect of the present work is the analysis of all the potential confounders that could affect the methylation status in the newborn cord blood. It is totally unexpected that previous studies on the same topic evaluating genome wide DNA methylation [10, 13–15] failed to correct for factors potentially affecting methylation status or considered only a small number of them. Therefore, given the complexity of the networks and of the phenotypic traits involved in pregnancy establishment, the causal relationship between the epigenetic status and ART needs to be evaluated with caution and controlling for potential confounders. The complexity of the phenotypic traits represents also another important issue; the correlation analysis performed among phenotypic traits revealed the existence of several hidden associations among variables, and this needs to be considered when adjusting for confounders in order to avoid multicollinearity.

Another aspect that is often disregarded is the potential role of ART techniques on placenta methylation status and the consequent effect on birth weight and on the epigenome of newborns. Recent studies conducted in animal models reported that ART has a predominant or exclusive effect on the placenta methylation status compared to that on the fetus [9, 41, 42]. An attractive hypothesis that comes from these data is that the higher incidence of premature birth and low birth weight observed in

ART-conceived children may be related to abnormal placental function resulting from genomic imprinting errors at multiple genes. Recently, Ghosh et al. reported evidence of placental methylation altered by ART procedures at repeated sequences (LINE1 elements) and CCGG sites [43]. Similarly, Choux et al. reported lower DNA methylation for two imprinted loci (*H19/IGF2* and *KCNQ1OT1* DMRs) and two transposon families (LINE-1Hs and ERVFRD-1) in the placenta of babies conceived by ART [44]. Interestingly, DNA methylation of the same imprinted genes DMRs and transposable elements in cord blood was not altered by ART procedures, thus confirming the main effect at the placental level as seen in animal experiments. A whole genome analysis of the methylation status of placenta samples from babies conceived by ART is needed in order to elucidate this crucial aspect.

A number of limitations need to be considered when interpreting our results. First, only DNA from cord blood was analyzed. Since cord blood is not necessarily representative of the epigenetic status of all tissues and cells in the newborn, additional studies on other tissues are mandatory to confirm these data. Second, the phenotypic data of the studied subjects did not include all the possible variables related to pregnancy and labor although a surrogate variables analysis was conducted to compensate for this deficiency. Third, although the number of subjects used for comparisons is of the same order of magnitude of previously conducted EWAS, we must underline that a larger sample size could better estimate normal ranges of DNA methylation in each locus. Confirming our results on a larger sample size would allow to exclude the possibility that small methylation differences have gone undetected. Fourth, these findings represent the experience relative to the ICSI procedure of a single IVF center and a single lab. Although we selected only ICSI procedures in order to analyze a homogeneous group of babies obtained using the more invasive technique, we cannot exclude that procedures done in different ways and with different technologies could result in different data. Moreover, it should be considered that when comparing naturally conceived and in vitro-conceived babies, there is a consistent number of inescapable differences between the two groups such as parents' infertility status that may represent an important selection bias. Finally, although the Infinium HumanMethylation450 BeadChips covers 99% of RefSeq genes, permitting a whole-genome analysis, the coverage of total CpG sites is low (around 2%). This means that sequencing-based methods should be adopted in the future in order to study other genomic features (e.g., enhancers) that have only small coverage in the present analysis.

Conclusions

The presented prospective study does not support that children born after ART have an increased risk of genome-wide changes in DNA methylation neither at specific loci neither randomly scattered throughout the genome. On the other hand, the study confirms that there are several environmental and behavioral conditions able to affect epigenetic variability in cord blood and leads to the conclusion that they need to be considered as potential confounders in investigations of this nature.

A reanalysis of previous data based on phenotypic traits of the parents and the babies potentially associated with epigenetic changes is warranted as well as a meta-analysis including all the data from genome-wide studies.

Methods
Study design and study population

This is a prospective study designed to avoid biases related to the improper selection of complicated pregnancies in one of the two groups. Women that underwent ICSI treatment were enrolled in the study at 20 weeks' gestation. These women were stimulated with standard ovulation induction drugs. Pregnant women who naturally conceived were also enrolled at 20 weeks' of gestation. The in vivo group had no history of infertility, and the index pregnancy was achieved without medications or treatments. None of the pregnancy ended in abortion, and all the patients were included in the study. Samples of cord blood from both ART-conceived pregnancies ($n = 23$) and naturally conceived pregnancies ($n = 41$) were obtained at the time of delivery by the midwives of the San Raffaele Hospital, Milano, Italy, by puncturing the umbilical vein while the placenta was in utero [45]. Patients were informed that cord blood would be used for research purposes and gave written consent. Approval for this study was granted by the local Human Institutional Investigation Committee (#PMAMET). Clinical information obtained for each pregnancy included demographic and obstetric factors, cause of infertility, details of the ART procedure as well as pregnancy, delivery, and neonatal outcomes. Multifetal gestations were excluded from both groups.

Sample size was calculated based on the analysis of parameters observed in a previous study in which more than 400 subjects were evaluated [12]. Mean and variance were estimated for all the CpG sites of the Infinium HumanMethylation 450 BeadChip array. The number of subjects to be enrolled has been calculated assuming an effect size taking into account a difference in the percentage of methylation between groups of at least 10%, by imposing a probability of type I error in the order of 10^{-7} (level of significance that takes into account the need to correct for multiple testing) and a power of 95%. A description of the study design is shown in Additional file 8: Figure S7.

In vitro fertilization procedures

Controlled ovarian stimulation was performed according to the clinical practice and as previously described [46–48]. Oocyte collection was performed 36 h after triggering of ovulation. After 2–3 h incubation in Human Serum Albumin (HSA)-supplemented Fertilization medium (Sage In-Vitro Fertilization, Inc. Trumbull, CT, USA) under oil, denudation of the cumulus oophorus was performed as previously described [46, 49, 50]. Injected oocytes were grouped-cultured in microdrops of equilibrated Serum Substitute Supplement (SSS, Irvine, CA, USA)-supplemented Cleavage medium (Sage In-Vitro Fertilization, Inc. Trumbull, CT, USA) under oil. Sixteen to 18 h after ICSI, all oocytes were checked for fertilization as previously described [46, 49, 50]. For a subgroup of patients ($n = 7$, 30.4%), embryos were cultured to blastocyst stage in SSS (Irvine, CA, USA)-supplemented Blastocyst medium (Sage In-Vitro Fertilization, Inc. Trumbull, CT, USA). All the incubation steps were conducted using low (5%) oxygen concentration incubators [49]. All the transfers were performed in fresh cycles [48]. All the patients underwent luteal phase support with progesterone 600 mg/d (Prometrium) administered vaginally and continued through week 12 of pregnancy.

DNA extraction and bisulphite treatment of the DNA

Genomic DNA was extracted from cord blood using the Wizard genomic DNA purification kit (PROMEGA, Madison WI, USA) as previously described [12]. Quality control and quantification of DNA were performed before and after bisulphite conversion. DNA was quantified with NanoDrop (NanoDrop Products Thermo Scientific, Wilmington, DE, USA) and quality was assessed by visualization of genomic DNA on 1% agarose gel electrophoresis. Only DNA samples not fragmented and with a concentration higher than 50 ng/µl were subsequently processed.

DNA methylation assay

4 µl of bisulfite-converted DNA was used for hybridization on Infinium HumanMethylation 450 BeadChip, following the Illumina Infinium HD Methylation protocol. This consists of a whole genome amplification step followed by enzymatic end-point fragmentation, precipitation, and resuspension. The resuspended samples were hybridized on HumanMethylation 450 BeadChips at 48 °C for 16 h. Then, unhybridized and non-specifically hybridized DNA were washed away followed by a single nucleotide extension using the hybridized bisulfite-treated DNA as a template. The nucleotides incorporated were labeled with biotin (ddCTP and ddGTP) and 2,4-dinitrophenol (DNP) (ddATP and ddTTP). After the single base extension, repeated rounds of staining were performed with a combination of antibodies that differentiate DNP and biotin by fixing them different fluorophores. Finally, the BeadChip was washed and protected in order to scan it. The Illumina HiScan SQ scanner is a two-color laser (532 nm/660 nm) fluorescent scanner with a 0.375 µm spatial resolution capable of exciting the fluorophores generated during the staining step of the protocol. Image intensities were extracted using GenomeStudio (2010.3). The methylation score for each CpG site was represented as β values according to the fluorescent intensity ratio between methylated and unmethylated probes. β values may range between 0 (unmethylated) and 1 (completely methylated).

Data management, pre-processing, normalization, and quality control

Illumina Methylation 450K raw data were analyzed using the RnBeads analysis software package [51]. Sites with overlapping SNPs were firstly removed from the analysis ($n = 4713$) as well as probes on sex chromosomes ($n = 11119$). Possible removal of probes and samples of highest impurity from the dataset was evaluated using the Greedycut algorithm. We considered every β value to be unreliable when its corresponding detection p value was not below the threshold ($T = 0.05$). In order to avoid an erroneous interpretation of stochastic epigenetic variations, probes with coordinates overlapping rare genetic variants annotated in 1000 genomes and EXAC databases were removed [52, 53]. After the quality control step, none of the samples was excluded for quality reasons while a total of 14208 probes were removed. The background was subtracted using the methylumi package (method "noob") [51]. The signal intensity values were normalized using the SWAN normalization method, as implemented in the minfi package. In addition to CpG sites, four sets of genomic regions were covered in the analysis (tiling, genes, promoters and CpG Islands).

Blood cell type counts

Proportions of CD8 T cells, CD4 T cells, NK cells, B cells, monocytes, and granulocytes were estimated using the "estimateCellCounts" function in the Bioconductor minfi package [54] with the reference data for cord blood provided by Bakulski et al. [55].

Differential methylation analysis

Differential methylation analysis was conducted both at site and region level according to the sample groups. p values were computed using the limma method for the site level analysis while a combined p value was calculated from all site p values for the region-based [51]. Regions were defined according to RnBeads definitions [51]:

- Genes and promoters: Ensembl [56] gene definitions were downloaded using the biomaRt package. A promoter was defined as the region spanning 1500 bases upstream and 500 bases downstream of the transcription start site of the corresponding gene.
- GpG islands: the CpG island track was downloaded from the dedicated FTP directory of the UCSC Genome Browser [57].
- Tiling regions: not overlapping tiling regions with a window size of 5 kb were defined over the whole genome.

In order to avoid potentially confounding factors, a multiple factor analysis (MFA) was performed based on phenotypic data (birth weight, birthweight centiles, mother's age, parity status, gestational age, cesarean section, sex of the baby, presence of adverse pregnancy outcomes, pre-gestational mother weight, parents' BMI and obesity status, gestational weight increase, smoking status, pre-post conception folate supplementation, CD8T, CD4T, NK cells, B cells, monocytes, granulocytes, season of birth). Variables were entered in the analysis as factorial or linear values. Chip batch and dimensions that were significantly associated with the case-control status were used as covariates in the differential methylation analysis. Adjustment for surrogate variables was conducted using the function directly provided in the package RnBeads, which can detect batch effects and other unwanted variation of unknown origin and annotate them in such a way that they can be controlled for as covariates [51].

Epigenetic variations detection

In order to identify stochastic epigenetic variations (SEVs), we used a method previously described by our group [12, 22]. Briefly, after the pre-processing step, the distribution and variability of methylation levels were studied in the populations for all the probes of the array using box and whiskers plots. At each CpG site, the methylation level of a subject that was extremely different from the rest of the population was counted as an epigenetic variation. Thus, for each locus, epigenetic variations were identified as the extreme outliers, with their methylation level that lied outside of $Q1 - (3 \times IQR)$ and $Q3 + (3 \times IQR)$. Finally, all the observed epigenetic variations were annotated in a new data matrix that allowed to calculate, for each subject, the total amount of epigenetic variations and their genomic position. The box and whiskers plot analysis was conducted using boxplot function in the R car package and confirmed using the outlier function in the R outliers package.

In addition to the previously described control population composed by 41 natural conceived babies, two other different reference populations have been used for this analysis:

1) Methylation row data from 60 subjects were obtained from the public functional genomics data repository GEO. We have selected two different datasets containing methylation data from cord blood samples (GSE54399, GSE30870), and we have extracted only methylation data from control subjects. This population (naturally conceived cord blood GEO data reference) represented our "external" control population. GEO and in house raw data were pre-processed following the same procedure.

2) Methylation row data from 350 healthy subjects with an age spanning from 1 to 107 years were also obtained from the Istituto Auxologico Italiano Epigenetic Database. This population represented a second reference population used for the estimation of epigenetic variations (general population whole blood reference).

A schematic description of the strategy used to obtain different estimations of the number of SEVs by using the various reference populations is shown is Additional file 9: Figure S8.

Briefly:

- In the first step, the analysis described above was applied on naturally conceived cord blood population. Samples were analyzed together, and the number of SEVs was calculated in each control subject.
- In a second step, all the samples in the case group were tested individually using the naturally conceived cord blood reference and the number of SEVs was calculated for each case subject.
- In the third step, the naturally conceived cord blood GEO data reference was used to calculate the number of SEVs both in cases and control subjects. Also in this step, each subject was tested individually.
- Finally, the general population whole blood reference was used to calculate the number of SEVs both in control and case subjects. Also in this step, each subject was tested individually.

Using three different reference populations, three different estimations of the number of SEVs were calculated for each subject. A test for over-representation of these probes was conducted, for each subject, using sliding windows and the hypergeometric cumulative function, obtaining the number of genomic regions that were enriched in SEVs [12].

Validation of the SEVs analysis

In order to confirm the power of this analytical approach to detect epigenetic variations, two separate tests were performed on positive controls. Three samples were analyzed in duplicates, and epigenetic variations found in each of them were compared. Results showed a mean correlation of 0.99 ($p < 0.01$) among the experiments. The duplicate samples underwent independent bisulfite conversion reactions, and this suggests that epigenetic variations are not significantly influenced by bisulfite conversion errors. In the second validation step, 48 whole blood DNA samples obtained from subjects affected by imprinting diseases (Beckwith-Wiedemann syndrome, Angelman syndrome and Silver Russel syndrome) who underwent diagnostic assays at Istituto Auxologico Italiano were analyzed. For these subjects, a medical report indicating the genomic position of their epigenetic alteration was already available. Briefly, after the identification of the outlier probes, a test for over-representation of these probes inside each gene was performed using the hypergeometric cumulative function. The analysis identified genes with enriched number of outliers probes (Bonferroni's corrected p value < 0.05) confirming the presence of the epigenetic alterations previously reported in the medical report.

Statistical tests

The "Shapiro.test" function provided in the R package "stats" was applied to test normality among variables. The "Wilcox.test" function provided in the R package "class" was used to test differences between cases and controls groups for all non-parametric data. Considering the presence of categorical variables, dimensional reduction was performed using the multiple factor analysis of mixed data approach and the "FAMD" function provided in the R package "FactoMineR." The univariate and multivariate linear regressions were conducted using the "Generalised Linear Model" function provided in the R "base" package. Bonferroni's correction was performed to correct for multiple testing. Correlation analysis between Dims and environmental and behavioral conditions has been performed using the hector function provided in the package "polycor."

Comparative analysis with previous EWAS

We conducted a systematic search of the literature focusing on studies that used a genome-wide approach (Illumina Infinium HumanMethylation27 BeadChip and Illumina Infinium Human Methylation 450K BeadChip) with the aim to compare cord blood methylation levels between in vitro and in vivo conceived babies. The four selected studies [10, 13–15] reported differentially methylated genes using different parameters for the selection.

Melamed et al. identifies genes that had at least two significantly differentially methylated CpG sites and genes with at least a CpG site showing a significant methylation difference ≥ 10% between ART and control groups [10]. A total of 33 genes were found. Estill et al. considered as significant all those genes with a minimum absolute average methylation change of 2.5% for the clusters of CpGs that were associated with a given gene (at least 75% of the cluster intersecting a gene body or promoter), with only the significant clusters that were considered in the average count [14]. The study reported a list of differentially methylated metastable epialleles, imprinted genes, and genes related to differentially methylated enhancers. A total of 87 genes as having significantly different methylation status emerged when comparing babies born with various ART techniques and naturally conceived. Castillo-Fernandez et al. reported a list of all the genes located near each differentially methylated CpGs between the two groups selected using a false discovery rate equal to 25% [13]. A total of 66 genes were found to be associated with the 46 reported differentially methylated regions. Finally, El Hajj et al. reported a list of 34 genes with a methylation difference of $\beta > \pm 0.03$ and an adjusted $p < 0.05$ observed in promoters, imprinting control regions and CpG islands [15].

Additional files

Additional file 1: Figure S1. Correlation analysis among phenotypic, behavioral and environmental features considered in the study. Degree and direction of correlations are highlighted by the color and dimension of squares. (TIF 307 kb)

Additional file 2: Table S1. Top 50 ranked hypomethylated or hypermethylated probes in babies born after ICSI. (XLS 41 kb)

Additional file 3: Figure S2. QQ plots obtained using (A) Dim1 and Dim3 resulted from the multiple factor analysis of mixed data. (B) Surrogate variable analysis (SVA), and Dim1 and Dim3 obtained from the multiple factor analysis of mixed data as covariates in the differential methylation analysis. The QQ plot obtained without data correction is illustrated in C. The elevated genomic inflation factor of unadjusted data suggests presence of potential confounders. (TIF 141 kb)

Additional file 4: Figure S3. Venn diagram illustrating the number of genes found in literature to be differentially methylated in cord blood of ART babies when compared to natural conceived babies and the overlapping of results among previous EWAS [10, 13–15]. (TIF 234 kb)

Additional file 5: Figure S4. For each subject, the total number of region enriched in SEVs was calculated using three different reference populations. Differences between cases and controls in the number and distribution of region enriched in SEVs are shown. In panels A and D, SEVs were computed using naturally conceived cord blood population as reference. In panels B and E, SEVs were computed using naturally conceived cord blood population obtained from GEO database as reference. In panels C and F, SEVs were computed using general population whole blood as reference. Number of region enriched in SEVs is reported in logarithmic scale. Outer limits of the box represent the interquartile range, while the outer limits of the whiskers represent values equal to Q1 − (3 × IQR) and Q3 + (3 × IQR). The central line in each box represents the median number of SEVs. (TIF 181 kb)

Additional file 6: Figure S5. Genomic regions under imprinting control carrying an epigenetic alteration in a control subject. In panel A, stochastic epigenetic variations (SEVs) detected in the cord blood of a single subject from the control population are represented in red while the differentially methylated regions (DMRs) reported by Court et al. [18] are represented in blue. The high number of reported SEVs suggested a defect in the establishment or maintenance of methylation imprints confirmed using MS-MLPA. Panel B illustrates the magnification of one of the DMRs. (TIF 1062 kb)

Additional file 7: Figure S6. Effect of folates supplementation, mother's obesity status, cesarean section, and season of birth on number of SEVs. Number of SEVs is reported in logarithmic scale. Outer limits of the box represent the interquartile range, while the outer limits of the whiskers represent values equal to Q1 − (3 × IQR) and Q3 + (3 × IQR). The central line in each box represents the median number of SEVs. (TIF 107 kb)

Additional file 8: Figure S7. Schematic representation of the study design. (TIF 1116 kb)

Additional file 9: Figure S8. Schematic description of the strategy used to estimate the number of SEVs. (TIF 982 kb)

Abbreviation

ART: Assisted reproduction technology; BMI: Body mass index; Dim: Dimension; DMR: Differentially methylated region; EWAS: Epigenome wide association study; ICSI: Intra citoplasmatic sperm injection; IVF: in vitro fertilization; NGS: Next generation sequencing; SEV: Stochastic epigenetic variation; SVA: Surrogate variable analysis

Authors' contributions

DG, ES, PG, LB, EP, MC, AMDB, and PV planned and implemented the study. LP and ER collected the data. DG does the statistical analyses. DG and PV wrote the first draft of the manuscript. All authors participated to the discussion of the findings and revised the manuscript. All authors read and approved the final manuscript.

Competing interests

Dr. Davide Gentilini, Dr. Luca Pagliardini, Dr. Elisa Rabellotti, Dr. Paolo Garagnani, Prof. Luisa Bernardinelli, Dr. Anna Maria Di Blasio, and Dr. Paola Vigano' declare no COIs in relation to the work described. Prof. Edgardo Somigliana declares no personal COIs. His institution received grants for research from Ferring, Merck Serono, and IBSA. Dr. Enrico Papaleo reports consultancies with MSD, Merck-Serono, Ferring, and IBSA Institut Biochimique SA; grants for institutional research from MSD, Merck-Serono, Ferring, and IBSA Institut Biochimique SA; honoraria from MSD, Merck-Serono; and travel expenses paid by MSD, Merck-Serono, Ferring, and IBSA Institut Biochimique SA. Prof. Candiani Massimo reports grants for institutional research from Merck-Serono, Astella Pharma, Roche Diagnostics, MSD Italia, Ferring.

Author details
[1]Istituto Auxologico Italiano IRCCS, 20095 Cusano Milanino, Italy. [2]Infertility Unit, Fondazione Ca' Granda, Ospedale Maggiore Policlinico, 20122 Milan, Italy. [3]Reproductive Sciences Laboratory, Division of Genetics and Cell Biology, IRCCS Ospedale San Raffaele, Via Olgettina 58, 20132 Milan, Italy. [4]Department of Experimental, Diagnostic and Specialty Medicine, University of Bologna, 40138 Bologna, Italy. [5]Department of Brain and Behavioral Sciences, University of Pavia, 27100 Pavia, Italy. [6]Obstetrics and Gynaecology Unit, IRCCS Ospedale San Raffaele, 20132 Milan, Italy.

References

1. Iliadou AN, Janson PC, Cnattingius S. Epigenetics and assisted reproductive technology. J Intern Med. 2011;270:414–20.
2. Lazaraviciute G, Kauser M, Bhattacharya S, Haggarty P, Bhattacharya S. A systematic review and meta-analysis of DNA methylation levels and imprinting disorders in children conceived by IVF/ICSI compared with children conceived spontaneously. Hum Reprod Update. 2014;20:840–52.
3. Song S, Ghosh J, Mainigi M, Turan N, Weinerman R, Truongcao M, et al. DNA methylation differences between in vitro- and in vivo-conceived children are associated with ART procedures rather than infertility. Clin Epigenetics. 2015;7:41–9.
4. Odom LN, Segars J. Imprinting disorders and assisted reproductive technology. Curr Opin Endocrinol Diabetes Obes. 2010;17:517–22.
5. Tierling S, Souren NY, Gries J, Loporto C, Groth M, Lutsik P, et al. Assisted reproductive technologies do not enhance the variability of DNA methylation imprints in human. J Med Genet. 2010;47:371–6.
6. De Waal E, Yamazaki Y, Ingale P, Bartolomei M, Yanagimachi R, McCarrey JR. Primary epimutations introduced during intracytoplasmic sperm injection (ICSI) are corrected by germline-specific epigenetic reprogramming. Proc Natl Acad Sci U S A. 2012;109:4163–8.
7. Batcheller A, Cardozo E, Maguire M, DeCherney AH, Segars JH. Are there subtle genome-wide epigenetic alterations in normal offspring conceived by assisted reproductive technologies? Fertil Steril. 2011;96: 1306–11.
8. Messerschmidt DM, Knowles BB, Solter D. DNA methylation dynamics during epigenetic reprogramming in the germline and preimplantation embryos. Genes Dev. 2014;28:812–28.
9. De Waal E, Mak W, Calhoun S, Stein P, Ord T, Krapp C, et al. In vitro culture increases the frequency of stochastic epigenetic errors at imprinted genes in placental tissues from mouse concepti produced through assisted reproductive technologies. Biol Reprod. 2014;90:22.
10. Melamed N, Choufani S, Wilkins-Haug LE, Koren G, Weksberg R. Comparison of genome-wide and gene-specific DNA methylation between ART and naturally conceived pregnancies. Epigenetics. 2015;10:474–83.
11. Arnaud P, Hata K, Kaneda M, Li E, Sasaki H, Feil R, et al. Stochastic imprinting in the progeny of Dnmt3L–/– females. Hum Mol Genet. 2006;15:589–98.
12. Gentilini D, Garagnani P, Pisoni S, Bacalini MG, Calzari L, Mari D, et al. Stochastic epigenetic mutations (DNA methylation) increase exponentially in human aging and correlate with X chromosome inactivation skewing in females. Aging. 2015;7:568–78.
13. Castillo-Fernandez JE, Loke YJ, Bass-Stringer S, Gao F, Xia Y, Wu H, et al. DNA methylation changes at infertility genes in newborn twins conceived by in vitro fertilisation. Genome Med. 2017;9:28.
14. Estill MS, Bolnick JM, Waterland RA, Bolnick AD, Diamond MP, Krawetz SA. Assisted reproductive technology alters deoxyribonucleic acid methylation profiles in bloodspots of newborn infants. Fertil Steril. 2016;106:629–39.
15. El Hajj N, Haertle L, Dittrich M, Denk S, Lehnen H, Hahn T, et al. DNA methylation signatures in cord blood of ICSI children. Hum Reprod. 2017;32: 1761–9.
16. Diplas AI, Lambertini L, Lee MJ, Sperling R, Lee YL, Wetmur J, et al. Differential expression of imprinted genes in normal and IUGR human placentas. Epigenetics. 2009;4:235–40.
17. Turan N, Ghalwash MF, Katari S, Coutifaris C, Obradovic Z, Sapienza C. DNA methylation differences at growth related genes correlate with birth weight: a molecular signature linked to developmental origins of adult disease? BMC Med Genet. 2012;5:10.
18. Joubert BR, Felix JF, Yousefi P, Bakulski KM, Just AC, Breton C, et al. DNA methylation in newborns and maternal smoking in pregnancy: genome-wide consortium meta-analysis. Am J Hum Genet. 2016;98:680–96.
19. Sharp GC, Salas LA, Monnereau C, Allard C, Yousefi P, Everson TM, et al. Maternal BMI at the start of pregnancy and offspring epigenome-wide DNA methylation: findings from the pregnancy and childhood epigenetics (PACE) consortium. Hum Mol Genet. 2017;26:4067–85.
20. Court F, Tayama C, Romanelli V, Martin-Trujillo A, Iglesias-Platas I, Okamura K, et al. Genome-wide parent-of-origin DNA methylation analysis reveals the intricacies of human imprinting and suggests a germline methylation-independent mechanism of establishment. Genome Res. 2014;24:554–69.

21. Rubino P, Viganò P, Luddi A, Piomboni P. The ICSI procedure from past to future: a systematic review of the more controversial aspects. Hum Reprod Update. 2016;22:194–227.

22. Gentilini D, Scala S, Gaudenzi G, Garagnani P, Capri M, Cescon M, et al. Epigenome-wide association study in hepatocellular carcinoma: identification of stochastic epigenetic mutations through an innovative statistical approach. Oncotarget. 2017;8:41890–902.

23. Haertle L, El Hajj N, Dittrich M, Müller T, Nanda I, Lehnen H, et al. Epigenetic signatures of gestational diabetes mellitus on cord blood methylation. Clin Epigenetics. 2017;9:28.

24. Maccani JZ, Koestler DC, Houseman EA, Marsit CJ, Kelsey KT. Placental DNA methylation alterations associated with maternal tobacco smoking at the RUNX3 gene are also associated with gestational age. Epigenomics. 2013;5(6):619–30.

25. Yuen RK, Jiang R, Peñaherrera MS, McFadden DE, Robinson WP. Genome-wide mapping of imprinted differentially methylated regions by DNA methylation profiling of human placentas from triploidies. Epigenetics Chromatin. 2011;4:10.

26. Chen D, Zhang A, Fang M, Fang R, Ge J, Jiang Y, et al. Increased methylation at differentially methylated region of GNAS in infants born to gestational diabetes. BMC Med Genet. 2014;15:108.

27. Soubry A, Murphy SK, Wang F, Huang Z, Vidal AC, Fuemmeler BF, et al. Newborns of obese parents have altered DNA methylation patterns at imprinted genes. Int J Obes. 2015;39:650–7.

28. Vidal AC, Benjamin Neelon SE, Liu Y, Tuli AM, Fuemmeler BF, Hoyo C, Murtha AP, et al. Maternal stress, preterm birth, and DNA methylation at imprint regulatory sequences in humans. Genet Epigenet. 2014;6:37–44.

29. McCullough LE, Mendez MA, Miller EE, Murtha AP, Murphy SK, Hoyo C. Associations between prenatal physical activity, birth weight, and DNA methylation at genomically imprinted domains in a multiethnic newborn cohort. Epigenetics. 2015;10:597–606.

30. Rotroff DM, Joubert BR, Marvel SW, Håberg SE, Wu MC, Nilsen RM, et al. A maternal smoking impacts key biological pathways in newborns through epigenetic modification in utero. BMC Genomics. 2016;17(1):976.

31. Chango A, Pogribny IP. Considering maternal dietary modulators for epigenetic regulation and programming of the fetal epigenome. Nutrients. 2015;7:2748–70.

32. Kahn HS, Morgan TM, Case LD, Dabelea D, Mayer-Davis EJ, Lawrence JM, et al. Association of type 1 diabetes with month of birth among U.S. youth: the SEARCH for diabetes in youth study. Diabetes Care. 2009;32:2010–5.

33. Vaiserman AM, Carstensen B, Voitenko VP, Tronko MD, Kravchenko VI, Khalangot MD, et al. Seasonality of birth in children and young adults (0-29 years) with type 1 diabetes in Ukraine. Diabetologia. 2007;50:32–5.

34. Li L, Boland MR, Miotto R, Tatonetti NP, Dudley JT. Replicating cardiovascular condition-birth month associations. Sci Rep. 2016;6:33166.

35. La Rosa F, Liso A, Bianconi F, Duca E, Stracci F. Seasonal variation in the month of birth in patients with skin cancer. Br J Cancer. 2014;111:1810–3.

36. Pazderska A, Fichna M, Mitchel AL, Napier CM, Gan E, Ruchała M, et al. Impact of month of birth on the risk of development of autoimmune Addison's disease. J Clin Endocrinol Metab. 2016;101:4214–8.

37. Doblhammer G, Vaupel JW. Lifespan depends on month of birth. Proc Natl Acad Sci U S A. 2001;98(5):2934–9.

38. Ueda P, Edstedt Bonamy AK, Granath F, Cnattingius S. Month of birth and mortality in Sweden: a nation-wide population-based cohort study. PLoS One. 2013;8:e56425.

39. Ueda P, Edstedt Bonamy AK, Granath F, Cnattingius S. Month of birth and cause-specific mortality between 50 and 80 years: a population-based longitudinal cohort study in Sweden. Eur J Epidemiol. 2014;29:89–94.

40. Gavrilov LA, Gavrilova NS. Season of birth and exceptional longevity: comparative study of american centenarians, their siblings, and spouses. J Aging Res. 2011;2011:104616.

41. De Waal E, Vrooman LA, Fischer E, Ord T, Mainigi MA, Coutifaris C, et al. The cumulative effect of assisted reproduction procedures on placental development and epigenetic perturbations in a mouse model. Hum Mol Genet. 2015;24:6975–85.

42. Li B, Chen S, Tang N, Xiao X, Huang J, Jiang F, et al. Assisted reproduction causes reduced fetal growth associated with downregulation of paternally expressed imprinted genes that enhance fetal growth in mice. Biol Reprod. 2016;94:45.

43. Ghosh J, Coutifaris C, Sapienza C, Mainigi M. Global DNA methylation levels are altered by modifiable clinical manipulations in assisted reproductive technologies. Clin Epigenetics. 2017;6:9–14.

44. Choux C, Binquet C, Carmignac V, Bruno C, Chapusot C, Barberet J, et al. The epigenetic control of transposable elements and imprinted genes in newborns is affected by the mode of conception: ART versus spontaneous conception without underlying infertility. Hum Reprod. 2018;33:331–40.

45. Solves P, Moraga R, Saucedo E, Perales A, Soler MA, Larrea L, et al. Comparison between two strategies for umbilical cord blood collection. Bone Marrow Transplant. 2003;31:269–73.

46. Restelli L, Paffoni A, Corti L, Rabellotti E, Mangiarini A, Vigano P, et al. The strategy of group embryo culture based on pronuclear pattern on blastocyst development: a two center analysis. J Assist Reprod Genet. 2014; 31:1629–34.

47. Intra G, Alteri A, Corti L, Rabellotti E, Papaleo E, Restelli L, et al. Application of failure mode and effect analysis in an assisted reproduction technology laboratory. Reprod BioMed Online. 2016;33:132–9.

48. Papaleo E, Pagliardini L, Vanni VS, Delprato D, Rubino P, Candiani M, et al. A direct healthcare cost analysis of the cryopreserved versus fresh transfer policy at the blastocyst stage. Reprod BioMed Online. 2017;34:19–26.

49. Calzi F, Papaleo E, Rabellotti E, Ottolina J, Vailati S, Vigano P, et al. Exposure of embryos to oxygen at low concentration in a cleavage stage transfer program: reproductive outcomes in a time-series analysis. Clin Lab. 2012;58: 997–1003.

50. Corti L, Papaleo E, Pagliardini L, Rabellotti E, Molgora M, La Marca A, et al. Fresh blastocyst transfer as a clinical approach to overcome the detrimental effect of progesterone elevation at hCG triggering: a strategy in the context of the Italian law. Eur J Obstet Gynecol Reprod Biol. 2013;171:73–7.

51. Assenov Y, Muller F, Lutsik P, Walter J, Lengauer T, Bock C. Comprehensive analysis of DNA methylation data with RnBeads. Nat Methods. 2014;11: 1138–40.

52. 1000 Genomes Project Consortium, Auton A, Brooks LD, Durbin RM, Garrison EP, Kang HM, et al. A global reference for human genetic variation. Nature. 2015;526:68–74.

53. Lek M, Karczewski KJ, Minikel EV, Samocha KE, Banks E, Fennell T, et al. Analysis of protein-coding genetic variation in 60,706 humans. Nature. 2016; 536:285–91.

54. Aryee MJ, Jaffe AE, Corrada-Bravo H, Ladd-Acosta C, Feinberg AP, Hansen KD, et al. Minfi: a flexible and comprehensive Bioconductor package for the analysis of Infinium DNA methylation microarrays. Bioinformatics. 2014;30: 1363–9.

55. Bakulski KM, Feinberg JI, Andrews SV, Yang J, Brown S, McKenney SL, et al. DNA methylation of cord blood cell types: applications for mixed cell birth studies. Epigenetics. 2016;11:354–62.

56. Ensembl. http://www.ensembl.org/index.html. Accessed 27 Nov 2017.

57. UCSC Genome Browser. http://genome.ucsc.edu/. Accessed 27 Nov 2017.

6

A new approach to epigenome-wide discovery of non-invasive methylation biomarkers for colorectal cancer screening in circulating cell-free DNA using pooled samples

María Gallardo-Gómez[1], Sebastian Moran[2], María Páez de la Cadena[1], Vicenta Soledad Martínez-Zorzano[1], Francisco Javier Rodríguez-Berrocal[1], Mar Rodríguez-Girondo[3,4], Manel Esteller[2], Joaquín Cubiella[5], Luis Bujanda[6], Antoni Castells[7], Francesc Balaguer[7], Rodrigo Jover[8] and Loretta De Chiara[1*]

Abstract

Background: Colorectal cancer is the fourth cause of cancer-related deaths worldwide, though detection at early stages associates with good prognosis. Thus, there is a clear demand for novel non-invasive tests for the early detection of colorectal cancer and premalignant advanced adenomas, to be used in population-wide screening programs. Aberrant DNA methylation detected in liquid biopsies, such as serum circulating cell-free DNA (cfDNA), is a promising source of non-invasive biomarkers. This study aimed to assess the feasibility of using cfDNA pooled samples to identify potential serum methylation biomarkers for the detection of advanced colorectal neoplasia (colorectal cancer or advanced adenomas) using microarray-based technology.

Results: cfDNA was extracted from serum samples from 20 individuals with no colorectal findings, 20 patients with advanced adenomas, and 20 patients with colorectal cancer (stages I and II). Two pooled samples were prepared for each pathological group using equal amounts of cfDNA from 10 individuals, sex-, age-, and recruitment hospital-matched. We measured the methylation levels of 866,836 CpG positions across the genome using the MethylationEPIC array. Pooled serum cfDNA methylation data meets the quality requirements. The proportion of detected CpG in all pools (> 99% with detection p value < 0.01) exceeded Illumina Infinium methylation data quality metrics of the number of sites detected. The differential methylation analysis revealed 1384 CpG sites (5% false discovery rate) with at least 10% difference in the methylation level between no colorectal findings controls and advanced neoplasia, the majority of which were hypomethylated. Unsupervised clustering showed that cfDNA methylation patterns can distinguish advanced neoplasia from healthy controls, as well as separate tumor tissue from healthy mucosa in an independent dataset. We also observed that advanced adenomas and stage I/II colorectal cancer methylation profiles, grouped as advanced neoplasia, are largely homogenous and clustered close together.

(Continued on next page)

* Correspondence: ldechiara@uvigo.es
[1]Department of Biochemistry, Genetics and Immunology, Centro Singular de Investigación de Galicia (CINBIO), University of Vigo, Campus As Lagoas-Marcosende s/n, 36310 Vigo, Spain
Full list of author information is available at the end of the article

(Continued from previous page)

Conclusions: This preliminary study shows the viability of microarray-based methylation biomarker discovery using pooled serum cfDNA samples as an alternative approach to tissue specimens. Our strategy sets an open door for deciphering new non-invasive biomarkers not only for colorectal cancer detection, but also for other types of cancers.

Keywords: Advanced adenomas, Circulating cell-free DNA, Colorectal cancer, DNA methylation, MethylationEPIC, Non-invasive diagnostic biomarkers, Pooled samples, Serum

Background

Colorectal cancer (CRC) is the fourth leading cause of cancer-related deaths worldwide, accounting for over 1.4 million new cases in 2012 [1, 2]. While diagnosis at early stages associates with good prognosis and reduced mortality rates, the detection and removal of premalignant advanced adenomas (AA) results in the reduction of CRC incidence [3]. Since neoplastic transformation can last decades, there is a broad time window for implementing screening strategies for the detection of advanced neoplasia (AN: CRC or AA) [3, 4].

Approaches for CRC screening can be divided into two groups. Invasive procedures like colonoscopy allow the examination of the entire colon and the removal of lesions (polypectomy); however, limitations of this strategy include considerably low participation rates and high cost [5]. On the other hand, non-invasive methods like fecal immunological test (FIT) have the advantage of increased acceptance and adequate specificity, though sensitivity for colorectal tumors, especially of proximal location, and AA is moderate to low [6, 7]. Blood-based markers are capable of improving CRC screening adherence, and a large number of candidates have been reported for CRC diagnosis, reviewed in [8]. Currently, the most promising is the *SEPT9* methylation assay, though its performance for the detection of early-stage tumors and AA needs to be improved [9]. Therefore, there is an imperative need of finding new non-invasive biomarkers for CRC screening.

Nowadays, it is well-established that not only genetic alterations but also epigenetic modifications are involved in CRC development and progression [10]. The abnormal methylation occurring during colorectal neoplasia is characterized by promoter hypermethylation and transcriptional silencing of tumor suppressor or DNA repair genes [11, 12], coexisting with a global loss of methylation that leads to chromosomal and microsatellite instability and oncogene activation [11, 13]. Both promoter hypermethylation and global hypomethylation are hallmarks of early stages of colorectal carcinogenesis [10, 14].

Several methodologies are suitable for genome-wide methylation biomarker discovery, including whole and reduced genome bisulfite sequencing and array-based genotyping technology [15, 16]. These epigenome-wide measurements allow a more successful identification of methylation alterations related to complex diseases compared to target studies. The main drawback is the large sample size needed, which increases project costs. DNA sample pooling strategies represent an affordable approach for biomarker discovery, resulting in reduced costs and increased amount of input DNA when small amounts are available. Additionally, it has been reported that pooled samples provide similar results to individual samples in both genome-wide [17, 18] and epigenome-wide [19] association studies.

During the last years, it has been demonstrated that circulating cell-free DNA (cfDNA) present in liquid biopsies reflects methylation changes originated in tumor cells [20–22]. Given the stability of DNA methylation in body fluids [23–25], the discovery of cfDNA methylation markers using serum samples seems a very attractive alternative to direct the search of non-invasive biomarkers.

Taking advantage of this fact, we hypothesized that an array-based epigenome-wide analysis using serum cfDNA as input could be a novel and affordable approach for the discovery of a methylation marker panel with greater diagnostic value, compared to other indirect strategies using tumor tissue and mucosa as input DNA. Therefore, in the present study, we aim to assess the feasibility of hybridizing pooled serum cfDNA to the MethylationEPIC array to detect differentially methylated patterns between patients with advanced neoplasia and individuals with no colorectal findings.

Methods

Study population and serum samples

Individuals were recruited from the following Spanish Hospitals: Hospital Donostia (San Sebastián), Complexo Hospitalario Universitario de Ourense (Ourense), Hospital Clínic de Barcelona (Barcelona), and Hospital General Universitario de Alicante (Alicante). Patients' characteristics are described elsewhere [26]. We carried out a stratified random sampling using colorectal finding and gender as stratifying variables. Moreover, age was restricted to 50–75 years and strata were matched by recruitment hospital and age. We selected from this multicenter cohort 20 individuals with no colorectal findings (NCF), 20 individuals with AA (adenomas ≥ 10 mm, with villous component or high-grade dysplasia), and 20 CRC cases (7 stage I and 13 stage II, according to the AJCC staging system [27]). Individuals were classified according to the most advanced lesion after colonoscopy. Lesions were considered "proximal" when located only proximal to the splenic flexure of the colon and "distal" when lesions were found only in the distal colon or in both distal and proximal colons. Advanced neoplasia (AN) was defined as AA or CRC.

Blood samples were obtained the same day of the colonoscopy, immediately prior to the procedure. Blood samples were coagulated and subsequently centrifuged according to the manufacturer's instruction for serum collection. Serum samples were stored at − 20 °C until used.

DNA extraction and sample pooling

We extracted cfDNA from 0.5–1.5 mL of serum using a phenol-chloroform protocol as described by Clemens et al. [28], with minor modifications, and resuspended in 20 μL sterile water. DNA concentration was determined for each individual sample using the Qubit dsDNA HS Assay Kit (Thermo Fisher Scientific, MA, USA), a fluorimetric assay specific for double-stranded DNA that gives an accurate measurement of DNA concentration. All cfDNA samples were stored at − 20 °C.

Two independent pooled samples were constructed for each pathological group (NCF, AA, and CRC) using equal amounts of cfDNA from 10 individuals per pool. The factors considered to match between pools were gender, age, and recruitment hospital. Table 1 shows epidemiologic and clinical data of each individual included in pool A and B (NCF), pool C and D (AA), and pool E and F (CRC).

Since the preparation of pooled samples is a critical step that requires high accuracy, cfDNA from each individual included in a pool was thawed, tempered, and re-quantified using the Qubit assay. As reported by previous DNA pooling protocols [18, 29], in order to avoid inaccuracies derived from pipetting small volumes, we decided to dilute by a factor of two samples with more than 10 ng/μL of DNA. Diluted DNA was measured again.

Once the actual concentration of all the individual samples of a pool was available, we determined the sample containing the limiting ng of cfDNA (based on measured concentration and volume). Based on this limiting nanogram, we calculated for each of the nine remaining samples the volume containing the same nanogram of cfDNA as the limiting sample. Finally, the pool was constructed by incorporating into the tube the corresponding volume of each of the 10 individual samples of the pool. The cfDNA

mixture was allowed to stand for 1 h, and then the DNA concentration was quantified with the Qubit Assay to ensure that the final DNA concentration of the pool was as expected according to the theoretical calculation:

$$\frac{(\text{limiting ng}) \cdot n}{(\text{total volume of the pool})}$$

where n is the number of individuals included in each pool (10). Pools were considered valid for the Infinium Methylation Assay protocol when the difference between expected and measured concentration (Qubit) was less than 5%. A graphical description of the pooling protocol is presented [see Additional file 1]. This protocol was followed for each of the pools included in the study. The six pooled cfDNA samples were stored at − 20 °C and were submitted to the Cancer Epigenetics and Biology Program (PEBC) facilities at the Bellvitge Biomedical Research Institute for processing.

Epigenome-wide methylation measurements

DNA methylation was analyzed with the Infinium MethylationEPIC BeadChip microarray (EPIC; Illumina Inc., CA, USA), that quantitatively measures the methylation levels of more than 850,000 CpG sites across the genome [30], located in promoter regions and gene bodies, and also in intergenic enhancer regions identified by the ENCODE [31, 32] and FANTOM5 [33] projects. Pooled samples were bisulfite treated in the same batch, and MethylationEPIC arrays were hybridized according to manufacturer's instructions.

Data preprocessing and differential methylation analysis

Data quality control was assessed with the GenomeStudio V2011.1, based on the internal control probes present on the array. The preprocessing, normalization, and correction steps were conducted using the R environment (versions 3. 3.3 and 3.4.0) with Bioconductor packages. The pipeline was a sequence of R functions adapted from the minfi [34] and ChAMP [35] Bioconductor packages. Our dataset was normalized using the Functional Normalization implemented in the minfi package. This algorithm does not rely on any biological assumption and therefore is suitable for cases where global changes in the methylation levels are expected, such as in cancer-normal comparisons [36].

Detection p values were computed with the minfi package, and mean detection p values were examined across all samples in order to identify any failed sample. Probes with a detection p value > 0.01 in at least one sample were discarded. We filtered out probes containing a single nucleotide polymorphism (SNP) at the CpG interrogation site and at the single nucleotide extension for any minor allele frequency (MAF), and probes containing a SNP at the probe body for a MAF >5 %,

Table 1 Epidemiologic and clinical characteristics of the individuals included in the pools

Pool[a]	Gender[b]	Age		Gender[b]	Age
Pool A-NCF	F	72	Pool B-NCF	F	63
	F	68		F	62
	F	61		F	59
	F	54		F	54
	F	54		F	54
	M	67		M	71
	M	67		M	68
	M	65		M	66
	M	62		M	60
	M	54		M	53

Pool[a]	Gender[b]	Age	Lesion description[c]	Lesion location[d]
Pool C-AA	F	72	10 mm, T, LGD	Distal
	F	68	25 mm, V, LGD	Distal
	F	65	10 mm, TV, LGD	Distal
	F	63	12 mm, T, LGD	Proximal
	F	54	10 mm, T, LGD	Distal
	M	71	10 mm, T, LGD	Distal
	M	66	10 mm, TV, LGD	Distal
	M	65	20 mm, T, LGD	Distal
	M	61	15 mm, T, LGD	Proximal
	M	58	3 mm, TV, LGD	Proximal
Pool D-AA	F	70	30 mm, T, LGD	Proximal
	F	67	20 mm, TV, LGD	Distal
	F	65	30 mm, TV, LGD	Proximal
	F	61	10 mm, TV, LGD	Distal
	F	59	10 mm, TV, LGD	Distal
	M	71	8 mm, TV, LGD	Distal
	M	71	10 mm, V, LGD	Proximal
	M	64	20 mm, V, LGD	Distal
	M	64	20 mm, T, LGD	Proximal
	M	54	5 mm, TV, LGD	Distal
Pool E-CRC	F	70	T3N0, WD	Distal
	F	67	T3N0, MD	Distal
	F	65	T3N0, MD	Distal
	F	59	T4N0, MD	Distal
	F	59	T3N0, WD	Distal
	M	72	T2N0, MD	Distal
	M	66	T2N0, NA	Distal
	M	62	T3N0, MD	Distal
	M	60	T1N0M0, WD	Distal
	M	51	T3N0, MD	Proximal
Pool F-CRC	F	72	T3N0, WD	Distal
	F	65	T3N0, WD	Distal

Table 1 Epidemiologic and clinical characteristics of the individuals included in the pools (Continued)

Pool[a]	Gender[b]	Age		Gender[b]	Age
	F	61	T2N0, MD	Distal	
	F	60	T3N0, MD	Proximal	
	F	55	T3N0, NA	Distal	
	M	67	T2N0M0, WD	Proximal	
	M	63	T2N0, MD	Distal	
	M	61	T3N0, MD	Distal	
	M	59	T3N0, WD	Distal	
	M	57	T2N0, MD	Distal	

[a]Identification of the pool (NCF no colorectal findings, AA advanced adenoma, CRC colorectal cancer)
[b]Gender (F female, M male)
[c]Lesion description for AA cases include size of adenoma (mm), histology (T tubular, TV tubulo-villous, V villous) and dysplasia (LGD low grade of dysplasia), lesion description for CRC cases include TNM classification and tumor differentiation grade (WD well-differentiated, MD moderately differentiated, NA not available)
[d]Lesion location refers to distal or proximal colon

because differential methylation levels can be confounded with actual polymorphisms in the DNA sequence. According to the list provided by Pidsley et al. [37], cross-reactive probes were removed. Probes targeting X and Y chromosomes were also discarded.

In accordance with Du et al. [38], methylation levels were expressed as beta and M values. Beta values were used for visualization and intuitive interpretation of the results, and M values were used for the differential methylation analysis.

Prior to differential methylation analysis, data was checked for batch effects across all array runs using the combat method implemented in the ChAMP package. Differentially methylated positions (DMP) between NCF and AN (AA or CRC) were detected with the dmpFinder function from the minfi package, which uses an F-test for categorical phenotype comparisons at a probe level. p values for each probe were corrected for multiple testing using the Benjamini-Hochberg procedure, with a false discovery rate (FDR) of 5% to determine significant DMPs.

In silico evaluation of differential methylation

We applied unsupervised clustering approaches to evaluate the differentially methylated patterns between AN and NCF pools in an independent dataset. The publicly available dataset GSE48684 that includes the methylation data of 64 colorectal tumor biopsies (adenocarcinomas) and 41 healthy mucosa biopsies, measured with the Infinium HumanMethylation450 BeadChip array (450K) [14], was used as a test cohort. This independent evaluation was limited to the probes shared by 450K and

EPIC arrays due to the absence of colorectal tumor and mucosa EPIC public datasets.

Results and discussion

DNA pooling methodology

To our knowledge, this is the first pooling-based study that analyzes the methylation patterns in cfDNA, aiming to assess the feasibility of liquid biopsy methylation biomarker discovery using microarray technology in a more affordable manner compared to individual samples.

DNA sample pooling has been reported as an efficient tool for genome-wide and high-throughput association studies [17, 18]. More recently, its potential utility was highlighted in microarray-based epigenome-wide association studies (EWAS), as Gallego-Fabrega et al. reported high correlation of the methylation levels between pools and individual DNA samples using the Infinium HumanMethylation450 BeadChip [19]. Taking into account the limitation that only mean methylation levels can be obtained from pooled samples, pooling strategy is an accurate and affordable alternative that can significantly reduce costs in large EWAS. DNA pooling is also an efficient alternative when small amounts of DNA are available and when working with precious samples.

For sample pooling, accurate construction is critical, and each DNA sample must be equally represented in the pool. To guarantee the most precise pool construction, we first tested two different pooling strategies: diluting all samples to a common concentration and then mixing equal volumes in a tube as in previous works [19, 29] or directly adding the same nanogram of DNA (calculated corresponding volume from each sample) into the tube. Once test pools were constructed and DNA concentration measured, we checked for discrepancies between the actual and the expected concentration. Variations inferior to 5% of the expected pooled DNA concentration were found when using the second protocol; therefore, sample pooling was performed as described [see Additional file 1].

We prepared two pooled samples for each pathological group (two pools of individuals with NCF, two pools of AA patients, and two pools of CRC patients stages I and II). We included 10 individuals per pool to ensure an acceptable amount of DNA input for the microarray analyses and also to reduce population stratification and the presence of unobserved confounding variables. The categories considered to match between pools were gender, age (median 63.5, range 51–72 years), and recruitment hospital. The age range was selected based on the USPSTF guideline recommendation for CRC screening, targeting individuals from 50 to 75 years [39]. No statistically significant difference was found in the mean age between pools (ANOVA, $p < 0.05$). The

final cfDNA concentration of the six pooled samples ranged from 135 to 250 ng.

Quality control of methylation data

The methylation levels of 866,836 CpG positions across the genome in the six pooled samples were measured using the MethylationEPIC BeadChip. The quality control based on the internal control probes present on the array, which include bisulfite conversion efficiency, hybridization, extension, and staining, among others, indicates that pooled serum cfDNA methylation data meets the quality requirements. The QC report is presented [see Additional file 2] and shows that the signals observed are much higher than the background signal, coinciding with what is expected for high-quality DNA. In relation to CpG detection, all the pools showed more than 99% of CpG detected correctly (only 2811 probes presented a detection p value > 0.01 at least in one sample, and were discarded). The number of probes detected in each pool was 866,497; 866,021; 865,865; 865,501; 865,778; and 866,463 for pools A, B, C, D, E, and F, respectively. These results are indicative of a uniform amplification and hybridization in all the pooled samples. The proportion of CpG detection observed in our samples exceeded Illumina Infinium methylation data quality metrics of the number of sites detected ($> 96\%$ for genomic DNA and $> 90\%$ for FFPE samples). A probable explanation could be the pooling design, as measuring methylation of 10 individuals in the same assay would increase the representation of each CpG in the input DNA. Therefore, no samples were discarded due to QC issues.

The distribution of methylation levels in pooled samples presented the expected bimodal distribution for both beta and M values, with the two peaks indicating fully methylated and unmethylated states characteristic of DNA methylation data (Fig. 1a). Then, we evaluated the distribution of beta values by type I and II probes separately. As observed in Fig. 1b, all the pools showed the distribution of type II probes shifted in relation to type I, as previously reported in the 450K and EPIC data [37, 40].

Differential methylation

Once the technical quality of the six pooled sample data is verified, we performed a differential methylation analysis. In order to detect differentially methylated positions (DMPs), we compared the two NCF pools (colonoscopically confirmed controls) with the two AA pools together with the two CRC pools (considered as AN). The differential methylation analysis was performed on the 703,653 probes left after the filtering step (see the "Methods" section). We first assessed the global methylation in the NCF and AN groups, and in the AA and CRC groups. As shown in Fig. 2a, a

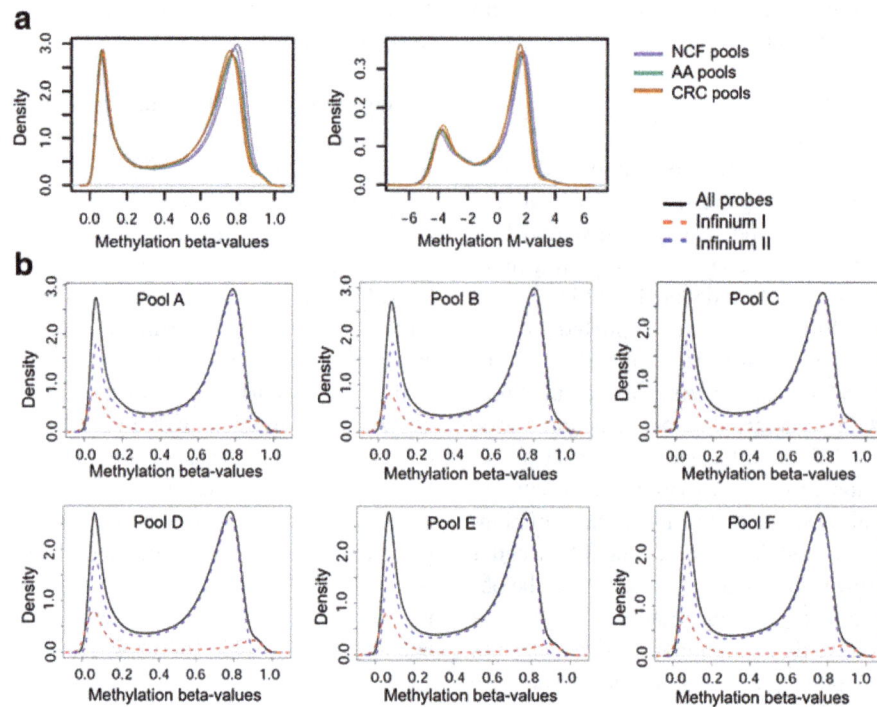

Fig. 1 Density distributions of methylation data. **a** Density distribution of the raw methylation beta and *M* values across the 866,836 CpG sites measured in the six pooled serum cfDNA pooled samples. **b** Density distribution of the beta values by probe type for all the interrogated CpG sites in pools A–F

lower content of global methylation was observed in AN, AA, and CRC compared to NCF. In addition, we found there is no difference in terms of global methylation between AA and CRC cfDNA pooled samples.

Since the purpose of screening programs include the detection of early stage CRC together with the identification and removal of premalignant AA [4], we grouped AA and CRC in the single group AN for the analyses. We found a total of 5808 significant DMPs between the NCF and AN groups, identified with a FDR of 5% (Fig. 2b). Of these, 1384 presented at least 10% difference in the methylation level between NCF and AN (|Δbeta| > 0.1): 135 (9.75%) were found hypermethylated in AN, while 1249 (90.25%) appeared hypomethylated (Fig. 2c). The distribution of the DMPs identified according to their location relative to CpG islands (CGI) and promoter regions is represented in Fig. 2d. The majority of the differentially hypomethylated CpGs in AN are located in opensea (78.08%), outside gene promoters, within regions with no enrichment in CpG content followed by CGI-shore (10.23%), CGI-shelf (7.50%), and CGI (4.19%).

DNA hypomethylation was the first aberrant methylation alteration described in several human cancers (reviewed in [41]). This global loss of genome-wide methylation was also described long time ago in both CRC and colorectal adenomas [42], indicating that

global hypomethylation is characteristic of early stages of colorectal carcinogenesis [10, 14, 43]. Large hypomethylated blocks were also identified by Timp and colleagues (2014) using the 450K array. Among the six different tumor types analyzed, colon cancer tissue showed the highest proportions of hypomethylation in opensea, CGI-shelf, CGI-shore, and CGI [44]. In our work, using pooled serum samples, we found that more than 90% of the DMPs appeared hypomethylated in AN, agreeing with these previous reports, and suggesting that perhaps efforts should be centered on hypomethylated candidates to accomplish a greater discrimination capacity.

Unsupervised clustering performed on DNA methylation values for the top 1384 DMPs identified is presented in Fig. 3a, b. These results highlight the differences between AN and NCF pooled samples and suggest that differential cfDNA methylation profiles obtained with pooled samples can discriminate AN from NCF controls.

We further evaluated the DMPs identified in our pooled serum cfDNA samples with dataset GSE48684 consisting of tumor and mucosa tissue samples [14] as a test cohort, restricting the analysis to the 518 DMPs between AN and NCF with |Δbeta| > 0.1 targeted by probes shared by 450K and EPIC arrays. The unsupervised clustering shown in Fig. 4, performed on tumor and mucosa samples from GSE48684 based on our DMPs, reveals that the differential methylation patterns found between AN and NCF

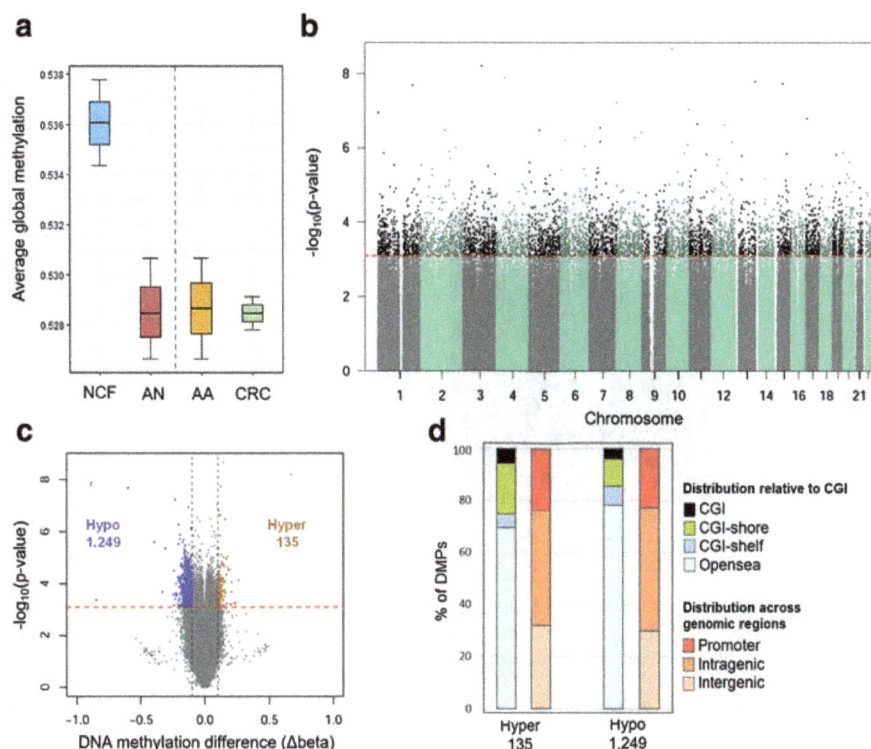

Fig. 2 Identification of differential methylation. **a** Boxplot of global cfDNA methylation in NCF, AN, AA, and CRC pools. Global methylation is expressed as the average methylation rate for each pooled sample. The box plot represents the median (line across the box), interquartile range, and maximum and minimum values (whiskers). **b** Manhattan plot showing $-\log_{10}(p$ value) resulting from the differential methylation analysis for all the CpGs considered (703,653). The p values are sorted by chromosome coordinates. Significant DMPs between AN and NCF pooled samples with a FDR < 5% (5808) appear highlighted in darker color, above the red dashed line. **c** Volcano plot of differential methylation $-\log_{10}(p$ value) versus differences in methylation levels (Δbeta: obtained by subtracting the DNA methylation levels (beta values) of NCF from AN). Significant DMPs appear above the red dashed line (FDR 5%). Significant DMPs with a difference in the methylation levels greater than 10% (1384) are highlighted in color (135 hypermethylated DMPs in AN, orange dots: Δbeta > 0.1 and FDR < 5%; 1249 hypomethylated DMPs in AN, blue dots: Δbeta < − 0.1 and FDR < 5%). **d** Relative distribution of the 1385 DMPs with absolute Δbeta > 0.1 in relation to CpG islands (CGI) and across different genomic regions. The EPIC array categorizes probes following a functional classification into three major groups: promoter regions (5'UTR, TSS200, TSS1500, and first exons), intragenic regions (gene body and 3'UTR), and intergenic regions. TSS200, TSS1500: 200 and 1500 bp upstream the transcription start site, respectively. CGI-shore: sequences 2 kb flanking the CGI, CGI-shelf: sequences 2 kb flanking shore regions, opensea: sequences located outside these regions [30]

cfDNA can also separate tumor tissue from healthy mucosa samples. It is worth to mention that 24 healthy mucosa samples from GSE48684 were normal colon concurrent with CRC and were obtained from the normal-appearing resection margin of the colorectal tumor biopsy [14], as represented in Fig. 4b. This can be related to the fact that a subcluster of mucosa samples partially overlaps with CRC samples. Though this in silico verification is limited, a considerable degree of concordance can be deduced. It should also be mentioned that discrepancy in the frequencies of methylation alterations have been reported in tumor and cfDNA, showing the latter considerably lower frequencies [45]. Hence, array-based strategies that rely on tissue samples for cfDNA methylation marker discovery have the inconvenience of resulting in decreased sensitivity of the selected candidate markers once tested in serum or plasma, limiting their

utility as non-invasive tests [46, 47]. An alternative approach for biomarker discovery was accomplished by Heiss et al. that used whole blood. However, these authors indicate that the methylation signature identified in leukocyte DNA may not be specific for CRC, reflecting immune responses [48].

The exploratory nature of this study, with a reduced number of samples, limits further analyses, but offers a new affordable strategy for biomarker discovery, providing an alternative approach to tissue biopsy, reducing costs in microarray-based EWAS. This work should be followed by new studies that include a greater number of pooled serum cfDNA samples and a greater range of colorectal pathologies, allowing a more robust comparison between methylation profiles. Furthermore, differential methylation profiles must be validated in independent serum cfDNA individual samples, using quantitative real-

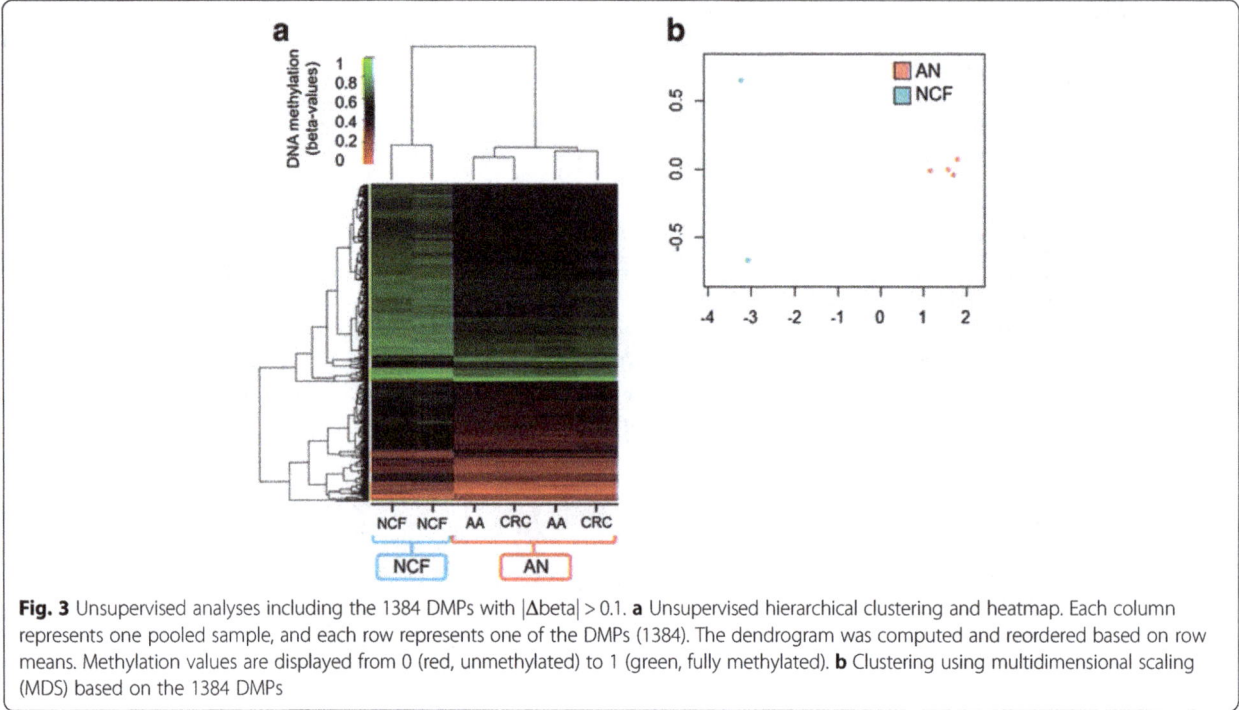

Fig. 3 Unsupervised analyses including the 1384 DMPs with |Δbeta| > 0.1. **a** Unsupervised hierarchical clustering and heatmap. Each column represents one pooled sample, and each row represents one of the DMPs (1384). The dendrogram was computed and reordered based on row means. Methylation values are displayed from 0 (red, unmethylated) to 1 (green, fully methylated). **b** Clustering using multidimensional scaling (MDS) based on the 1384 DMPs

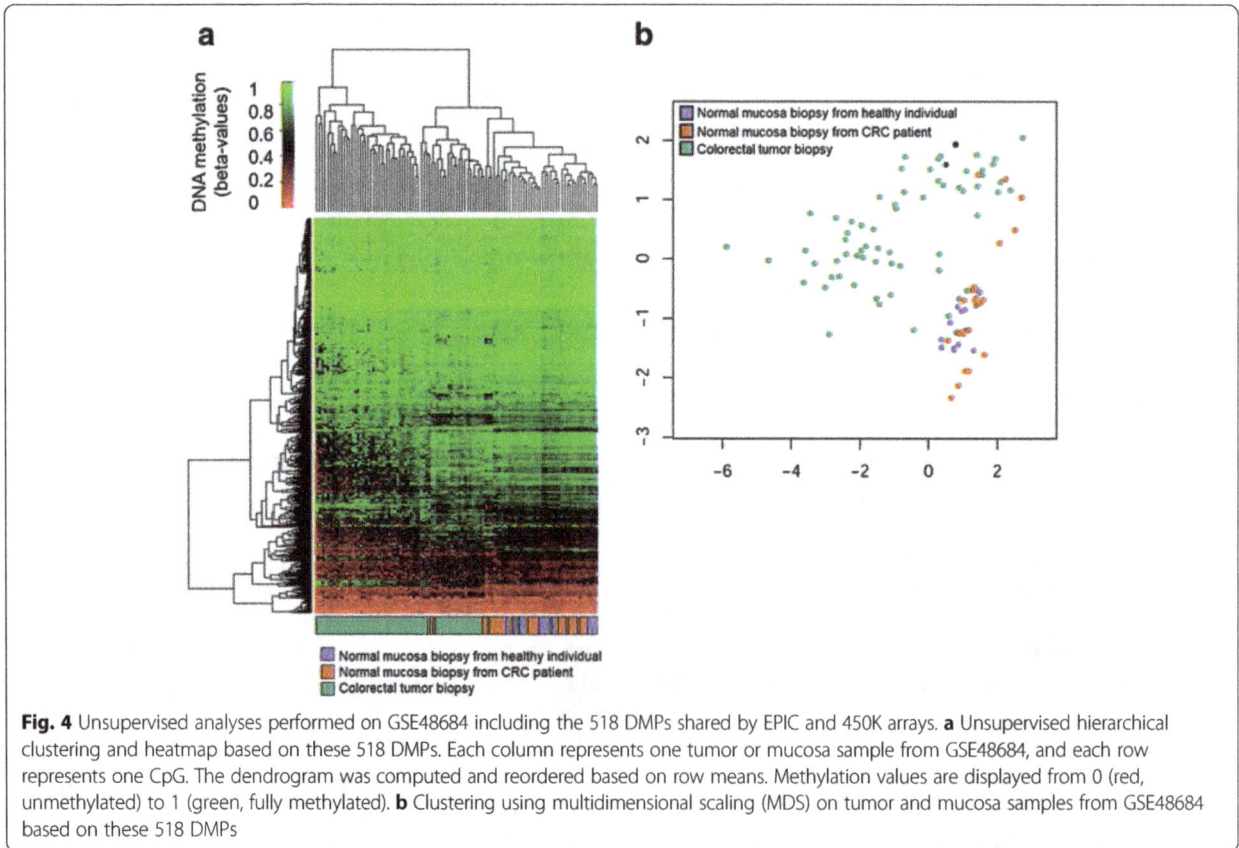

Fig. 4 Unsupervised analyses performed on GSE48684 including the 518 DMPs shared by EPIC and 450K arrays. **a** Unsupervised hierarchical clustering and heatmap based on these 518 DMPs. Each column represents one tumor or mucosa sample from GSE48684, and each row represents one CpG. The dendrogram was computed and reordered based on row means. Methylation values are displayed from 0 (red, unmethylated) to 1 (green, fully methylated). **b** Clustering using multidimensional scaling (MDS) on tumor and mucosa samples from GSE48684 based on these 518 DMPs

time techniques, with the aim of finding a serum methylation panel for CRC diagnosis and screening.

Conclusion

As far as we are concerned, this proof-of-principle study is the first to evaluate pooled serum cfDNA profiling on an epigenome-wide scale for CRC biomarker discovery using the MethylationEPIC array. Our data, although preliminary, revealed that the whole epigenome is represented in pooled serum cfDNA samples and that differentially methylated cfDNA profiles can discriminate NCF controls from AN cases (AA or CRC). These results suggest that a pooling strategy using cfDNA may be a valuable source of novel non-invasive methylation biomarkers for CRC early detection and screening. Also, our approach can be translated to the search of biomarkers for other types of tumors, as an affordable alternative approach to tissue biopsy.

Abbreviations

AA: Advanced adenoma; AN: Advanced neoplasia; cfDNA: Circulating cell-free DNA; CRC: Colorectal cancer; DMP: Differentially methylated position; FDR: False discovery rate; NCF: No colorectal findings

Acknowledgements

We would like to thank Leticia Barcia for her support in daily laboratory work and also Dr. Jezabel Varadé for her advice and tips about the results presentation.

Funding

This work received funding from *Plan Nacional I +D +I 2015-2018* (Acción Estratégica en Salud) Instituto de Salud Carlos III (Spain)-FEDER (PI15/02007), "Fundación Científica de la Asociación Española contra el Cáncer" (GCB13131592CAST), and support from Centro Singular de Investigación de Galicia (Consellería de Cultura, Educación e Ordenación Universitaria) (ED431G/02, Xunta de Galicia and FEDER-European Union). María Gallardo-Gómez is supported by a predoctoral fellowship from Ministerio de Educación, Cultura y Deporte (Spanish Government) (FPU15/02350).

Authors' contributions

LD, VSMZ, and SM conceived and designed the study. LD, MP, FJRB, and ME supervised the study. JC, LB, AC, FB, and RJ clinical advise for the study design, collection, and management of clinical data. MGG, MRG, and MP contributed to the experimental design. MGG, LD, and SM contributed to the sample preparation and data acquisition. LD, MGG, VSMZ, and SM performed the analysis and interpretation of data. MGG, LD, FJRB, and MP prepared the manuscript. All authors critically reviewed and approved the final manuscript.

Author details

[1]Department of Biochemistry, Genetics and Immunology, Centro Singular de Investigación de Galicia (CINBIO), University of Vigo, Campus As Lagoas-Marcosende s/n, 36310 Vigo, Spain. [2]Cancer Epigenetics and Biology Program (PEBC), Bellvitge Biomedical Research Institute (IDIBELL), Barcelona, Spain. [3]Department of Medical Statistics and Bioinformatics, Leiden University Medical Centre, Leiden, The Netherlands. [4]SiDOR Research Group and Centro de Investigaciones Biomédicas (CINBIO), Faculty of Economics and Business Administration, University of Vigo, Vigo, Spain. [5]Department of Gastroenterology, Complexo Hospitalario Universitario de Ourense, Instituto de Investigación Biomédica Galicia Sur, Centro de Investigación Biomédica en Red de Enfermedades Hepáticas y Digestivas (CIBERehd), Ourense, Spain. [6]Department of Gastroenterology, Instituto Biodonostia, Centro de Investigación Biomédica en Red de Enfermedades Hepáticas y Digestivas (CIBERehd), Universidad del País Vasco (UPV/EHU), San Sebastián, Spain. [7]Gastroenterology Department, Hospital Clínic, IDIBAPS, CIBERehd, University of Barcelona, Barcelona, Spain. [8]Department of Gastroenterology, Hospital General Universitario de Alicante, Alicante, Spain.

References

1. Ferlay J, Soerjomataram I, Dikshit R, Eser S, Mathers C, Rebelo M, et al. Cancer incidence and mortality worldwide: sources, methods and major patterns in GLOBOCAN 2012. Int J Cancer. 2015;136:E359–86.
2. Arnold M, Sierra MS, Laversanne M, Soerjomataram I, Jemal A, Bray F. Global patterns and trends in colorectal cancer incidence and mortality. Gut. 2017; 66:683–91. https://doi.org/10.1136/gutjnl-2015-310912.
3. Ng SC, Lau JYW, Chan FKL, Suen BY, Leung WK, Tse YK, et al. Increased risk of advanced neoplasms among asymptomatic siblings of patients with colorectal cancer. Gastroenterology. 2013;144:544–50.
4. Brenner H, Stock C, Hoffmeister M. Colorectal cancer screening: the time to act is now. BMC Med. 2015;13:262. https://doi.org/10.1186/s12916-015-0498-x.
5. Salas Trejo D, Portillo Villares I, Espinàs Piñol JA, Ibáñez Cabanell J, Vanaclocha Espí M, Pérez Riquelme F, et al. Implementation of colorectal cancer screening in Spain. Eur J Cancer Prev. 2017;26:17–26. https://doi.org/10.1097/CEJ.0000000000000232.
6. Castro I, Cubiella J, Rivera C, González-Mao C, Vega P, Soto S, et al. Fecal immunochemical test accuracy in familial risk colorectal cancer screening. Int J Cancer. 2014;134:367–75. https://doi.org/10.1002/ijc.28353.
7. Kim NH, Yang H-J, Park S-K, Park JH, Park DI, Sohn CI, et al. Does low threshold value use improve proximal neoplasia detection by fecal immunochemical test? Dig Dis Sci. 2016;61:2685–93. https://doi.org/10.1007/s10620-016-4169-3.
8. Shah R, Jones E, Vidart V, Kuppen PJK, Conti JA, Francis NK. Biomarkers for early detection of colorectal cancer and polyps: systematic review. Cancer Epidemiol Biomark Prev. 2014;23:1712–28. https://doi.org/10.1158/1055-9965.EPI-14-0412.
9. Song L, Li Y. Progress on the clinical application of the SEPT9 gene methylation assay in the past 5 years. Biomark Med. 2017;11:415–8. https://doi.org/10.2217/bmm-2017-0091.
10. Lao VV, Grady WM. Epigenetics and colorectal cancer. Nat Rev Gastroenterol Hepatol. 2012;8:686–700.
11. Bariol C, Suter C, Cheong K, Ku SL, Meagher A, Hawkins N, et al. The relationship between hypomethylation and CpG island methylation in colorectal neoplasia. Am J Pathol. 2003;162:1361–71.
12. Øster B, Thorsen K, Lamy P, Wojdacz TK, Hansen LL, Birkenkamp-Demtröder K, et al. Identification and validation of highly frequent CpG island hypermethylation in colorectal adenomas and carcinomas. Int J Cancer. 2011; 129:2855–66.
13. Beggs AD, Jones A, El-Bahrawy M, Abulafi M, Hodgson SV, Tomlinson IPM. Whole-genome methylation analysis of benign and malignant colorectal tumours. J Pathol. 2013;229:697–704.
14. Luo Y, Wong CJ, Kaz AM, Dzieciatkowski S, Carter KT, Morris SM, et al. Differences in DNA methylation signatures reveal multiple pathways of progression from adenoma to colorectal cancer. Gastroenterology. 2014;147: 418–29. https://doi.org/10.1053/j.gastro.2014.04.039.
15. Laird PW. Principles and challenges of genome-wide DNA methylation analysis. Nat Rev Genet. 2010;11:191–203. https://doi.org/10.1038/nrg2732.
16. Fan S, Chi W. Methods for genome-wide DNA methylation analysis in human cancer. Brief Funct Genomics. 2016;15:elw010. https://doi.org/10.1093/bfgp/elw010.
17. Norton N, Williams NM, O'Donovan MC, Owen MJ. DNA pooling as a tool for large-scale association studies in complex traits. Ann Med. 2004;36:146–52.
18. Pearson JV, Huentelman MJ, Halperin RF, Tembe WD, Melquist S, Homer N, et al. Identification of the genetic basis for complex disorders by use of pooling-based genomewide single-nucleotide–polymorphism association studies. Am J Hum Genet. 2007;80:126–39. https://doi.org/10.1086/510686.

19. Gallego-Fabrega C, Carrera C, Muiño E, Montaner J, Krupinski J, Fernandez-Cadenas I. DNA methylation levels are highly correlated between pooled samples and averaged values when analysed using the Infinium HumanMethylation450 BeadChip array. Clin Epigenetics. 2015;7:78. https://doi.org/10.1186/s13148-015-0097-x.

20. Schwarzenbach H, Hoon DSB, Pantel K. Cell-free nucleic acids as biomarkers in cancer patients. Nat Rev Cancer. 2011;11:426–37. https://doi.org/10.1038/nrc3066.

21. Krishnamurthy N, Spencer E, Torkamani A, Nicholson L. Liquid biopsies for cancer: coming to a patient near you. J Clin Med. 2017;6:3. https://doi.org/10.3390/jcm6010003.

22. Zhai R, Zhao Y, Su L, Cassidy L, Liu G, Christiani DC. Genome-wide DNA methylation profiling of cell-free serum DNA in esophageal adenocarcinoma and Barrett esophagus. Neoplasia. 2012;14:29–33. https://doi.org/10.1593/neo.111626.

23. Bosch LJW, Mongera S, sive Droste JST, Oort FA, van Turenhout ST, Penning MT, et al. Analytical sensitivity and stability of DNA methylation testing in stool samples for colorectal cancer detection. Cell Oncol. 2012;35:309–15. https://doi.org/10.1007/s13402-012-0092-6.

24. Forat S, Huettel B, Reinhardt R, Fimmers R, Haidl G, Denschlag D, et al. Methylation markers for the identification of body fluids and tissues from forensic trace evidence. PLoS One. 2016;11:e0147973. https://doi.org/10.1371/journal.pone.0147973.

25. Galanopoulos M, Tsoukalas N, Papanikolaou IS, Tolia M, Gazouli M, Mantzaris GJ. Abnormal DNA methylation as a cell-free circulating DNA biomarker for colorectal cancer detection: a review of literature. World J Gastrointest Oncol. 2017;9:142–52. https://doi.org/10.4251/wjgo.v9.i4.142.

26. Quintero E, Castells A, Bujanda L, Cubiella J, Salas D, Lanas Á, et al. Colonoscopy versus fecal immunochemical testing in colorectal-cancer screening. N Engl J Med. 2012;366:697–706. https://doi.org/10.1056/NEJMoa1108895.

27. Edge SB, Compton CC. The American Joint Committee on Cancer: the 7th edition of the AJCC cancer staging manual and the future of TNM. Ann Surg Oncol. 2010;17:1471–4. https://doi.org/10.1245/s10434-010-0985-4.

28. Clemens H, Markus S, Martin M, Roland G, Richard G. A modified phenol-chloroform extraction method for isolating circulating cell free DNA of tumor patients. J Nucleic Acids Investig. 2013;4:1.

29. Sham P, Bader JS, Craig I, O'Donovan M, Owen M. DNA pooling: a tool for large-scale association studies. Nat Rev Genet. 2002;3:862–71.

30. Moran S, Arribas C, Esteller M. Validation of a DNA methylation microarray for 850,000 CpG sites of the human genome enriched in enhancer sequences. Epigenomics. 2016;8:389–99. https://doi.org/10.2217/epi.15.114.

31. ENCODE Project Consortium. An integrated encyclopedia of DNA elements in the human genome. Nature. 2012;489:57–74. https://doi.org/10.1038/nature11247.

32. Siggens L, Ekwall K. Epigenetics, chromatin and genome organization: recent advances from the ENCODE project. J Intern Med. 2014;276:201–14.

33. Lizio M, Harshbarger J, Shimoji H, Severin J, Kasukawa T, Sahin S, et al. Gateways to the FANTOM5 promoter level mammalian expression atlas. Genome Biol. 2015;16:22. https://doi.org/10.1186/s13059-014-0560-6.

34. Aryee MJ, Jaffe AE, Corrada-Bravo H, Ladd-Acosta C, Feinberg AP, Hansen KD, et al. Minfi: a flexible and comprehensive bioconductor package for the analysis of Infinium DNA methylation microarrays. Bioinformatics. 2014;30:1363–9.

35. Morris TJ, Butcher LM, Feber A, Teschendorff AE, Chakravarthy AR, Wojdacz TK, et al. ChAMP: 450k chip analysis methylation pipeline. Bioinformatics. 2014;30:428–30.

36. Fortin J-P, Labbe A, Lemire M, Zanke BW, Hudson TJ, Fertig EJ, et al. Functional normalization of 450k methylation array data improves replication in large cancer studies. Genome Biol. 2014;15:503. https://doi.org/10.1186/s13059-014-0503-2.

37. Pidsley R, Zotenko E, Peters TJ, Lawrence MG, Risbridger GP, Molloy P, et al. Critical evaluation of the Illumina MethylationEPIC BeadChip microarray for whole-genome DNA methylation profiling. Genome Biol. 2016;17:208. https://doi.org/10.1186/s13059-016-1066-1.

38. Du P, Zhang X, Huang C-C, Jafari N, Kibbe WA, Hou L, et al. Comparison of beta-value and M-value methods for quantifying methylation levels by microarray analysis. BMC Bioinformatics. 2010;11:587. https://doi.org/10.1186/1471-2105-11-587.

39. Bibbins-Domingo K, Grossman DC, Curry SJ, Davidson KW, Epling JW, García FAR, et al. Screening for colorectal cancer. JAMA. 2016;315:2564–75. https://doi.org/10.1001/jama.2016.5989.

40. Dedeurwaerder S, Defrance M, Calonne E, Denis H, Sotiriou C, Fuks F. Evaluation of the Infinium methylation 450K technology. Epigenomics. 2011;3:771–84.

41. Ehrlich M. DNA hypomethylation in cancer cells. Epigenomics. 2009;1: 239–59. https://doi.org/10.2217/epi.09.33.

42. Goelz SE, Vogelstein B, Hamilton SR, Feinberg AP. Hypomethylation of DNA from benign and malignant human colon neoplasms. Science. 1985;228: 187–90. https://doi.org/10.1126/SCIENCE.2579435.

43. Okugawa Y, Grady WM, Goel A. Epigenetic alterations in colorectal cancer: emerging biomarkers. Gastroenterology. 2015;149:1204–1225.e12. https://doi.org/10.1053/j.gastro.2015.07.011.

44. Timp W, Bravo HC, McDonald OG, Goggins M, Umbricht C, Zeiger M, et al. Large hypomethylated blocks as a universal defining epigenetic alteration in human solid tumors. Genome Med. 2014;6 https://doi.org/10.1186/s13073-014-0061-y.

45. Jung K, Fleischhacker M, Rabien A. Cell-free DNA in the blood as a solid tumor biomarker—a critical appraisal of the literature. Clin Chim Acta. 2010; 411:1611–24. https://doi.org/10.1016/j.cca.2010.07.032.

46. Roperch JP, Incitti R, Forbin S, Bard F, Mansour H, Mesli F, et al. Aberrant methylation of NPY, PENK, and WIF1 as a promising marker for blood-based diagnosis of colorectal cancer. BMC Cancer. 2013;13:566.

47. Barault L, Amatu A, Siravegna G, Ponzetti A, Moran S, Cassingena A, et al. Discovery of methylated circulating DNA biomarkers for comprehensive non-invasive monitoring of treatment response in metastatic colorectal cancer. Gut. 2017;0:1–11. https://doi.org/10.1136/gutjnl-2016-313372.

48. Heiss JA, Brenner H. Epigenome-wide discovery and evaluation of leukocyte DNA methylation markers for the detection of colorectal cancer in a screening setting. Clin Epigenetics. 2017;9:24. https://doi.org/10.1186/s13148-017-0322-x.

7

Methylation of *BRCA1* and *MGMT* genes in white blood cells are transmitted from mothers to daughters

Nisreen Al-Moghrabi[1*], Maram Al-Showimi[2], Nujoud Al-Yousef[1], Bushra Al-Shahrani[2], Bedri Karakas[1], Lamyaa Alghofaili[3], Hannah Almubarak[1], Safia Madkhali[4] and Hind Al Humaidan[5]

Abstract

Background: Constitutive methylation of tumor suppressor genes are associated with increased cancer risk. However, to date, the question of epimutational transmission of these genes remains unresolved. Here, we studied the potential transmission of *BRCA1* and *MGMT* promoter methylations in mother-newborn pairs.

Methods: A total of 1014 female subjects (cancer-free women, $n = 268$; delivering women, $n = 295$; newborn females, $n = 302$; breast cancer patients, $n = 67$; ovarian cancer patients, $n = 82$) were screened for methylation status in white blood cells (WBC) using methylation-specific PCR and bisulfite pyrosequencing assays. In addition, *BRCA1* gene expression levels were analyzed by quantitative real-time PCR.

Results: We found similar methylation frequencies in newborn and adults for both *BRCA1* (9.9 and 9.3%) and *MGMT* (12.3 and 13.1%). Of the 290 mother-newborn pairs analyzed for promoter methylation, 20 mothers were found to be positive for *BRCA1* and 29 for *MGMT*. Four mother-newborn pairs were positive for methylated *BRCA1* (20%) and nine pairs were positive for methylated *MGMT* (31%). Intriguingly, the delivering women had 26% lower *BRCA1* and *MGMT* methylation frequencies than those of the cancer-free female subjects. *BRCA1* was downregulated in both cancer-free woman carriers and breast cancer patients but not in newborn carriers. There was a statistically significant association between the *MGMT* promoter methylation and late-onset breast cancers.

Conclusions: Our study demonstrates that *BRCA1* and *MGMT* epimutations are present from the early life of the carriers. We show the transmission of *BRCA1* and *MGMT* epimutations from mother to daughter. Our data also point at the possible demethylation of *BRCA1* and *MGMT* during pregnancy.

Keywords: BRCA1, MGMT, Methylation, Transmission, Blood, Breast cancer, Ovarian cancer

Background

Defects in epigenetic manipulation, which results in the atypical transcriptional silencing of active genes and/or reactivation of silent genes, are defined as "Epimutation" [1]. This non-genetic change is a potent mechanism responsible for the suppression of various tumor suppressor genes; hence, it is considered as a mechanism for cancer predisposition [2]. The presence of epimutation in all animal tissues could be either germ line, with evidence of inheritance, or constitutional, with no evidence of inheritance [3–5]. DNA repair genes have been reported to be inactivated in many cancer types by epigenetic silencing mechanism. Deficiencies in these genes usually lead to genetic instability, which is an important mechanism in cancer initiation and/or progression.

BRCA1 is a DNA repair gene that is expressed in all mammalian cells. This gene plays an important role in the error-free pathway of homologous recombination [6], which repairs double-strand breaks. Cells that lack BRCA1 protein are prone to acquire mutations and chromosomal rearrangements, which can lead to carcinogenesis. It is well established that germline *BRCA1* mutations are responsible for many familial cancer types including breast and ovarian cancers [7]. Similarly,

* Correspondence: nisreen@kfshrc.edu.sa
[1]Head of Cancer Epigenetic Section, Molecular Oncology Department, King Faisal Specialist Hospital and Research Centre, PO BOX 3354, Riyadh 11211, Kingdom of Saudi Arabia

methylation in the *BRCA1* promoter is a mechanism for *BRCA1* inactivation during early carcinogenesis. Constitutive *BRCA1* methylation has been found to be associated with a 3.5-fold increase in the risk of developing early-onset breast cancer and a major predisposition factor for serous ovarian cancer [8–13]. This renders the constitutive *BRCA1* promoter methylation as a potential predictive biomarker for breast and ovarian cancer predisposition [12].

MGMT is another DNA repair gene that is also inactivated in human cancers by promoter methylation [14, 15]. It is involved in the removal of an alkyl group from the O^6 position of the guanine nucleotide [16]. The loss of *MGMT* activity leads to G>A transition due to the inability of removing the mutagenic adducts from guanine [17] resulting in DNA aberrations and tumor progression [18]. It has been reported that *MGMT* methylation is a common mechanism in triple negative breast cancers (TNBC) where it has been detected in 83.1% of the cases with a weak association with advanced age [19]. Furthermore, *MGMT* promoter methylation and the lack of *MGMT* expression were found to be associated with the mucinous and clear cell subtypes of epithelial ovarian cancer [20]. To date, the prevalence of *MGMT* methylation in cancer-free individuals and its potential inheritance have not been studied.

Transgenerational epigenetic inheritance is the passage of epigenetic markers, such as DNA methylation, through germline from one generation to the next. Evidences of epimutation inheritance have been reported for the DNA mismatch repair genes *MLH1* and *MSH2* [21–23]. Since no association has been found between the presence of *BRCA1* methylation in peripheral blood cells and age [9, 10], it has been also suggested that *BRCA1* epimutation might be inherited. However, up to date, the question of germ line *BRCA1*epimutation inheritance remains unresolved.

In this study, we investigated the prevalence of *BRCA1* and *MGMT* promoter methylations in white blood cells (WBC) from cancer-free women and newborn females. In addition, we investigated the potential transmission of the epimutation of the two genes from mother to daughter in mother-newborn female pairs.

Results

Cancer-free women and newborns have similar frequencies of WBC *BRCA1* promoter methylation

To investigate the potential transmission of methylated *BRCA1* promoter from mother to daughter, we examined the *BRCA1* promoter methylation status in DNA from WBC using MSP assay in a cohort of 865 female subjects (cancer-free women, $n = 268$; delivering women, $n = 295$; newborn females, $n = 302$). The cohort of the mothers and newborns included 290 mother-newborn

pairs. We detected the *BRCA1* promoter methylation in 25 of 268 (9.3%) cancer-free women and in 20 of 295 (6.8%) delivering women (Fig. 1a and Table 1). Interestingly, 30 of 302 (9.9%) newborns were positive for the methylated *BRCA1* promoter. This shows that cancer-free women and newborns have similar frequencies of *BRCA1* promoter methylation in their WBC.

Cancer-free woman and newborn carriers have similar levels and pattern of WBC *BRCA1* promoter CpG Island methylation

To further elucidate the *BRCA1* promoter methylation status in newborn carriers as compared to woman carriers, we analyzed the level and the pattern of the *BRCA1* promoter methylation in their WBC. The methylation levels and patterns were studied by sodium bisulfite pyrosequencing in 10 CpG sites located in the *BRCA1* promoter at the 5′ flanking region. This region is known to have a strong promoter activity. Both women and newborns' WBC DNA showed a distinct pattern of *BRCA1* methylation wherein – 134 and – 37 sites showed higher levels of methylation compared to other sites (Fig. 2a, b). Furthermore, both DNA types contained similar levels of methylation across the 10 CpG sites. This indicates that the level and pattern of WBC *BRCA1* promoter methylation are similar in woman and newborn carriers.

BRCA1 epimutation is transmitted from mother to daughter

Interestingly, we found four out of the 20 mothers (20%), who were tested positive for *BRCA1* methylation, had *BRCA1* methylation-positive daughters (Fig. 1c, d). This result is the first indication of the transmission of *BRCA1* epimutation from mother to daughter. To further verify the methylation in the positive mother-newborn pairs, the promoter region was analyzed by pyrosequencing in three pairs (Fig. 2g). Importantly, both mothers and newborns' WBC DNA showed similar pattern and levels of methylation across the CpG sites analyzed. Importantly, we found one of the newborn carriers, who have a *BRCA1* methylation-negative mother, has also a *BRCA1* methylation negative father.

MGMT promoter is methylated in both cancer-free women and newborns

We have previously shown that the *MGMT* gene is methylated in WBC of cancer-free *BRCA1* methylation carriers [24]. Thus, in this study, we sought to investigate whether there is an association between the presence of *BRCA1* and *MGMT* promoter methylations in WBC. To this end, we analyzed the *MGMT* promoter methylation in WBC using MSP assay in the same cohort of 865 cancer-free females. We detected the *MGMT* methylation in 35 of 268 (13.1%) cancer-free women, in 29 of 295 (9.8%) delivering women, and in 37 of 302

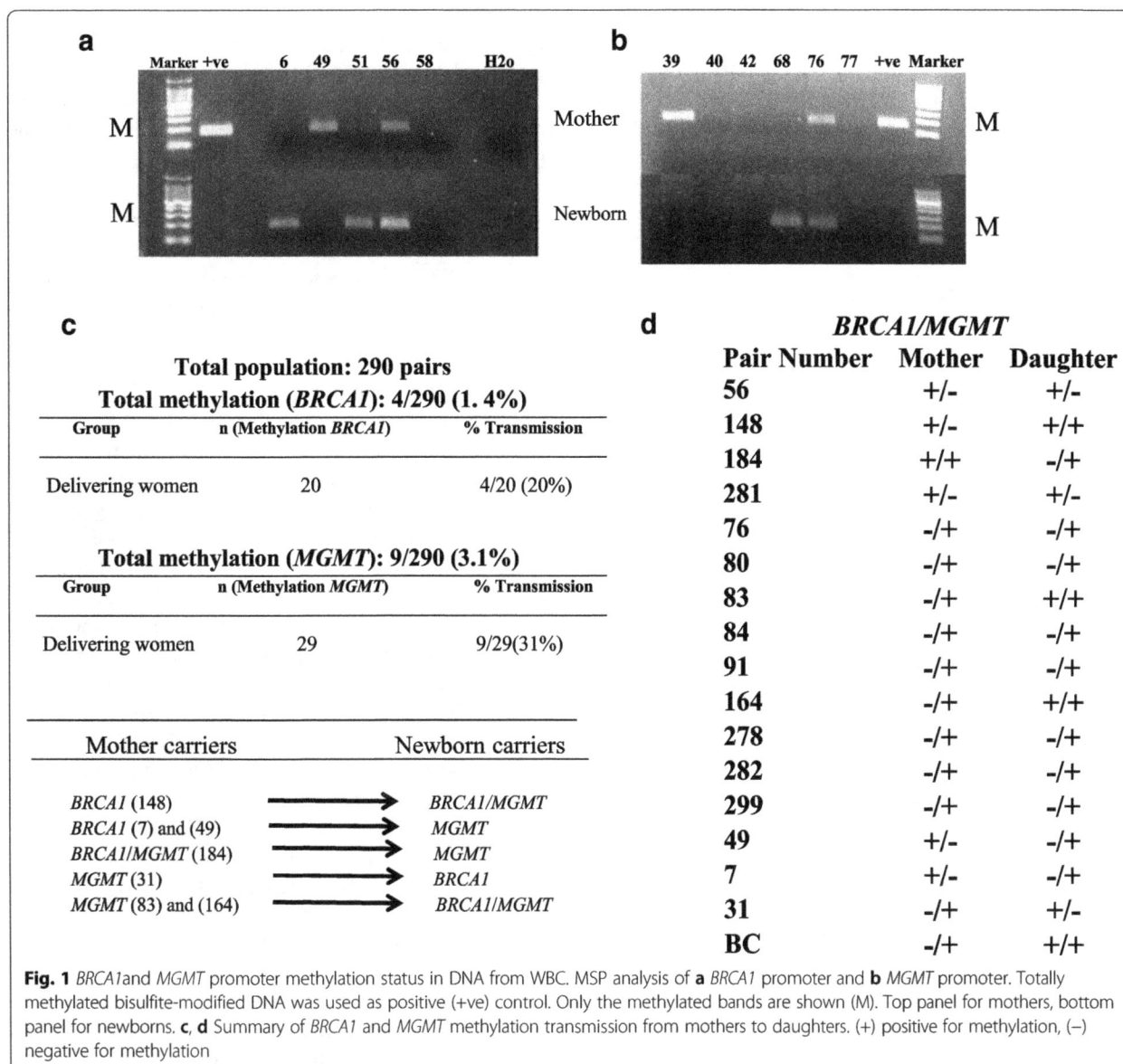

Fig. 1 *BRCA1* and *MGMT* promoter methylation status in DNA from WBC. MSP analysis of **a** *BRCA1* promoter and **b** *MGMT* promoter. Totally methylated bisulfite-modified DNA was used as positive (+ve) control. Only the methylated bands are shown (M). Top panel for mothers, bottom panel for newborns. **c, d** Summary of *BRCA1* and *MGMT* methylation transmission from mothers to daughters. (+) positive for methylation, (−) negative for methylation

(12.3%) newborns (Fig. 1b and Table 1). These results show a high prevalence of methylated *MGMT* promoter in both adult and newborns. Importantly, we found six women (24%), two delivering women (10%), and three newborns (10%) to be positive for paired *BRCA1/MGMT* methylation (Table 1).

MGMT epimutation is transmitted from mother to daughter
Interestingly, nine out of the 29 mothers (31%), who were tested positive for *MGMT* methylation, had *MGMT* methylation-positive daughters (Fig. 1c, d). This is also the first reported result suggesting the transmission of *MGMT* epimutation from mother to daughter. Additionally interesting, we found two *BRCA1* methylation-positive mothers having *MGMT* methylation-positive daughters and vice versa (Fig. 1c, d). Notably, the mother of a *BRCA1* woman

carrier was a breast cancer patient who was positive for methylated *MGMT* (Fig. 1d).

MGMT promoter methylation is associated with ovarian cancer and the late onset of breast cancer
In order to value the epimutation of *MGMT* and *BRCA1* in WBC from cancer-free women and newborns, we investigated the prevalence of the methylated *BRCA1* and *MGMT* promoters in breast and ovarian cancer patients. To this end, we screened 67 breast and 82 ovarian cancer patients using MSP assay. We found that 5 out of 67 (7.5%) breast and 13 out of 82 (15.8%) ovarian cancer patients tested positive for *BRCA1* promoter methylation (Table 1). Moreover, 10 of 67 (15%) breast and 17 of 82 (20.7%) ovarian cancer patients were positive for *MGMT* methylation (Table 1). We did not detect

Table 1 Percentage of WBC DNA *BRCA1* and *MGMT* methylations

	Total population (n = 1014)	
Gene	Group	Promoter methylation (%)
BRCA1	Control women	25/268 (9.3)
	Delivering women	20/295 (6.8)
	Newborns	30/302 (9.9)
	Breast cancer	5/67 (7.5)
	Ovarian cancer	13/82 (15.8)
MGMT	Control women	35/268 (13.1)
	Delivering women	29/295 (9.8)
	Newborns	37/302 (12.3)
	Breast cancer	10/67 (15)
	Ovarian cancer	17/82 (20.7)
	Group	Methylation (%)
BRCA1/MGMT	Control women	6/25 (24)
	Delivering women	2/20 (10)
	Newborns	3/30 (10)
	Breast cancer	0
	Ovarian cancer	5/17 (29.4)

any case with both *BRCA1* and *MGMT* methylations in breast cancer patients. However, in a cohort of 17 breast cancer patients who were tested positive for *BRCA1* methylation in our previous study [24], four patients (23.5%) were found to be positive for *MGMT* methylation (Table 2). Interestingly, we found that the mean age for the onset of breast cancer in the *BRCA1* methylation-positive patients was 40.3 ± 6.4 (95%CI 37.1–43.4) years compared to 50.9 ± 12.7 (95%CI 41.8–60) years for methylated *MGMT* and 56 ± 14.1(95%CI 33.8–78.7) years for both *BRCA1/MGMT*-methylated patients ($p = 0.0044$). This indicates a significant association between the *MGMT* methylation and late onset of the disease, ($p = 0.0253$) for *MGMT* alone and ($p = 0.0157$) for paired *BRCA1/MGMT*. Importantly, five of the 13 (38.5%) *BRCA1* methylation-positive ovarian cancer patients had methylated *MGMT* gene. However, no association was found between the *MGMT* methylation and the onset of the disease (Table 3).

BRCA1 expression is reduced in breast cancer patients and woman carriers but not in newborn carriers

Next, we sought to assess the expression of *BRCA1*, at the level of mRNA, in WBC. To this end, we analyzed the expression level of the *BRCA1* gene by real-time RT-PCR in the newborn carriers, woman carriers, and *BRCA1* methylation-positive breast cancer patients. Interestingly, we did not find any reduction in the expression level of the *BRCA1* in six highly methylated newborns as compared to unmethylated controls (Fig. 2a, d). However, in woman carriers, the expression level was reduced by two folds in three out of five woman carriers (Fig. 2b, e).

Furthermore, we found a considerable reduction in the expression level of the *BRCA1* in six out of nine breast cancer patients (Fig. 2c, f). Interestingly, the fold change of the *BRCA1* expression level in breast cancer patients highly correlated ($R = 0.89$) with patient's age in eight out of nine cases (Fig. 2h). We were not able to analyze the expression level of *BRCA1* in ovarian cancer patients due to lack of RNA samples. However, we found extensive disorganization in the pattern and levels of methylation across the 23 CpG sites in the promoter region as compared to that in cancer-free woman and newborn carriers (Fig. 2i).

Discussion and conclusions

In this study, we have screened a total of 865 females for their WBC *BRCA1* and *MGMT* promoters' methylation status by the MSP assay. The overall frequencies were 8.7% for the *BRCA1* and 11.7% for the *MGMT* gene promoter. Remarkably, we found the frequency of *BRCA1* methylation to be similar in both newborns and adult females and are analogous to our previously reported frequencies [11, 24]. Importantly, both newborn and adult samples showed identical pattern and levels of methylation across all the studied CpG sites in the *BRCA1* promoter. This indicates that constitutional epimutation of the *BRCA1* gene is present from the early life of the carriers, as opposed to the belief that it is acquired later on during the lifetime of the individual.

The frequencies of *BRCA1* and *MGMT* methylations in delivering women were about 26% lower than that of both adult and newborn females, suggesting that the *BRCA1* and *MGMT* promoters are demethylated in women during pregnancy. Indeed, it has been reported that pregnancy reprograms the epigenome as a protective mechanism against breast cancer in women [25]. In addition, it was found that the IGF acid labile subunit, which is responsible for transporting the IGF1 protein in the blood circulation, is activated by hypomethylation whereas the IGF1R is silenced by hypermethylation [26]. Thus, the epigenetic modifications of these two genes could contribute to the protective outcome of early pregnancy and parity against breast cancers. Hence, it is plausible that in a portion of the delivering women, the *BRCA1* and *MGMT* promoters are demethylated due to either parity or early pregnancy as a protective mechanism against breast and ovarian cancers. However, further studies with larger sample size are needed to verify this.

Our group is the first to report the transmission of the *BRCA1* and *MGMT* epimutations from mothers to daughters. Although the overall frequency of inheritance was low, 1.4% for *BRCA1* and 3.1% for *MGMT*, it accounted for a high proportion of the mother carriers. In a recent report, the authors have concluded that *BRCA1* methylation is not transmitted from mother to

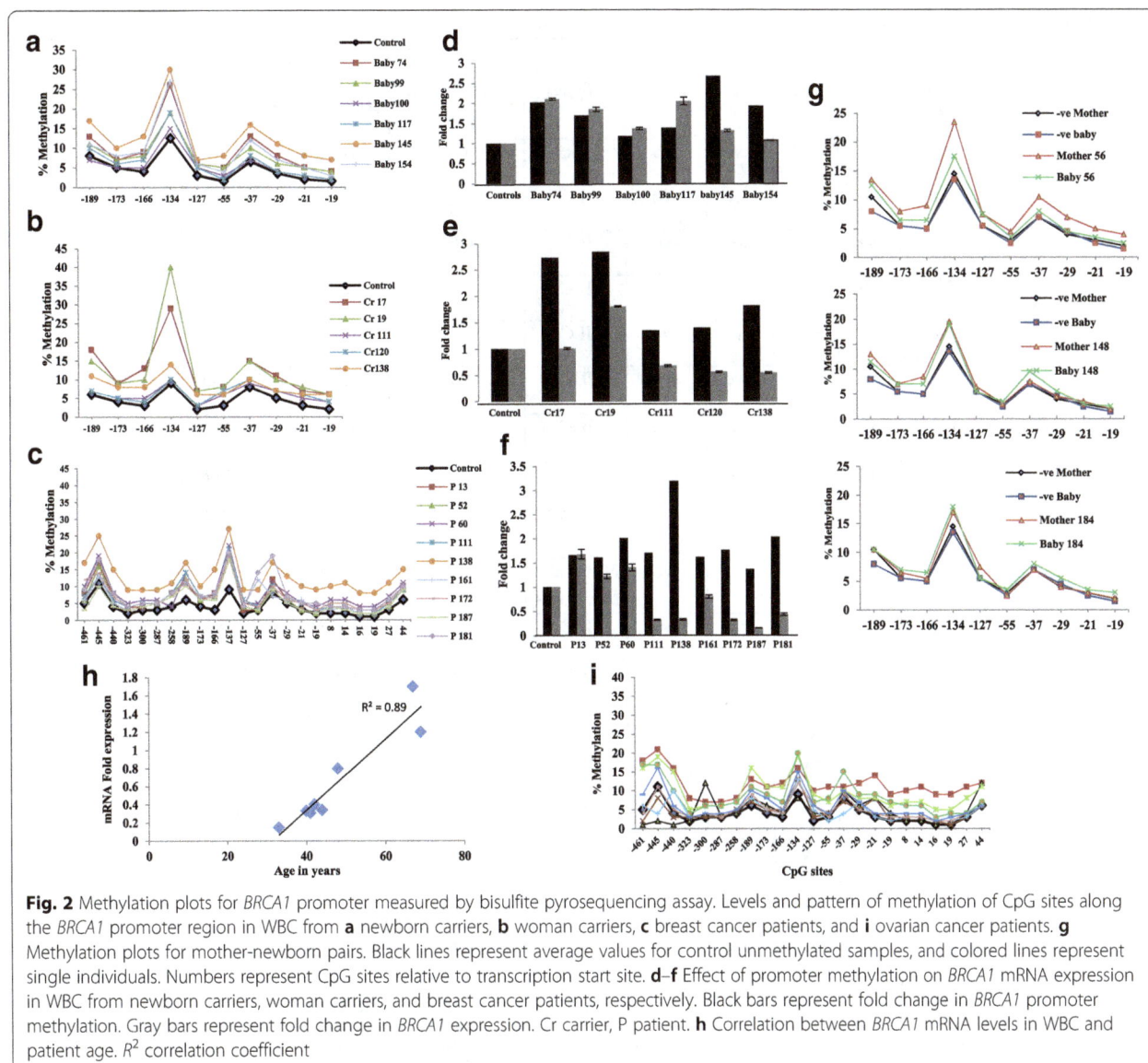

Fig. 2 Methylation plots for *BRCA1* promoter measured by bisulfite pyrosequencing assay. Levels and pattern of methylation of CpG sites along the *BRCA1* promoter region in WBC from **a** newborn carriers, **b** woman carriers, **c** breast cancer patients, and **i** ovarian cancer patients. **g** Methylation plots for mother-newborn pairs. Black lines represent average values for control unmethylated samples, and colored lines represent single individuals. Numbers represent CpG sites relative to transcription start site. **d–f** Effect of promoter methylation on *BRCA1* mRNA expression in WBC from newborn carriers, woman carriers, and breast cancer patients, respectively. Black bars represent fold change in *BRCA1* promoter methylation. Gray bars represent fold change in *BRCA1* expression. Cr carrier, P patient. **h** Correlation between *BRCA1* mRNA levels in WBC and patient age. R^2 correlation coefficient

daughter [27]. The discordance between the two studies could be due to the sample sizes, 6 mother-daughter pairs versus 290 pairs in our study. Although, in our study, *BRCA1* methylation was not transmitted from father to daughter, we cannot rule out the potential inheritance through paternal germ line as only one father was tested. However, we can conclude from this result that the majority of *BRCA1* epimutation appears to occur during early development, which could be due to an exposure to environmental insults. The finding that *BRCA1* mother carriers have *MGMT* newborn carriers, and vice versa may indicate a possible link between the constitutional epimutation of these two genes. Additionally important, it does rule out the possibility of contamination of maternal blood in cord samples.

The inheritance of methylated cancer-associated genes has been previously reported [21, 22]. As constitutive methylation of *BRCA1* and *MGMT* has been found to associate with an increased risk of cancer development [8–13, 28], it is conceivable to believe that the affected daughter has a high risk for developing these cancers. Indeed, it has been reported that a mother with constitutional *MLH1* and who had Lynch syndrome has transmitted *MLH1* epimutation to two of her children who developed also early colonic tumors [23].

It is still not clear whether epimutational inheritance occurs per se or it arises due to cross linkage to cis-acting genetic lesions. Several studies have revealed the constitutional epimutation of tumor suppressor genes to be linked to *cis*-acting genetic lesions [29–31]. As no such genetic lesion has been found in the promoter of *BRCA1* to explain its methylation [13], the inheritance of *BRCA1* methylation, we report in this study, may support the concept of transgenerational epigenetic inheritance.

Table 2 Clinical characterizations of *BRCA1*- and *MGMT*-methylated breast cancer-positive cases

Patient #	Age	ER	PR	HER-2	Type	Histological grade	BRCA1	MGMT
13	67	+ve	+ve	-ve	ILC	GI	Meth	Meth
138	40	+ve	+ve	-ve	IDC	GII	Meth	Meth
176	49	-ve	-ve	-ve	IDC	GIII	Meth	Meth
52	69	+ve	+ve	-ve	ILC	GI	Meth	Meth
54	39	+ve	+ve	-ve	ILC	GII	Meth	Un Meth
142	56	+ve	+ve	-ve	IDC	GII	Meth	Un meth
195	33	+ve	-ve	-ve	IDC	GIII	Meth	Un Meth
197	40	-ve	-ve	-ve	IDC	GIII	Meth	Un Meth
202	44	+ve	+ve	-ve	IDC	GII	Meth	Un Meth
101	53	-ve	-ve	-ve	Metastatic carcinoma	ND	Un Meth	Meth
112	75	+ve	+ve	-ve	IPC	ND	Un Meth	Meth
155	59	+ve	+ve	-ve	IDC	GII	Un Meth	Meth
162	36	+ve	+ve	+ve	IDC	GIII	Un Meth	Meth
191	38	+ve	+ve	-ve	IDC	GII	Un Meth	Meth
200	54	-ve	-ve	+ve	IDC	GIII	Un Meth	Meth
7	33	+ve	+ve	eqa	IDC	GIII	Un Meth	Meth
12	51	+ve	+ve	-ve	ILC	GI	Un Meth	Meth
20	46	+ve	+ve	eqa	IDC	GII	Un Meth	Meth
35	64	+ve	+ve	-ve	IDC	GII	Un Meth	Meth

Shaded area specifies patients identified in our previous study (reference [24])
ILC invasive lobular carcinoma, *IDC* invasive ductal carcinoma, *ND* no data

In this study, we report a high frequency of constitutional *BRCA1* and *MGMT* methylation in breast and ovarian cancer. The detection of methylated *BRCA1* in WBC from ovarian cancer was reported previously in 20 out of 154 cases [32]. Although several studies have shown high frequencies of methylated *MGMT* promoter in breast and ovarian tumor tissues, our study is the first in finding the methylated *MGMT* in patients' peripheral WBC [19, 20, 33, 34] suggesting that as in *BRCA1*, *MGMT* epigenetic modification in WBC also predispose women to breast and ovarian cancer. While we found a significant association between constitutional *BRCA1* methylation and early onset breast cancers (≤ 40 years) [11, 24], the constitutional *MGMT* methylation was significantly associated with late onset (≥ 50 years). Our results are in concordance with a previous study where a weak association was found between *MGMT* methylation with advanced age in triple negative breast cancers [19].

The analysis of the pattern and levels of methylation across the CpG sites in the *BRCA1* promoter region revealed that this pattern was very well-defined in the newborn and adult carriers but it was highly disorganized in the breast and ovarian cancer patients. Although in newborn carriers, we found high methylation levels in a region known to have strong promoter activity; this did not decrease the *BRCA1* expression. This is in accord with the argument that constitutional methylation is mono allelic [35]; consequently, only one allele of the *BRCA1* gene is methylated in the newly born carriers. However, according to the Knudson's two-hit hypothesis, in the breast cancer patients, the two alleles are affected through the progress

Table 3 Clinical characterizations of *BRCA1*- and *MGMT*-methylated ovarian cancer patients

Patient no.	Age	Type	Grade	BRCA1	MGMT
2	54	Clear cell carcinoma	Advanced	Meth	Meth
13	54	Serous carcinoma	High	Meth	Meth
36	55	Ovarian serous carcinoma	High	Meth	Meth
50	43	Ovarian serous carcinoma.	High	Meth	Meth
23	40	Serous carcinoma	High	Mut/Meth	Meth
38	54	Serous carcinoma	ND	Mut/Meth	Un Meth
7	57	Papillary serous carcinoma	High	Meth	Un Meth
24	53	Serous adenocarcinoma	3	Meth	Un Meth
27	47	Serous carcinoma involving uterus	High	Meth	Un Meth
52	67	ovarian adenocarcinoma	High	Meth	Un Meth
59	53	ovarian serous carcinoma	High	Meth	Un Meth
71	38	Ovarian serous carcinoma	ND	Meth	Un Meth
29	47	Carcinoma of the right ovary	High	Meth	Un Meth
6	58	Papillary serous carcinoma	High	Mut	Meth
14	34	Serous adenocarcinoma	High	Mut	Meth
47	65	Poorly differentiated adenocarcinoma	ND	Mut	Meth
17	66	serous ovarian carcinoma	ND	Mut	Meth
69	41	Ovarian serous carcinoma	ND	Mut	Meth
4	38	Clear cell carcinoma	GII	WT	Meth
9	46	papillary serous cancer	High	WT	Meth
16	67	Serous adenocarcinoma	High	WT	Meth
44	88	Metastatic granulosa cell tumor	ND	WT	Meth
55	43	serous carcinoma	High	WT	Meth
60	49	Granulosa cell tumor	ND	WT	Meth
79	44	Mucinous cyst adenocarcinoma	ND	WT	Meth

Meth methylated, *Mut* mutated, *WT* wild type, *ND* no data

of the patient's life [36]. Indeed, in the woman carriers, a twofold decrease in the expression level of the *BRCA1* mRNA was found in three out of five individuals, while the highest level of reduction in *BRCA1* expression was detected in breast cancer cases, which, interestingly, correlated highly ($R = 0.89$) with patient's age reflecting the association between *BRCA1* promoter methylation and the early onset of the disease. Importantly, lower *BRCA1* expression was detected in blood leukocytes from healthy unaffected *BRCA1*mutation carriers as compared to that in controls [37] indicating the similarity between the effect of methylated and mutated *BRCA1*.

In conclusion, we have clearly shown:

1- The transmission of both *BRCA1* and *MGMT* epimutations from mother to daughter.
2- The frequencies of *BRCA1* and *MGMT* epimutations in female newborns are similar to that of cancer-free women.

3- Our data point at the possible demethylation of *BRCA1* and *MGMT* through reprograming of the epigenome during pregnancy.
4- *MGMT* epimutation is associated with ovarian cancer and the late onset of breast cancer.
Our study sheds some light on the potential use of epimutations in cord blood as predictive biomarkers for cancer.

Methods
Study population
The study was approved by the Human Research Ethics Committee of the King Faisal Specialist Hospital and Research Centre according to the Declaration of Helsinki. All participants provided written consent before participation. Ten milliliters of cord blood and 10 ml of maternal peripheral blood were collected at the time of delivery at Al Yamamah Hospital (Riyadh), age of mothers range 19–46 years. Additionally, 10 ml of fresh peripheral blood was collected from cancer-free females, age range

Table 4 Bisulfite pyrosequencing and real-time PCR primers

	Primers sequences	No. of CpG sites	Annealing temp
F1 R1Bio Sequencing	GGTATTGGATGTTTTTTTTTATAAGATTAT CCAATCCCCCACTCTTTC ATTATAGTTTTTAAGGAATATTGTG	3	56
F2 R2 Sequencing	GAAAGAGTGGGGGATTGGGATT AAAATACCTACCCTCTAACCTCTACT ACCTCTACTCTTCCA	4	60
F3 R3 Bio Sequencing	AGGGTAGGTATTTTATGGTAAATTTAGGT TATCTAAAAAACCCCACAACCTATCC ATGGTAAATTTAGGTAGAATTTT	5	60
F4 R4Bio Sequencing	AGATTGGGTGGTTAATTTAGAGT TCTAAAAAACCCCACAACCTATCC GGAAAAGAGAGGGAATTATAGATAA	6	58
F5 R5 Bio Sequencing	GGGGTAGATTGGGTGGTTAA TTATCTAAAAAACCCCACAACCTATC GAGAGGTTGTTGTTTAG	5	58
BRCA1	F 5′–TGTAGGCTCCTTTTGGTTATATCATTC–3′ R 5′–CATGCTGAAACT TCTCAACCAGAA–3′		59 °C
β- *Actin*	F 5′–TCC CTG GAG AAG AGC TAC GA–3′ R 5′–TGA AGG TAG TTT CGT GGA TGC–3′		59 °C

F forward, *R* reverse

15–50 years, and from breast and ovarian cancer patients coming to the oncology department in King Faisal Specialist Hospital and Research Centre in Riyadh, Saudi Arabia. Clinicopathological data (age, histological grade, and ER and PR status) were provided by the Department of Pathology. All blood samples were collected into EDTA tubes.

Blood DNA and RNA isolation

Blood samples were immediately centrifuged at 2000×*g* for 10 min at 4 °C, and WBCs were carefully collected and transferred into two 2-ml Eppendorf tubes, one containing 900 ml RBC Lysis solution for subsequent DNA extraction using the Gentra Puregene Blood Kit and the other tube contained 1.2 ml RNALater solution for subsequent RNA extraction using RiboPure Blood Kit (Ambion).

Methylation-specific PCR

DNA was treated with sodium bisulfate DNA and purified using EpiTect Bisulfite Kit (Qiagen) following the manufacturer's recommendations. The DNA was then amplified using published PCR primers for *BRCA1* and *MGMT* [38, 39] that distinguish methylated and unmethylated DNA. PCR products were electrophoresed on 2% agarose gels and stained with Ethidium bromide. Totally methylated bisulfite-treated DNA was used as positive control. All the PCR reactions were repeated at least twice.

Bisulfite pyrosequencing

DNA methylation was quantified by bisulfite pyrosequencing. Five different assays were designed using the PyroMark Assay Design software (Qiagen) in order to analyze the methylation status of 23 CpG sites across the *BRCA1* promoter. All the primers used in PCR

amplifications and sequencings are listed in Table 4. The PCR and pyrosequencing reactions were performed using PyroMark products and reagents (Qiagen) as previously described [40]. Methylation quantification was performed using PyroMark Q24 software (Qiagen).

Real-time PCR

cDNA was generated from RNA by Superscript III (Invitrogen) reverse transcriptase and random hexomers. Quantitative real-time PCR was then performed with primer pairs specific for *BRCA1* transcript using *Actin* as an internal control. Primers are listed in Table 4. PCR was performed with SYBR green using CFX96 Real-Time System (Bio-Rad). The relative *BRCA1* expression was calculated based on the threshold cycle (Ct) value using the $2^{-\Delta\Delta ct}$ method. The fold change of mRNA expression was done relative to unmethylated cancer-free women for breast cancer patients and woman carriers and relative to unmethylated babies for the newly born baby carriers.

Statistical analysis

General linear regression (GLM) was performed to determine the statistical significance for the association between *BRCA1* and *MGMT* promoter methylation and age of patients. All observed differences were considered to be significant when associated with a *p* value < 0.05.

Acknowledgements
We are grateful to the mothers, patients, and controls who participated in this study. We would like to acknowledge Dr. Abdelilah Aboussekhra for revising the article.

Funding
This work was supported by The National Comprehensive Plan for science and Technology, project number 14-MED2307-20.

Authors' contributions

NM conceived and designed the study. NM, MS, NY, and BS performed the data analysis. LA, SM, and HH contributed to the sample and data collection. NM drafted the manuscript with the help from BK and HA. All authors read and approved the final manuscript.

Author details

[1]Head of Cancer Epigenetic Section, Molecular Oncology Department, King Faisal Specialist Hospital and Research Centre, PO BOX 3354, Riyadh 11211, Kingdom of Saudi Arabia. [2]Cancer Epigenetic section, Department of Molecular Oncology, King Faisal Specialist Hospital and Research Centre, PO BOX 3354, Riyadh 11211, Kingdom of Saudi Arabia. [3]Al Faisal University College of Medicine, PO BOX 50927, Riyadh 11533, Kingdom of Saudi Arabia. [4]King Saud bin Abdulaziz University for Health Sciences, PO BOX 22490, Riyadh 3130, Kingdom of Saudi Arabia. [5]Department of pathology and Laboratory Medicine, King Faisal Specialist Hospital and Research Centre, PO BOX 3354, Riyadh 11211, Kingdom of Saudi Arabia.

References

1. Cropley JE, Martin DI, Suter CM. Germline epimutation in humans. Pharmacogenomics. 2008;9(12):1861–8.
2. Jones PA, Baylin SB. The fundamental role of epigenetic events in cancer. Nat Rev Genet. 2002;3(6):415–28.
3. Chong S, Youngson NA, Whitelaw E. Heritable germline epimutation is not the same as transgenerational epigenetic inheritance. Nat Genet. 2007;39(5):574–5. author reply 575-576
4. Horsthemke B. Heritable germline epimutations in humans. Nat Genet. 2007;39(5):573–4. author reply 575-576
5. Suter CM, Martin DI. Inherited epimutation or a haplotypic basis for the propensity to silence? Nat Genet. 2007;39(5):573. author reply 576
6. Jacinto FV, Esteller M. Mutator pathways unleashed by epigenetic silencing in human cancer. Mutagenesis. 2007;22(4):247–53.
7. Welcsh PL, King MC. BRCA1 and BRCA2 and the genetics of breast and ovarian cancer. Hum Mol Genet. 2001;10(7):705–13.
8. Matros E, Wang ZC, Lodeiro G, Miron A, Iglehart JD, Richardson AL. BRCA1 promoter methylation in sporadic breast tumors: relationship to gene expression profiles. Breast Cancer Res Treat. 2005;91(2):179–86.
9. Iwamoto T, Yamamoto N, Taguchi T, Tamaki Y, Noguchi S. BRCA1 promoter methylation in peripheral blood cells is associated with increased risk of breast cancer with BRCA1 promoter methylation. Breast Cancer Res Treat. 2011;129(1):69–77.
10. Kontorovich T, Cohen Y, Nir U, Friedman E. Promoter methylation patterns of ATM, ATR, BRCA1, BRCA2 and p53 as putative cancer risk modifiers in Jewish BRCA1/BRCA2 mutation carriers. Breast Cancer Res Treat. 2009;116(1):195–200.
11. Al-Moghrabi N, Al-Qasem AJ, Aboussekhra A. Methylation-related mutations in the BRCA1 promoter in peripheral blood cells from cancer-free women. Int J Oncol. 2011;39(1):129–35.
12. Wong EM, Southey MC, Fox SB, Brown MA, Dowty JG, Jenkins MA, Giles GG, Hopper JL, Dobrovic A. Constitutional methylation of the BRCA1 promoter is specifically associated with BRCA1 mutation-associated pathology in early-onset breast cancer. Cancer Prev Res (Phila). 2011;4(1):23–33.
13. Hansmann T, Pliushch G, Leubner M, Kroll P, Endt D, Gehrig A, Preisler-Adams S, Wieacker P, Haaf T. Constitutive promoter methylation of BRCA1 and RAD51C in patients with familial ovarian cancer and early-onset sporadic breast cancer. Hum Mol Genet. 2012;21(21):4669–79.
14. Cho YH, Yazici H, Wu HC, Terry MB, Gonzalez K, Qu M, Dalay N, Santella RM. Aberrant promoter hypermethylation and genomic hypomethylation in tumor, adjacent normal tissues and blood from breast cancer patients. Anticancer Res. 2010;30(7):2489–96.
15. Cho YH, McCullough LE, Gammon MD, Wu HC, Zhang YJ, Wang Q, Xu X, Teitelbaum SL, Neugut AI, Chen J, et al. Promoter hypermethylation in white blood cell DNA and breast cancer risk. J Cancer. 2015;6(9):819–24.
16. Daniels DS, Woo TT, Luu KX, Noll DM, Clarke ND, Pegg AE, Tainer JA. DNA binding and nucleotide flipping by the human DNA repair protein AGT. Nat Struct Mol Biol. 2004;11(8):714–20.
17. Gerson SL. MGMT: its role in cancer aetiology and cancer therapeutics. Nat Rev Cancer. 2004;4(4):296–307.

18. Kim JI, Suh JT, Choi KU, Kang HJ, Shin DH, Lee IS, Moon TY, Kim WT. Inactivation of O6-methylguanine-DNA methyltransferase in soft tissue sarcomas: association with K-ras mutations. Hum Pathol. 2009;40(7):934–41.
19. Fumagalli C, Pruneri G, Possanzini P, Manzotti M, Barile M, Feroce I, Colleoni M, Bonanni B, Maisonneuve P, Radice P, et al. Methylation of O6-methylguanine-DNA methyltransferase (MGMT) promoter gene in triple-negative breast cancer patients. Breast Cancer Res Treat. 2012;134(1):131–7.
20. Roh HJ, Suh DS, Choi KU, Yoo HJ, Joo WD, Yoon MS. Inactivation of O(6)-methylguanine-DNA methyltransferase by promoter hypermethylation: association of epithelial ovarian carcinogenesis in specific histological types. J Obstet Gynaecol Res. 2011;37(7):851–60.
21. Hitchins MP, Wong JJ, Suthers G, Suter CM, Martin DI, Hawkins NJ, Ward RL. Inheritance of a cancer-associated MLH1 germ-line epimutation. N Engl J Med. 2007;356(7):697–705.
22. Morak M, Schackert HK, Rahner N, Betz B, Ebert M, Walldorf C, Royer-Pokora B, Schulmann K, von Knebel-Doeberitz M, Dietmaier W, et al. Further evidence for heritability of an epimutation in one of 12 cases with MLH1 promoter methylation in blood cells clinically displaying HNPCC. Eur J Hum Genet. 2008;16(7):804–11.
23. Crepin M, Dieu MC, Lejeune S, Escande F, Boidin D, Porchet N, Morin G, Manouvrier S, Mathieu M, Buisine MP. Evidence of constitutional MLH1 epimutation associated to transgenerational inheritance of cancer susceptibility. Hum Mutat. 2012;33(1):180–8.
24. Al-Moghrabi N, Nofel A, Al-Yousef N, Madkhali S, Bin Amer SM, Alaiya A, Shinwari Z, Al-Tweigeri T, Karakas B, Tulbah A, et al. The molecular significance of methylated BRCA1 promoter in white blood cells of cancer-free females. BMC Cancer. 2014;14:830.
25. Katz TA. Potential mechanisms underlying the protective effect of pregnancy against breast cancer: a focus on the IGF pathway. Front Oncol. 2016;6:228.
26. Katz TA, Liao SG, Palmieri VJ, Dearth RK, Pathiraja TN, Huo Z, Shaw P, Small S, Davidson NE, Peters DG, et al. Targeted DNA methylation screen in the mouse mammary genome reveals a parity-induced hypermethylation of Igf1r that persists long after parturition. Cancer Prev Res (Phila). 2015;8(10):1000–9.
27. Wojdacz TK, Harari F, Vahter M, Broberg K. Discordant pattern of BRCA1 gene epimutation in blood between mothers and daughters. J Clin Pathol. 2015;68(7):575–7.
28. Shen L, Kondo Y, Rosner GL, Xiao L, Hernandez NS, Vilaythong J, Houlihan PS, Krouse RS, Prasad AR, Einspahr JG, et al. MGMT promoter methylation and field defect in sporadic colorectal cancer. J Natl Cancer Inst. 2005;97(18):1330–8.
29. Hitchins MP, Rapkins RW, Kwok CT, Srivastava S, Wong JJ, Khachigian LM, Polly P, Goldblatt J, Ward RL. Dominantly inherited constitutional epigenetic silencing of MLH1 in a cancer-affected family is linked to a single nucleotide variant within the 5'UTR. Cancer Cell. 2011;20(2):200–13.
30. Ligtenberg MJ, Kuiper RP, Chan TL, Goossens M, Hebeda KM, Voorendt M, Lee TY, Bodmer D, Hoenselaar E, Hendriks-Cornelissen SJ, et al. Heritable somatic methylation and inactivation of MSH2 in families with Lynch syndrome due to deletion of the 3' exons of TACSTD1. Nat Genet. 2009;41(1):112–7.
31. Candiloro IL, Dobrovic A. Detection of MGMT promoter methylation in normal individuals is strongly associated with the T allele of the rs16906252 MGMT promoter single nucleotide polymorphism. Cancer Prev Res (Phila). 2009;2(10):862–7.
32. Dobrovic A, Mikeska T, Alsop K, Candiloro I, George J, Mitchell G, Bowtell D. Constitutional BRCA1 methylation is a major predisposition factor for high-grade serous ovarian cancer. [abstract]. In: Proceedings of the 105th Annual Meeting of the American Association for Cancer Research; 2014 Apr 5-9; San Diego, CA. Philadelphia (PA): AACR; Cancer Res 2014;74(19 Suppl): Abstract nr 290. https://doi.org/10.1158/1538-7445.AM2014-290.
33. Munot K, Bell SM, Lane S, Horgan K, Hanby AM, Speirs V. Pattern of expression of genes linked to epigenetic silencing in human breast cancer. Hum Pathol. 2006;37(8):989–99.
34. Sharma G, Mirza S, Parshad R, Srivastava A, Gupta SD, Pandya P, Ralhan R. Clinical significance of promoter hypermethylation of DNA repair genes in tumor and serum DNA in invasive ductal breast carcinoma patients. Life Sci. 2010;87(3–4):83–91.
35. Wojdacz TK, Thestrup BB, Overgaard J, Hansen LL. Methylation of cancer related genes in tumor and peripheral blood DNA from the same breast cancer patient as two independent events. Diagn Pathol. 2011;6:116.
36. Knudson AG. Hereditary cancer: two hits revisited. J Cancer Res Clin Oncol. 1996;122(3):135–40.

8

H3K27 acetylation and gene expression analysis reveals differences in placental chromatin activity in fetal growth restriction

N. D. Paauw[1,6]*, A. T. Lely[1], J. A. Joles[2], A. Franx[1], P. G. Nikkels[3], M. Mokry[4] and B. B. van Rijn[1,5,6]*

Abstract

Background: Posttranslational modification of histone tails such as histone 3 lysine 27 acetylation (H3K27ac) is tightly coupled to epigenetic regulation of gene expression. To explore whether this is involved in placenta pathology, we probed genome-wide H3K27ac occupancy by chromatin immunoprecipitation sequencing (ChIP-seq) in healthy placentas and placentas from pathological pregnancies with fetal growth restriction (FGR). Furthermore, we related specific acetylation profiles of FGR placentas to gene expression changes.

Results: Analysis of H3K27ac occupancy in FGR compared to healthy placentas showed 970 differentially acetylated regions distributed throughout the genome. Principal component analysis and hierarchical clustering revealed complete segregation of the FGR and control group. Next, we identified 569 upregulated genes and 521 downregulated genes in FGR placentas by RNA sequencing. Differential gene transcription largely corresponded to expected direction based on H3K27ac status. Pathway analysis on upregulated transcripts originating from hyperacetylated sites revealed genes related to the HIF-1-alpha transcription factor network and several other genes with known involvement in placental pathology (LEP, FLT1, HK2, ENG, FOS). Downregulated transcripts in the vicinity of hypoacetylated sites were related to the immune system and growth hormone receptor signaling. Additionally, we found enrichment of 141 transcription factor binding motifs within differentially acetylated regions. Of the corresponding transcription factors, four were upregulated, SP1, ARNT2, HEY2, and VDR, and two downregulated, FOSL and NR4A1.

Conclusion: We demonstrate a key role for genome-wide alterations in H3K27ac in FGR placentas corresponding with changes in transcription profiles of regions relevant to placental function. Future studies on the role of H3K27ac in FGR and placental-fetal development may help to identify novel targets for therapy of this currently incurable disease.

Keywords: ChIP-seq, Growth restriction, H3K27ac, Epigenetics, Histone acetylation, Placenta, Placental pathology, RNA-seq

Background

The dynamics of histone 3 lysine 27 acetylation (H3K27ac) in DNA regulatory regions is one of the components playing a fundamental role in the precise timing and level of gene transcription [1, 2]. Consequently, aberrant H3K27ac has been suggested to be involved in disease pathology by eliciting pathological gene expression programs [3, 4]. H3K27ac marks both active promoters and distal enhancers, the most important and best understood regulatory domains. To study involvement of this regulatory level/layer in placental pathology, we mapped H3K27ac occupancy in healthy placentas and placentas from pregnancies with fetal growth restriction (FGR).

FGR, a condition in which the fetus is unable to achieve its full growth potential through inadequate supply of nutrients and growth factors, occurs in approximately 5% of pregnancies [5]. FGR imposes a major risk of perinatal morbidity and mortality [6] and programs the health of the fetus throughout life, by being associated with a future risk of type 2 diabetes and

* Correspondence: n.d.paauw-2@umcutrecht.nl; b.b.vanrijn@umcutrecht.nl
[1]Department of Obstetrics, Wilhelmina Children's Hospital Birth Center, University Medical Center Utrecht, Utrecht, the Netherlands
Full list of author information is available at the end of the article

cardiovascular and renal disease [7, 8]. At the histopathological level, FGR placenta exhibit signs of disrupted placental development characterized by increased infarction area, increased syncytial knotting, inflammation, and impaired trophoblast invasion into the spiral arteries of the uterus due to inappropriate maternal-fetal immune interaction [9–11].

Previous studies of placentas of FGR pregnancies have reported differences in gene transcription across many regions across the genome. Pathways associated with altered placental gene expression in FGR include angiogenesis, immune modulation, energy production, and growth signaling [12–15]. Most adaptive responses of the placenta, e.g., to support restricted fetal growth, are thought to result from changes in epigenetic regulation [16–18]. Recently, DNA methylation has been mapped in the human placenta [19] and a number of studies have suggested differences in genome-wide methylation profiles in FGR placentas [20–22]. We assume that disruptions in other epigenetic systems (e.g., histone modifications and other posttranslational chromatin modifications) regulating placenta gene expression are also likely to be involved [23, 24].

In this study, we mapped differential H3K27ac profiles in DNA regulatory regions in relation to disrupted development of the placenta, by exploring the presence of H3K27ac using chromatin immunoprecipitation sequencing (ChIP-seq) in FGR and control placentas. Next, we performed RNA-seq to examine whether differences in H3K27ac also reflects gene expression levels. With this approach, we identified previously unstudied alterations in promoter and enhancer activity related to placenta pathology.

Results
Detection of regions with differential H3K27ac occupancy
First, we performed genome-wide analysis of H3K27ac by ChIP-seq on placental tissue from control ($n = 4$) and FGR pregnancies ($n = 5$) and identified 30,288 H3K27ac peaks that were present in at least two independent samples. Of these, 970 regions showed differential H3K27ac levels in FGR compared to controls with 366 being hyperacetylated and 604 regions being hypoacetylated in FGR (Fig. 1a, full list supplied in Additional file 1: Table S1). Based on the differentially acetylated regions, the FGR and healthy placentas could be clearly segregated using both supervised and unsupervised analysis (Fig. 1b–c, Additional file 2) These findings indicate clear distinction between the two groups and suggest a specific and highly reproducible H3K27ac pattern in FGR placentas. Differentially acetylated regions were distributed throughout the whole genome as shown by Manhattan plot (Fig. 1d). Regions containing differentially acetylated peaks correspond with known H3K27ac positions derived from ENCODE databases (Fig. 1e).

Genes annotated to within 20 kb of differentially acetylated regions
To identify the biological relevance of differentially acetylated peaks, we annotated genes to the hyper- and hypoacetylated sites using a window of ± 20 kb from transcription start site (TSS). We annotated 368 genes corresponding to hyperacytelated sites and 313 genes associated with hypoacetylated sites (Additional file 1: Table S2). Several of these annotated genes are known to be involved in placental development. For instance, we found hyperacetylation of regions near HK2, FLT1, and LEP, previously reported to be upregulated in other placental disorders [25, 26], and hypoacetylation of regions near CH2 and CDLN1, which are involved in growth and endothelial cell-to-cell adhesions. The individual peaks of selected regions of interest are presented in Fig. 2a (near HK2) and Fig. 2b (near Flt-1, LEP, CDLN1, and CH1). These figures show that sites identified to be differentially acetylated are highly similar across each of the replicates.

Pathway analysis of differential acetylated regions in FGR placentas
Next, we aimed to assign biological significance to genes annotated to differentially acetylated peaks by pathway analysis using GREAT software. The software annotated 515 genes to hyperacetylated regions in FGR. Although no enrichment for GO biological process or for pathways was identified using this approach, the annotated genes were enriched for genes that are transcriptionally regulated by HIF-1-alfa/hypoxia within the MSigDB perturbation ontology (full output supplied in Additional file 1: Table S3). Other functional pathways related to hyperacetylated regions include pathways involved in cancer and immune response. Nearby the differential hypoacetylated regions, GREAT identified 868 genes. GO biological processes and pathways related to these genes consisted of angiogenesis, response to external signals, and immune activation (Fig. 3a, b, full output supplied in Additional file 1: Table S3). Interestingly, many of these pathways are known to be disrupted in FGR, especially angiogenesis, HIF-1-alpha signaling, and the immune environment/response [27–29].

Cross-validation of functional effects by combining H3K27ac and mRNA profiles
To cross-validate functional meaning of the differentially acetylated peaks and to examine whether hyper- or hypoacetylated state of H3K27 was also accompanied by differential gene expression, we performed RNA-seq. We identified 569 upregulated genes and 521 downregulated genes in FGR vs. control (full list supplied in Additional file 1: Table S4, heatmap and MA and V plots in Additional file 3). These gene expression profiles

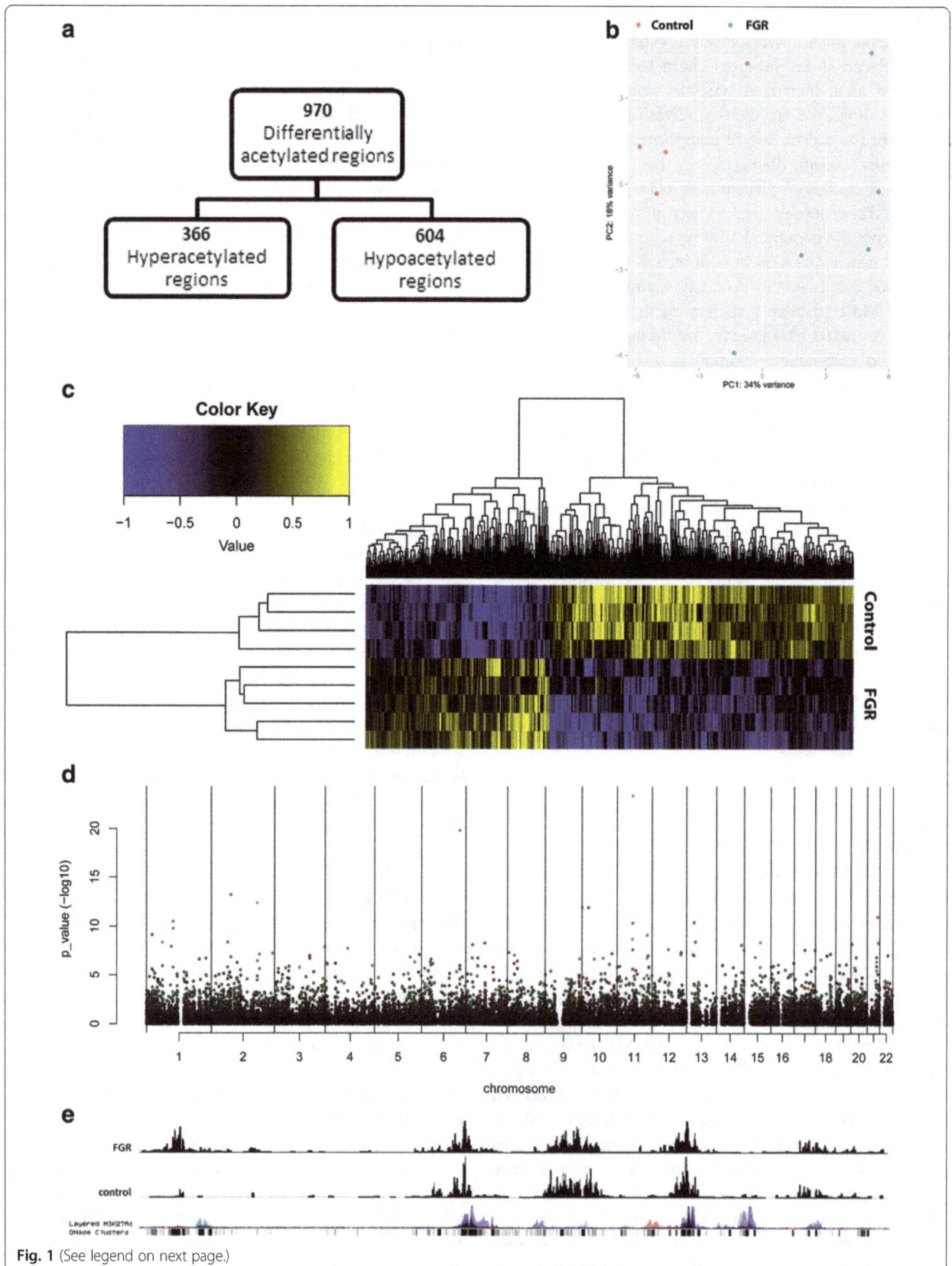

Fig. 1 (See legend on next page.)

(See figure on previous page.)
Fig. 1 Detection of H3K27ac occupancy in placentas of FGR and controls by CHIP-seq. **a** Flowchart of differentially acetylated region in FGR vs. control placentas (adjusted $p < 0.05$). **b** Heatmap of differentially acetylated regions between FGR and controls. **c** PCA clustering of the 500 most variable acetylated regions based on H3K27ac ChIP-seq signal between FGR and controls. **d** Manhattan plot depicting distribution of differentially H3K27 acetylated regions in FGR vs. controls: non-significant regions (black), hyperacetylated regions (green), and hypoacetylated regions (red). **e** Selected peaks from Chr11 showing hypoacetylation in FGR vs. controls with ENCODE as reference

largely overlapped with findings from earlier gene expression studies in FGR placentas using microarrays [12–15]. This is also reflected in the biological processes and pathways associated with the up- and downregulated genes supplied in Additional file 1: Table S5. These findings confirm disruption of gene expression in placenta from FGR pregnancies involved in important processes of placental development in angiogenesis and immune modulation.

To investigate whether the direction of transcription change corresponds with differential acetylation, we investigated the distribution transcriptional direction of all genes and that of the genes annotated within 20 kb to hyperacetylated and hypoacetylated regions. Despite multiple levels/layers involved in regulation of the mRNA levels, we found a clear correlation between differential H3K27ac levels and gene expression changes (Fig. 4a). Next, we identified genes that overlapped in the gene annotation derived from differentially acetylated regions with the up- and downregulated transcripts to inspect acetylation sites that most likely influenced gene expression. We identified 34 upregulated genes in close vicinity of hyperacetylated sites and 26 downregulated genes near hypoacetylated regions (Fig. 4b). These

lists contain many candidates known to be involved in the pathophysiology of FGR, such as Flt-1 and LEP, which have been described in up to one third of the studies using placentas derived from pregnancies complicated by preeclampsia [26], a placental disorder frequently associated with FGR. Other identified candidate genes included FOS, ENG (upregulated transcripts), and GH2 (downregulated transcripts).

Identification of pathways by combining H3K27ac profiles and gene expression levels

Pathway with TOPPfun on upregulated genes near hyperacetylated sites revealed genes to be related to the HIF-1-alpha transcription factor network (Fig. 4c, Additional file 1: Table S6). In addition, the downregulated transcripts and hypoacetylated regions could be grouped as genes encoding secreted soluble factors, extracellular matrix proteins, and molecules involved in growth hormone receptor signaling (Fig. 4c, Additional file 1: Table S6).

Transcription factor binding motif analysis

To further investigate functional properties of the differential H3K27ac peaks, we tested whether the peaks contained enricanalysishment of transcription factor binding

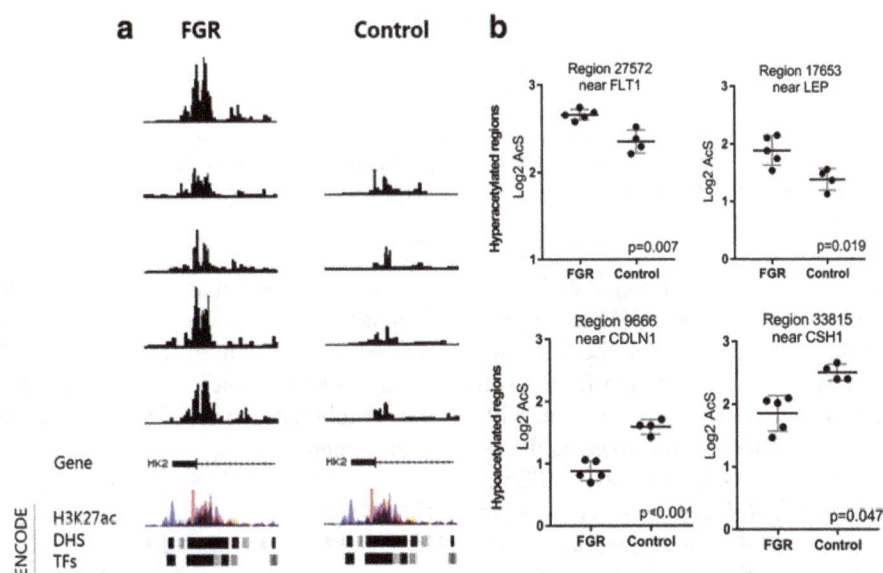

Fig. 2 Selected regions of differentially acetylated regions in FGR placentas and related pathways. **a** A selected acetylated region near the HK2 gene in each individual sample using the USC Genome Browser showing similarity of patterns between each replicate in both groups. **b** Dot plots of four differently acetylated regions related to genes known to be involved in placental development (mean ± SD, adjusted p value shown)

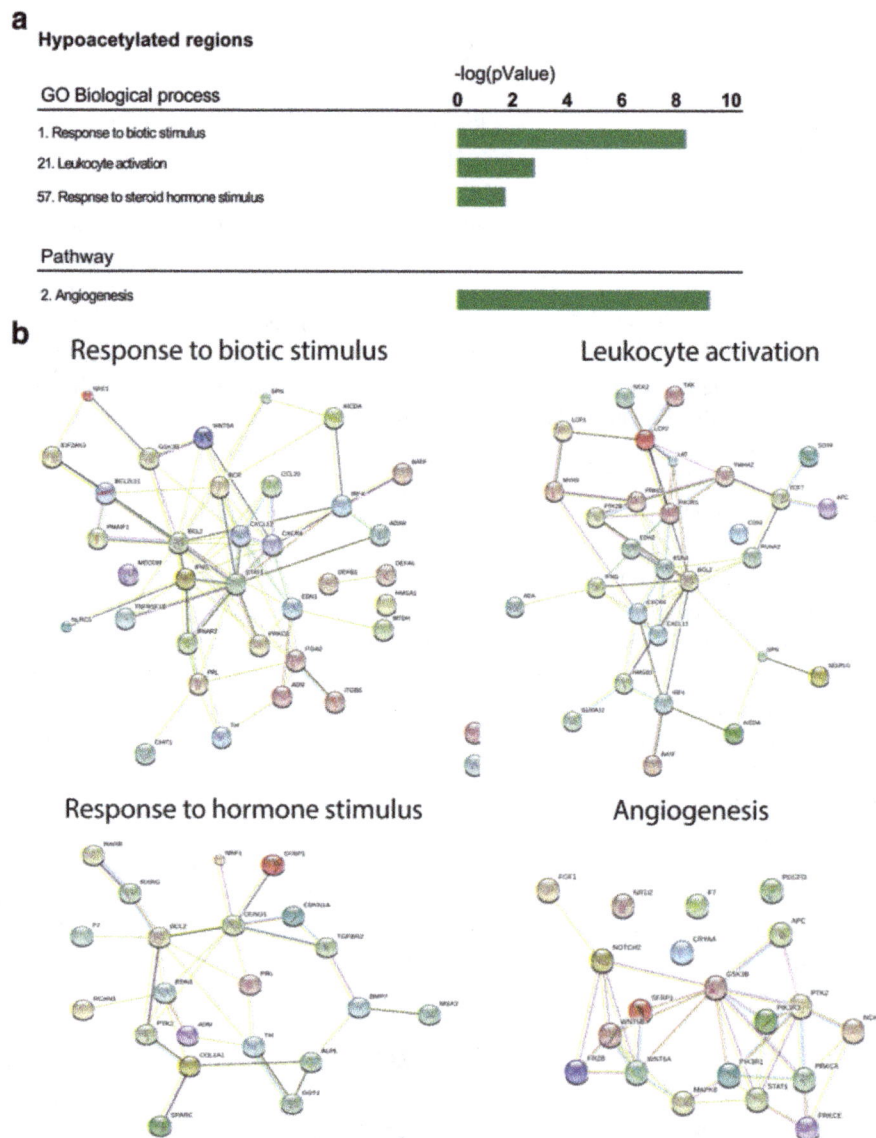

Fig. 3 GREAT pathway analysis using differentially acetylated regions. **a** Identification of GO biological processes and pathways related to differentially acetylated regions in FGR using GREAT software. **b** Detection of interacting proteins by STRING protein database using genes annotated to biological processes and pathways related to enriched differentially acetylated regions. Only the highest confidence interactions are displayed. Disconnected nodes were removed

motifs (TFBM) using AME [30]. We detected 86 hyperacetylated and 55 hypoacetylated TFBM (Additional file 1: Table S7). Combining these motifs with the RNA-seq, we identified four upregulated transcription factors with enriched H3K27ac in their DNA binding domains (SP1, ARNT2, HEY2, and VDR) and two downregulated transcription factors with lower H3K27ac peaks (FOSL1, NR4A1) (Fig. 5). Of these, ARNT2 and HEY2 were previously shown to be upregulated under hypoxic conditions [31, 32]. Moreover similar changes in gene expression of VDR have been reported previously in preeclamptic placenta pathways [33], and FOSL1 was previously showed to be important for the establishment of

the maternal-fetal interface [34, 35]. Collectively, these findings point towards TFs linking differentially transcribed genes with differentially acetylated regulatory chromosomal regions. Thus, transcriptional and epigenetic regulations are intricately connected in placental development.

Discussion

In this study, we used ChIP-seq and RNA-seq to perform an in-depth analysis of DNA regions with differential chromatin activity in healthy human placentas and pathological placentas of pregnancies affected by FGR. With this combined approach, we were able to identify

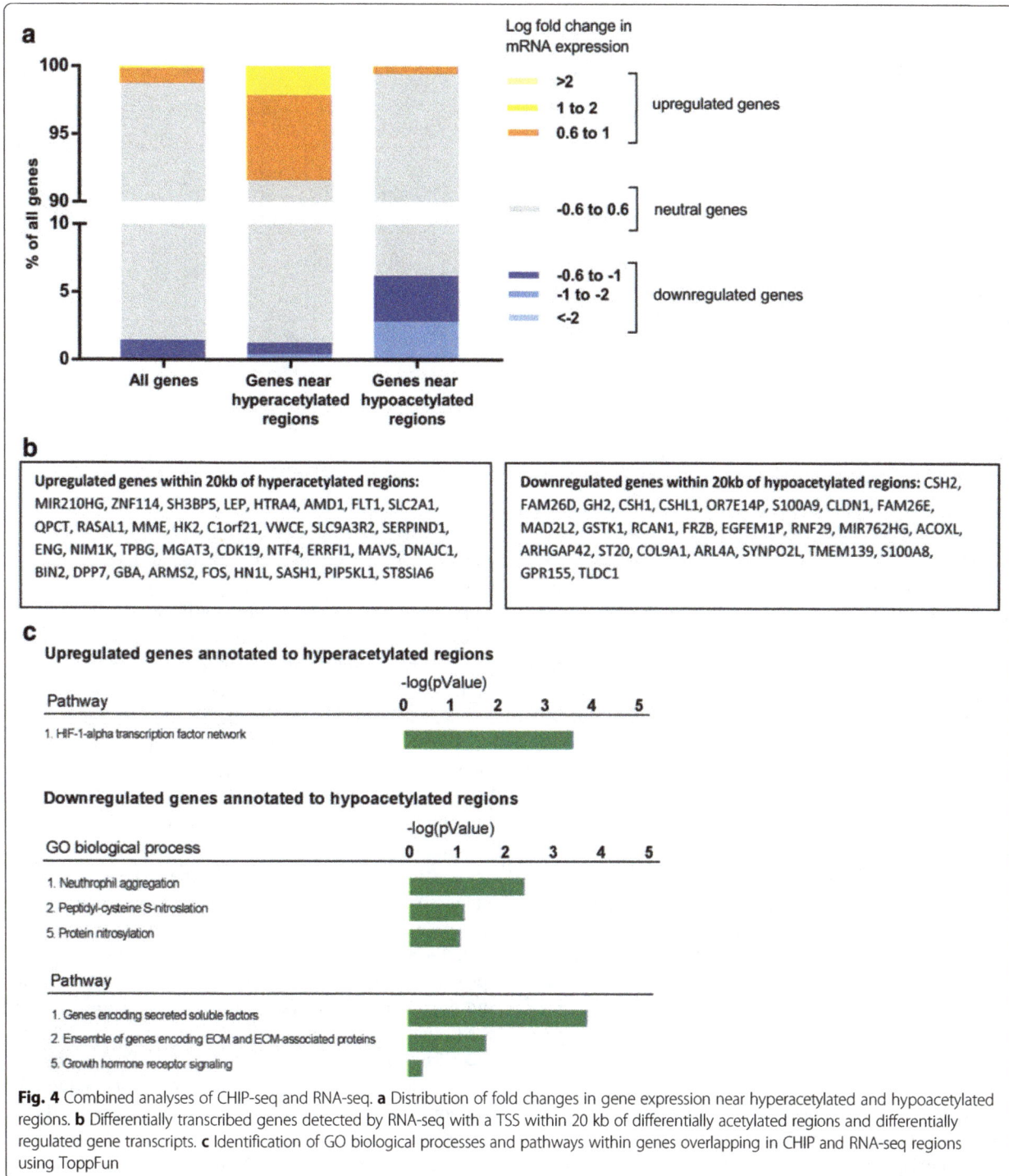

Fig. 4 Combined analyses of CHIP-seq and RNA-seq. **a** Distribution of fold changes in gene expression near hyperacetylated and hypoacetylated regions. **b** Differentially transcribed genes detected by RNA-seq with a TSS within 20 kb of differentially acetylated regions and differentially regulated gene transcripts. **c** Identification of GO biological processes and pathways within genes overlapping in CHIP and RNA-seq regions using ToppFun

H3K27 acetylation as a key additional layer involved in epigenetic regulation of gene expression in placental function which in turn might be related to impaired fetal growth.

In summary, our findings confirm that, in FGR, the placenta exhibits substantial genome-wide alterations in H3K27 acetylation, with corresponding changes in transcription profiles in several regions pertinent to placental development and presumably function. The identified acetylation patterns show a clear distinction between FGR and healthy placentas, and the genes annotated to differentially acetylated regions are involved in pathways known to be affected in FGR [27–29]. We confirmed functionality of the differentially acetylated regions by showing a clear correlation between the acetylation profiles with differential gene expression. In-depth analyses of the differences in FGR placenta that revealed

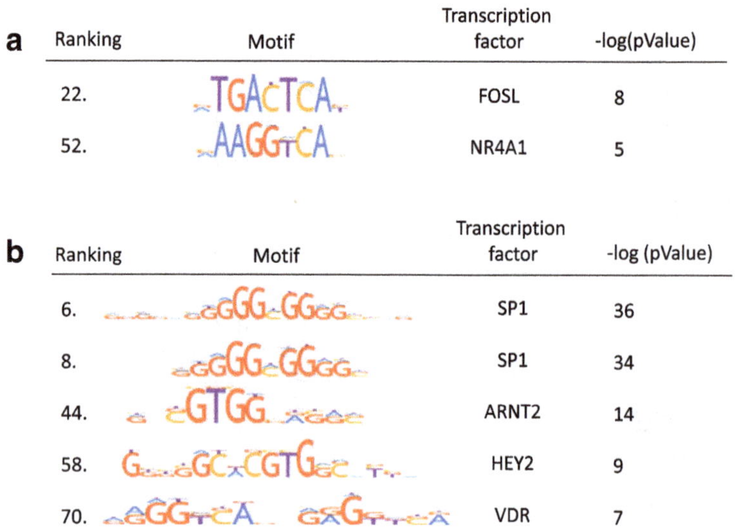

Fig. 5 Differentially acetylated transcription factor binding motifs (TFBMs). **a** TFBMs with upregulated transcripts of their corresponding TFs. **b** TFBMs with downregulated transcripts of their corresponding TFs

candidate genes and pathways that fit previously reported histopathological and protein data. For example, we found hyperacetylation and higher mRNA of the sFlt-1 region in FGR placentas, consistent with studies reporting upregulation of sFlt-1 protein in FGR placentas [36, 37]. Furthermore, sFlt-1 is known to be enriched in syncytial knots, which are also observed in FGR placenta [38]. Similarly, the leptin protein was showed to be upregulated in FGR placentas [39, 40] and GH and CSH proteins are often downregulated in FGR placentas [41, 42]. Additionally, we unmasked an interplay between differentially transcribed transcription factors with enriched TFBM within the differentially acetylated regions. Together, our data suggest an important role of H3K27ac as an additional layer/level in the regulation of placental gene expression. Our findings confirm that a combined ChIP-seq and RNA-seq approach may provide a useful approach to probe the pathophysiology of placental disease and discover novel targets to improve placental health and thus support fetal growth and development.

To date, we are not aware of any previous reports on histone modification in FGR placentas. Other groups have focused attention on epigenetic regulation of placentas in FGR involving DNA methylation. Genome-wide methylation studies in placenta of FGR suggest involvement of pathways associated with lipid metabolism, transcription, and cadherin and Wnt signaling [20–22]. Others have reported on DNA methylation of imprinted loci, since unbalanced placental expression of imprinted genes has been reported in FGR placenta [12, 43–45]. However, methylation actually fluctuates very little at these loci [45]. While DNA methylation

may contribute to placental gene regulation, it can only in part explain differences in gene expression [23, 24]. Together with our results, this emphasizes the need to include other epigenetic processes to fully appreciate the complexity of mechanisms underlying placental gene expression and (primary or secondary adaptive) gene responses during (disrupted) early human development.

Mechanisms involved in differential acetylation of histones within the human placenta have not been studied. In view of the "fetal origins of adult disease" hypothesis (also known as the *Barker hypothesis*), i.e., the concept that exposure to intrauterine conditions may have long-lasting effects on fetal development, these epigenetic alterations might well be the result of changes in the intrauterine environment associated with FGR [8]. One of the intrauterine factors that might play a role in changes in epigenetic profiles in the placenta of FGR is the timing and degree of hypoxia. For example, it was showed previously that the proliferation of trophoblasts is highly dependent on the crosstalk between HIFs and histone deacetylases (HDACs) in response to hypoxia [46]. In addition, differences in histone acetylation may be the in part driven by variation in the genetic code itself, e.g., single-nucleotide polymorphisms, that shape chromatin architecture and thereby disrupt normal placental development [47, 48]. Considering potential intervention, it is of great interest to study the contribution of both environmental and intrinsic factors in more detail.

Our study has several strengths. First, our data provide new and comprehensive information on epigenetic regulation of placental gene expression in FGR. Our data suggest that H3K27ac profiles have a role in genome-wide regulation of gene expression in FGR placenta and point towards disruptions in important pathways involved in placental development. Histone modifications represent mid-long-term effects [49] and are likely more stable and independent of sample moment compared to RNA, and by combining CHIP-seq data with RNA-seq data, we were able to relate epigenetic marks to functional gene expression patterns, confirming relevance of identified pathways. Another strength is our careful collection and detailed phenotyping of FGR placentas during Cesarean sections, excluding those women who have labored. Thus, we avoided confounding effects of temporal changes associated with parturition [50].

There are some limitations in our approach that also need to be addressed. First, we could not avoid the limitation of the use of nearest gene approach for functional annotation. Here, we used a 20-kb window to annotate genes which, although quite wide, still allowed identification of specific pathways and genes that corresponded with previous literature. With regard to the collected material, there were unavoidable difference in gestational ages in material from FGR and control due to the severity of the selected FGR cases. It is possible that gestational age in itself has an effect on H3K27ac and gene expression as shown in early mouse placenta [51] and for other epigenetic marks such as methylation as shown in human placenta [21]. While gestational age might be a confounder, the strongest determinant in our cohort is likely to be the disease, given that all placentas were from third trimester pregnancies while majority of gene expression changes occur earlier in development [52] and the confirmed disease-specific pathways. In addition, largest differences in epigenetics in the third trimester are mainly induced by parturition [50], which we ruled out by collecting samples from C-sections only.

With this study, we show that genome-wide H3K27ac profiles might be useful to better understand pathophysiology of FGR. Therefore, we would recommend future studies to confirm the identified acetylation targets in a larger population as this might be helpful to address association of the differentially acetylated regions with different subtypes of FGR, gestational-age specific effects on acetylation within the third trimester of healthy and FGR pregnancy, and, most importantly, to explore cause-effect relationships. The latter might be very valuable as the plasticity of histone marks form an attractive strategy for intervention, especially since no therapy is currently available to improve placental function. In addition, it will be valuable to study the combination of other epigenetic marks, such as DNA methylation and other histone marks, to better discriminate promoters from enhancers (H3K4me3, H3K4me1) or repressed chromatin (H3K27me3) [53]. Moreover, since placental samples represent an average state across different cellular compartments with trophoblast being the predominant cell type [54], newer techniques looking at subpopulations of cells might help to unravel cell-specific deregulated pathways [55].

Conclusions

We demonstrate involvement of H3K27ac in key regions related to the placental function and placental pathology associating with impaired fetal growth. Our findings underscore that an approach using combined CHIP-seq and RNA-seq analyses facilitates discovery of novel genes involved in FGR, and identification of molecular pathways and processes associated with the placental function and early (disrupted) human growth and development. Future studies on unraveling the role of H3K27ac in FGR pregnancies and placental-fetal development may help to identify novel targets for therapy of this currently incurable disease.

Methods

Study design and sample collection

Placenta biopsies were collected immediately after birth from women with a FGR pregnancy and women with uncomplicated pregnancy. Each placenta was sampled at four random locations. For this study, we only included women undergoing a primary Cesarean section. We defined FGR as an estimated fetal weight <p3 and only included cases with pulsatility index of the uterine artery >p97.5 since we were particularly interested in cases with FGR based on placenta insufficiency. Controls were included when planned for Cesarean section because of either breech presentation or history of Caesarian section. Additional file 4 provides an overview of characteristics from the pregnancies of which the placenta were derived. The material was snap-frozen directly after sampling and stored at − 80 °C. Before further processing, all four biopsies per placenta were pooled and ground into powder using mortar and pestle cooled with liquid nitrogen.

ChIP-sequencing for H3K27ac occupancy

The powdered samples, two scoops diluted in 700 µl sPBS, were used for chromatin isolation using the MAGnify™ Chromatin Immunoprecipitation System kit (Life Technologies, Thermo Fisher Scientific, Carlsbad, CA) according to manufacturer's instructions. In brief, the tissue was crosslinked with 1% formaldehyde and the crosslinking was stopped by adding 1.25 M glycine. Cells were lysed using the kit provided lysis buffer, and nuclei were sonicated using Covaris microTUBE (duty cycle 5%, intensity 2, 200 cycles per burst, 60 s cycle time, 10 cycles). We aimed for DNA fragments of 200–2000 bp long. We continued with one fifth of the volume, and the sheared chromatin was diluted and then incubated with 1 µl anti-H3K27ac antibody (ab4729, Abcam) pre-coupled to magnetic beads for 2 h at 4 °C. Beads were extensively washed, and crosslinking was reversed by the kit-provided reverse crosslinking buffer with proteinase K. DNA was purified using ChIP DNA Clean & Concentrator kit (Zymo Research). Libraries were prepared using the NEXTflex™ Rapid DNA Sequencing Kit (Bioo Scientific). Samples were PCR-amplified and checked for the proper size range and for the absence of adaptor dimers on a 2% agarose gel, and barcoded libraries were sequenced 75 bp single-end on Illumina NextSeq500 sequencer (Utrecht Sequencing Facility).

Mapping of ChIP-sequencing reads

Sequencing reads were mapped against the reference genome (hg19 assembly, GRCh37) using BWA package (mem −t 7 −c 100 −M −R) [56]. Multiple reads mapping to the same location and strand have been collapsed to single reads, and only uniquely placed reads were used for peak/region calling. Regions were called using Cisgenome 2.0 (−e 150 -maxgap 200 −minlen 200) [57]. Subsequently, to obtain a common reference, region coordinates from all FGR and control samples were stretched to at least 2000 bp and collapsed into a single common list. Overlapping regions were merged based on their outmost coordinates. Only the autosomal regions supported by at least two independent datasets were further analyzed. Sequencing reads from each ChIP-seq library were overlapped with the common region list, to set the H3K27ac occupancy for every region-sample pair.

ChIP data analysis

Regions with differential H3K27ac occupancy between FGR samples and controls were identified using DESeq2 ($p < 0.05$ by Wald test) [58] and are referred to as "differentially acetylated regions." Hierarchical clustering based on differentially acetylated regions was performed with quantile-normalized, log2-transformed, and median-centered read counts per common region. To avoid log2 transformation of zero values, one read was added to each region. A Manhattan plot was created representing the distribution of regions detected to be differentially acetylated in FRG vs. controls across autosomal chromosomes. The unsupervised PCA analysis was performed for the top 500 most variable regions using DESeq2. Based on the initial analysis, we excluded one control sample because of being an extreme outlier in the PCA analysis and continued the analysis with $n = 5$ FGR and $n = 4$ control samples.

To assign biological meaning to differentially acetylated peaks, we used three approaches. First, we annotated genes to the differentially acetylated sites in silico using a window of ± 20 kb from transcription start site

(TSS). Second, GREAT software (Stanford) was used to assign biological meaning to a set of non-coding genomic regions by analyzing the annotations of genes flanking differentially acetylated regions [59]. GREAT incorporates annotations from 20 ontologies and accounts for the length of gene regulatory domains. ToppFun was used for gene list enrichment analysis and candidate gene prioritization based on functional annotations and protein interaction networks (accessed in March 2017). In addition, we identified whether the differentially acetylated regions contain enrichment of specific transcription factor binding domains by overlapping the differentially hypo- and hyperacetylated regions in the FGR vs. control group to placenta DNAse hypersensitivity site (DHS) datasets obtained from the ENCODE database (ENCFF203HVV, ENCFF249GZW, ENCFF919NRH). The genomic sequence of overlapping DHS was repeat masked, and the enrichment of TFBM was calculated against a random set of non-overlapping DHS sequences using the Analysis Motif of Enrichment (AME tool) of the MEME Suite with default settings using human (HOCOMOCO v9) motif database.

RNA sequencing

Total RNA was extracted from placental powder using RNeasy® (Qiagen, Hilden, Germany) according to the manufacturer's instructions by which all RNA molecules longer than 200 nucleotides are purified. Polyadenylated mRNA fraction was isolated using Poly(A) Beads (NEXTflex, San Jose, CA), and sequencing libraries were constructed using the Rapid Directional RNA-seq kit (NEXTflex, San Jose, CA). Libraries were sequenced on the Nextseq500 platform (Illumina, San Diego, CA), producing single-end reads of 75 bp (Utrecht Sequencing Facility). Reads were aligned to the human reference genome GRCh37 using STAR version 2.4.2a. Picard's AddOrReplaceReadGroups (v1.98) was used to add read groups to the BAM files, which were sorted with Sambamba v0.4.5, and transcript abundances were quantified with HTSeq-count version 0.6.1p1 using the union mode. Subsequently, reads per kilobase million reads sequenced (RPKMs) were calculated with edgeR's RPKM function.

RNA-seq data analysis

Differentially expressed genes were identified using the DESeq2 package with standard settings. Genes with padj < 0.05 were considered as differentially expressed. Again, ToppFun was used for gene list enrichment analysis and candidate gene prioritization (accessed in March 207). The list of up- and downregulated genes were tested separately using probability density function p value calculation, FDR B&H correction, p value cutoff 0.05.

ChIP-seq and RNA-seq overlap analyses

To validate functional consequences of differentially acetylated regions, we overlapped the genes annotated to differentially hyperacetylated regions with upregulated genes derived from the mRNA-seq and genes annotated to differentially hypoacetylated regions with downregulated genes derived from the mRNA-seq. Functional pathway analysis with TOPPFUN were performed on both sets of overlapping genes. In addition, we searched the up- and downregulated genes for transcription factors (TF) with enriched TFBM within the differentially acetylated regions.

Statistical analysis

Data are shown as mean ± SD or median (range) and analyzed with Student's t test or χ^2 test.

Acknowledgements
The authors acknowledge N. van Dungen and N. Lansu for their technical support.

Funding
This study was funded by Fonds Gezond Geboren (personal grant awarded to BBR) and Dutch Kidney Foundation (15O141).

Authors' contributions
BBR, AF, and ATL contributed to the research idea. BBR and ATL contributed to the study design and sample collection. NDP contributed to the sample processing. MM and NDP contributed to the analysis of data. MM contributed to the statistics. NDP contributed to the drafting of the manuscript. BBR, PN, ATL, JAJ, MM, and AF contributed to the editing of the manuscript. All authors read and approved the final manuscript.

Author details
[1]Department of Obstetrics, Wilhelmina Children's Hospital Birth Center, University Medical Center Utrecht, Utrecht, the Netherlands. [2]Department of Nephrology and Hypertension, University Medical Center Utrecht, Utrecht, the Netherlands. [3]Department of Pathology, University Medical Center Utrecht, Utrecht, the Netherlands. [4]Division of Pediatrics, University Medical Center Utrecht, Utrecht, the Netherlands. [5]Academic Unit of Human Development and Health, University of Southampton, Southampton, UK. [6]Division Woman and Baby, University Medical Center Utrecht, Postbus 85090, 3508 AB Utrecht, the Netherlands.

References

1. Ernst J, Kheradpour P, Mikkelsen TS, Shoresh N, Ward LD, Epstein CB, et al. Mapping and analysis of chromatin state dynamics in nine human cell types. Nature. 2011;473:43–9.
2. Creyghton MP, Cheng AW, Welstead GG, Kooistra T, Carey BW, Steine EJ, et al. Histone H3K27ac separates active from poised enhancers and predicts developmental state. Proc Natl Acad Sci U S A. 2010;107:21931–6.
3. Mirabella AC, Foster BM, Bartke T. Chromatin deregulation in disease. Chromosoma. 2016;125:75–93.
4. Hnisz D, Abraham BJ, Lee TI, Lau A, Saint-Andre V, Sigova AA, et al. Super-enhancers in the control of cell identity and disease. Cell. 2013;155:934–47.
5. Romo A, Carceller R, Tobajas J. Intrauterine growth retardation (IUGR): epidemiology and etiology. Pediatr Endocrinol Rev. 2009;6(3):332–6.
6. Bernstein IM, Horbar JD, Badger GJ, Ohlsson A, Golan A. Morbidity and mortality among very-low-birth-weight neonates with intrauterine growth restriction. The Vermont Oxford Network. Am J Obstet Gynecol. 2000;182(1 1):198–206.
7. Barker DJ, Osmond C, Golding J, Kuh D, Wadsworth ME. Growth in utero, blood pressure in childhood and adult life, and mortality from cardiovascular disease. BMJ. 1989;298:564–7.
8. Kermack AJ, Van Rijn BB, Houghton FD, Calder PC, Cameron IT, Macklon NS. The "developmental origins" hypothesis: relevance to the obstetrician and gynecologist. J Dev Orig Health Dis. 2015;6:415–24.
9. Chaddha V, Viero S, Huppertz B, Kingdom J. Developmental biology of the placenta and the origins of placental insufficiency. Semin Fetal Neonatal Med. 2004;9:357–69.
10. Veerbeek JHW, Brouwers L, Koster MPH, Koenen SV, van Vliet EOG, Nikkels PGJ, et al. Spiral artery remodeling and maternal cardiovascular risk: the spiral artery remodeling (SPAR) study. J Hypertens. 2016;34:1570–7.
11. Veerbeek JHW, Nikkels PGJ, Torrance HL, Gravesteijn J, Post Uiterweer ED, Derks JB, et al. Placental pathology in early intrauterine growth restriction associated with maternal hypertension. Placenta. 2014;35:696–701.
12. McMinn J, Wei M, Schupf N, Cusmai J, Johnson EB, Smith AC, et al. Unbalanced placental expression of imprinted genes in human intrauterine growth restriction. Placenta. 2006;27:540–9.
13. McCarthy C, Cotter FE, McElwaine S, Twomey A, Mooney EE, Ryan F, et al. Altered gene expression patterns in intrauterine growth restriction: potential role of hypoxia. Am J Obstet Gynecol. 2007;196:70.e1–6.
14. Struwe E, Berzl G, Schild R, Blessing H, Drexel L, Hauck B, et al. Microarray analysis of placental tissue in intrauterine growth restriction. Clin Endocrinol. 2010;72:241–7.
15. Madeleneau D, Buffat C, Mondon F, Grimault H, Rigourd V, Tsatsaris V, et al. Transcriptomic analysis of human placenta in intrauterine growth restriction. Pediatr Res. 2015;77:799–807.
16. Nelissen ECM, van Montfoort APA, Dumoulin JCM, Evers JLH. Epigenetics and the placenta. Hum Reprod Update. 2011;17:397–417.
17. Bianco-Miotto T, Mayne BT, Buckberry S, Breen J, Rodriguez Lopez CM, Roberts CT. Recent progress towards understanding the role of DNA methylation in human placental development. Reproduction. 2016;152:R23–30.
18. Lewis RM, Cleal JK, Hanson MA. Review: placenta, evolution and lifelong health. Placenta. 2012;33:S28–32. https://doi.org/10.1016/j.placenta.2011.12.003.
19. Schroeder DI, Blair JD, Lott P, Yu HOK, Hong D, Crary F, et al. The human placenta methylome. Proc Natl Acad Sci U S A. 2013;110:6037–42.
20. Roifman M, Choufani S, Turinsky AL, Drewlo S, Keating S, Brudno M, et al. Genome-wide placental DNA methylation analysis of severely growth-discordant monochorionic twins reveals novel epigenetic targets for intrauterine growth restriction. Clin Epigenetics. 2016;8:70. https://doi.org/10.1186/s13148-016-0238-x.
21. Hillman SL, Finer S, Smart MC, Mathews C, Lowe R, Rakyan VK, et al. Novel DNA methylation profiles associated with key gene regulation and transcription pathways in blood and placenta of growth-restricted neonates. Epigenetics. 2015;10:50–61. https://doi.org/10.4161/15592294.2014.989741.
22. Lambertini L, Lee T-L, Chan W-Y, Lee M-J, Diplas A, Wetmur J, et al. Differential methylation of imprinted genes in growth-restricted placentas. Reprod Sci. 2011;18:1111–7.
23. Joo JE, Hiden U, Lassance L, Gordon L, Martino DJ, Desoye G, et al. Variable promoter methylation contributes to differential expression of key genes in human placenta-derived venous and arterial endothelial cells. BMC Genomics. 2013;14:475.
24. Lopez-Abad M, Iglesias-Platas I, Monk D. Epigenetic characterization of CDKN1C in placenta samples from non-syndromic intrauterine growth restriction. Front Genet. 2016;7:62.
25. Kaartokallio T, Cervera A, Kyllonen A, Laivuori K, Kere J, Laivuori H. Gene expression profiling of pre-eclamptic placentae by RNA sequencing. Sci Rep. 2015;5:14107.
26. Kleinrouweler CE, van Uitert M, Moerland PD, Ris-Stalpers C, van der Post JAM, Afink GB. Differentially expressed genes in the pre-eclamptic placenta: a systematic review and meta-analysis. PLoS One. 2013;8;e68991.
27. Gourvas V, Dalpa E, Konstantinidou A, Vrachnis N, Spandidos DA, Sifakis S. Angiogenic factors in placentas from pregnancies complicated by fetal growth restriction (review). Mol Med Rep. 2012;6:23–7.
28. Kimura C, Watanabe K, Iwasaki A, Mori T, Matsushita H, Shinohara K, et al. The severity of hypoxic changes and oxidative DNA damage in the placenta of early-onset preeclamptic women and fetal growth restriction. J Matern Fetal Neonatal Med. 2013;26:491–6.

29. Prins JR, Faas MM, Melgert BN, Huitema S, Timmer a HMN, et al. Altered expression of immune-associated genes in first-trimester human decidua of pregnancies later complicated with hypertension or foetal growth restriction. Placenta. 2012;33:453–5. https://doi.org/10.1016/j.placenta.2012.02.010.

30. McLeay RC, Bailey TL. Motif enrichment analysis: a unified framework and an evaluation on ChIP data. BMC Bioinformatics. 2010;11:165.

31. Mandl M, Depping R. Hypoxia-inducible aryl hydrocarbon receptor nuclear translocator (ARNT) (HIF-1beta): is it a rare exception? Mol Med. 2014;20:215–20.

32. Diez H, Fischer A, Winkler A, Hu C-J, Hatzopoulos AK, Breier G, et al. Hypoxia-mediated activation of Dll4-Notch-Hey2 signaling in endothelial progenitor cells and adoption of arterial cell fate. Exp Cell Res. 2007;313:1–9.

33. Ma R, Gu Y, Zhao S, Sun J, Groome LJ, Wang Y. Expressions of vitamin D metabolic components VDBP, CYP2R1, CYP27B1, CYP24A1, and VDR in placentas from normal and preeclamptic pregnancies. Am J Physiol Endocrinol Metab. 2012;303:E928–35.

34. Kent LN, Rumi MAK, Kubota K, Lee D-S, Soares MJ. FOSL1 is integral to establishing the maternal-fetal interface. Mol Cell Biol. 2011;31:4801–13.

35. Soares MJ, Chakraborty D, Renaud SJ, Kubota K, Bu P, Konno T, et al. Regulatory pathways controlling the endovascular invasive trophoblast cell lineage. J Reprod Dev. 2012;58:283–7.

36. Nevo O, Many A, Xu J, Kingdom J, Piccoli E, Zamudio S, et al. Placental expression of soluble FMS-like tyrosine kinase 1 is increased in singletons and twin pregnancies with intrauterine growth restriction. J Clin Endocrinol Metab. 2008;93:285–92.

37. Hoeller A, Ehrlich L, Golic M, Herse F, Perschel FH, Siwetz M, et al. Placental expression of sFlt-1 and PlGF in early preeclampsia vs. early IUGR vs. age-matched healthy pregnancies. Hypertens pregnancy. 2017;36:151–60.

38. Rajakumar A, Cerdeira AS, Rana S, Zsengeller Z, Edmunds L, Jeyabalan A, et al. Transcriptionally active syncytial aggregates in the maternal circulation may contribute to circulating soluble FMS-like tyrosine kinase 1 in preeclampsia. Hypertens (Dallas, Tex 1979). 2012;59:256–64.

39. Schrey S, Kingdom J, Baczyk D, Fitzgerald B, Keating S, Ryan G, et al. Leptin is differentially expressed and epigenetically regulated across monochorionic twin placenta with discordant fetal growth. Mol Hum Reprod. 2013;19:764–72.

40. Li RHW, Poon SCS, Yu MY, Wong YF. Expression of placental leptin and leptin receptors in preeclampsia. Int J Gynecol Pathol. 2004;23:378–85.

41. Velegrakis A, Sfakiotaki M, Sifakis S. Human placental growth hormone in normal and abnormal fetal growth. Biomed reports. 2017;7:115–22.

42. Mannik J, Vaas P, Rull K, Teesalu P, Laan M. Differential placental expression profile of human growth hormone/chorionic somatomammotropin genes in pregnancies with pre-eclampsia and gestational diabetes mellitus. Mol Cell Endocrinol. 2012;355:180–7.

43. Diplas AI, Lambertini L, Lee M-J, Sperling R, Lee YL, Wetmur J, et al. Differential expression of imprinted genes in normal and IUGR human placentas. Epigenetics. 2009;4:235–40.

44. Iglesias-Platas I, Martin-Trujillo A, Petazzi P, Guillaumet-Adkins A, Esteller M, Monk D. Altered expression of the imprinted transcription factor PLAGL1 deregulates a network of genes in the human IUGR placenta. Hum Mol Genet. 2014;23:6275–85.

45. Camprubi C, Iglesias-Platas I, Martin-Trujillo A, Salvador-Alarcon C, Rodriguez MA, Barredo DR, et al. Stability of genomic imprinting and gestational-age dynamic methylation in complicated pregnancies conceived following assisted reproductive technologies. Biol Reprod. 2013;89:50.

46. Maltepe E, Krampitz GW, Okazaki KM, Red-Horse K, Mak W, Simon MC, et al. Hypoxia-inducible factor-dependent histone deacetylase activity determines stem cell fate in the placenta. Development. 2005;132:3393–403.

47. Handy DE, Castro R, Loscalzo J. Epigenetic modifications: basic mechanisms and role in cardiovascular disease. Circulation. 2011;123:2145–56.

48. Miguel-Escalada I, Pasquali L, Ferrer J. Transcriptional enhancers: functional insights and role in human disease. Curr Opin Genet Dev. 2015;33:71–6.

49. Turner BM. Defining an epigenetic code. Nat Cell Biol. 2007;9:2–6.

50. Lee KJ, Shim SH, Kang KM, Kang JH, Park DY, Kim SH, et al. Global gene expression changes induced in the human placenta during labor. Placenta. 2010;31:698–704.

51. Tuteja G, Chung T, Bejerano G. Changes in the enhancer landscape during early placental development uncover a trophoblast invasion gene-enhancer network. Placenta. 2016;37:45–55.

52. Uusküla L, Männik J, Rull K, Minajeva A, Kõks S, Vaas P, et al. Mid-gestational gene expression profile in placenta and link to pregnancy complications. PLoS One. 2012;7:e49248.

53. Karlic R, Chung H-R, Lasserre J, Vlahovicek K, Vingron M. Histone modification levels are predictive for gene expression. Proc Natl Acad Sci U S A. 2010;107: 2926–31.

54. Bonet B, Brunzell JD, Gown AM, Knopp RH. Metabolism of very-low-density lipoprotein triglyceride by human placental cells: the role of lipoprotein lipase. Metabolism. 1992;41:596–603.

55. Gormley M, Ona K, Kapidzic M, Garrido-Gomez T, Zdravkovic T, Fisher SJ. Preeclampsia: novel insights from global RNA profiling of trophoblast subpopulations. Am J Obstet Gynecol. 2017;217(2):200.e1–200.e17.

56. Li H, Durbin R. Fast and accurate short read alignment with Burrows-Wheeler transform. Bioinformatics. 2009;25:1754–60.

57. Ji H, Jiang H, Ma W, Johnson DS, Myers RM, Wong WH. An integrated software system for analyzing ChIP-chip and ChIP-seq data. Nat Biotechnol. 2008;26:1293–300.

58. Love MI, Huber W, Anders S. Moderated estimation of fold change and dispersion for RNA-seq data with DESeq2. Genome Biol. 2014;15:550.

59. McLean CY, Bristor D, Hiller M, Clarke SL, Schaar BT, Lowe CB, et al. GREAT improves functional interpretation of cis-regulatory regions. Nat Biotechnol. 2010;28:495–501.

9

Effects of novel HDAC inhibitors on urothelial carcinoma cells

Aline Kaletsch[1], Maria Pinkerneil[1], Michèle J. Hoffmann[1]●, Ananda A. Jaguva Vasudevan[1]●, Chenyin Wang[2]●, Finn K. Hansen[2]●, Constanze Wiek[3], Helmut Hanenberg[3], Christoph Gertzen[2]●, Holger Gohlke[2]●, Matthias U. Kassack[2]●, Thomas Kurz[2]●, Wolfgang A. Schulz[1]*● and Günter Niegisch[1]●

Abstract

Background: Histone deacetylase inhibitors (HDACi) are promising anti-cancer drugs that could also be employed for urothelial carcinoma (UC) therapy. It is unclear, however, whether inhibition of all 11 zinc-dependent HDACs or of individual enzymes is more efficacious and specific. Here, we investigated the novel HDACi 19i (LMK235) with presumed preferential activity against class IIA HDAC4/5 in comparison to the pan-HDACi vorinostat (SAHA) and the HDAC4-specific HDACi TMP269 in UC cell lines with basal expression of HDAC4 and characterized two HDAC4-overexpressing UC cell lines.

Methods: Cytotoxic concentrations 50% (CC_{50}s) for HDACi were determined by MTT assay and high-content analysis-based fluorescent live/dead assay in UC cell lines with different expression of HDAC4 and as well as in normal urothelial cell cultures, HBLAK and HEK-293 cell lines. Effects of HDACis were analyzed by flow cytometry; molecular changes were followed by qRT-PCR and Western blots. UC lines overexpressing HDAC4 were established by lentiviral transduction. Inhibitor activity profiles of HDACi were obtained by current state in vitro assays, and docking analysis was performed using an updated crystal structure of HDAC4.

Results: In UC cell lines, 19i CC_{50}s ranged around 1 μM; control lines were similarly or less sensitive. Like SAHA, 19i increased the G2/M-fraction, disturbed mitosis, and elicited apoptosis or in some cells senescence. Thymidylate synthase expression was diminished, and p21^{CIP1} was induced; global histone acetylation and α-tubulin acetylation also increased. In most cell lines, 19i as well as SAHA induced HDAC5 and HDAC4 mRNAs while rather repressing HDAC7. UC cell lines overexpressing HDAC4 were not significantly less sensitive to 19i. Reevaluation of the in vitro HDAC isoenzyme activity inhibition profile of 19i and its docking to HDAC4 using current assays suggested rather low activity against class IIA HDACs. The specific class IIA HDAC inhibitor TMP269 impeded proliferation of UC cell lines only at concentrations > 10 μM.

Conclusions: Anti-neoplastic effects of 19i on UC cells appear to be exerted by targeting class I HDACs. In fact, HDAC4 may rather impede UC growth. Our results suggest that targeting of class IIA HDACs 4/5 may not be optimal for UC therapy. Moreover, our investigation provides further evidence for cross-regulation of class IIA HDACs by class I HDACs.

Keywords: Histone deacetylase HDAC4, Class IIA HDACs, Histone deacetylase inhibitor, Urothelial bladder cancer, Cell cycle arrest

* Correspondence: wolfgang.schulz@uni-duesseldorf.de
[1]Department of Urology, Medical Faculty, Heinrich Heine University, Moorenstr. 5, 40225 Duesseldorf, Germany
Full list of author information is available at the end of the article

Background

Histone deacetylase inhibitors (HDACi) are being developed for the treatment of a broad range of diseases, prominently cancer. Human histone deacetylases are classified into classes I, IIA, IIB, III, and IV. Class I HDACs (HDACs 1, 2, 3, and 8) are essential for global acetylation patterns in the nucleus and the epigenetic regulation of gene expression [1]. Increased expression of these isoenzymes is observed in a variety of malignant tumors and often correlates with a worse patient outcome [2–5]. As class I HDACs typically promote cellular proliferation in tumors, while inhibiting differentiation and apoptosis, they are the primary targets of treatment by HDACi [2, 6]. However, many HDACi under development or already used in clinical practice inhibit HDACs from other classes as well. This broader specificity may be beneficial in some cases. For instance, class IIB HDACs like HDAC6 may enhance stress resistance of cancer cells, thereby facilitating metastatic spread [7]. In other cases, though, more selective inhibitors may be superior for therapy and may elicit fewer adverse effects [8, 9].

A particularly difficult issue in cancer therapy is whether inhibition of class IIA HDACs is useful or counterproductive. These enzymes, the HDACs 4, 5, 7, and 9, compared to class I enzymes, possess limited enzymatic activity on their own. Rather, as components of multiprotein complexes, they act primarily as transcriptional corepressors at specific genes [10, 11]. In addition, they may function as transcriptional co-activators, as SUMO-E3 ligases, as components of DNA repair complexes and in cell cycle regulation [12]. Class IIA HDACs are expressed in a more tissue-specific pattern and interact with tissue-specific transcription factors to regulate organogenesis and cell differentiation [13–15]. Consequently, overexpression of HDAC4 and HDAC5 has been shown to be anti-proliferative in some cancer types, whereas pharmacological inhibition of their enzymatic function or siRNA-mediated downregulation has been proposed as an efficacious treatment approach in others [16]. For example, homozygous deletion of HDAC4 is a frequent event in malignant melanoma, whereas inhibition of HDAC4 expression by miR-125a-5p was anti-neoplastic in breast cancer cells and HDAC4 promotes proliferation of gastric cancer cell lines [17–19].

Our group studies HDACs in urothelial carcinoma (UC), the most common histological subtype of bladder cancer, with the aim of defining an optimal profile of targets for treatment by HDACi in this cancer type [20]. So far, we have identified HDAC1 and HDAC2 as promising [21] and excluded HDAC6 and HDAC8 as relevant targets [22, 23]. Here, we aimed to address whether inhibiting HDAC4 might contribute to the therapeutic efficacy of HDACi in urothelial carcinoma. HDAC4 is likely the main class IIA HDAC in the urinary bladder. For instance, in a comprehensive proteome analysis of various human tissues [24], HDAC4 was strongly expressed in the colon, testis, urinary bladder, and ovary and less strongly in the cortex and T cells. HDAC5 was most strongly expressed in the retina and in B cells, HDAC7 was largely restricted to immune cells, and HDAC9 was expressed at very low levels throughout [24]. This tissue distribution is in keeping with substantial experimental evidence on the functions of HDAC5 and HDAC7 in the nervous system and lymphocyte differentiation, respectively [25–27]. Moreover, in a previous screen of HDAC4 expression, we observed strong expression of the protein in normal urothelial cells, but diminished expression in some, albeit not all urothelial carcinoma cell lines (UCCs). Likewise, according to our qRT-PCR measurements and published microarray expression data, HDAC4 mRNA expression was often decreased in UC tissues [28]. In contrast, frequent overexpression of HDAC4 protein was reported in an immunohistochemical study by others [29]. Taken together, these observations suggest that HDAC4 expression in UC is highly variable.

To assess the suitability of HDAC4 as a therapeutic target in UC, we made use of novel hydroxamic acid HDAC inhibitors, 19i (LMK235), 19h (LMK233), and 19e (LMK225), which had been reported to exhibit preferential activity towards HDAC4/5 in older in vitro assays [30]. In addition, 19i had been found to inhibit class I HDAC1 and HDAC2 as well as class IIB HDAC6 at sub-micromolar concentrations. The inhibitors 19h and 19e displayed similar inhibition activity profiles [30].

Here, we report that 19i, 19h, and 19e indeed inhibited proliferation of all tested UCCs at low micromolar concentrations with 19i being the most efficient component. In UCCs, the biological characteristics of 19i action, i.e., cell cycle disturbances and induction of apoptosis, resembled that of the pan-HDAC inhibitor SAHA [21] in many regards and were overall compatible with a predominant effect on class I HDACs. Overexpression of HDAC4 did not protect against 19i, but impeded the proliferation of one UC cell line with low endogenous HDAC4 expression. Interestingly, treatment with 19i or SAHA strongly affected the expression of class IIA HDAC mRNAs. Corrected inhibitor activity profiles of 19i, 19h, and 19e obtained by current state in vitro assays and docking analysis using an updated crystal structure of HDAC4 were in keeping with a main effect on class I HDACs.

Methods

Cell culture, compounds, and treatment

For most experiments, three different UCCs with different expression of HDAC4 (VM-CUB1—low, UM-UC-3—normal, 639-V—moderately increased [28]) were used. Further experiments were performed in VM-CUB1 and UM-UC-3 cells overexpressing HDAC4 (see below). Standard UCCs were obtained from the DSMZ (Braunschweig, Germany) and Dr. H.B. Grossmann HB (Houston, USA). For comparison, we investigated the spontaneously immortalized normal human bladder cell line HBLAK (provided by CELLnTEC, Bern, Switzerland) [31] and the immortalized human embryonic kidney cell line HEK-293 (provided by Dr. V. Kolb-Bachofen, Duesseldorf, Germany). Cells were cultured and treated in DMEM GlutaMAX-I (Gibco, Darmstadt, Germany; UCCs and HEK-293) supplemented with 10% fetal calf serum (Biochrom, Berlin, Germany), except for HBLAK cultured in CnT-Prime Epithelial Culture Medium (CELLnTEC, Bern, Switzerland; HBLAK), at 37 °C and 5% CO_2. STR (short tandem repeat) profiling via DNA fingerprint analysis was performed for all cell lines. Primary cultures of normal urothelial cells (UP) were established from healthy ureters removed during tumor nephrectomy and cultured as described [31]. These cultures were used with informed consent of the patients and approval by the Ethics Committee of the Medical Faculty of the Heinrich-Heine-University, study number 1788. All inhibitors were dissolved in DMSO and stored as 10 mM stocks. One day after seeding, cells were incubated with a single defined dose of 19i, 19h, or 19e [30], the carboxylic acid derivative of 19i, the pan-inhibitor vorinostat (SAHA, suberoylanilide hydroxamic acid; #1009929, Cayman Chemicals, Ann Arbor, MI) or the specific class IIA inhibitor TMP269 (Selleck Chemicals, Munich, Germany) for 24, 48, or 72 h with a maximal 0.1% DMSO concentration in the treatment medium. The pan-HDACi inhibitor SAHA previously studied in detail [21, 22, 28, 32] was used for comparison. Solvent control cells were treated with equal amounts of DMSO.

Determining in vitro HDAC inhibitor activity profiles of 19i, 19h, and 19e

The in vitro inhibitory activity of compounds 19i, 19h, and 19e against each HDAC isoform was re-assessed at Reaction Biology Corp. (Malvern, PA) with fluorescence-based assays according to the company's standard operating procedures. The IC_{50} values were determined using 10 different concentrations ranging from 0.003 to 100 μM with threefold serial dilution. TMP269 was used as reference compound for class IIA HDACs, and trichostatin A served as control for all other HDAC isoforms. IC_{50} values were obtained by fitting the data to the four-parameter logistic equation using Prism 4.0 from GraphPad. Details for the experimental procedures can be obtained from Reaction Biology Corp.

Generation of HDAC4-overexpressing and control vector UC cell lines

HDAC4 cDNA from the pcDNA-HDAC4-FLAG plasmid kindly provided by Tso-Pang Yao (Addgene plasmid # 30485) was cloned into the lentiviral vector puc2-CL12IPwo using standard techniques, thereby creating the vector puc2CL12IPwo-HDAC4-FLAG (Additional file 1: Figure S1). Integrity of the HDAC4 coding sequence was verified by sequencing. Lentivirus production and cell transduction were performed as previously described [33, 34]. In brief, to produce replication-deficient lentiviruses, HEK-293T cells were transfected with helper plasmid expression construct (pCD/NL-BH [35]), envelope vector (pczVSV-G [36]), and the vector plasmids puc2CL12IPwo or puc2CL12IPwo-HDAC4-FLAG. Viral particles were harvested 48 h after transfection and used to transduce VM-CUB1 and UM-UC-3 cells using 8 μg/ml polybrene (Sigma Aldrich, St. Louis, MO). Twenty-four hours after transduction, the supernatant containing viral particles was removed and the transduced cells were selected with 4 (VM-CUB1) or 1 (UM-UC-3) μg/ml puromycin (Invitrogen, Carlsbad, CA) for 7 days. Stable overexpression of HDAC4 was confirmed by Western blot analysis of cells from several passages.

Determination of mean cytotoxic concentrations (CC_{50}) and time-dependent viability in cell lines

For the determination of cellular mean cytotoxic concentration (CC_{50}), UCCs, non-malignant control cells, and HDAC4-overexpressing clones were seeded in a 96-well format and treated once with a range of defined concentrations of the HDAC inhibitors. After 72 h, viability was quantified by NAD(P)H-dependent 3-(4,5-dimethylthiazol-2-yl)-2,5-diphenyltetrazolium bromide dye reduction assay (MTT, Sigma Aldrich, St. Louis, MO). CC_{50} values were estimated from three independent experiments by non-linear regression analysis (four-parameter logistic equation) using Prism 4.0 (Graph Pad) or Origin 8.0 (Origin Lab, Northhampton, GB). For time-dependent proliferation experiments, viability of untreated or inhibitor-treated cells was measured after 24, 48, and 72 h.

High-content analysis-based fluorescent live/dead assay

Live and dead cells were assayed by high-content analysis (HCA). Briefly, cells were treated with various concentrations of 19i or TMP269 in 96-well plates. After 72 h of treatment, cells were stained with a mixture of Hoechst 33342 (Sigma Aldrich, St. Louis, MO), calcein AM (Merck Millipore, Germany), and propidium iodide (Santa Cruz Biotechnology, Heidelberg) for cell nuclei, live and dead cells. The staining solution was replaced by PBS after 20 min. Images were acquired using ArrayScan XTI Live High Content Platform (Thermo Fisher Scientific Inc., USA) using excitation filters of 386, 485, and 560 nm for Hoechst 33342, calcein AM, and propidium iodide, respectively. The results were analyzed using HCS Studio Cellomics Scan (Thermo Fisher Scientific Inc., USA).

Clonogenicity assay and Giemsa staining

For clone formation assays, cells were treated for 24 or 48 h with inhibitors (as a rule 2 µM 19i, 2.5 µM SAHA). Then, depending on the cell line, 500–1000 cells were seeded in 6-cm plates, and 10 to 15 days later, colonies were washed with PBS, fixed in methanol, and stained with Giemsa (Merck Millipore, Darmstadt, Germany).

Determination of caspase activity

Caspase activity after inhibitor treatment was quantified by the Caspase-Glo 3/7 assay and normalized to cell viability measured by CellTiter-Glo® reagent (Promega, Mannheim, Germany) as previously described [21]. Briefly, following exposure to inhibitors, defined aliquots of trypsinized cells were transferred to 96-well plates for viability and caspase-3/7 measurements according to the manufacturer's protocol.

Cell cycle analysis by flow cytometry

Cell cycle analyses were performed with UCCs or non-malignant control cells treated with 2 µM 19i, 2.5 µM SAHA, or DMSO for 24 or 48 h as previously described [21]. Trypsinized cells and floating cells collected from the supernatant were stained with Nicoletti-buffer (50 µg/µl propidium iodide (PI), 0.1% sodium citrate and 0.1% Triton X-100 [37]), and their cell cycle profiles were measured with a Miltenyi MACSQuant® Analyzer (Milteny Biotec GmbH, Bergisch Gladbach, Germany) using the MACSQuantify software.

Senescence assay via β-galactosidase staining

Cells exposed to 19i, SAHA, or DMSO for 24 and 48 h were stained for β-galactosidase as previously described [21]. Briefly, PBS-washed cells were fixed with 2% formaldehyde and 0.2% glutaraldehyde for 5 min at RT. After another washing step, cells were incubated overnight with fresh β-Gal staining solution (1 mg/ml X-Gal (5-bromo-4-chloro-3-indolyl-beta-D-galacto-pyranoside; Merck, Darmstadt, Germany), 150 mM NaCl, 2 mM $MgCl_2$, 5 mM $K_3Fe(CN)_6$, 5 mM $K_4Fe(CN)_6$) at 37 °C. Documentation of stained cells was performed with a Nikon Eclipse TE2000-S microscope (Nikon, Tokyo, Japan).

RNA isolation, cDNA synthesis, and qRT-PCR

Total cell RNA was isolated by the Qiagen RNeasy Mini Kit (Qiagen, Hilden, Germany) according to the manufacturer's protocol, and cDNA was synthesized using QuantiTect Reverse Transcription Kit (Qiagen, Hilden, Germany) with an extended incubation time of 30 min at 42 °C as previously described [21, 23, 32]. Target mRNA expression was measured by qRT-PCR with QuantiTect SYBR Green RT-PCR Kit (Qiagen, Hilden, Germany) on the LightCycler® 96 Real-Time PCR system with software version 1.1 (Roche Diagnostics, Rotkreuz, Switzerland). All used primers, comprising QuantiTect Primer assays (Qiagen, Hilden, Germany), self-designed target primers, and primers for the reference housekeeping gene TBP (TATA-box binding protein), are listed in Additional file 2: Table S1.

Total protein extraction, purification of histones, and Western blot analysis

Total protein extraction, purification of histones, and Western blot analysis were performed as previously described [21, 23, 32]. Briefly, cells were incubated for 30 min on ice in RIPA-buffer (150 mM NaCl, 1% Triton X-100, 0.5% desoxycholate, 1% Nonidet P-40, 0.1% SDS, 1 mM EDTA, 50 mM TRIS (pH 7.6)) containing 10 µl/ml protease inhibitor cocktail (#P-8340, Sigma Aldrich, St. Louis, MO). Histones were extracted for detection of histone H3 and H4 acetylation by a modified published protocol employing sulfuric acid extraction and TCA-precipitation [38]. Concentrations of total protein and histones were determined by BCA protein assay (Thermo Fisher Scientific, Carlsbad, CA). Subsequently, total cell proteins (15 µg) or extracted histones (2 µg) were separated by SDS-PAGE (total proteins 10–12% gels, histones 15% gels), transferred to PVDF membranes (Merck Millipore, Berlin, Germany), and were incubated with primary antibodies (at RT for 1 h or 4 °C overnight, see Additional file 3: Table S2) following blocking with 5% non-fat milk or BSA (bovine serum albumin) in TBST (150 mM NaCl, 10 mM TRIS, pH 7.4 and 0.1% Tween-20). For signal detection, membranes were incubated with a suitable horseradish peroxidase-conjugated secondary antibody (see Additional file 2: Table S1) at RT for 1 h and signals were visualized by SuperSignal™ West Femto (Thermo Fisher Scientific, Carlsbad, CA) and WesternBright Quantum kit (Biozym, Hessisch Oldendorf, Germany).

Nuclear morphology analysis and quantification

Analysis of nuclear morphology was performed after treatment of UCCs or VM-CUB1 and UM-UC-3 clones with 2 µM 19i, 2.5 µM SAHA, or DMSO for 24 and 48 h. As previously described [21, 32], after fixation with 4% formaldehyde, cells were permeabilized (0.3% Triton X100 in PBS, 10 min, RT), blocked (1% BSA in PBS, 30 min, RT), and subsequently incubated for 1 h at RT with 14 nM Rhodamine Phalloidin in blocking solution. Following counter-staining of nuclei with 1 µg/ml DAPI (4′,6-diamidino-2-phenylindole), cells were mounted with fluorescence mounting medium (DAKO, Glostrup, Denmark). For each treatment option and sample, 500 cells were counted and the amount of mitosis and micronuclei was quantified using a Nikon Eclipse 400 microscope (Nikon, Tokyo, Japan).

Statistical analysis

P values between different groups were determined by the Student's *t* test; asterisks denote significant (* < 0.05) differences; error bars indicate SD. Concentration-effect curves were obtained by fitting the data to the four-parameter logistic equation using Prism 4.0 from GraphPad or Origin 8.0 (Origin Lab, Northhampton, GB).

Results

Proliferation and cell cycle following treatment with novel HDAC inhibitors

Initially, the effects of the three inhibitors 19i, 19h, and 19e on cell viability were determined by MTT assay in three UC cell lines differing in HDAC4 expression (VM-CUB1—low, UM-UC-3—normal, 639-V—moderate, according to [28]), after 72 h of treatment. 19i was the most potent compound with cellular CC_{50}s between 0.82 and 1.03 µM. By comparison, CC_{50} values for the other two compounds 19h and 19e were two- to three-fold higher (CC_{50} 2.20–3.27 µM; Table 1). Notably, we often observed a slight increase in cell viability at low concentrations, especially after shorter treatment for 24 or 48 h. The cytotoxic effects of higher concentrations of the compounds usually became discernible after 24 h, increasing over time (Fig. 1a). The carboxylic acid derivative of 19i, which is the most likely metabolite, did not reach CC_{50} in any UC cell line at concentrations up to 100 µM (data not shown).

Since we observed a stronger anti-neoplastic effect of 19i than of 19h and 19e in clone formation assays as well (data not shown), we focused on 19i as the most potent compound in further experiments. Additionally, we used HEK-293, immortalized from embryonal kidney cells, and HBLAK, a spontaneously immortalized urothelial cell line. Interestingly, HEK-293 was at least as sensitive to 19i as the UC cell lines, with a CC_{50} value of 0.61 µM after 72 h. HBLAK cells were more resistant with a CC_{50} value above 5 µM (Table 1). As in some UC cells, low doses of 19i increased HBLAK viability (Fig. 1b). Based on the results from the MTT assays, in the following experiments, cells were usually treated with 2 µM 19i or with 2.5 µM SAHA. Treatment with 2 µM 19i impaired the clonogenic potential of UC cells comparably to treatment with the pan-HDACi SAHA. This was also the case for HEK-293 cells, but HBLAK again were less sensitive (Fig. 1c).

To confirm the results obtained using MTT assays, a high-content analysis-based fluorescent live/dead assay, which allows direct counting of the numbers of live and dead cells, was conducted for 19i. In these assays, we also included primary cultures of normal urothelial cells as an additional control (Additional file 4: Figure S2). After 72 h of treatment, this assay yielded comparable CC_{50} values as the MTT assay of below 1 µM for the three UCCs, but was more informative for HBLAK cells. The number of these cells decreased at relatively low concentrations of 19i, but less cell death was observed than in cancer cells. This effect was even pronounced in cultured normal urothelial cells, in which even low concentrations of 19i led to decreased cell numbers, but only very high concentrations induced significant cell death. These findings indicate that 19i induces proliferation arrest rather than cell death in normal control cells.

Efficacious concentrations of 19i elicited an increased fraction of cells in the G2/M phase in UC cells and in the non-urothelial HEK-293 cells. The changes in cell cycle distribution developed gradually over time and resembled those caused by the pan-HDAC inhibitor SAHA. However, 19i caused a more profound increase in the G2/M fraction. In HBLAK cells, no significant effects on cell cycle distribution could be observed after treatment with HDACi at 2 µM 19i (Fig. 1d).

Apoptosis and senescence following 19i treatment

Morphologically, both features of cellular apoptosis and senescence were observed in UCCs treated with 19i. Many cells became elongated and occasionally apoptotic cells were seen. Over time, cells became larger and flatter, indicative of cellular senescence (Additional file 5: Figure S3). Indeed, some 19i-treated cells, especially from the VM-CUB1 cell line, stained positive for senescence-associated β-galactosidase (Additional file 5: Figure S3). As indicators of apoptosis, in 19i-treated UC cells, caspase 3/7 activity was significant, albeit moderately increased and PARP cleavage was augmented, especially in 639-V (Fig. 2a, b). The number of mitoses, as revealed by staining with DAPI and rhodamine phalloidin, decreased sharply in VM-CUB1 and UM-UC-3

Table 1 CC_{50} values for novel HDAC inhibitors in urothelial carcinoma cell lines

	19e	19h	19i
VM-CUB1	2.35	2.24	0.97
UM-UC-3	2.54	2.20	0.82
639-V	2.86	3.27	1.03
HBLAK	n.d.	n.d.	> 5
HEK-293	n.d.	n.d.	0.61
VM-CUB1-LV	n.d.	n.d.	0.95
VM-CUB-HDAC4	n.d.	n.d.	0.63
UM-UC-3-LV	n.d.	n.d.	0.79
UM-UC-3-HDAC4	n.d.	n.d.	0.74

CC_{50} values following 72 h of incubation with the indicated inhibitors are given in micromolar. Data shown are mean from $n = 4$

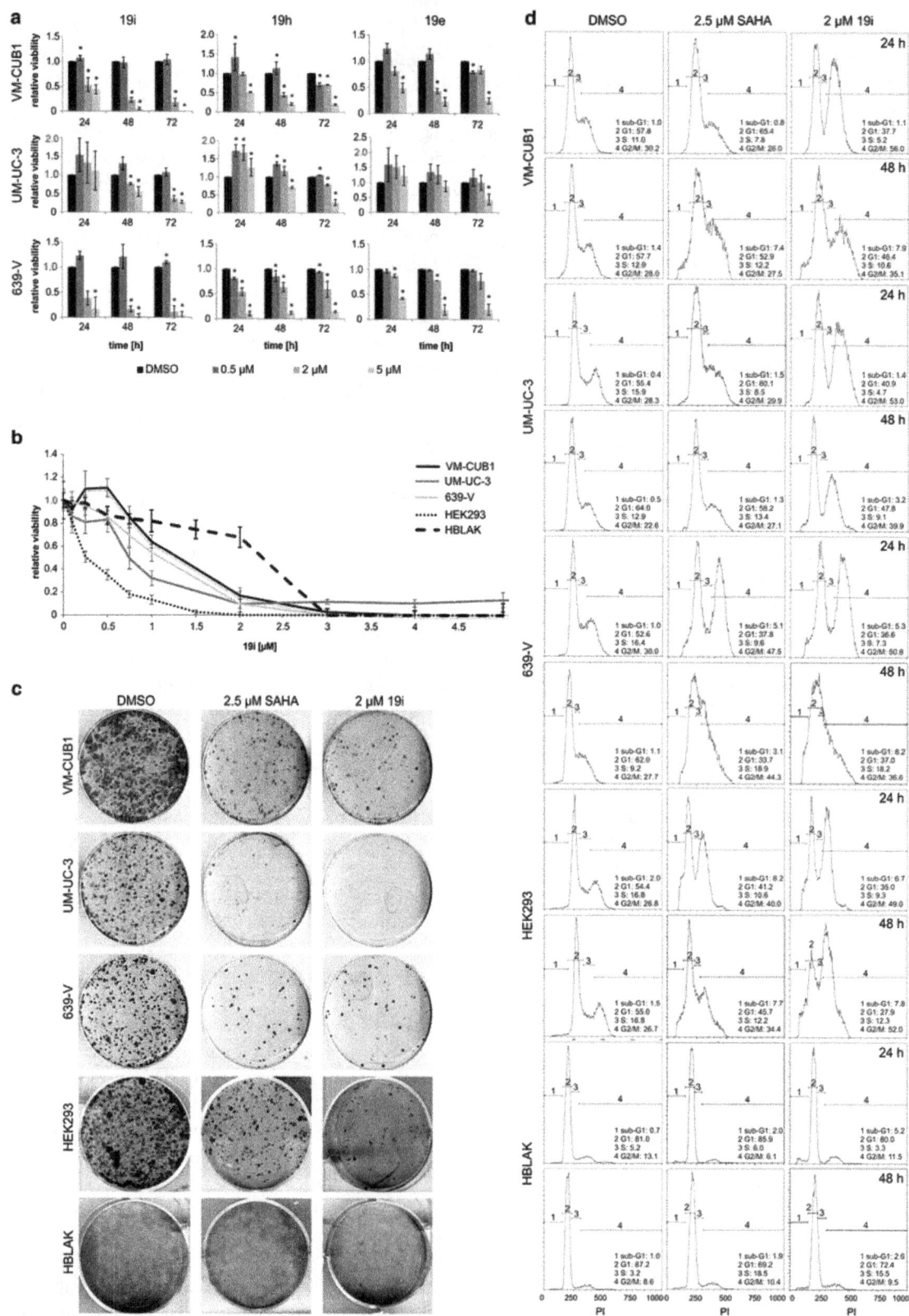

Fig. 1 (See legend on next page.)

(See figure on previous page.)
Fig. 1 Effects of HDACi 19e, 19h, and 19i on urothelial carcinoma and control cell lines. HDACi were applied to UC cell lines VM-CUB1, UM-UC-3, and 639-V as well as control cell lines HEK293 (non-urothelial) and HBLAK (urothelial). **a** Dose-response curves after 24, 48, and 72 h of treatment of UCCs with 0.5, 2, und 5 μM of each HDACi. The calculated significances refer to the DMSO solvent control (*$p < 0.05$). Data shown are mean from $n = 3$. **b** Dose-response curve of UCCs VM-CUB1, UM-UC-3, 639-V, HEK293, and HBLAK after 72 h of treatment with 0.5–5 μM 19i. Data shown are mean from $n = 4$. **c** Clonogenicity following 19i treatment of VM-CUB1, UM-UC-3, 639-V, HEK293, and HBLAK. Cells were treated with DMSO, 2.5 μM SAHA, or 2 μM 19i for 48 h, replated at clonal density, cultured for 2 weeks, and stained with Giemsa. **d** Changes in cell cycle distribution after 24 or 48 h of treatment with 19i. Cell cycle changes and amount of apoptotic cells (as sub-G1 fraction) determined by flow cytometry following 2 μM 19i or 2.5 μM SAHA treatment in VM-CUB1 UM-UC-3, 639-V, HEK293, and HBLAK. DMSO is the solvent control. Data shown are representative of triplicates

cells upon treatment with 19i, whereas the percentage of cells with micronuclei increased (Fig. 2c).

Marker expression and acetylation changes following 19i treatment

In response to treatment with 19i for 24 or 48 h, expression of thymidylate synthase (TS) mRNA decreased and p21^{CIP1} mRNA expression increased in all three UCCs in a similar manner as during treatment with SAHA (Fig. 3a, Additional file 6: Figure S4A). Expression of p21 protein was more prominently induced by 19i than by SAHA (Additional file 6 Figure S4). Acetylation of α-tubulin, which depends mainly on class IIB HDAC6 activity, was strongly induced both after 19i and SAHA treatment

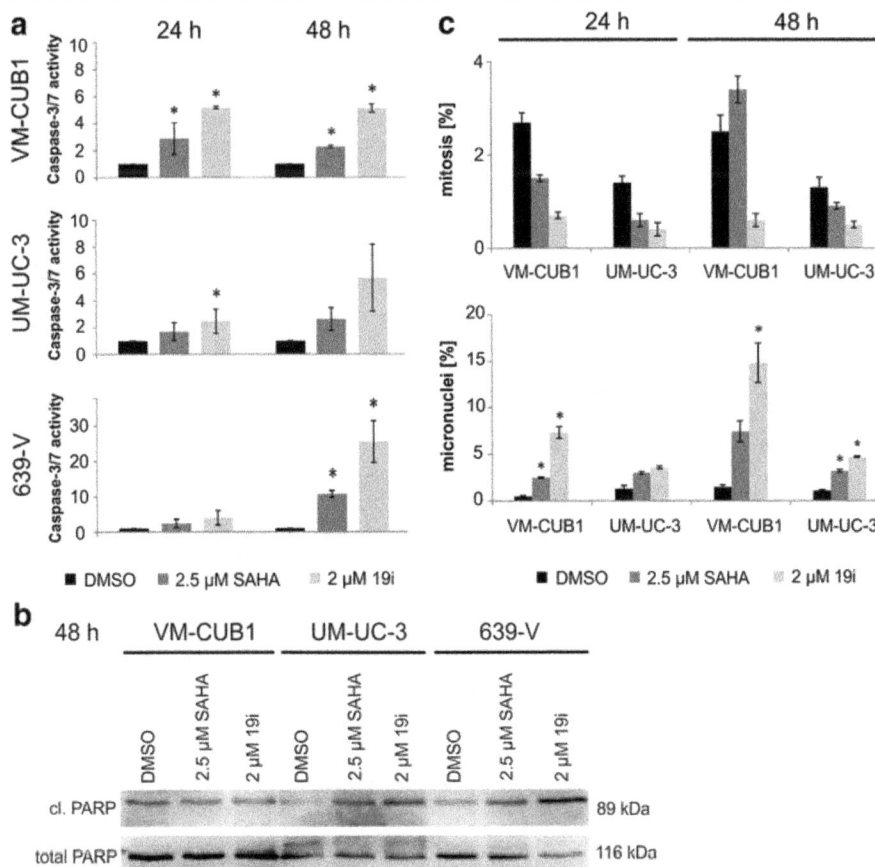

Fig. 2 Cellular effects of 19i treatment in urothelial carcinoma cell lines. **a** Caspase 3/7 activity (24 and 48 h) and **b** cleaved PARP (48 h) were monitored in UCCs VM-CUB1, UM-UC-3, and 639-V after treatment with 19i (2 μM) or SAHA (2.5 μM). **c** Quantitative analysis of nuclear morphology, based on DAPI stainings, in UCCs VMCUB1 and UM-UC-3. The percentages of mitoses and micronuclei are shown after treatment with HDACi 19i (2 μM), SAHA (2.5 μM), or DMSO for 24 or 48 h. The calculated significances refer to the DMSO solvent control (*$p < 0.05$). Data in **a** and **c** are mean from $n = 3$; the blot in **b** shows a representative experiment

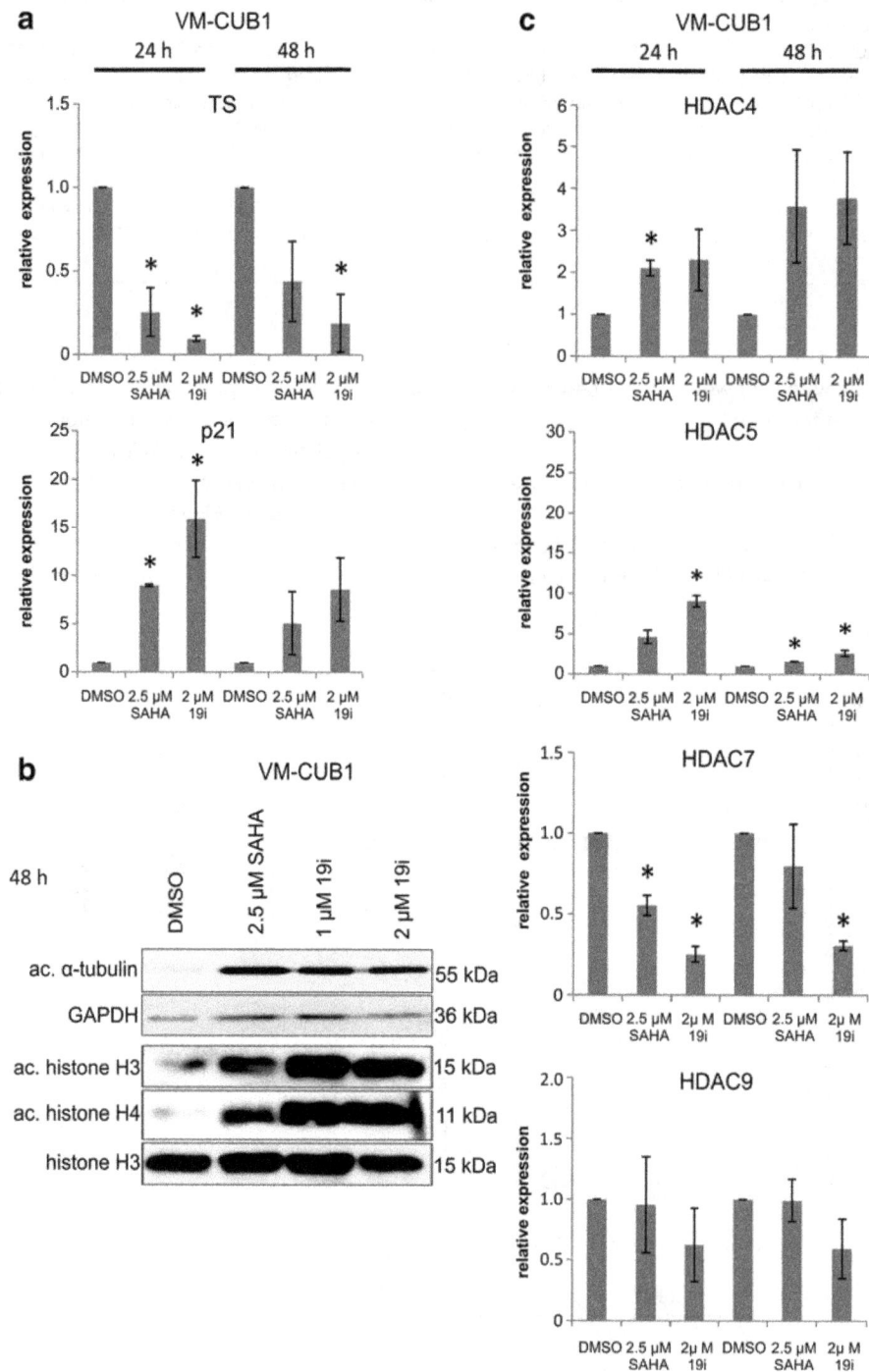

Fig. 3 Effects of 19i treatment on gene expression and protein acetylation in VM-CUB1. Effects on mRNA and protein expression levels in VM-CUB1 following treatment with 19i (2 μM), SAHA (2.5 μM), or DMSO as solvent control. **a** Expression of thymidylate synthase (*TS*) and p21^CIP1^(*CDKN1A*) mRNAs after 24 and 48 h of treatment as measured by qRT-PCR. **b** Acetylation of α-tubulin and histones H3 and H4 after 48 h of treatment with 2.5 μM SAHA, 1 or 2 μM 19i, or DMSO; ac acetylated. **c** HDAC4, HDAC5, HDAC7, and HDAC9 mRNA expression after 24 or 48 h of treatment. In **a** and **c**, all values indicate relative expression compared to a standard for each gene and adjusted to TBP as a reference gene. Significance levels refer to the DMSO solvent control (*$p < 0.05$). Data in **a** and **c** are mean from $n = 3$; the blot in **b** shows a representative experiment

(Fig. 3b, Additional file 6: Figure S4B). Global acetylation of histones H3 and H4 was likewise enhanced following 19i treatment (Fig. 3b, Additional file 6: Figure S4B).

Intriguingly, mRNA expression of class IIA HDACs was affected by treatment with 19i as well as SAHA (Fig. 3c, Additional file 6: Figure S4C). Most prominently, HDAC5 was induced by the HDAC inhibitors in VM-CUB1 and UM-UC-3 cells after 24 h of treatment, whereas HDAC4 responded significantly only in VM-CUB1 cells. In contrast, HDAC7 mRNA tended to decrease upon inhibitor treatment. HDAC9 mRNA expression remained very low. Only minor and transient increases were observed in the expression of HDAC1, HDAC2, and HDAC6 mRNAs following treatment with 19i or SAHA (Additional file 7: Figure S5).

To investigate whether the changes in HDAC4, HDAC5, and HDAC7 mRNA expression are reflected in persistent changes at their protein levels, these were determined in the three UCCs by Western blotting following treatment with 19i or SAHA for 48 h (Additional file 6: Figure S4D). In VM-CUB1 cells, HDAC4 protein remained essentially undetectable and HDAC5 likewise very low, whereas HDAC7 decreased in accord with its mRNA level following treatment with either inhibitor. The same decrease was observed for HDAC7 in UM-UC3 and 639-V. Interestingly, HDAC5 protein was diminished in 639-V and HDAC4 protein in both UM-UC-3 and 639-V by either HDACi. Variable effects were observed on HDAC6 expression. HDAC9 protein was not investigated because of its very low mRNA expression level.

Experimental overexpression of HDAC4 in UC cell lines

Next, we generated VM-CUB1 and UM-UC-3 cell lines overexpressing HDAC4-FLAG by lentiviral transduction (designated VM-CUB1-HDAC4 and UM-UC-3-HDAC4). As a control, cells were transduced with an empty vector (designated VM-CUB1-LV and UM-UC-3-LV). The HDAC4-transduced cells expressed strongly increased levels of HDAC4 mRNA (Fig. 4a) and protein stably over many cell passages (Fig. 4b). The HDAC4-overexpressing cells were morphologically indistinguishable from the parental or LV cells (Additional file 5: Figure S3C). VM-CUB1-HDAC4, but not UM-UC-3-HDAC4, cells grew more slowly than the parental cell line or LV cells (Fig. 4c). Accordingly, VM-CUB1-HDAC4 required less frequent passaging and their clonogenic potential was impaired, which was not the case in UM-UC-3-HDAC4 cells (Fig. 4d).

Effects of 19i on UCCs overexpressing HDAC4

The increased expression of HDAC4 did not severely affect the sensitivity of the UC cell lines to 19i in short-term assays (72 h). In UM-UC-3 cells, no significant difference was observed, whereas the CC_{50} of 19i was

diminished to 0.63 μM in VM-CUB1-HDAC4 cells compared to 0.95 μM in VM-CUB1-LV cells (Fig. 5a, Table 1). Both VM-CUB1-HDAC4 and UM-UC-3-HDAC4 cells formed fewer colonies after treatment with 19i (Fig. 5b).

In untreated VM-CUB1-HDAC4 cells, the number of mitoses was decreased and more micronuclei were discernible compared to VM-CUB1-LV and parental cells. Upon treatment with 19i, the number of mitoses decreased in VM-CUB1-HDAC4 as well as VM-CUB1-LV, but in contrast to the controls, fewer micronuclei were detectable in VM-CUB1-HDAC4. In UM-UC-3-HDAC4 treated with 19i, disturbances of mitosis were seen as in the controls with a decreased number of mitoses but increased number of micronuclei (Fig. 5c). As in the parental cells, 19i treatment induced evident morphological changes in the HDAC4-overexpressing cell lines (Additional file 5: Figure S3C).

In VM-CUB1-HDAC4 cells, in addition to HDAC4 mRNA, HDAC7 mRNA was significantly increased by about threefold, whereas changes in other class IIA HDACs were minor. No significant changes in the expression of other class IIA HDACs were observed in UM-UC-3-HDAC4 cells (Fig. 6a). Treatment with HDAC inhibitors, either with SAHA or 19i, induced expression changes in $p21^{CIP1}$, TS (Fig. 6b), and class IIA HDAC mRNAs (Additional file 8: Figure S6) in the HDAC4-overexpressing UC lines analogous to those in the parental or control vector-transduced cell lines. Notably, expression of HDAC4 was further increased by treatment with the inhibitors, although its expression was driven by a viral promoter, suggesting posttranscriptional regulation (Additional file 8: Figure S6). Increases in the acetylation of α-tubulin and the histones H3 and H4 were also analogous to those in the parental and vector only cell lines (Fig. 6c).

Reevaluation of inhibitor activity profiles of 19i, 19h, and 19e

As the effects of 19i on UC cell lines resembled those of SAHA which has little activity towards class IIA HDACs and because HDAC4-overexpressing UC lines did not become less sensitive to 19i, the HDAC inhibitory profiles of 19i, 19h, and 19e in vitro were re-measured using current state in vitro assays, in comparison to the novel class IIa-specific compound TMP269 [39] and the broad-range inhibitor trichostatin A (Table 2). These control compounds displayed the expected profiles. Likewise, newly measured IC_{50}s of 19i, 19h, and 19e for class I and class IIB HDACs were similar to those reported previously [30]. However, inhibitory activity of 19i, 19h, and 19e against HDACs 4, 5, and 7 was weak with IC_{50}s well above 10 μM.

In addition, docking analysis using an updated crystal structure of HDAC4 was performed. The method and

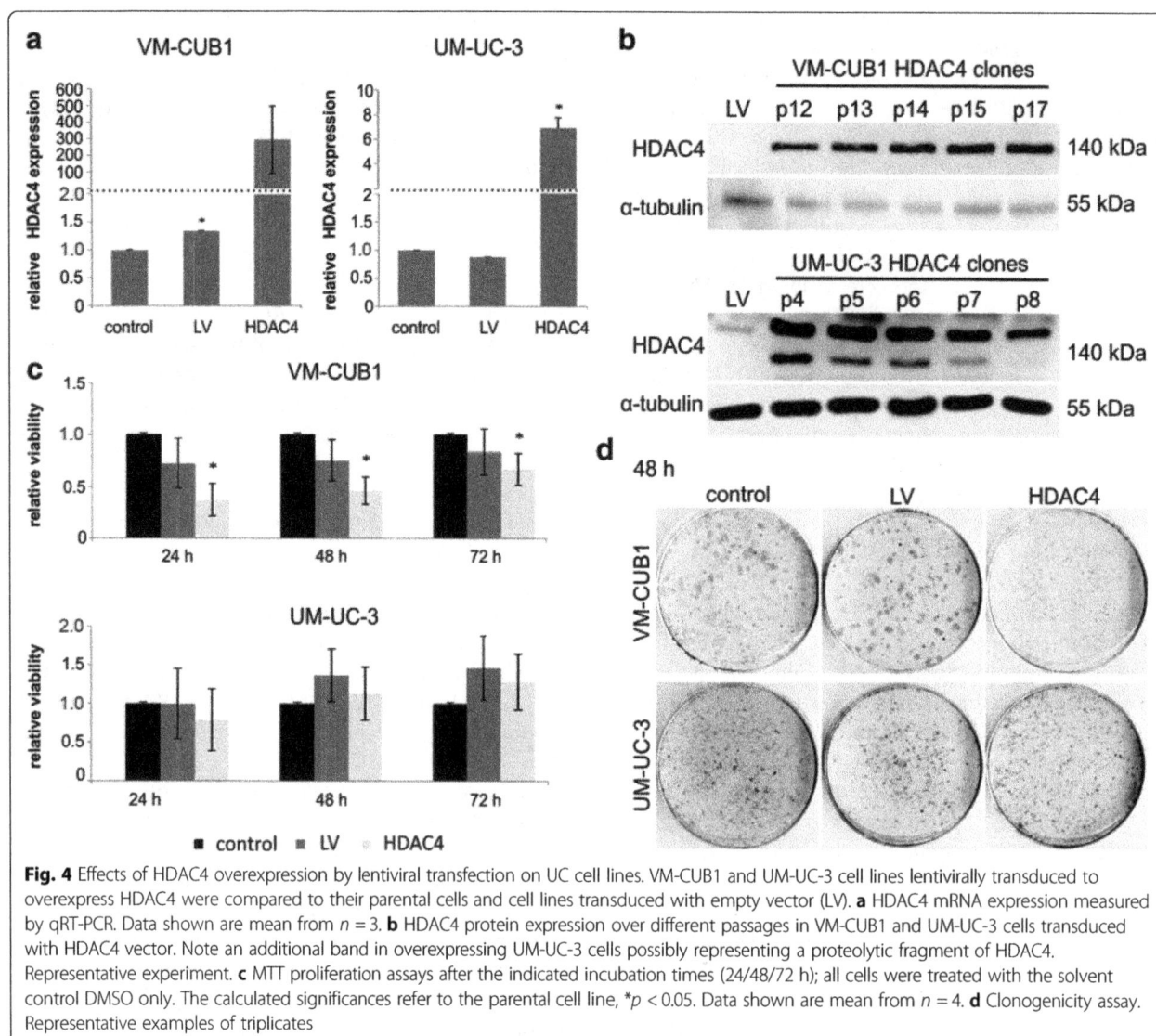

Fig. 4 Effects of HDAC4 overexpression by lentiviral transfection on UC cell lines. VM-CUB1 and UM-UC-3 cell lines lentivirally transduced to overexpress HDAC4 were compared to their parental cells and cell lines transduced with empty vector (LV). **a** HDAC4 mRNA expression measured by qRT-PCR. Data shown are mean from $n = 3$. **b** HDAC4 protein expression over different passages in VM-CUB1 and UM-UC-3 cells transduced with HDAC4 vector. Note an additional band in overexpressing UM-UC-3 cells possibly representing a proteolytic fragment of HDAC4. Representative experiment. **c** MTT proliferation assays after the indicated incubation times (24/48/72 h); all cells were treated with the solvent control DMSO only. The calculated significances refer to the parental cell line, *$p < 0.05$. Data shown are mean from $n = 4$. **d** Clonogenicity assay. Representative examples of triplicates

results are described in detail in Additional file 9. In summary, docking of 19i into the X-ray crystal structure of the WT of HDAC4 did not reveal a valid binding mode, which agrees with the data from biological evaluation that shows no binding of 19i to HDAC4.

Effect of HDAC class IIA-specific inhibitor TMP269 on UC cell lines and normal urothelial cells

As 19i turned out to be a weak inhibitor of HDAC4 and the novel compound TMP269 specifically inhibiting class IIA HDACs has recently become available [39], we tested its effect on UC cell lines using MTT and high-content analysis-based fluorescent live/dead cell assays (Fig. 7). Only high concentrations exceeding 10 μM were effective; CC_{50}s on cell lines derived from MTT and high-content analysis (Table 3) were about two

orders of magnitude higher than in vitro HDAC inhibitory concentrations (Table 2). Interestingly, the lowest CC_{50} for TMP269 was measured in HBLAK immortalized urothelial cells and normal urothelial cells reacted even more sensitively (Additional file 10: Figure S7).

Discussion

Whereas class I HDACs are well established as valid targets for anti-tumor drugs, the functions of class IIA HDACs in cancer development and their potential as drug targets are much less clear. One reason for that uncertainty is that to date only few drugs specifically or at least preferentially target class IIA enzymes. A second reason may be that class IIA HDACs are expressed in a more cell-type-specific manner, implying likewise cancer-type-specific functions. Yet another reason could

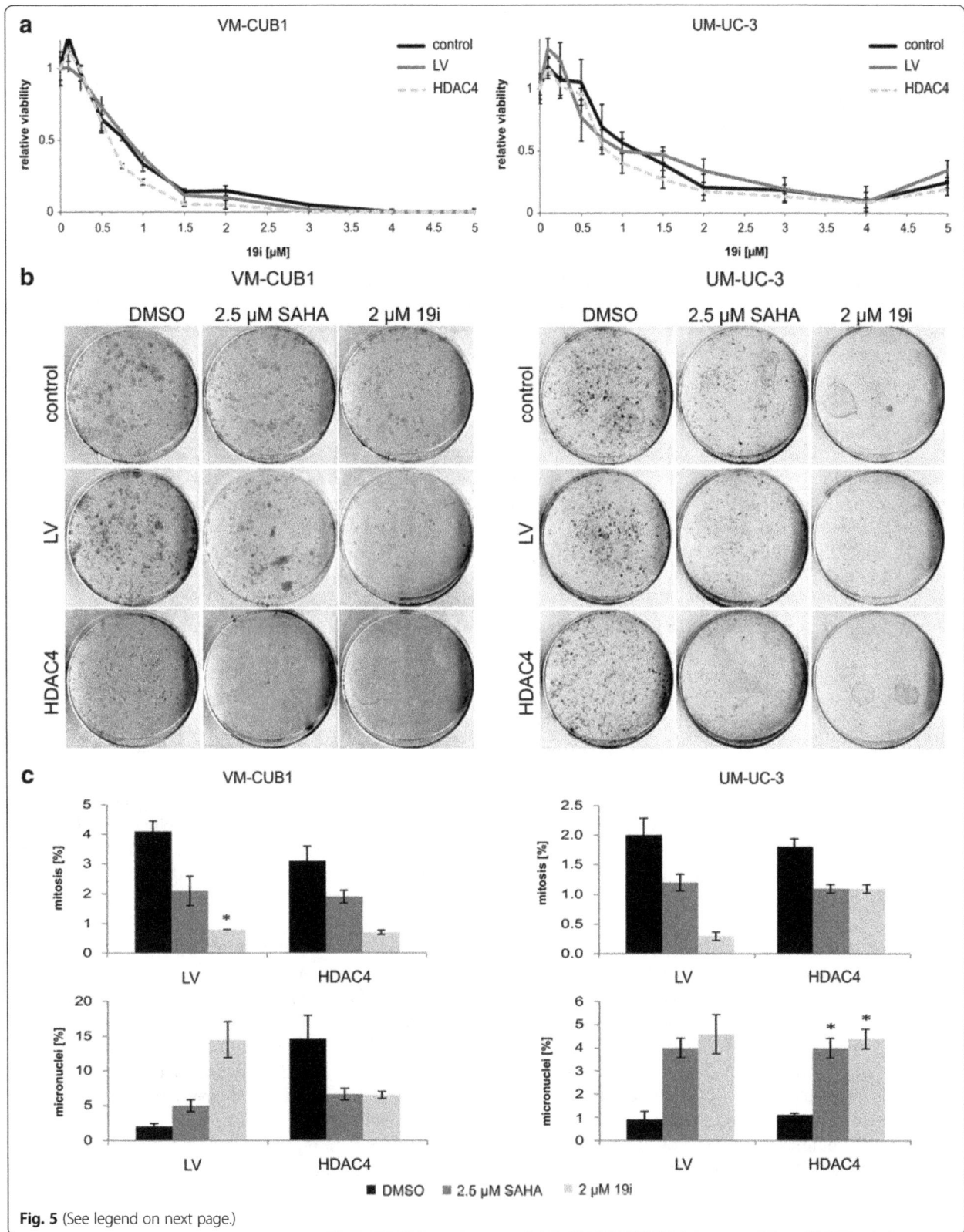

Fig. 5 (See legend on next page.)

(See figure on previous page.)
Fig. 5 Cellular effects of 19i on HDAC4-overexpressing UCCs. Cellular effects of 19i on VM-CUB1 and UM-UC-3 cell lines lentivirally transduced to overexpress HDAC4 compared to the parental cells and cell lines transduced with empty vector (LV). **a** Dose-response curves of UC cell lines treated with increasing concentrations of 19i (0.1–5 µM) for 72 h. Data shown are mean from $n = 4$. **b** Clonogenicity of cells treated with DMSO, 2 µM 19i, or 2.5 µM SAHA for 48 h. Note smaller colonies in VM-CUB1-HDAC4 DMSO-treated controls. Representative examples of triplicates. **c** Analysis of nuclear morphology, based on DAPI staining. The percentage amount of mitoses and micronuclei are shown after treatment with HDACi 19i (2 µM), SAHA (2.5 µM), or DMSO for 48 h. The calculated significances refer to the DMSO solvent control (*$p < 0.05$). Data shown are mean from $n = 3$

be that class IIA HDACs are less directly involved in the control of cell proliferation than class I HDACs and may rather influence cancer growth indirectly through their effects on cell differentiation and cell metabolism. The present study was initiated to explore some of these issues in the context of urothelial carcinoma.

The novel hydroxamic acid HDAC inhibitors, 19i (LMK235), 19h (LMK233), and 19e (LMK225), were thought to inhibit HDAC4/5 with in vitro IC_{50}s in the nanomolar range, whereas their in vitro IC_{50}s for HDAC1/2 range between 0.3 and 1.4 µM [30]. Of note, all compounds also inhibit the class IIB HDAC6 with in vitro IC_{50}s below 1 µM. Applied to urothelial carcinoma cell lines, 19i consistently yielded the lowest CC_{50} values and was therefore selected for closer investigation of its mechanism of action. Notably, the main metabolite of 19i, its corresponding carboxylic acid, was completely inactive on the UC cells, making it likely that 19i itself was the active compound within the cells. For all three compounds, the CC_{50} values against UC cells were in the low micromolar range (approximately 1 µM for 19i), i.e., about two orders of magnitude higher than their presumed in vitro IC_{50}s for HDAC4/5. For other hydroxamic acid HDAC inhibitors such as SAHA, in vitro IC_{50}s for class I HDACs are relatively similar to their CC_{50} values on tumor cells. Assuming that cellular uptake and metabolism are likewise not limiting the action of the novel hydroxamic acid compounds, the discrepancy between their in vitro IC_{50}s for HDAC4/5 and their CC_{50} values on tumor cells suggests that inhibition of class IIA HDACs may not be responsible for the observed inhibition of cell proliferation. Instead, their CC_{50} values correspond rather well to their in vitro IC_{50}s for HDAC1/2. Very likely, the compounds also inhibit HDAC6 in the tumor cells, as evidenced by a prominent increase in α-tubulin acetylation. However, even specific inhibitors or knockdown of HDAC6 exert only limited effects on UC cell lines [22], and therefore, this inhibitory activity is unlikely to contribute substantially to the anti-neoplastic activity of 19i.

Several further findings support the interpretation that the anti-neoplastic activity of 19i derives primarily from its activity against class I HDACs. UC cell lines react in

a characteristic fashion to specific inhibition of class I HDACs which includes accumulation in G2/M-phase, mitotic disturbances, a limited increase in apoptosis, induction of p21[CIP1], and downregulation of thymidylate synthase [21, 32]. These changes, which gradually appear over time, were also evident following treatment with 19i. Moreover, 19i increased overall histone acetylation like the more HDAC1/2-specific inhibitors romidepsin and givinostat. In many respects, thus, the action of 19i at low micromolar concentrations resembled that of the pan-HDAC inhibitor SAHA at higher concentrations. This conclusion prompted us to have the complete inhibitor activity profile of the new HDACi reevaluated by current assays for HDAC class IIA enzyme activities, which are more difficult to measure in vitro than class I activities. Indeed, whereas the in vitro inhibition constants against class I enzymes and HDAC6 were similar to the previously reported values, inhibitory activity against class IIA enzymes was much weaker than originally reported [30] and was particularly low against HDAC4. Thus, 19i is a compound with similar overall action as SAHA, albeit active at lower concentrations against UC cell lines.

The data from the biological and biochemical characterization agree well with the new molecular docking analysis of 19i. In contrast to the previously used gain-of-function mutant structure, docking into the HDAC4 wildtype structure did not yield a binding pose in which the zinc-binding group of 19i would complex the zinc ion of HDAC4. This result shows that a pronounced conformational difference by one amino acid can impact a docking result, even if all other amino acids in the binding site region are identical. Our results implicate that the greatly enhanced activity of the variant might not only result from the additional hydrogen bonding by the mutant tyrosine residue [40], but also from the restriction of the conformational freedom of the lysine inside the catalytic center. The increased conformational freedom of the 19i zinc-binding group in the wildtype HDAC4 compared to the gain-of-function variant might also apply to the acetylated lysine substrates, with similar steric conformation and flexibility.

An important finding was that 19i and SAHA affected the expression of the mRNAs for class IIA HDACs,

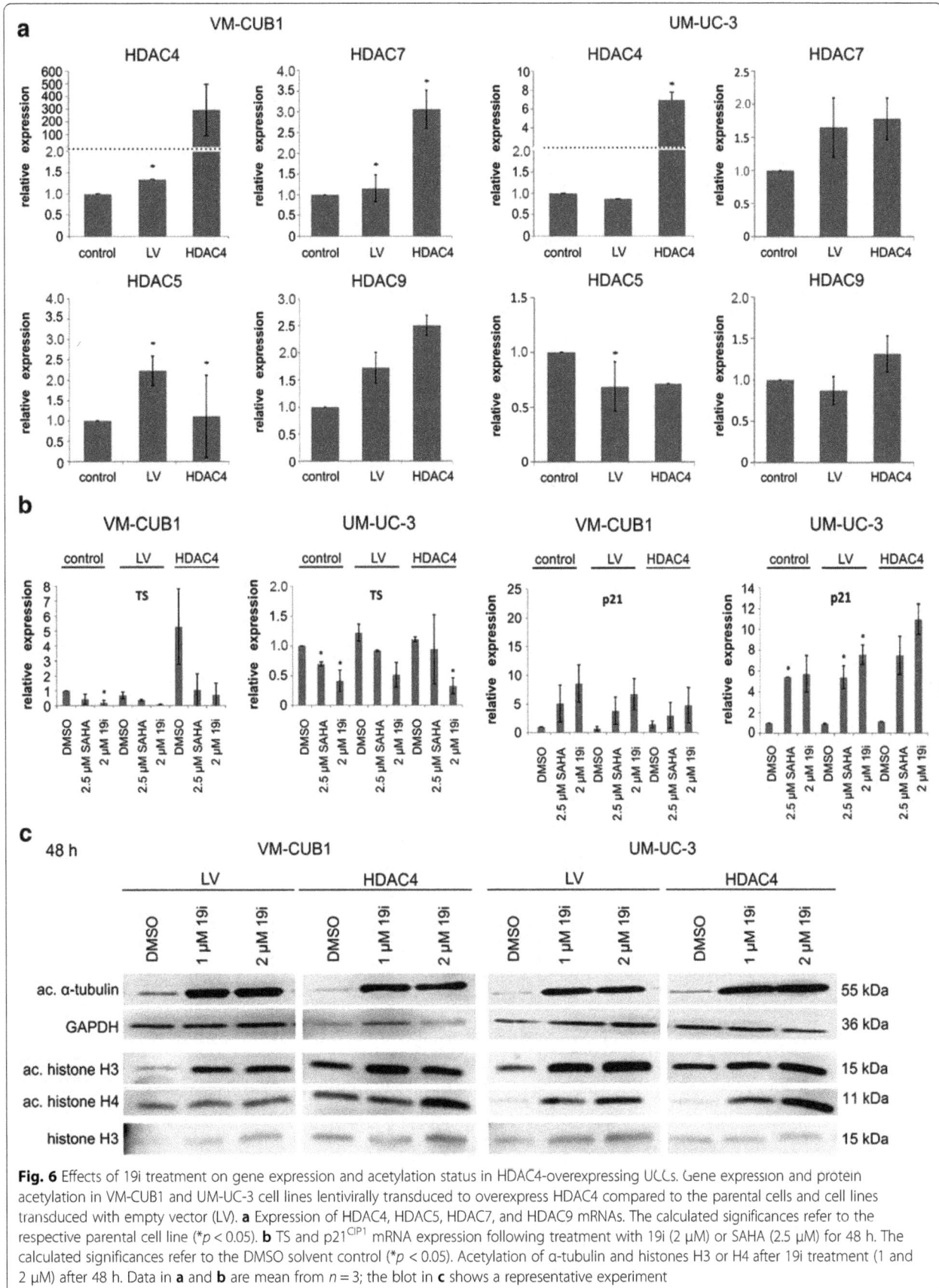

Fig. 6 Effects of 19i treatment on gene expression and acetylation status in HDAC4-overexpressing UCCs. Gene expression and protein acetylation in VM-CUB1 and UM-UC-3 cell lines lentivirally transduced to overexpress HDAC4 compared to the parental cells and cell lines transduced with empty vector (LV). **a** Expression of HDAC4, HDAC5, HDAC7, and HDAC9 mRNAs. The calculated significances refer to the respective parental cell line (*$p < 0.05$). **b** TS and p21^{CIP1} mRNA expression following treatment with 19i (2 µM) or SAHA (2.5 µM) for 48 h. The calculated significances refer to the DMSO solvent control (*$p < 0.05$). Acetylation of α-tubulin and histones H3 or H4 after 19i treatment (1 and 2 µM) after 48 h. Data in **a** and **b** are mean from $n = 3$; the blot in **c** shows a representative experiment

Table 2 Inhibitor activity profiles of 19i, 19h, and 19e in vitro

Compound	HDAC1	HDAC2	HDAC3	HDAC4	HDAC5	HDAC6	HDAC7	HDAC8	HDAC9	HDAC10	HDAC11
19i	0.315	0.402	0.236	>100	45.6	0.032	131	2.84	198	0.491	109
19h	0.586	2.24	n.d.	263	51.9	0.038	n.d.	1.92	n.d.	n.d.	147
19e	0.399	1.38	n.d.	184	37.6	0.020	n.d.	1.50	n.d.	n.d.	66.4
TSA	0.020	0.048	0.032	n.d.	n.d.	0.006	n.d.	0.423	n.d.	0.073	5.30
TMP269	n.d.	n.d.	n.d.	0.282	0.101	n.d.	0.101	n.d.	0.032	n.d.	n.d.

Inhibitor activity profiles of novel HDAC inhibitors using current assays; TSA and TMP269 were tested for comparison. All IC_{50} values are given in micromolar. The experiment was performed once

n.d. not done

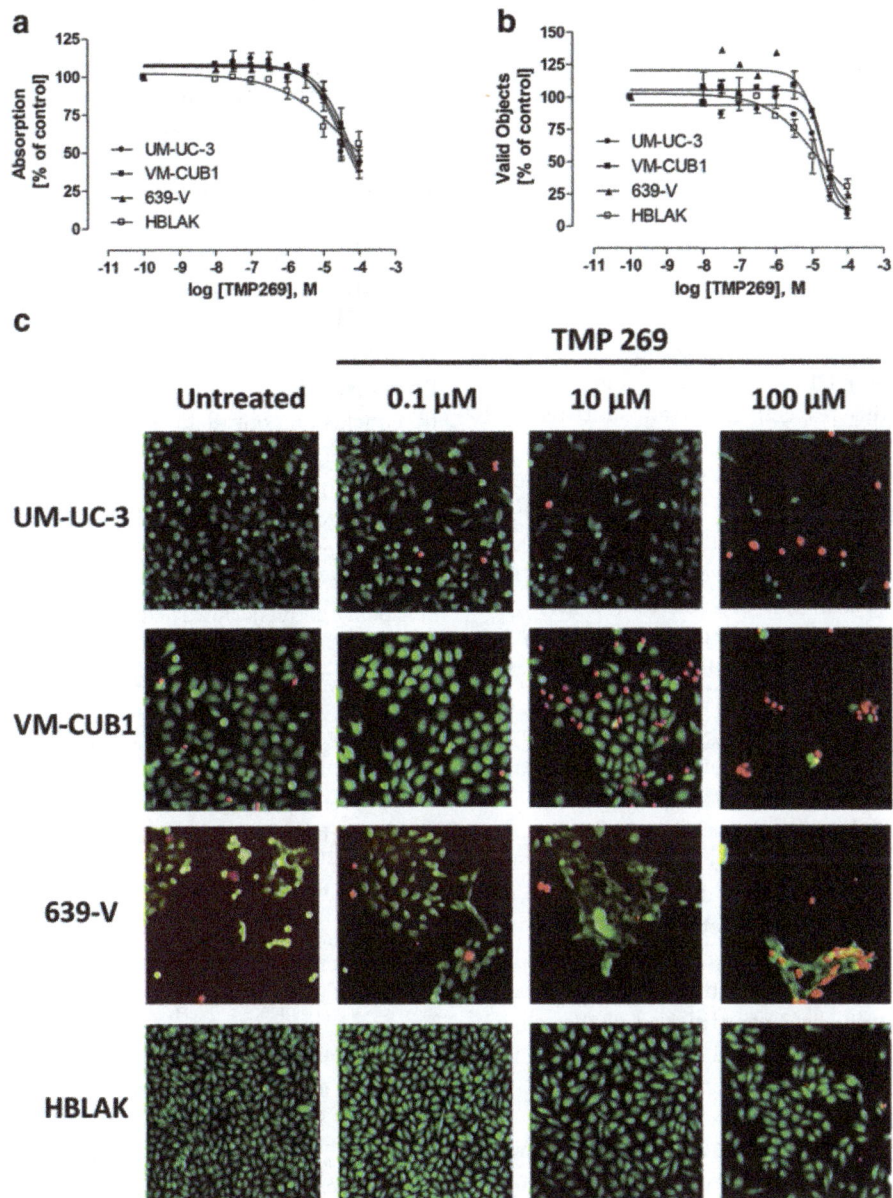

Fig. 7 Effects of HDACi TMP269 on urothelial carcinoma cell lines. **a** Concentration-response curves after 72 h of treatment with TMP269 in UCC cells using MTT assays. Data shown are mean ± SEM of the three independent experiments. **b** Concentration-response curves after 72 h of treatment with TMP269 in UCC cells using high-content analysis-based fluorescent live/dead assay. Data shown are mean ± SEM of the three independent experiments. **c** Staining of live (calcein-AM, green) and dead (PI, red) UCC cells after 72 h of treatment with TMP269. Data shown are a representative experiment of a set of 3

albeit to varying extents between the UC cell lines. In general, HDAC4 and HDAC5 mRNAs tended to become upregulated, whereas HDAC7 mRNA was rather downregulated. Changes in HDAC1, 2, and 6 mRNA expression were weaker and more transient. Interestingly, some of the changes at the mRNA level, but not others, resulted in according changes in protein levels. Thus, upregulation of HDAC7, but not of HDAC4 protein, was observed following the HDACi treatment. These observations

could be seen as another indication of potential compensatory mechanisms against HDAC inhibition (as discussed in [21]). In particular, it suggests regulation of class IIA by class I HDACs. Hints at this phenomenon have been obtained by others [41, 42] and its underlying mechanisms clearly deserve further investigation.

In the clinical application of HDAC inhibitors, tumor selectivity is crucial. While adverse effects on rapidly and continuously proliferating cells in the gut, skin, and

Table 3 CC_{50} values of TMP269 in urothelial carcinoma cell lines estimated after 24, 48, and 72 h of incubation

Assay	Incubation time (h)	UM-UC-3	VMCub1	639-V	HBLAK
MTT	24	110	115	96.1	
MTT	48	73.8	115	65.8	
MTT	72	32.3	45.9	39.4	48.7
HCA	72	14.6	20.1	16.5	10.6

CC_{50} values following the indicated incubation times are given in micromolar. Data shown are mean from $n = 3$

hematopoietic system are major concerns, inhibition of urothelial regeneration should be considered for drugs targeting UC. Class I HDAC-specific inhibitors are not very selective in this respect; CC_{50}s for short-term effects are similar, but, importantly, non-cancerous urothelial cells retain the potential for long-term growth, presumably by properly activating G1 checkpoints [20]. By comparison, immortalized HBLAK urothelial cells were less sensitive to 19i even in short-term assays. Like normal urothelial cells, they reacted to relatively low concentrations of 19i, but induction of cell death occurred only at high levels of the drug, as observed with other HDAC inhibitors in previous studies [21, 32]. Another control cell line, HEK-293, which was immortalized from fetal kidney by viral genes, was however as sensitive as the cancer cells in both types of assays. The mechanisms underlying this difference is unknown, but we note that HEK-293 are also more sensitive to a new compound, 4SC-202, which inhibits HDAC1/2 and HDAC3 as well as the histone demethylase LSD1/KDM1A and potentially WNT and hedgehog signaling [32]. In fact, the use of HEK-293 as a benign control cell line in pharmacological studies has been criticized, as the cell line is aneuploid and forms tumors in immune-deficient mice [43]. Our results buttress this argument, as HEK-293 reacts like UC cancer cell lines to HDACi treatment.

The functions of class IIA HDACs in normal urothelium and in urothelial carcinoma are essentially unknown. As a first step to address this issue, we have generated HDAC4-overexpressing VM-CUB1 and UM-UC3 cells by lentiviral transduction. These cell lines were also employed to investigate whether HDAC4 was a critical target of 19i. In keeping with the argument expounded above, overexpression of HDAC4 did not protect the cells from the inhibitor; if anything, the cells became more sensitive.

HDAC4-overexpressing UC cell lines did not discernibly differ morphologically from untransduced cells or cells transduced with control vector. However, VM-CUB1 cells overexpressing HDAC4 grew more slowly and formed fewer and smaller colonies, while proliferation of UM-UC-3 cells, with higher basal HDAC4 expression than VM-CUB1, was not diminished by HDAC4 overexpression. While the mechanisms underlying the subtle

growth impediment in VM-CUB1 require further investigation in detail, it is evident that HDAC4 overexpression does not regularly promote proliferation of UC cells, likewise supporting the argument that targeting of HDAC4 by HDAC inhibitors is unlikely to be helpful in the treatment of UC. This conclusion is supported by the weak effect of TMP269, a new class IIA HDAC-specific inhibitor. Effects of HDAC4 overexpression on other properties of these two and further UC cell lines, such as metabolic properties, differentiation, and response to stress, will have to be addressed in a future study.

Conclusions

In conclusion, our data suggest that at least HDAC4, among the class IIA HDACs, does not significantly contribute to proliferation and survival of common urothelial carcinoma cell lines. The new HDACi 19i, upon reassessment, was found to not act via class IIA HDAC inhibition, but rather in a similar manner as SAHA, albeit being active at lower concentrations.

Additional files

Additional file 1: Figure S1. Lentiviral vector used for HDAC4 overexpression. (JPG 2487 kb)

Additional file 2: Table S1. Primers used for PCR. (DOCX 21 kb)

Additional file 3 Table S2. Antibodies and conditions used for Western blotting. (DOCX 15 kb)

Additional file 4: Figure S2. Effects of 72 h treatment with 19i on UCC cells using High Content Analysis-based fluorescent live/dead assay. (A) Percentage of control cell counts of UM-UC-3, VM-CUB1, 639-V, HBLAK and primary normal urothelial cells after 72 h treatment with 19i using High Content Analysis-based fluorescent live/dead assay. (B) Staining of live (calcein-AM, green) and dead (PI, red) UCC cells and urothelial control cells (culture # UP281) after 72 h treatment with 19i. Data shown are mean from $n = 3$. (JPG 3640 kb)

Additional file 5: Figure S3. Morphological changes following treatment with 2.5 μM SAHA or 2 μM 19i. (A, C) Morphology of indicated cell lines and (B) staining for SA-β-galactosidase in VM-CUB1 and UM-UC-3 after 19i or SAHA treatment for 48 h. Exemplary photographs. (JPG 3608 kb)

Additional file 6: Figure S4. Effects of 19i treatment on gene expression, protein expression and protein acetylation in UM-UC-3 and 639-V. Effects on mRNA and protein expression levels in UM-UC-3 and 639-V following treatment with 19i (2 μM), SAHA (2.5 μM) or DMSO as solvent control. (A) Expression of thymidylate synthase (TS) and p21^{CIP1}(CDKN1A) mRNAs after 24 and 48 h treatment as measured by qRT-PCR. (B) Acetylation of α-tubulin and histones H3 and H4 after 48 h treatment with 2.5 μM SAHA, 1 or 2 μM 19i, or DMSO; ac: acetylated. (C) HDAC4, HDAC5, HDAC7 und HDAC9 mRNA expression after 24 h or 48 h treatment. (D) Expression of HDAC4, HDAC5, HDAC7, HDAC6 and p21^{CIP1} protein in VM-CUB1, UM-UC-3 and 639-V following HDACi treatment; α-tubulin was used as a loading control. In (A) and (C) all values indicate relative expression compared to a standard for each gene, adjusted to TBP as a reference gene and set as 1 for the solvent control value of each cell line. Significance levels refer to DMSO solvent controls (* = $p < 0.05$). qRT-PCR data shown are mean from $n = 3$, western blots are representative experiments. (JPG 4401 kb)

Additional file 7: Figure S5. Expression of HDAC1, HDAC2 and HDAC6 mRNA following treatment of UCCs with 19i or SAHA. Effects of 24 and 48 h treatment with 19i (2 μM), SAHA (2.5 μM) or DMSO as solvent control on mRNA expression of HDAC1, HDAC2 and HDAC6 in VM-CUB1, UM-UC-3 and 639-V cells. All values indicate relative expression compared to a standard for each gene, adjusted to TBP as a reference gene and set as 1 for the solvent control. Significance levels likewise refer to the solvent control (* = $p < 0.05$). Data shown are mean from $n = 3$. (PDF 105 kb)

Additional file 8: Figure S6. Effect of 19i treatment on the expression of class IIA HDAC mRNAs in HDAC4 overexpressing cell lines. Effects of 24 and 48 h treatment with 19i (1 or 2 μM), SAHA (2.5 μM) or DMSO as solvent control on mRNA expression of HDAC4, HDAC5 and HDAC7 in VM-CUB1, VM-CUB1-LV, VM-CUB1-HDAC4, UM-UC-3, UM-UC-3-LV and UM-UC-3-HDAC4 cells. All values indicate relative expression compared to a standard for each gene, adjusted to TBP as a reference gene and set as 1 for the solvent control in the respective parental cell lines. Significance levels refer to the solvent control for each subline (* = $p < 0.05$). Data shown are mean from $n = 3$. (JPG 5738 kb)

Additional file 9: Docking of 19i to HDAC4. (DOCX 1064 kb)

Additional file 10: Figure S7. Effects of treatment with 19i on primary normal urothelial cells using High Content Analysis-based fluorescent live/dead assay. Percentage of control cell counts of primary urothelial cells (culture # UP281) after 72 h treatment with TMP269 using High Content Analysis-based fluorescent live/dead assay. Data shown are mean from $n = 3$. (JPG 1137 kb)

Abbreviations
DAPI: 4,6-Diamidine-2-phenylindol; DMSO: Dimethyl sulfoxide; FITC: Fluorescein isothiocyanate; HCA: High-content analysis; HDAC: Histone deacetylase; HDACi: HDAC inhibitors; PI: Propidium iodide; PVDF: Polyvinylidene fluoride; SAHA: Suberoylanilide hydroxamic acid; UC: Urothelial carcinoma; UCCs: Urothelial cancer cell lines; ZBG: Zinc-binding group

Funding
This work was supported by grants from the Deutsche Forschungsgemeinschaft (NI 1398/1-1), from the Forschungskommission der Medizinischen Fakultät der Heinrich-Heine-Universität (42/2015), and from the Dr.-Brigitte-& Constanze-Wegener-Stiftung (Project #11) to GN. The Deutsche Forschungsgemeinschaft (DFG) is further acknowledged for funds used to purchase the ArrayScan XTI Live High Content Platform used in this research (INST 208/690-1).

Authors' contributions
FKH, MJH, TK, MUK, WAS, and GN conceived the study. AK, MP, MJH, CoW, MUK, WAS, and GN designed the experiments and analyzed the data. AK, MP, MJH, AAJV, CoW, ChW, CG, and HG performed and evaluated the experiments. FKH, HH, and TK provided the essential materials. AK, MP, WAS, MUK, and GN wrote the manuscript and assembled the figures and tables. All authors read and approved the final version of the manuscript.

Author details
[1]Department of Urology, Medical Faculty, Heinrich Heine University, Moorenstr. 5, 40225 Duesseldorf, Germany. [2]Institute for Pharmaceutical and Medical Chemistry, Heinrich Heine University, Duesseldorf, Germany. [3]Department of Otorhinolaryngology and Head and Neck Surgery, Medical Faculty, Heinrich Heine University, Duesseldorf, Germany.

References
1. Moser MA, Hagelkruys A, Seiser C. Transcription and beyond: the role of mammalian class I lysine deacetylases. Chromosoma. 2014;123:67–78.
2. Witt O, Deubzer HE, Milde T, Oehme I. HDAC family: what are the cancer relevant targets? Cancer Lett. 2009;277:8–21.
3. Weichert W. HDAC expression and clinical prognosis in human malignancies. Cancer Lett. 2009;280:168–76.
4. Montezuma D, Henrique RM, Jeronimo C. Altered expression of histone deacetylases in cancer. Crit Rev Oncog. 2015;20:19–34.
5. Nakagawa M, Oda Y, Eguchi T, Aishima S, Yao T, Hosoi F, et al. Expression profile of class I histone deacetylases in human cancer tissues. Oncol Rep. 2007;18:769–74.
6. Reichert N, Choukrallah MA, Matthias P. Multiple roles of class I HDACs in proliferation, differentiation, and development. Cell Mol Life Sci. 2012;69: 2173–87.
7. Yang PH, Zhang L, Zhang YJ, Zhang J, Xu WF. HDAC6: physiological function and its selective inhibitors for cancer treatment. Drug Discov Ther. 2013;7:233–42.
8. Thaler F, Minucci S. Next generation histone deacetylase inhibitors: the answer to the search for optimized epigenetic therapies? Expert Opin Drug Discov. 2011;6:393–404.
9. Subramanian S, Bates SE, Wright JJ, Espinoza-Delgado I, Piekarz RL. Clinical toxicities of histone deacetylase inhibitors. Pharmaceuticals. 2010;3:2751.
10. Fischle W, Dequiedt F, Hendzel MJ, Guenther MG, Lazar MA, Voelter W, et al. Enzymatic activity associated with class II HDACs is dependent on a multiprotein complex containing HDAC3 and SMRT/N-CoR. Mol Cell. 2002;9:45–57.
11. Lahm A, Paolini C, Pallaoro M, Nardi MC, Jones P, Neddermann P, et al. Unraveling the hidden catalytic activity of vertebrate class IIa histone deacetylases. Proc Natl Acad Sci USA. 2007;104:17335–40.
12. Martin M, Kettmann R, Dequiedt F. Class IIa histone deacetylases: regulating the regulators. Oncogene. 2007;26:5450–67.
13. Martin M, Kettmann R, Dequiedt F. Class IIa histone deacetylases: conducting development and differentiation. Int J Dev Biol. 2009;53:291–301.
14. Parra M. Class IIa HDACs—new insights into their functions in physiology and pathology. FEBS J. 2015;282:1736–44.
15. Haberland M, Montgomery RL, Olson EN. The many roles of histone deacetylases in development and physiology: implications for disease and therapy. Nat Rev Genet. 2009;10:32–42.
16. Clocchiatti A, Florean C, Brancolini C. Class IIa HDACs: from important roles in differentiation to possible implications in tumourigenesis. J Cell Mol Med. 2011;15:1833–46.
17. Hsieh TH, Hsu CY, Tsai CF, Long CY, Chai CY, Hou MF, et al. miR-125a-5p is a prognostic biomarker that targets HDAC4 to suppress breast tumorigenesis. Oncotarget. 2015;6:494–509.
18. Kang ZH, Wang CY, Zhang WL, Zhang JT, Yuan CH, Zhao PW, et al. Histone deacetylase HDAC4 promotes gastric cancer SGC-7901 cells progression via p21 repression. PLoS One. 2014;9:e98894.
19. Stark M, Hayward N. Genome-wide loss of heterozygosity and copy number analysis in melanoma using high-density single-nucleotide polymorphism arrays. Cancer Res. 2007;67:2632–42.
20. Pinkerneil M, Hoffmann MJ, Schulz WA, Niegisch G. HDACs and HDAC inhibitors in urothelial carcinoma—perspectives for an antineoplastic treatment. Curr Med Chem. 2017;24:4151–65.
21. Pinkerneil M, Hoffmann MJ, Deenen R, Kohrer K, Arent T, Schulz WA, et al. Inhibition of class I histone deacetylases 1 and 2 promotes urothelial carcinoma cell death by various mechanisms. Mol Cancer Ther. 2016;15: 299–312.
22. Rosik L, Niegisch G, Fischer U, Jung M, Schulz WA, Hoffmann MJ. Limited efficacy of specific HDAC6 inhibition in urothelial cancer cells. Cancer Biol Ther. 2014;15:742–57.
23. Lehmann M, Hoffmann MJ, Koch A, Ulrich SM, Schulz WA, Niegisch G. Histone deacetylase 8 is deregulated in urothelial cancer but not a target for efficient treatment. J Exp Clin Cancer Res. 2014;33:59.
24. Kim MS, Pinto SM, Getnet D, Nirujogi RS, Manda SS, Chaerkady R, et al. A draft map of the human proteome. Nature. 2014;509:575–81.
25. Kasler HG, Young BD, Mottet D, Lim HW, Collins AM, Olson EN, et al. Histone deacetylase 7 regulates cell survival and TCR signaling in CD4/CD8 double-positive thymocytes. J Immunol. 2011;186:4782–93.
26. Cho Y, Sloutsky R, Naegle KM, Cavalli V. Injury-induced HDAC5 nuclear export is essential for axon regeneration. Cell. 2013;155:894–908.

27. Renthal W, Maze I, Krishnan V, Covington HE 3rd, Xiao G, Kumar A, et al. Histone deacetylase 5 epigenetically controls behavioral adaptations to chronic emotional stimuli. Neuron. 2007;56:517–29.
28. Niegisch G, Knievel J, Koch A, Hader C, Fischer U, Albers P, et al. Changes in histone deacetylase (HDAC) expression patterns and activity of HDAC inhibitors in urothelial cancers. Urol Oncol. 2013;31:1770–9.
29. Xu XS, Wang L, Abrams J, Wang G. Histone deacetylases (HDACs) in XPC gene silencing and bladder cancer. J Hematol Oncol. 2011;4:17.
30. Marek L, Hamacher A, Hansen FK, Kuna K, Gohlke H, Kassack MU, et al. Histone deacetylase (HDAC) inhibitors with a novel connecting unit linker region reveal a selectivity profile for HDAC4 and HDAC5 with improved activity against chemoresistant cancer cells. J Med Chem. 2013;56:427–36.
31. Hoffmann MJ, Koutsogiannouli E, Skowron MA, Pinkerneil M, Niegisch G, Brandt A, et al. The new immortalized uroepithelial cell line HBLAK contains defined genetic aberrations typical of early stage urothelial tumors. Bladder Cancer. 2016;2:449–63.
32. Pinkerneil M, Hoffmann MJ, Kohlhof H, Schulz WA, Niegisch G. Evaluation of the therapeutic potential of the novel isotype specific HDAC inhibitor 4SC-202 in urothelial carcinoma cell lines. Target Oncol. 2016;11:783–98.
33. Wiek C, Schmidt EM, Roellecke K, Freund M, Nakano M, Kelly EJ, et al. Identification of amino acid determinants in CYP4B1 for optimal catalytic processing of 4-ipomeanol. Biochem J. 2015;465:103–14.
34. Schmidt EM, Wiek C, Parkinson OT, Roellecke K, Freund M, Gombert M, et al. Characterization of an additional splice acceptor site introduced into CYP4B1 in Hominoidae during evolution. PLoS One. 2015;10:e0137110.
35. Mochizuki H, Schwartz JP, Tanaka K, Brady RO, Reiser J. High-titer human immunodeficiency virus type 1-based vector systems for gene delivery into nondividing cells. J Virol. 1998;72:8873–83.
36. Pietschmann T, Heinkelein M, Heldmann M, Zentgraf H, Rethwilm A, Lindemann D. Foamy virus capsids require the cognate envelope protein for particle export. J Virol. 1999;73:2613–21.
37. Nicoletti I, Migliorati G, Pagliacci MC, Grignani F, Riccardi C. A rapid and simple method for measuring thymocyte apoptosis by propidium iodide staining and flow cytometry. J Immunol Methods. 1991;139:271–9.
38. Shechter D, Dormann HL, Allis CD, Hake SB. Extraction, purification and analysis of histones. Nat Protoc. 2007;2:1445–57.
39. Lobera M, Madauss KP, Pohlhaus DT, Wright QG, Trocha M, Schmidt DR, et al. Selective class IIa histone deacetylase inhibition via a nonchelating zinc-binding group. Nat Chem Biol. 2013;9:319–25.
40. Bottomley MJ, Lo Surdo P, Di Giovine P, Cirillo A, Scarpelli R, Ferrigno F, et al. Structural and functional analysis of the human HDAC4 catalytic domain reveals a regulatory structural zinc-binding domain. J Biol Chem. 2008;283: 26694–704.
41. Ajamian F, Salminen A, Reeben M. Selective regulation of class I and class II histone deacetylases expression by inhibitors of histone deacetylases in cultured mouse neural cells. Neurosci Lett. 2004;365:64–8.
42. Dokmanovic M, Perez G, Xu W, Ngo L, Clarke C, Parmigiani RB, et al. Histone deacetylase inhibitors selectively suppress expression of HDAC7. Mol Cancer Ther. 2007;6:2525–34.
43. Stepanenko AA, Dmitrenko VV. HEK293 in cell biology and cancer research: phenotype, karyotype, tumorigenicity, and stress-induced genome-phenotype evolution. Gene. 2015;569:182–90.

miR-29c plays a suppressive role in breast cancer by targeting the TIMP3/STAT1/FOXO1 pathway

Wan Li[1,2†], Jie Yi[3†], Xiangjin Zheng[1,2], Shiwei Liu[4], Weiqi Fu[1,2], Liwen Ren[1,2], Li Li[2], Dave S. B. Hoon[5], Jinhua Wang[1,2*] and Guanhua Du[1,2*]

Abstract

Background: miR-29c has been associated with the progression of many cancers. However, the function and mechanism of miR-29c have not been well investigated in breast cancers.

Methods: Real-time quantitative PCR was used to assess expression of miR-29c and DNMT3B mRNA. Western blot and immunochemistry were used to examine the expression of DNA methyltransferase 3B (DNMT3B) protein in breast cancer cells and tissues. The functional roles of miR-29c in breast cancer cells such as proliferation, migration, invasion, colony formation, and 3D growth were evaluated using MTT, transwell chambers, soft agar, and 3D Matrigel culture, respectively. In addition, the luciferase reporter assay was used to check if miR-29c binds the 3'UTR of DNMT3B. The effects of miR-29c on the DNMT3B/TIMP3/STAT1/FOXO1 pathway were also examined using Western blot and methyl-specific qPCR. The specific inhibitor of STAT1, fludarabine, was used to further check the mechanism of miR-29c function in breast cancer cells. Studies on cell functions were carried out in DNMT3B siRNA cell lines.

Results: The expression of miR-29c was decreased with the progression of breast cancers and was closely associated with an overall survival rate of patients. Overexpression of miR-29c inhibited the proliferation, migration, invasion, colony formation, and growth in 3D Matrigel while knockdown of miR-29c promoted these processes in breast cancer cells. In addition, miR-29c was found to bind 3'UTR of DNMT3B and inhibits the expression of DNMT3B, which was elevated in breast cancers. Moreover, the protein level of TIMP3 was reduced whereas methylation of TIMP3 was increased in miR-29c knockdown cells compared to control. On the contrary, the protein level of TIMP3 was increased whereas methylation of TIMP3 was reduced in miR-29c-overexpressing cells compared to control. Knockdown of DNMT3B reduced the proliferation, migration, and invasion of breast cancer cell lines. Finally, our results showed that miR-29c exerted its function in breast cancers by regulating the TIMP3/STAT1/FOXO1 pathway.

Conclusion: The results suggest that miR-29c plays a significant role in suppressing the progression of breast cancers and that miR-29c may be used as a biomarker of breast cancers.

Keywords: Breast cancer, miR-29c, DNMT3B, methylation, and STAT1/FOXO1

* Correspondence: wjh@imm.ac.cn; dugh@imm.ac.cn
†Equal contributors
[1]The State Key Laboratory of Bioactive Substance and Function of Natural Medicines, Beijing, China
Full list of author information is available at the end of the article

Background

Cancer is a major public health problem worldwide and is the second leading cause of death in China and the USA [1, 2]. Breast cancer is the most commonly diagnosed female cancer in the world. It is extremely important to elucidate the mechanisms of breast cancer development and progression and to facilitate early diagnosis.

In the last decades, studies have focused on the epigenetic changes in the development and progression of breast cancers. Epigenetic changes include DNA methylation, histone modifications, abnormal expression of non-coding RNAs, and chromatin remodeling [3]. microRNAs are conserved small non-coding RNAs that regulate gene expression at the translational or post-transcriptional level by repressing or degrading target messenger RNAs [4]. miRNAs are widely expressed in normal tissues and are often miss-regulated in disease states [5]. There is increasing evidence that miRNAs play critical roles in tumorigenesis by functioning as oncogenes or tumor suppressors [6]. Recently, miRNAs have emerged as novel biomarkers in the diagnosis, therapy, and prevention of breast cancer. The miR-29 family consists of miR-29a, miR-29b, and miR-29c. They regulate a series of biological processes, including cell proliferation [7], epigenetic modification [8], intracellular signaling [9], and cell movement [10]. The expression of miR-29c is decreased in many cancers including hepatocellular carcinoma [11], leukemia [12], glioma [13], bladder cancer [14], gastric carcinoma [15], breast cancer [16, 17], and melanoma [18].

DNA methylation is an epigenetic modification that is involved in many of the vital biological functions, such as embryonic development [19], regulation of gene expression [20], imprinting [21], and X-chromosome inactivation [22]. DNMT3B, one of the major DNA methyltransferases, is thought to function in de novo methylation of DNA [23]. DNA methylation of promoter CpG dinucleotides is associated with the suppression of gene expression in cancers. Several studies have shown that DNMT3B is frequently upregulated and plays an important role in many cancers [24, 25]. It is unclear if there is an association between miR-29c and DNMT3B, and what regulatory mechanisms of miR-29c and DNMT3B occur in breast cancer cells.

In this study, we investigated the expression of miR-29c in breast cancer at different clinicopathological stages to identify any association with clinical staging and overall patient survival. We also studied the effects of miR-29c overexpression in cell growth, migration, invasion, and colony formation. The binding of miR-29c to the 3′UTR of DNMT3B was examined, and the effects of knockdown of DNMT3B on proliferation, migration, and invasion were investigated in breast cancer cell lines. The expression of DNMT3B, TIMP3, STAT1, and FOXO1 was assessed by Western blot in miR-29c overexpression cells, miR-29c knockdown cells, and DNMT3B siRNA cells. Together, the results demonstrate a suppressive role of miR-29c by targeting the TIMP3/STAT1/FOXO1 pathway in breast cancer cell proliferation, migration and invasion, and suggest that the loss of miR-29c might be a novel biomarker related to the progression of breast cancer.

Methods

Cell culture

MCF-7, MDA-MB-231, and MDA-MB-436 breast cancer cell lines were purchased from the Cell Bank of the Chinese Academy of Sciences (Beijing, China). All cells lines were authenticated using the Short Tandem Repeat (STR) method, performed by this cell bank. MCF-7 cells were maintained in RPMI 1640 (Thermo Fisher Scientific, Carlsbad, CA) while MDA-MB-231 and MDA-MB-436 cells were cultured in Dulbecco's modified Eagle medium (DMEM, Thermo Fisher Scientific). The complete culture medium was prepared by adding 10% fetal bovine serum (FBS, Thermo Fischer Scientific). Cells were cultured at 37 °C in a humidified incubator containing 5% CO_2.

For drug treatment, cells were treated with fludarabine 2 μM, a STAT1 inhibitor for 24 h and used in specific cell culture experiments.

Breast cancer tissues

The use of human tissues was approved by the Institutional Review Board at the Peking Union Medical College Hospital, Beijing, China. Breast cancer tissues were diagnosed at a different stage and obtained from the Peking Union Medical College Hospital Pathology Department.

miRNA was extracted from serums

Serum samples were collected from 20 healthy females and 79 breast cancer patients at a different stage. The use of serums was also approved by the Institutional Review Board at the Peking Union Medical College Hospital, Beijing, China. Cell-free total RNA including primary miRNA and other small RNA was purified from serum by using miRNeasy Serum/Plasma Kit (Cat No 217184, QIAGEN, Hilden, China).

Transfection

MCF-7, MDA-MB-231, and MDA-MB-436 cells were plated in 60-mm dishes at 80% confluence before transfection. Anti-miR-29c (Cat# AM17000, Thermo Fisher Scientific, Waltham, MA USA) was transfected into MCF-7 cells, and miR-29c mimic (Cat# 4464066, Thermo Fisher Scientific, Waltham, MA, USA) was transfected into MDA-MB-231 and MDA-MB-436 cells using the Lipofectamine™ 3000 transfection reagent (Invitrogen, Grand Island, NY). After transfection for 48 h, the cells were collected and used for the in vitro functional analysis.

MDA-MB-231 miR-29c cells (after transfection of miR-29c mimic for 48 h) were transfected with DNMT3B expression plasmid, and the functions of cells with high DNMT3B were evaluated in following experiments including migration, invasion, colony formation, and 3D Matrigel growth assays.

DNMT3B siRNA 1 and DNMT3B siRNA 2 (Integrated DNA Technologies, Inc., Coralville, IA) were also transfected into MDA-MB-231 and MDA-MB-436 cells. Sequences of DNMT3B siRNA 1 and 2 can be seen in Additional file 1: Table S1. After transfection for 48 h, cells were collected and used for the in vitro cell culture experiments listed below.

Cell proliferation assay

Cells which were transfected with anti-miR-29c and miR-29c mimic (Origene, Rockville, MD) were seeded in 96-well plates at 2×10^3/well, respectively, and cultured for 24, 48, 72, and 96 h. Ten microliters CCK-8 (Dojindo, Kumamoto, Japan) was added to the cells for 3–4 h, and their viability was measured at 450 nm using SpectraMax M5 Microplate Reader, according to the manufacturer's instructions.

Cell migration and invasion assays

Briefly, 10^4 cells were plated on the top of transwells with 8.0-μm pore polycarbonate membrane inserts (Corning, New York, NY) for the migration assay. For the invasion assay, the inserts were coated with a thin layer of Matrigel basement membrane matrix (BD Biosciences San Diego, CA). Serum (10%) was used as the chemoattractant. After 24 h, the cells on the lower surface of the inserts were fixed with methanol for 15 min, stained with 1% crystal violet solution for 15 min, and counted using a light microscope.

Soft agar colony formation assay and 3D Matrigel culture

The soft agar colony formation assay was performed using 6-well plates. Each well contained 2 mL of 0.7% agar in complete medium as the bottom layer and 1 mL of 0.35% agar in complete medium containing 3000 cells as the top layer. Cultures were then maintained under standard culture conditions for 3–4 weeks. After culture, the colonies were stained with MTT solution (200 μL/well), and the number of clones was counted. The 3D cell culture was performed using Matrigel matrix (BD Biosciences, San Diego, CA) in 96-well plates. Each well contained a mixture of 50 μL complete medium containing 1000 cells and 50 μL Matrigel matrix.

In silicon assay

To explore the expression of DNMT3B in breast cancer, in silicon assay was carried out using data from Oncomine (www.oncomine.org) and TCGA. The database from Oncomine is very useful for investigating genes that are expressed in multiple cancer datasets to validate the relationship between transcription and disease. More advanced analyses were used to check the expression of genes in a small fraction of samples of a cancer type using different filters.

To explore if survival rate of patients with breast cancers was associated with miR-29c or DNMT3B. Data online (OncoLnc: linking TCGA survival data to mRNAs, miRNAs, and lncRNAs) was used. OncoLnc is available at http://www.oncolnc.org. The plot of Kaplan-Meier was automatically given using TCGA data when the special gene was decided and values of lower and higher percentiles were input [26].

Western blot

Whole cell extracts were prepared from MCF-7 control and MCF-7 transfected with anti-miR-29c, MDA-MB-231 control and MDA-MB-231 transfected with miR-29c mimic, and MDA-MB-436 control and MDA-MB-436 transfected with miR-29c mimic and MDA-MB-231 transfected with DNMT3B siRNAs. In brief, cells were lysed in radioimmunoprecipitation assay (RIPA) lysis buffer at 4 °C for 30 min. The cell lysate was centrifuged at 12,000 rpm for 10 min at 4 °C, and supernatant was collected. Protein concentrations were determined by using the BCA Kit (Beyotime, Guangzhou, China). Cell extracts were resolved by 10% SDS-PAGE, and the separated proteins were transferred to a polyvinylidene difluoride membrane (Millipore, Billerica, MA). The membranes were blocked in 5% fat-free milk in TBS containing 0.1% Tween 20 for 1 h and then immunoblotted with primary antibodies with appropriate dilutions overnight at 4 °C. The primary antibodies for staining included DNMT3B (Abcam, Cambridge, MA), TIMP3 (EMD Millipore, Billerica, MA), STAT1 (Cell Signal, Boston, MA), and FOXO1 (Cell Signal, Boston, MA). After immunoblotting, the membranes were washed three times with phosphate-buffered saline with Tween (PBST) and followed by 1-h incubation with horseradish peroxidase-conjugated goat anti-rabbit Ab (1:5000, Santa Cruz Biotech, Santa Cruz, CA) or horseradish peroxidase-conjugated rabbit anti-mouse Ab (1:5000, Santa Cruz). The densities of protein bands were quantified by Alpha Ease FCTM software (Version 3.1.2, Alpha Innotech Corp, San Leandro, CA).

Quantitative reverse transcription PCR

Total extracted RNA (1 μg) was used for cDNA synthesis, with Oligo(dT) 20 primers (Invitrogen, Grand Island, NY). The cDNA was added to a quantitative reverse transcription-PCR mixture that contained 1× SYBR Green PCR master mix (Quanta Biosciences, Gaithersburg, MD) and 500 nmol/L gene-specific primers. Assays were performed in triplicate on a CFX thermocycler (Bio-Rad, Hercules, CA). The primers are listed in Additional file 1: Table S2.

Quantitative real-time methylation-specific PCR

The extraction of genomic DNA from breast cancer cells (1×10^6) was performed using a QIAamp DNA Mini Kit (Qiagen, Hilden, Germany) according to the manufacturer's protocol. Bisulfite modification was strictly carried out according to the manufacturer's instructions (Qiagen). The methylation status of TIMP3 in specimens was assessed by quantitative real-time methylation-specific PCR (qMSP) using two sets of primers designed for methylated (M) or unmethylated (U) DNA sequences using bisulfite-modified DNA. The methylation-specific primers and unmethylated-specific primers for the TIMP3 gene were designed according to the standard methods as described previously [27] and are listed in Additional file 1: Table S3.

Immunohistochemistry

Five-micrometer paraffin-embedded tissue sections (35 tissues of breast cancers and 20 adjacent normal tissues) were deparaffinized and rehydrated, antigens were retrieved, and IHC procedures were performed as reported previously [28]. Briefly, the deparaffinized sections were immersed in boiled 10 mM sodium citrate buffer (pH 6.0) and maintained at sub-boiling temperature for 20 min. After that, peroxidase activity was inactivated by incubation with 3% H_2O_2 solution for 10 min at room temperature. Then, the sections were incubated with primary DNMT3B antibody (1:50 dilution; Abcam, Cambridge, MA) in a moist chamber at 4 °C overnight. Negative controls were conducted by the exchange of primary antibody for PBS. Slides were incubated with biotinylated anti-rabbit immunoglobulins for 60 min at room temperature and treated with streptavidin-peroxidase (DAKO, Woodbridge, VA). Staining was achieved by 3,3-diaminobenzidine (DAB; Vectastain, Vector Laboratories, Inc., Linaris GmbH), and the slides were counterstained with hematoxylin. Photographs were taken with equal exposure on a Nikon Eclipse Ti microscope coupled with NIS elements software (Nikon, Melville, NY) for Windows. Three visual fields were randomly selected for the quantitative analysis which was performed independently by two pathologists. The semi-quantitative analysis of the stained sections was done by light microscopy according to the immunoreactive score of Remmele and Stegner (IRS) [29, 30].

Luciferase reporter assay

DNMT3B luciferase reporters containing DNMT3B wild-type 3′UTR (CUCUUCUUACUGGUGCUA) or mutant 3′UTR (CUCUUCUUACUCCUCCUA) were purchased from SWITCH Gear Genomics Company (Menlo Park, CA). MDA-MB-231 cells were co-transfected with the 50 ng luciferase reporter, 1 ng Renilla luciferase reporter (pRL-CMV vector, Promega, Madison, WI), or/and 100 nM mimic miR-29c by Lipofectamine 3000 (Invitrogen, Grand Island, NY), respectively. After transfection for 24 h, cells were lysed and centrifuged at 12000 rpm for 10 min. The supernatant was collected following centrifuging, and luciferase activities were measured using the Dual-Luciferase Assay System (Promega, Madison, WI). The activity of Renilla luciferase was normalized to that of firefly luciferase.

Statistical analysis

The results are given as mean ± SD. Student's t test was used to calculate the differences between the two study groups. One-way ANOVA followed by LSD test was used to calculate the differences among multiple study groups. Fisher's exact test was used to calculate the proportional differences of immunoreactive scores between normal and tumor samples. Differences were considered statistically significant at $P < 0.05$.

Results

The expression level of miR-29c was reduced in breast cancer and was positively correlated with patient survival rate

To assess the expression of miR-29c in breast cancer and normal tissues, we extracted mRNA from breast cancer tissues and normal tissues and checked the expression of miR-29c by qRT-PCR. As shown in Fig. 1a, the expression of miR-29c was much lower in breast cancers than in normal tissues. We also examined the expression of miR-29c in serum from breast cancer patients at different stages and found that the expression of miR-29c in the serum was decreased with the progression of breast cancers (Fig. 1b). Furthermore, Kaplan-Meier meta-analyses of miR-29c using online TCGA data (http://www.oncolnc.org) showed that patients with high miR-29c expression had a higher survival rate than patients with low miR-29c expression, respectively (Fig. 1c).

Level of DNMT3B expression was upregulated in breast cancer tissues and negatively correlated with the survival rate

To investigate the expression of DNMT3B mRNA in breast cancer tissues, publicly available expression data for DNMT3B were retrieved from Oncomine and TCGA. Results showed that the expression level of DNMT3B mRNA was upregulated in invasive breast carcinoma (Fig. 2a, b), ductal breast carcinoma (Fig. 2c), and invasive ductal breast carcinoma (Fig. 2d).

The expression of DNMT3B mRNA and protein in eight breast cancer tissues and eight adjacent non-tumor tissues was assessed by qRT-PCR and Western blot. As shown in Fig. 3a, b and Additional file 1: Figure S1, the

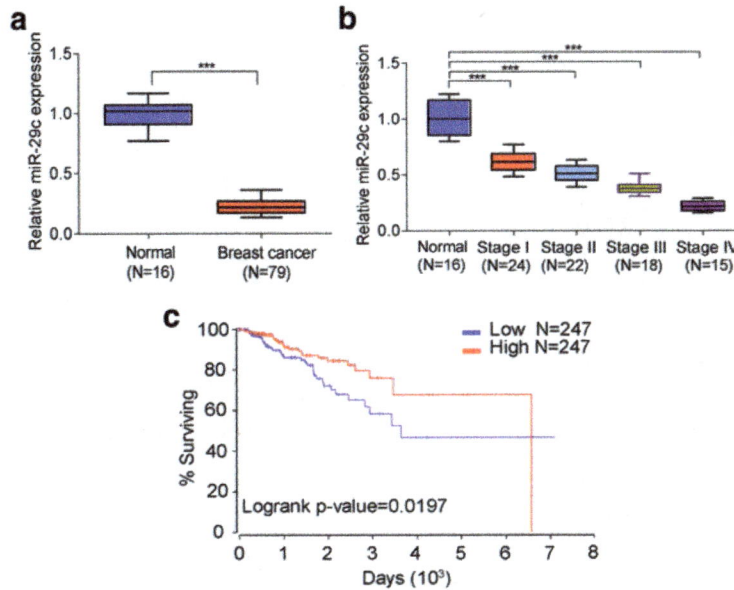

Fig. 1 The expression of miR-29c was reduced in breast cancers and was positively correlated with the survival rate of breast cancer patients. **a** The expression of miR-29c in normal tissues and breast cancer tissues was checked by qRT-PCR. **b** The expressions of miR-29c in the serum of normal controls and breast cancer patients at different stages were evaluated by qRT-PCR. **c** Kaplan-Meier analysis of overall survival curves for breast cancer patients with low versus high expressions of miR-29. Data were presented as mean ± SD, ***P < 0.001

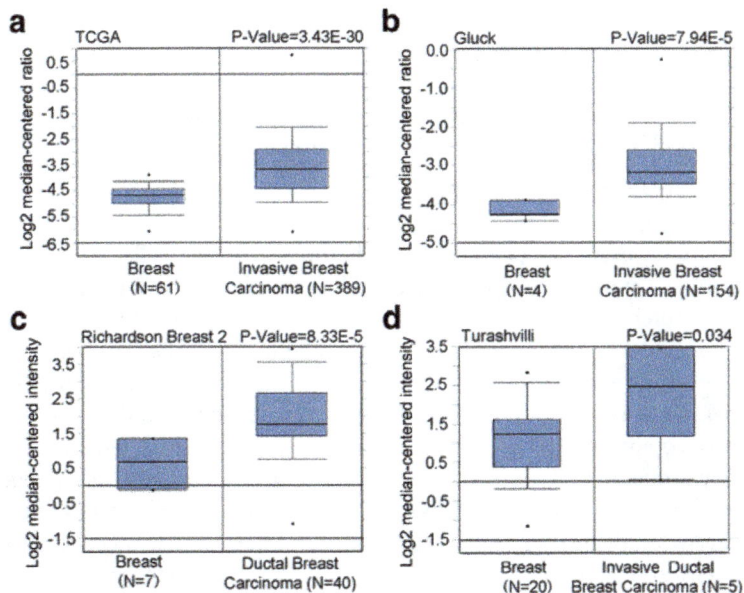

Fig. 2 The data retrieved from Oncomine and TCGA showed that the expression of DNMT3B mRNA was increased in breast cancers. **a** Comparison of the mRNA levels of DNMT3B in normal breast tissues (N = 61) and invasive breast carcinoma tissues (N = 389) using TCGA data retrieved from the Oncomine database. **b** Comparison of the mRNA levels of DNMT3B in normal breast tissues (N = 4) and invasive breast carcinoma tissues (N = 154) using Gluck's data retrieved from the Oncomine database. **c** Comparison of the mRNA levels of DNMT3B in normal breast tissues (N = 7) and ductal breast carcinoma tissues (N = 40) using Richardson's data retrieved from the Oncomine database. **d** Comparison of the mRNA levels of DNMT3B in normal breast tissues (N = 20) and invasive ductal breast carcinoma tissues (N = 5) using Turashvili's data retrieved from the Oncomine database

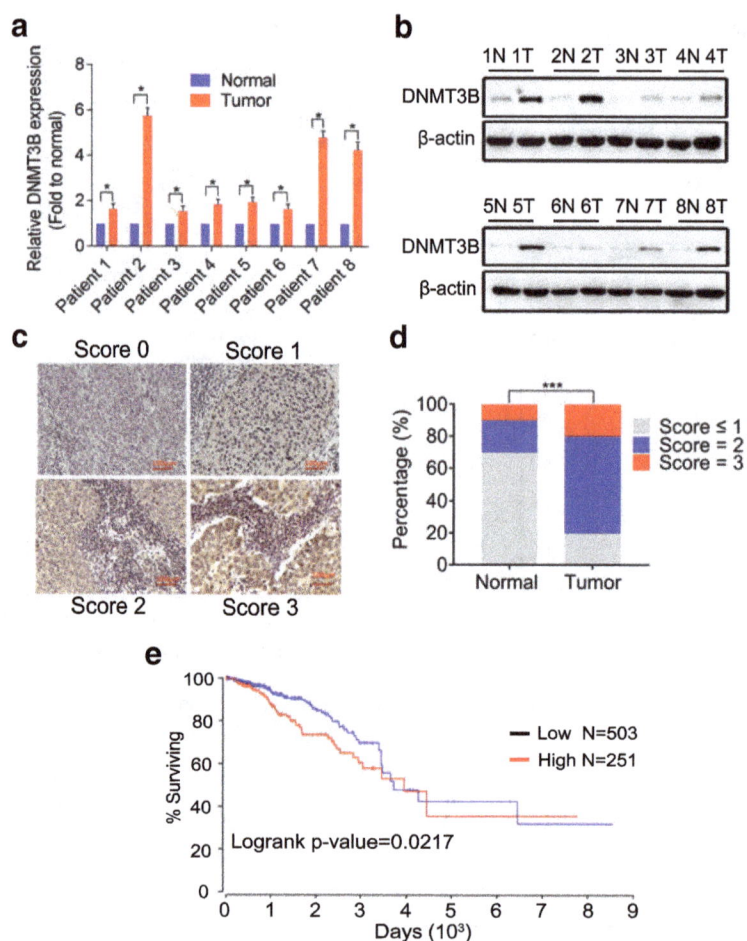

Fig. 3 DNMT3B expression was upregulated in breast cancers and was negatively correlated with the survival rate of breast cancer patients. **a** mRNA levels of DNMT3B detected by qRT-PCR in eight breast cancer tissues were higher than that in their adjacent normal tissues. **b** Comparison of the protein levels of DNMT3B in eight paired breast cancer and adjacent non-tumor tissues by Western blotting. **c** Immunohistochemistry representative photos of DNTM3B expression in normal and different immunoreactive scores breast cancer tissues. **d** Immunoreactive scores of DNMT3B in breast cancer and the adjacent normal tissues. **e** Kaplan-Meier analysis of overall survival curves for breast cancer patients with low versus high expression of DNMT3B. Data were presented as mean ± SD, $*P < 0.05$, $***P < 0.001$

expression level of DNMT3B mRNA and protein, respectively, was higher in breast cancers than in normal breast tissues. To check the protein expression in breast cancer tissues, IHC was carried out, and the results showed that DNMT3B expression was higher in breast cancers than that in normal breast tissues (Fig. 3c, d). In addition, we performed in silico analysis using an online TCGA database (http://www.oncolnc.org) and found that breast cancer patients with high DNMT3B mRNA expression had a lower survival rate than patients with low DNMT3B mRNA expression (Fig. 3e).

miR-29c inhibited the proliferation, migration, and invasion of breast cancer cells, which could be reversed by the overexpression of DNMT3B

To explore the functional role of miR-29c in breast cell lines, we performed loss- and gain-of-function analysis

in breast cancer cells. The knockdown of miR-29c in MCF-7 cells increased cell proliferation (Fig. 4a) and promoted the migration and invasion of cells (Fig. 4b, Additional file 1: Figure S2). In contrast, the overexpression of miR-29c in MDA-MB-231 and MDA-MB-436 cells reduced cell proliferation (Fig. 4c and Additional file 1: Figure S3) and inhibited the migration and invasion of cells (Fig. 4d, Additional file 1: Figures S2 and S3).

To determine whether miR-29c-induced inhibition of cell migration and invasion could be reversed by restoration of DNMT3B expression, we performed gain-of-function analysis in MDA-MB-231 miR-29c cells. Results showed that the overexpression of DNMT3B in MDA-MB-231 miR-29c cells promoted cell migration and invasion of cells (Additional file 1: Figure S4), which suggested that miR-29c-induced inhibition of cell migration and invasion could be reversed by the overexpression of DNMT3B.

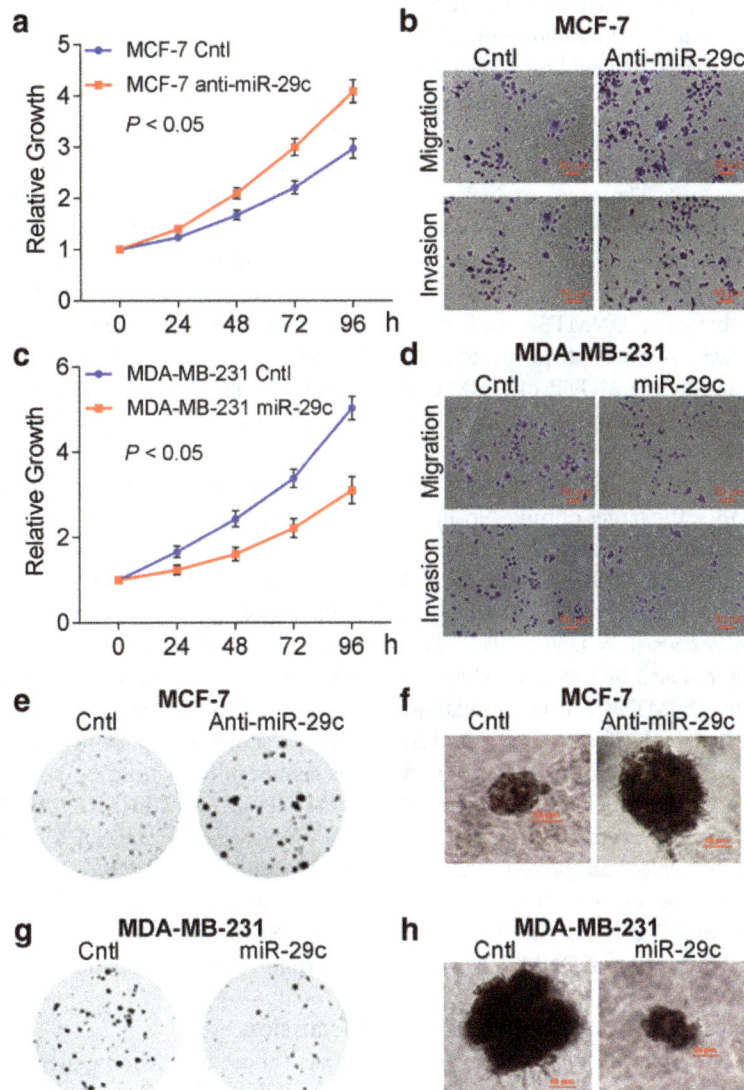

Fig. 4 miR-29c inhibited the proliferation, migration and invasion, colony formation, and growth in 3D Matrigel of breast cancer cells. **a** Proliferation of MCF-7 anti-miR-29c is higher than that of MCF-7 Cntl by CCK8 proliferation assay. **b** Migration and invasion of MCF-7 anti-miR-29cis higher than that of MCF-7 Cntl. **c** Proliferation of MDA-MB-231 miR-29c mimic is lower than that MDA-MB-231 Cntl by CCK8 proliferation assay. **d** Migration and invasion assays of MDA-MB-231 miR-29c mimic are lower than that MDA-MB-231 Cntl. **e** Colony formations of MCF-7 anti-miR-29c are more than that of MCF-7 Cntl in Soft agar assays. **f** Growth of MCF-7 anti-miR-29c is more than that of MCF-7 Cntl in 3D Matrigel culture. **g** Colony formations of MDA-MB-231 miR-29c mimic are less than that of MDA-MB-231 Cntl in soft agar assays. **h** Growth of MDA-MB-231 miR-29c mimic is less than that of MDA-MB-231 Cntl in 3D Matrigel culture. Data are presented as mean ± SD from three independent experiments, and every experiment was repeated three times, *$P < 0.05$

miR-29c inhibited colony formation and growth in breast cancer cells

To investigate the role of miR-29c in the tumorigenesis of breast cancer cells, soft agar and 3D Matrigel culture of MCF-7 Cntl, MCF-7 anti-miR-29c, MDA-MB-231 Cntl, MDA-MB-231 miR-29c, MDA-MB-436Cntl, and MDA-MB-436 miR-29c were carried out. Results showed that the knockdown of miR-29c in MCF-7 cells facilitated the colony formation and growth (Fig. 4e, f and Additional file 1: Figure S5), whereas the overexpression of miR-29c in MDA-MB-231 and MDA-MB-436 cells reduced the colony formation and growth in both soft agar (Fig. 4g, Additional file 1: Figures S3 and S5) and 3D Matrigel cultures (Fig. 4h and Additional file 1: Figure S3).

To determine whether miR-29c-induced the inhibition of tumorigenesis could be reversed by restoration of DNMT3B expression, we performed gain-of-function analysis in MDA-MB-231 miR-29c cells. The overexpression of DNMT3B in MDA-MB-231 miR-29c cells facilitated the colony formation and growth in both soft agar and 3D Matrigel cultures (Additional file 1: Figure S4), which suggested that miR-29c-induced inhibition of colony formation and growth in 3D Matrigel could be reversed by the overexpression of DNMT3B.

DNMT3B is directly targeted by miR-29c

Previous study showed that miR-29c was negatively correlated with the expression of DNMT3B in melanoma in our group [18]. In breast cancers, DNMT3B was also post-transcriptionally regulated by miRNAs [17, 31]. To explore the relationship between DNMT3B and miR-29c, an in silico assay was performed to investigate whether miR-29c could bind to the 3′UTR of DNMT3B (http://www.targetscan.org/, http://www.mirbase.org). This analysis identified a conserved sequence UGGUGCU is the 3′UTR as a potential binding site for miR-29c (Fig. 5a). To further verify that DNMT3B is the target of miR-29c, luciferase reporter plasmids containing conserved or mutated sequences UCCUCCU of DNMT3B were co-transfected with miR-29c mimic in MDA-MB-231 cells. As shown in Fig. 5b, the luciferase activity caused by DNMT3B 3′UTR (wild-type) was significantly reduced by miR-29c, while the luciferase activity caused by DNMT3B 3′UTR (mutation) was not reduced by miR-29c. The luciferase assay was also carried out in MCF-7 cell, and similar results were found (shown in Additional file 1: Figure S6). The expression of DNMT3B protein was reduced by overexpression of miR-29c while the expression of DNMT3B protein was increased by inhibition of miR-29c expression (Fig. 5c, e). These results suggest that miR-29c binds the 3′UTR of DNMT3B and regulates the expression of DNMT3B.

miR-29c inhibits breast cancer cells by targeting the DNMT3B/TIMP3/STAT1/FOXO1 pathway

TIMP3 plays a role as a tumor suppressor in many cancers. Methylation of TIMP3 has been found in several cancers [32, 33]. Since DNMT3B is a major DNA methyltransferase, regulated by miR-29c, we investigated TIMP3 methylation and the expression in MDA-MB-231 cells with miR-29c overexpression and MCF-7 cells with miR-29c knockdown. Methylation of TIMP3 was increased, whereas the protein level of TIMP3 was reduced in MCF-7 cells with miR-29c knockdown compared to control (Fig. 5c, d, Additional file 1: Figure S7B). On the contrary, methylation of TIMP3 was reduced, and the protein level of TIMP3 was increased in MDA-MB-231 with miR-29c overexpression compared to control (Fig. 5e, f, Additional file 1: Figure S7F). STAT1 and FOXO1 are downstream targets of TIMP3. To confirm that miR-29c exerts its function on breast cancer by STAT1/FOXO1 pathway, the protein levels of STAT1 and FOXO1 were checked in MDA-MB-231 cells with miR-29c overexpression and MCF-7 cells with miR-29c knockdown. As shown in Fig. 5c, e and Additional file 1: Figures S7C and S5D, the

protein expression of STAT1 was increased while the expression of FOXO1 was reduced in MCF-7 cells with miR-29c knockdown compared to control. On the contrary, the protein expression of STAT1 was reduced while the protein expression of FOXO1 was increased in MDA-MB-231 with miR-29c overexpression compared to control (Fig. 5c, e, Additional file 1: Figures S7G and S7H). In addition, pretreatment of cells with fludarabine, a specific inhibitor of STAT1 activation but not of other STATs, abrogated the increment of migration and invasion caused by miR-29c inhibition in MCF-7 cells (Fig. 5g, h). Furthermore, pretreatment of fludarabine blocked the changes in expression of STAT1 and FOXO1 caused by miR-29c inhibition in MCF-7 cells (Fig. 5i). All together, these results suggest that miR-29c inhibits breast cancer by targeting the DNMT3B/TIMP3/STAT1/FOXO1 pathway (Fig. 7).

Knockdown of DNMT3B by siRNA reduced the proliferation, migration, and invasion

To check whether DNMT3B protein expression affected cell proliferation, migration, and invasion, MDA-MB-231 and MDA-MB-436 were transfected with DNMT3B siRNAs. As shown in Fig. 6a–d, DNMT3B protein expression was significantly reduced by both DNMT3B siRNA 1 and DNMT3B siRNA 2 in MDA-MB-231 and MDA-MB-436 cells. Knockdown of DNMT3B by siRNA reduced proliferation, migration, and invasion of MDA-MB-231 and MDA-MB-436 cells, respectively (Fig. 6e–h, Additional file 1: Figure S8). These results suggest that DNMT3B played an important role in the functions of breast cancer cells.

Discussion

Breast cancer is a heterogeneous disease, both biologically and clinically. More and more evidence supports the notion that microRNAs (miRNAs) play a critical role as oncogenes or as tumor suppressor genes in cancers. miR-29c is significantly downregulated in many cancers including breast cancer, suggesting that miR-29c acts as a suppressor miRNA in cancers. However, the functional role and underlying mechanism of miR-29c action in breast cancer have not been elucidated. In this study, we investigated the function of miR-29c and explored its underlying mechanism in breast cancers. We firstly reported that miR-29c plays a significant role in suppressing the progression of breast cancers by targeting the TIMP3/STAT1/FOXO1 pathway. Our results also showed there was a lower miR-29c expression in breast cancers than that in normal tissues and that overexpression of miR-29c inhibited cell proliferation, migration and invasion of cells, colony formation, and growth in 3D Matrigel. In addition, we identified that miR-29c directly targets DNMT3B and inhibited expression of DNMT3B which was associated with methylation of TIMP3.

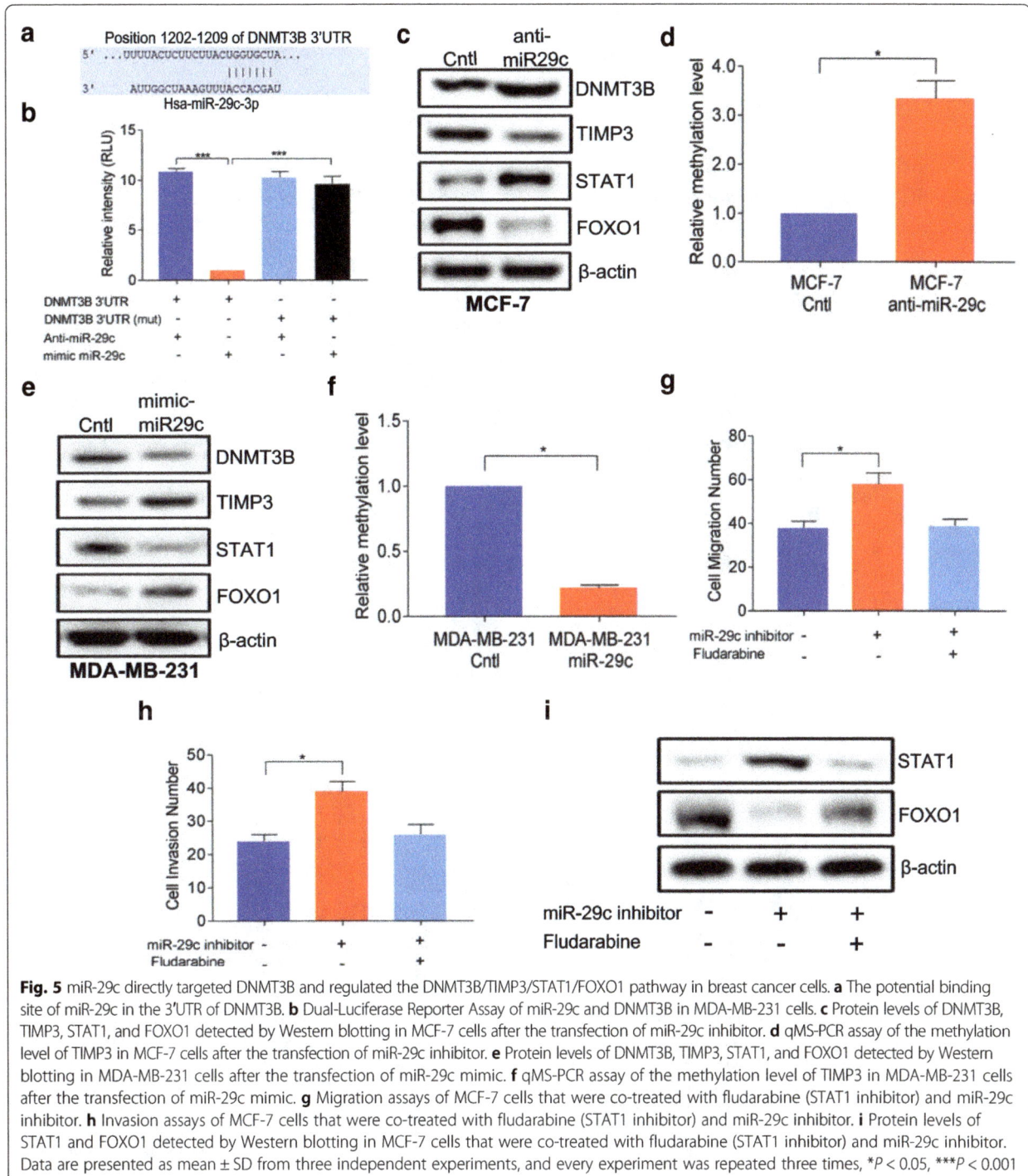

Fig. 5 miR-29c directly targeted DNMT3B and regulated the DNMT3B/TIMP3/STAT1/FOXO1 pathway in breast cancer cells. **a** The potential binding site of miR-29c in the 3'UTR of DNMT3B. **b** Dual-Luciferase Reporter Assay of miR-29c and DNMT3B in MDA-MB-231 cells. **c** Protein levels of DNMT3B, TIMP3, STAT1, and FOXO1 detected by Western blotting in MCF-7 cells after the transfection of miR-29c inhibitor. **d** qMS-PCR assay of the methylation level of TIMP3 in MCF-7 cells after the transfection of miR-29c inhibitor. **e** Protein levels of DNMT3B, TIMP3, STAT1, and FOXO1 detected by Western blotting in MDA-MB-231 cells after the transfection of miR-29c mimic. **f** qMS-PCR assay of the methylation level of TIMP3 in MDA-MB-231 cells after the transfection of miR-29c mimic. **g** Migration assays of MCF-7 cells that were co-treated with fludarabine (STAT1 inhibitor) and miR-29c inhibitor. **h** Invasion assays of MCF-7 cells that were co-treated with fludarabine (STAT1 inhibitor) and miR-29c inhibitor. **i** Protein levels of STAT1 and FOXO1 detected by Western blotting in MCF-7 cells that were co-treated with fludarabine (STAT1 inhibitor) and miR-29c inhibitor. Data are presented as mean ± SD from three independent experiments, and every experiment was repeated three times, *$P < 0.05$, ***$P < 0.001$

It was reported that miR-29c-5p expression was upregulated in breast cancers with the luminal subtypes [34]. Elizabeth Poli et al. reported that MicroRNA-29c (miR-29c) has been shown to be significantly downregulated in basal-like breast tumors and to be involved in cell invasion and sensitivity to chemotherapy [16]. Study showed that there was significantly reduced expression of miR-29c in basal-like breast cancers compared to other breast cancer molecular subtypes and that miR-29c was associated with DNMT3B and methylation of genes [17]. Study showed that miR-29c efficiently downregulated B7-H3 expression and the expression of miR-29c correlated with survival rate of breast cancer patients, suggesting a tumor suppressive role of miR-29c [35]. Our results showed that there

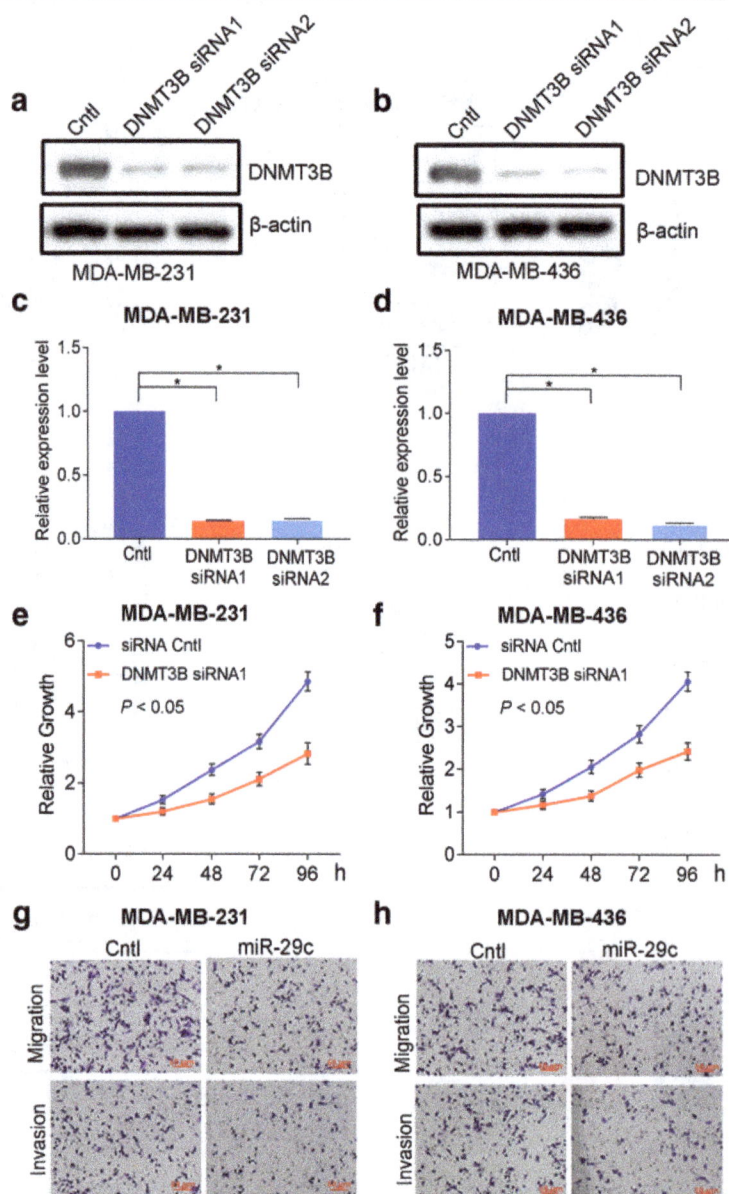

Fig. 6 Knockdown of DNMT3B inhibited the proliferation, migration, and invasion in MDA-MB-231 and MDA-MB-436 cells. **a** Protein levels of DNMT3B detected by Western blotting in MDA-MB-231 cells after the transfection of DNMT3B siRNA 1 and 2. **b** Protein levels of DNMT3B detected by Western blotting in MDA-MB-436 cells after the transfection of DNMT3B siRNA 1 and 2. **c** Quantification of DNMT3B protein levels in MDA-MB-231 cells after the transfection of DNMT3B siRNA 1 and 2. **d** Quantification of DNMT3B protein levels in MDA-MB-436 cells after the transfection of DNMT3B siRNA 1 and 2. **e** CCK-8 proliferation assays of MDA-MB-231 cells after the transfection of DNMT3B siRNA. **f** CCK-8 proliferation assays of MDA-MB-436 cells after the transfection of DNMT3B siRNA. **g** Migration and invasion assays of MDA-MB-231 cells after the transfection of DNMT3B siRNA. **h** Migration and invasion assays of MDA-MB-436 cells after the transfection of DNMT3B siRNA. Data are presented as mean ± SD from three independent experiments, and every experiment was repeated three times

was a different expression level of miR-29c in breast cancer cells with different subtypes. MCF-7 is a breast cancer cell line with ER positive. MDA-MB-231 is a breast cancer cell line with ER negative, PR negative, and HER2 negative). Our results further confirmed that the expression of miR-29c was associated with the subtype of breast cancers, grades of cancer, methylation of genes in breast cancers, and survival rate of patients with breast cancers. miR-29c

was found to exert a suppressive role in the development of breast cancers. These results can be very useful to identify miR-29c as a biomarker of diagnosis and therapy in breast cancers.

DNA methyltransferases, including DNMT1, DNMT3A, and DNMT3B, are enzymes that catalyze DNA methylation. DNMT3A and DNMT3B are mainly involved in de novo DNA methylation, whereas DNMT1 is required for the maintenance of pre-existing methylation [36]. In cancer tissues, DNMT3B is expressed more frequently compared to DNMT1 and DNMT3A [37]. In breast cancer, DNMT3B is also frequently overexpressed [24, 25]. We did in silico analysis using the Oncomine database (www.oncomine.org) and found that the expression level of DNMT3B was higher in invasive ductal breast carcinomas than in normal tissues, confirming previous results. miRNAs, acting as post-transcriptional regulators, can directly degrade target mRNAs and/or repress their translation in a sequence-specific manner [38]. Our previous study showed that miR-29c was negatively correlated with the expression of DNMT3B in melanoma [18]. Here, we demonstrated that miR-29c targeted the 3′UTR of DNMT3B and inhibited its expression, and that both miR-29c expression and DNMT3B expression were associated with the survival rate of patients with breast cancer.

Methylation of gene promoters increases with the progression of cancers [39, 40]. DNMT3B is overexpressed and is involved in the methylation of genes in cancers [18]. One of the major mechanisms of the carcinogenesis process is thought to be the inactivation of tumor suppressor genes by the methylation of their promoter regions. Abnormal expression of DNMT3B is related to the hypermethylation of the tumor suppressor genes. TIMP3 is an inhibitor of extracellular matrix metalloproteinase that can suppress angiogenesis [41, 42], tumor growth [43, 44], and invasion and migration [43–45]. It has been reported that in many common tumors, CpG islands of TIMP3 undergo methylation frequently [46, 47] and that in the primary tumors, the methylation of the TIMP3 promoter can lead to the loss of its protein expression [48]. Moreover, treating methylated human gastric cancer cell lines with 5-aza can even rescue the defective expression of TIMP3 [49]. These studies suggest that epigenetic changes in tumors may play an important role in regulating TIMP3 expression [50]. miR-29c regulated DNMT3B which was associated with methylation of genes in breast cancers [17]. There is a lower level of miR-29c expression in hypermethylator breast cancer cell lines than non-hypermethylator breast cancer cell lines. The expression of miR-29c correlated inversely with methylation-sensitive gene expression and directly with the methylation status of these genes [31]. In this study, methylation of the TIMP3 promoter and changes in expression of TIMP3 and DNMT3B were all affected by miR-29c regulation. In addition, the direct binding of miR-29c to the wild-type 3′UTR of DNTM3B indicates that miR-29c is the direct post-transcriptional regulator of DNMT3B, which is elevated in breast cancer and methylates the promoter of the

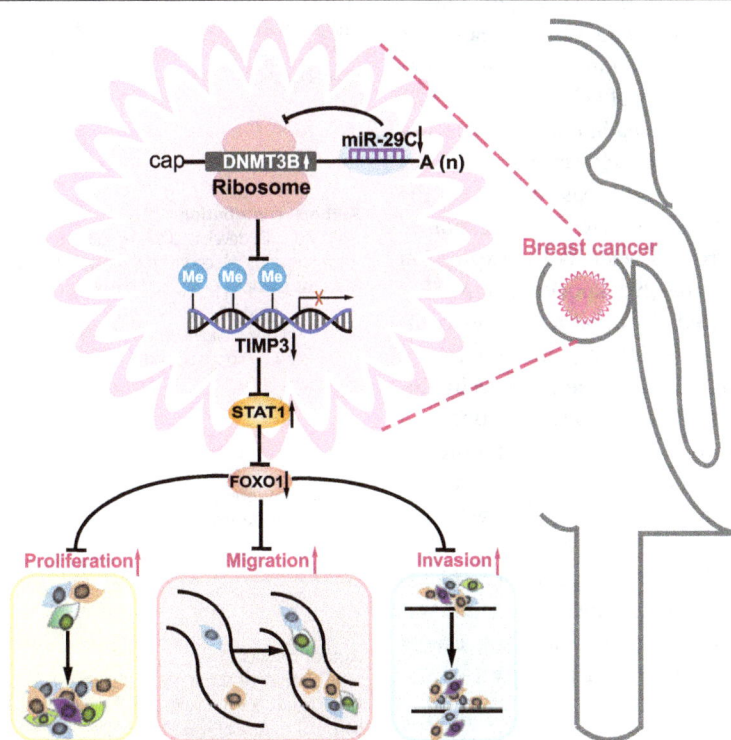

Fig. 7 Proposed mechanistic scheme: miR-29c suppresses breast cancer by the TIMP3/STAT1/FOXO1 pathway. The expression of miR-29c was decreased in breast cancer, which leading to the elevated expression of DNMT3B that is critical for promoter methylation and decreases the expression of TIMP3. As a result, the expression of STAT1 was increased, and it inhibits the expression of FOXO1, leading to proliferation, migration, and invasion of breast cancer cells

TIMP3 gene. Taken together, our results support the concept that the expression of TIMP3 is ultimately regulated by miR-29c.

Signal transducer and activator of transcription 1 (STAT1) is a member of the STAT protein family, which plays important roles in cancer inflammation. STAT1 was associated with cancers, especially in breast cancers [51]. In tumor microenvironment, tumor-induced stromal STAT1 increased the progression of breast cancer via deregulating tissue homeostasis [52]. STAT1 can promote the growth of breast cancer by inhibiting immunity [53]. Inhibition of STAT1 signaling reduced the primary growth and progression of breast cancer cells [54]. When activated via phosphorylation at the Tyr701 site, STAT1 binds specific regulatory elementary and regulates the transcription of its target genes [55]. Forkhead box protein O1 (FOXO1) belongs to the forkhead family of transcription factors which are characterized by a distinct forkhead domain and play many important roles in cancers [56]. FOXO1 was considered as tumor suppressor gene. The RNA-binding protein Quaking (QKI) resulted in low levels of FOXO1 expression in breast cancer cells [57]. Astrocyte-elevated gene-1 (AEG-1) inhibited the expression of FOXO1 and promoted the progression of breast cancer [58]. Acylglycerol kinase was reported to promote the growth of cells and tumorigenicity in breast cancer by inhibiting the expression of FOXO1 [59]. TIMP3 is a versatile extracellular regulator in cancers [60]. The loss of TIMP3 can lead to diabetic kidney disease in both human and mouse via the interplay of FOXO1 and STAT1 [61]. In addition, miR-29c is involved in diabetic nephropathy by targeting tristetraprolin [62]. However, it is unclear that TIMP3 inhibits the progress of breast cancer via the FOXO1/STAT1 pathway. We show that the expression of TIMP3 and FOXO1 is decreased whereas the expression of STAT1 is increased in miR-29c knockdown MCF-7 cells. STAT1 has been reported to exhibit a negative regulatory effect on FOXO1 transcription in pancreatic β cells [61] and bladder cancer [63]. Fludarabine is a specific inhibitor of STAT1 [64]. Fludarabine inhibited the decrease of FOXO1 expression caused by knockdown of miR-29c and abrogated the increment of cell migration and invasion caused by knockdown of miR-29c. We firstly illustrated that miR-29c exerted its regulatory function in breast cancers by activating the TIMP3/STAT1/FOXO1 pathway. This is firstly reported that miR-29c inhibited the proliferation, migration, invasion colony, and 3D growth of breast cancer cells by targeting TIMP3/STAT1/FOXO1 pathway.

Conclusion

In conclusion, we found that the expression of miR-29c is correlated with the progress and prognosis of breast cancers. DNMT3B is a direct target of miR-29c. DNMT3B expression increases as miR-29c expression decreases in cells. Upregulated DNMT3B is critical for promoter methylation and decreased expression of TIMP3, which could promote progression of breast cancer via the TIMP3/STAT1/FOXO1 pathway (Fig. 7). These results suggest that miR-29c could be used as a potential biomarker of diagnosis and therapy in breast cancers.

Abbreviations
DNMT: DNA methyltransferases; FBS: Fetal bovine serum; FOXO1: Forkhead box protein O1; IHC: Immunohistochemistry; MTT: 3-(4,5-Dimethylthiazol-2-yl)-2, 5-diphenyltetrazolium bromide; qRT-PCR: Quantitative real-time polymerase chain reaction; STAT1: Signal transducer and activator of transcription 1; STR: Short tandem repeat; TIMP3: Tissue inhibitor of metalloproteinases 3; UTR: Untranslated region

Acknowledgements
We thank Dr. Min Yang (Institute of Materia Medica, Chinese Academy of Medical Science and Peking Union Medical College) for her analysis of the immunochemistry staining. We also thank Dr. Ian Hutchinson for his editorial review.

Funding
This work was supported by the National Natural Science Foundation of China (No. 81573454 for JINHUA WANG, No. 81703565 for WEIQI FU, and No. 81703536 for WAN LI), CAMS Innovation Fund for Medical Sciences (CIFMS) (2016-I2M-3-007), and Natural Science Foundation of Beijing (7172142).

Authors' contributions
JHW and GHD developed the hypothesis, designed the experiments, and revised the manuscript. WL conducted most of the functional experiments and wrote the main manuscript. JY collected breast cancer tissues and performed the qPCR. XJZ, SWL, DSBH, and WQF performed the immunochemistry and luciferase reporter assay. LWR downloaded and analyzed the public data. LL performed the statistical analyses. All authors read and approved the final manuscript.

Competing interests
The authors declare that they have no competing interests.

Author details
[1]The State Key Laboratory of Bioactive Substance and Function of Natural Medicines, Beijing, China. [2]Key Laboratory of Drug Target Research and Drug Screen, Institute of Materia Medica, Chinese Academy of Medical Science and Peking Union Medical College, Beijing 100050, China. [3]Department of Clinical Laboratory, Peking Union Medical College Hospital, Beijing 100730, China. [4]Department of Endocrinology, Shanxi DAYI Hospital, Shanxi Medical University, Taiyuan 030002, Shanxi, China. [5]Department of Translational Molecular Medicine, John Wayne Cancer Institute (JWCI) at Providence Saint John's Health Center, Santa Monica, CA 90404, USA.

References

1. Chen W, Zheng R, Baade PD, Zhang S, Zeng H, Bray F, Jemal A, Yu XQ, He J. Cancer statistics in China, 2015. CA Cancer J Clin. 2016;66(2):115–32.

2. Siegel RL, Miller KD, Jemal A. Cancer statistics, 2017. CA Cancer J Clin. 2017; 67(1):7–30.

3. Perri F, Longo F, Giuliano M, Sabbatino F, Favia G, Ionna F, Addeo R, Della Vittoria Scarpati G, Di Lorenzo G, Pisconti S. Epigenetic control of gene expression: potential implications for cancer treatment. Crit Rev Oncol Hematol. 2017;111:166–72.

4. Bartel DP. MicroRNAs: target recognition and regulatory functions. Cell. 2009;136(2):215–33.

5. Lu J, Getz G, Miska EA, Alvarez-Saavedra E, Lamb J, Peck D, Sweet-Cordero A, Ebert BL, Mak RH, Ferrando AA, et al. MicroRNA expression profiles classify human cancers. Nature. 2005;435(7043):834–8.

6. Wozniak M, Mielczarek A, Czyz M. miRNAs in melanoma: tumor suppressors and oncogenes with prognostic potential. Curr Med Chem. 2016;23(28):3136–53.

7. Li Z, Jiang R, Yue Q, Peng H. MicroRNA-29 regulates myocardial microvascular endothelial cells proliferation and migration in association with IGF1 in type 2 diabetes. Biochem Biophys Res Commun. 2017;487(1):15–21.

8. Palmbos PL, Wang L, Yang H, Wang Y, Leflein J, Ahmet ML, Wilkinson JE, Kumar-Sinha C, Ney GM, Tomlins SA, et al. ATDC/TRIM29 drives invasive bladder cancer formation through miRNA-mediated and epigenetic mechanisms. Cancer Res. 2015;75(23):5155–66.

9. Rostas JW 3rd, Pruitt HC, Metge BJ, Mitra A, Bailey SK, Bae S, Singh KP, Devine DJ, Dyess DL, Richards WO, et al. microRNA-29 negatively regulates EMT regulator N-myc interactor in breast cancer. Mol Cancer. 2014;13:200.

10. Cui H, Wang L, Gong P, Zhao C, Zhang S, Zhang K, Zhou R, Zhao Z, Fan H. Deregulation between miR-29b/c and DNMT3A is associated with epigenetic silencing of the CDH1 gene, affecting cell migration and invasion in gastric cancer. PLoS One. 2015;10(4):e0123926.

11. Wang CM, Wang Y, Fan CG, Xu FF, Sun WS, Liu YG, Jia JH. miR-29c targets TNFAIP3, inhibits cell proliferation and induces apoptosis in hepatitis B virus-related hepatocellular carcinoma. Biochem Biophys Res Commun. 2011;411(3):586–92.

12. Zhou K, Yu Z, Yi S, Li Z, An G, Zou D, Qi J, Zhao Y, Qiu L. miR-29c down-regulation is associated with disease aggressiveness and poor survival in Chinese patients with chronic lymphocytic leukemia. Leukemia & lymphoma. 2014;55(7):1544–50.

13. Wang Y, Li Y, Sun J, Wang Q, Sun C, Yan Y, Yu L, Cheng D, An T, Shi C, et al. Tumor-suppressive effects of miR-29c on gliomas. Neuroreport. 2013;24(12): 637–45.

14. Xu F, Zhang Q, Cheng W, Zhang Z, Wang J, Ge J. Effect of miR-29b-1* and miR-29c knockdown on cell growth of the bladder cancer cell line T24. The Journal of international medical research. 2013;41(6):1803–10.

15. Saito Y, Suzuki H, Imaeda H, Matsuzaki J, Hirata K, Tsugawa H, Hibino S, Kanai Y, Saito H, Hibi T. The tumor suppressor microRNA-29c is downregulated and restored by celecoxib in human gastric cancer cells. Int J Cancer. 2013;132(8):1751–60.

16. Poli E, Zhang J, Nwachukwu C, Zheng Y, Adedokun B, Olopade OI, Han YJ. Molecular subtype-specific expression of microRNA-29c in breast cancer is associated with CpG dinucleotide methylation of the promoter. PLoS One. 2015;10(11):e0142224.

17. Sandhu R, Rivenbark AG, Mackler RM, Livasy CA, Coleman WB. Dysregulation of microRNA expression drives aberrant DNA hypermethylation in basal-like breast cancer. Int J Oncol. 2014;44(2):563–72.

18. Nguyen T, Kuo C, Nicholl MB, Sim MS, Turner RR, Morton DL, Hoon DS. Downregulation of microRNA-29c is associated with hypermethylation of tumor-related genes and disease outcome in cutaneous melanoma. Epigenetics. 2011;6(3):388–94.

19. Wu TP, Wang T, Seetin MG, Lai Y, Zhu S, Lin K, Liu Y, Byrum SD, Mackintosh SG, Zhong M, et al. DNA methylation on N(6)-adenine in mammalian embryonic stem cells. Nature. 2016;532(7599):329–33.

20. Zemach A, McDaniel IE, Silva P, Zilberman D. Genome-wide evolutionary analysis of eukaryotic DNA methylation. Science. 2010; 328(5980):916–9.

21. Nakao M, Sasaki H. Genomic imprinting: significance in development and diseases and the molecular mechanisms. J Biochem. 1996;120(3):467–73.

22. Panning B, Jaenisch R. RNA and the epigenetic regulation of X chromosome inactivation. Cell. 1998;93(3):305–8.

23. Okano M, Bell DW, Haber DA, Li E. DNA methyltransferases Dnmt3a and Dnmt3b are essential for de novo methylation and mammalian development. Cell. 1999;99(3):247–57.

24. Roll JD, Rivenbark AG, Jones WD, Coleman WB. DNMT3b overexpression contributes to a hypermethylator phenotype in human breast cancer cell lines. Mol Cancer. 2008;7:15.

25. Girault I, Tozlu S, Lidereau R, Bieche I. Expression analysis of DNA methyltransferases 1, 3A, and 3B in sporadic breast carcinomas. Clin. Cancer Res. 2003;9(12):4415–22.

26. Anaya J. OncoLnc: linking TCGA survival data to mRNAs, miRNAs, and lncRNAs. Peerj Computer Science. 2016;2(2):e67.

27. Li LC, Dahiya R. MethPrimer: designing primers for methylation PCRs. Bioinformatics. 2002;18(11):1427–31.

28. Wang J, Huang SK, Marzese DM, Hsu SC, Kawas NP, Chong KK, Long GV, Menzies AM, Scolyer RA, Izraely S, et al. Epigenetic changes of EGFR have an important role in BRAF inhibitor-resistant cutaneous melanomas. J Invest Dermatol. 2015;135(2):532–41.

29. Kaemmerer D, Peter L, Lupp A, Schulz S, Sanger J, Baum RP, Prasad V, Hommann M. Comparing of IRS and Her2 as immunohistochemical scoring schemes in gastroenteropancreatic neuroendocrine tumors. Int J Clin Exp Pathol. 2012;5(3):187–94.

30. Specht E, Kaemmerer D, Sanger J, Wirtz RM, Schulz S, Lupp A. Comparison of immunoreactive score, HER2/neu score and H score for the immunohistochemical evaluation of somatostatin receptors in bronchopulmonary neuroendocrine neoplasms. Histopathology. 2015; 67(3):368–77.

31. Sandhu R, Rivenbark AG, Coleman WB. Loss of post-transcriptional regulation of DNMT3b by microRNAs: a possible molecular mechanism for the hypermethylation defect observed in a subset of breast cancer cell lines. Int J Oncol. 2012;41(2):721–32.

32. Lim Y, Wan Y, Vagenas D, Ovchinnikov DA, Perry CF, Davis MJ, Punyadeera C. Salivary DNA methylation panel to diagnose HPV-positive and HPV-negative head and neck cancers. BMC Cancer. 2016;16(1):749.

33. Guilleret I, Losi L, Chelbi ST, Fonda S, Bougel S, Saponaro S, Gozzi G, Alberti L, Braunschweig R, Benhattar J. DNA methylation profiling of esophageal adenocarcinoma using Methylation Ligation-dependent Macroarray (MLM). Biochem Biophys Res Commun. 2016;479(2):231–7.

34. Haakensen VD, Nygaard V, Greger L, Aure MR, Fromm B, Bukholm IR, Luders T, Chin SF, Git A, Caldas C, et al. Subtype-specific micro-RNA expression signatures in breast cancer progression. Int J Cancer. 2016;139(5):1117–28.

35. Nygren MK, Tekle C, Ingebrigtsen VA, Makela R, Krohn M, Aure MR, Nunes-Xavier CE, Perala M, Tramm T, Alsner J, et al. Identifying microRNAs regulating B7-H3 in breast cancer: the clinical impact of microRNA-29c. Br J Cancer. 2014;110(8):2072–80.

36. Roscigno G, Quintavalle C, Donnarumma E, Puoti I, Diaz-Lagares A, Iaboni M, Fiore D, Russo V, Todaro M, Romano G, et al. MiR-221 promotes stemness of breast cancer cells by targeting DNMT3b. Oncotarget. 2016;7(1):580–92.

37. Robertson KD, Uzvolgyi E, Liang G, Talmadge C, Sumegi J, Gonzales FA, Jones PA. The human DNA methyltransferases (DNMTs) 1, 3a and 3b: coordinate mRNA expression in normal tissues and overexpression in tumors. Nucleic Acids Res. 1999;27(11):2291–8.

38. Bartel DP. MicroRNAs: genomics, biogenesis, mechanism, and function. Cell. 2004;116(2):281–97.

39. Kanda M, Tanaka C, Kobayashi D, Tanaka H, Shimizu D, Shibata M, Takami H, Hayashi M, Iwata N, Niwa Y, et al. Epigenetic suppression of the immunoregulator MZB1 is associated with the malignant phenotype of gastric cancer. Int J Cancer. 2016;139(10):2290–8.

40. Liu Y, Jin X, Li Y, Ruan Y, Lu Y, Yang M, Lin D, Song P, Guo Y, Zhao S, et al. DNA methylation of claudin-6 promotes breast cancer cell migration and invasion by recruiting MeCP2 and deacetylating H3Ac and H4Ac. J Exp Clin Cancer Res. 2016;35(1):120.

41. Wang CY, Liou JP, Tsai AC, Lai MJ, Liu YM, Lee HY, Wang JC, Pan SL, Teng CM. A novel action mechanism for MPT0G013, a derivative of arylsulfonamide, inhibits tumor angiogenesis through up-regulation of TIMP3 expression. Oncotarget. 2014;5(20):9838–50.

42. Das AM, Seynhaeve AL, Rens JA, Vermeulen CE, Koning GA, Eggermont AM, Ten Hagen TL. Differential TIMP3 expression affects tumor progression and angiogenesis in melanomas through regulation of directionally persistent endothelial cell migration. Angiogenesis. 2014;17(1):163–77.

43. Liu W, Li M, Chen X, Zhang D, Wei L, Zhang Z, Wang S, Meng L, Zhu S, Li B. Erratum: MicroRNA-373 promotes migration and invasion in human esophageal squamous cell carcinoma by inhibiting TIMP3 expression. Am J Cancer Res. 2016;6(6):1458–9.

44. Liu W, Li M, Chen X, Zhang D, Wei L, Zhang Z, Wang S, Meng L, Zhu S, Li B. MicroRNA-373 promotes migration and invasion in human esophageal squamous cell carcinoma by inhibiting TIMP3 expression. Am J Cancer Res. 2016;6(1):1–14.

45. Das AM, Bolkestein M, van der Klok T, Oude Ophuis CM, Vermeulen CE, Rens JA, Dinjens WN, Atmodimedjo PN, Verhoef C, Koljenovic S, et al. Tissue inhibitor of metalloproteinase-3 (TIMP3) expression decreases during melanoma progression and inhibits melanoma cell migration. Eur J Cancer. 2016;66:34–46.

46. Hoque MO, Begum S, Brait M, Jeronimo C, Zahurak M, Ostrow KL, Rosenbaum E, Trock B, Westra WH, Schoenberg M, et al. Tissue inhibitor of metalloproteinases-3 promoter methylation is an independent prognostic factor for bladder cancer. J Urol. 2008;179(2):743–7.

47. Wisman GB, Nijhuis ER, Hoque MO, Reesink-Peters N, Koning AJ, Volders HH, Buikema HJ, Boezen HM, Hollema H, Schuuring E, et al. Assessment of gene promoter hypermethylation for detection of cervical neoplasia. Int J Cancer. 2006;119(8):1908–14.

48. Bachman KE, Herman JG, Corn PG, Merlo A, Costello JF, Cavenee WK, Baylin SB, Graff JR. Methylation-associated silencing of the tissue inhibitor of metalloproteinase-3 gene suggest a suppressor role in kidney, brain, and other human cancers. Cancer Res. 1999;59(4):798–802.

49. Kang SH, Choi HH, Kim SG, Jong HS, Kim NK, Kim SJ, Bang YJ. Transcriptional inactivation of the tissue inhibitor of metalloproteinase-3 gene by dna hypermethylation of the 5'-CpG island in human gastric cancer cell lines. Int J Cancer. 2000;86(5):632–5.

50. Liu WB, Cui ZH, Ao L, Zhou ZY, Zhou YH, Yuan XY, Xiang YL, Liu JY, Cao J. Aberrant methylation accounts for cell adhesion-related gene silencing during 3-methylcholanthrene and diethylnitrosamine induced multistep rat lung carcinogenesis associated with overexpression of DNA methyltransferases 1 and 3a. Toxicol Appl Pharmacol. 2011;251(1):70–8.

51. Zhang M. Novel function of STAT1 in breast cancer. Oncoimmunology. 2013;2(8):e25125.

52. Zellmer VR, Schnepp PM, Fracci SL, Tan X, Howe EN, Zhang S. Tumor-induced stromal STAT1 accelerates breast cancer via deregulating tissue homeostasis. Mol. Cancer Res. 2017;15(5):585–97.

53. Hix LM, Karavitis J, Khan MW, Shi YH, Khazaie K, Zhang M. Tumor STAT1 transcription factor activity enhances breast tumor growth and immune suppression mediated by myeloid-derived suppressor cells. J Biol Chem. 2013;288(17):11676–88.

54. Airoldi I, Cocco C, Sorrentino C, Angelucci D, Di Meo S, Manzoli L, Esposito S, Ribatti D, Bertolotto M, Iezzi L, et al. Interleukin-30 promotes breast cancer growth and progression. Cancer Res. 2016;76(21):6218–29.

55. Khodarev NN, Roizman B, Weichselbaum RR. Molecular pathways: interferon/stat1 pathway: role in the tumor resistance to genotoxic stress and aggressive growth. Clin. Cancer Res. 2012;18(11):3015–21.

56. Coomans de Brachene A, Demoulin JB. FOXO transcription factors in cancer development and therapy. Cell. Mol. Life Sci. 2016;73(6):1159–72.

57. Yu F, Jin L, Yang G, Ji L, Wang F, Lu Z. Post-transcriptional repression of FOXO1 by QKI results in low levels of FOXO1 expression in breast cancer cells. Oncol Rep. 2014;31(3):1459–65.

58. Li J, Yang L, Song L, Xiong H, Wang L, Yan X, Yuan J, Wu J, Li M. Astrocyte elevated gene-1 is a proliferation promoter in breast cancer via suppressing transcriptional factor FOXO1. Oncogene. 2009;28(36):3188–96.

59. Wang X, Lin C, Zhao X, Liu A, Zhu J, Li X, Song L. Acylglycerol kinase promotes cell proliferation and tumorigenicity in breast cancer via suppression of the FOXO1 transcription factor. Mol Cancer. 2014;13:106.

60. Jackson HW, Defamie V, Waterhouse P, Khokha R. TIMPs: versatile extracellular regulators in cancer. Nat Rev Cancer. 2017;17(1):38–53.

61. Fiorentino L, Cavalera M, Menini S, Marchetti V, Mavilio M, Fabrizi M, Conserva F, Casagrande V, Menghini R, Pontrelli P, et al. Loss of TIMP3 underlies diabetic nephropathy via FoxO1/STAT1 interplay. EMBO molecular medicine. 2013;5(3):441–55.

62. Guo J, Li J, Zhao J, Yang S, Wang L, Cheng G, Liu D, Xiao J, Liu Z, Zhao Z. MiRNA-29c regulates the expression of inflammatory cytokines in diabetic nephropathy by targeting tristetraprolin. Sci Rep. 2017;7(1):2314.

63. Jiang G, Wu AD, Huang C, Gu J, Zhang L, Huang H, Liao X, Li J, Zhang D, Zeng X, et al. Isorhapontigenin (ISO) inhibits invasive bladder cancer formation in vivo and human bladder cancer invasion in vitro by targeting STAT1/FOXO1 axis. Cancer Prev Res. 2016;9(7):567–80.

64. Berentsen S, Randen U, Oksman M, Birgens H, Tvedt THA, Dalgaard J, Galteland E, Haukas E, Brudevold R, Sorbo JH, et al. Bendamustine plus rituximab for chronic cold agglutinin disease: results of a Nordic prospective multicenter trial. Blood. 2017;

11

MEST mediates the impact of prenatal bisphenol A exposure on long-term body weight development

Kristin M. Junge[1†], Beate Leppert[1†], Susanne Jahreis[1,2], Dirk K. Wissenbach[3,4], Ralph Feltens[3], Konrad Grützmann[1,5,6,7], Loreen Thürmann[1,18], Tobias Bauer[8], Naveed Ishaque[8,15], Matthias Schick[9], Melanie Bewerunge-Hudler[7], Stefan Röder[1], Mario Bauer[1], Angela Schulz[10], Michael Borte[11], Kathrin Landgraf[12,13], Antje Körner[12,13], Wieland Kiess[12,13], Martin von Bergen[3,14], Gabriele I. Stangl[15,16], Saskia Trump[1†], Roland Eils[17,18,19†], Tobias Polte[1,2†] and Irina Lehmann[1,20*†]

Abstract

Background: Exposure to endocrine-disrupting chemicals can alter normal physiology and increase susceptibility to non-communicable diseases like obesity. Especially the prenatal and early postnatal period is highly vulnerable to adverse effects by environmental exposure, promoting developmental reprogramming by epigenetic alterations. To obtain a deeper insight into the role of prenatal bisphenol A (BPA) exposure in children's overweight development, we combine epidemiological data with experimental models and BPA-dependent DNA methylation changes.

Methods: BPA concentrations were measured in maternal urine samples of the LINA mother-child-study obtained during pregnancy ($n = 552$), and BPA-associated changes in cord blood DNA methylation were analyzed by Illumina Infinium HumanMethylation450 BeadChip arrays ($n = 472$). Methylation changes were verified by targeted MassARRAY analyses, assessed for their functional translation by qPCR and correlated with children's body mass index (BMI) z scores at the age of 1 and 6 years. Further, female BALB/c mice were exposed to BPA from 1 week before mating until delivery, and weight development of their pups was monitored ($n \geq 8$/group). Additionally, human adipose-derived mesenchymal stem cells were treated with BPA during the adipocyte differentiation period and assessed for exposure-related epigenetic, transcriptional and morphological changes ($n = 4$).

Results: In prenatally BPA-exposed children two CpG sites with deviating cord blood DNA-methylation profiles were identified, among them a hypo-methylated CpG in the promoter of the obesity-associated mesoderm-specific transcript (*MEST*). A mediator analysis suggested that prenatal BPA exposure was connected to cord blood *MEST* promoter methylation and *MEST* expression as well as BMI z scores in early infancy. This effect could be confirmed in mice in which prenatal BPA exposure altered *Mest* promoter methylation and transcription with a concomitant increase in the body weight of the juvenile offspring. An experimental model of in vitro differentiated human mesenchymal stem cells also revealed an epigenetically induced *MEST* expression and enhanced adipogenesis following BPA exposure.

(Continued on next page)

* Correspondence: irina.lehmann@bihealth.de
†Equal contributors
[1]Department of Environmental Immunology, Helmholtz Centre for Environmental Research (UFZ), Leipzig, Germany
[20]Unit for Molecular Epidemiology, Berlin Institute of Health (BIH) and Charité - Universitätsmedizin Berlin, Berlin, Germany
Full list of author information is available at the end of the article

(Continued from previous page)

Conclusions: Our study provides evidence that *MEST* mediates the impact of prenatal BPA exposure on long-term body weight development in offspring by triggering adipocyte differentiation.

Keywords: EDC, Prenatal exposure, Infants, Obesity, LINA, Mice, Mesenchymal stem cells, Epigenetics, DNA methylation, Adipogenesis,

Background

Exposure to endocrine-disrupting chemicals (EDCs) during critical windows in development can permanently alter normal physiology and increase susceptibility to diseases like obesity, asthma, or cancer later in life [1]. Especially the prenatal and early postnatal period is highly vulnerable to EDC exposure as it is the time of developmental programming important for organogenesis and tissue differentiation [2]. The growing knowledge about the human epigenome emphasized the importance of environmental exposure-related epigenetic modifications predisposing an individual to the development of disease. Understanding the underlying effects leading to a disruption in epigenetic programming by EDCs during fetal development is important and might aid future prevention strategies for such diseases.

One EDC with a well-described impact on the human epigenome during development is bisphenol A (BPA). BPA is a chemical used in the manufacturing of polycarbonate plastics and epoxy resins contained in a variety of consumer products. It is readily released to the environment leading to extensive human exposure in industrialized countries [3, 4]. BPA has been detected in human blood, urine, adipose tissue, breastmilk, and also in placental tissue and amniotic fluid [3], suggesting that exposure already starts during the sensitive prenatal phase. BPA is classified as an endocrine disruptor because of its ability to mimic hormone activity, for example, through estrogen-, and peroxisome proliferator-activated receptor gamma (PPARγ) signaling [5, 6]. After oral administration BPA is rapidly biotransformed to glucuronidated BPA in the liver via UDP-glucuronosyl-transferase (UGT) and is eliminated by urinary excretion within 24 h [7, 8]. Complementary, studies in rats suggest that BPA metabolism might change during pregnancy due to alterations in UGT isoforms and expression level [9]. In addition, decreased UGT levels in fetal liver can lower the excretion capacity for BPA, making the fetus even more vulnerable to environmental pollutant EDC exposure [10–12]. So far, data on human BPA metabolism during pregnancy or early childhood are missing, but it seems reasonable to assume that also in pregnant women and in the developing fetus a lower excretion capacity might increase their vulnerability to BPA exposure with potential consequences for children's later disease development.

In this context, BPA is highly discussed in terms of increasing the risk for obesity pathology but only few controversial studies on human prenatal BPA exposure exist so far [13–15]. Although animal studies are available to a greater extent, derived results are inconsistent and mechanistic investigations, for example, regarding underlying BPA-related epigenetic changes, are lacking. Epigenetic alterations related to BPA exposure have previously been associated with an increased risk of carcinogenesis [16–18] in rodent models of hepatic and prostate cancer. So far, no data on BPA-induced epigenetic modifications leading to overweight development exist.

Therefore, the aim of the present study was to analyze epigenetic alterations in the cord blood of prenatally exposed children and their potential link to overweight development as part of the German prospective LINA mother-child cohort. Findings from our epidemiological study were validated by applying an experimental mouse model for prenatal BPA exposure and an in vitro stem cell differentiation model demonstrating the impact of BPA exposure on adipocyte development.

Methods

LINA study design and sample collection

The LINA cohort study (Lifestyle and environmental factors and their Influence on Newborns Allergy risk) recruited 622 pregnant mothers (629 mother-child-pairs) between May 2006 and December 2008 in Leipzig, Germany, to investigate how environmental factors in the pre- and postnatal period influence disease risks later in children's life [19–21]. Mothers suffering from immune or infectious diseases during pregnancy were excluded from the study.

Six hundred six mother-child-pairs participated in the year 1, 420 in the year 6 follow-up. Standardized questionnaires were administered during pregnancy (34th week of gestation) and annually thereafter, collecting general information about study participants, about housing and environmental conditions as well as about personal lifestyle. At the age of 1 and 6 years, height and body weight of the children were assessed during clinical visits. BMI z score were calculated according to the WHO references [22]. All questionnaires were self-administered by the parents. Participation in the study was voluntary and written informed consent was obtained from all participants. The study was approved by the Ethics Committee of the

University of Leipzig (file ref. # 046–2006, #206–12-02072012).

Analyses of urinary bisphenol A concentration in human samples

BPA quantification was carried out for 552 maternal urine samples (34th week of gestation) using a multianalyte procedure as described by Feltens et al. [23] and in more detail in the supplementary material. Absolute concentrations of BPA were calculated based on calibration curves and normalized to urinary creatinine concentrations as previously described [24].

In vivo mouse model

BALB/c mice (6–8 weeks of age) were obtained from the Elevage Janvier Laboratory (Le Genest St Isle, France). Mice were bred and maintained in the animal facility at the University of Leipzig (Germany) and housed under conventional conditions with 23 °C room temperature, 60% humidity, and 12 h day/night rhythm. Cages were bedded with LIGNOCEL® bedding material (fine particles < 200 μm 0.2%). Mice received phytoestrogen-free diet (C1000 from Altromin, Lage, Germany) and water ad libitum from custom-built glass bottles to avoid contamination with BPA. All animal experiments involved groups of 4–6 mice/cage and were performed according to institutional and state guidelines. The Committee on Animal Welfare of Saxony approved animal protocols used in this study.

Dams were exposed to 5 μg/ml BPA (Sigma Aldrich, Munich, Germany) via the drinking water 1 week before mating until delivery of the offspring. For each exposure group (control or BPA), the exposure protocol was performed at least two times in at least three dams (each with 2–5 pups). Serum was collected from dams at the end of the BPA exposure. 1 week after delivery, pups were weighed two times per week and a mean weight per week was calculated for each mouse. At the end of the observation period (10 weeks), whole body composition (fat mass and lean mass) was determined in awake mice based on nuclear magnetic resonance technology using an EchoMRI700™ instrument (Echo Medical Systems, Houston, TX, USA) in the offspring of control and BPA exposed dams. Further, DNA-methylation analysis (MassARRAY) as well as gene expression analysis was performed in visceral fat tissue as described below in 10-week-old offspring. For measurement of fat mass/lean mass, MassARRAY and gene expression analysis, we used at least four mice per group from two to four dams (to avoid litter effects), but in any case with an equal number of male and female mice.

Murine BPA ELISA

BPA concentration in serum was detected with BPA Assay Kit (Immuno-Biological Laboratories, Hamburg, Germany).

Serum samples, enzyme-labeled BPA and anti-BPA serum were added to a pre-coated microtiter plate with anti-rabbit IgG and incubated for 1 h at room temperature. After washing, TMB was added as substrate and color reaction was detected at 450 nm. BPA serum concentration was calculated from a standard curve with a detection range from 0.3 to 100 ng/ml. Measured BPA serum levels in adult mice reached 19 ng/ml.

In vitro adipocytes model

Human adipose-derived mesenchymal stem cells (MSC; ATCC®, PCS-500-011; #59753760) and culture media were purchased from LGC Standards (Wesel, Germany). For adipocyte differentiation MSCs at passage 1–3 were seeded at 9600 cells/cm^2 and were cultured with Adipocyte Differentiation Initiation Medium (ADIM; ATCC Adipocyte Differentiation Toolkit PCS-500-050) for 4 days. Thereafter, Adipocyte Maintenance Medium (ADMM; ATCC® Adipocyte Differentiation Toolkit PCS-500-050) was applied for the subsequent 11 days. Media was changed every 2 to 4 days according to the manufacturer's instructions. During the entire differentiation period, cells were exposed to 10 or 50 μM BPA (Sigma Aldrich, Munich, Germany) or a solvent control (0.05% ethanol); freshly added after every medium change. The differentiation process was monitored in real-time by the impedance-based xCELLigence SP System (ACEA Biosciences Inc., San Diego, USA) on a microelectrode 96 well E-View-Plate (ACEA Biosciences Inc.). The growth rate was monitored every 10 min by electrical impedance measurements that were paused for media changes and a Cell Index was calculated, by normalization to a blank value for each well. After differentiation, cells were stained with Oil Red O for 45 min for triglyceride depots and mRNA was extracted (see supplementary material).

A MTT assay (3-(4,5-Dimethylthiazol-2-yl)-2,5-diphenyl-tetrazoliumbromid) was applied to a BPA concentration series to identify appropriate non-toxic concentrations for the in vitro assay. For details, see supplementary material.

DNA methylation analysis via 450 K array

Genomic DNA was isolated from cord blood samples using the QIAmp DNA Blood Mini Kit (Qiagen, Hilden, Germany) followed by bisulfite conversion using the EZ-96 DNA Methylation Kit (Zymo Research Corporation, Orange, USA) according to the manufacturer's recommendations. All samples subsequently subjected to DNA methylation analyses passed the initial quality control check (n = 472).

A genome-wide DNA methylation screen was performed based on the Infinium HumanMethylation450 BeadChip (Illumina, San Diego, USA) array (see supplementary material). Data were normalized using the SWAN (subset-quantile within array normalization) method of the minfi R package [25]. DNA methylation values, described as beta values (β), were recorded for each locus in each sample. For statistical analyses β values were logit transformed to M values [26].

To account for potential differences in cell composition, we used publically available FACS data of sorted cord blood cells [27] implemented in the R package *FlowSorted.CordBloodNorway.450 k: Illumina Human-Methylation data on sorted cord blood cell populations* (version 1.4.0) [28] and the estimateCellCounts-function of the minfi R package. The resulting information on CD4+ T cells, CD8+ T cells, natural killer cells, B cells, granulocytes, and monocyte proportions were used as confounders in the subsequent regression analysis. In addition, previously identified factors with an impact on cord blood methylation were considered as confounders including the maternal vitamin D level [29], prenatal benzene exposure, maternal smoking [30, 31], and maternal stress during pregnancy [32]. Differentially methylated CpGs were determined by applying logistic regression models on methylation M values [33] adjusted for the confounders mentioned above. A Bonferroni correction was applied on obtained p values resulting in a significance level of $p < 2.37E-7$. For details, see supplementary material.

MassARRAY validation of DNA methylation

A quantitative DNA methylation analysis of the human *MEST* promoter was performed in cord blood samples of the LINA cohort and in in vitro adipocytes using Sequenom's MassARRAY platform as described previously [31]. Briefly, a PCR amplicon was designed on the reverse strand covering chr7: 130,132,068-130,132,287 including cg17580798 (Fig. 1, *MEST* forward primer: aggaagagagTTTAGAGGTAGTTTTAGTTYGG, reverse primer: cagtaatacgactcactatagggagaaggctCCRCTACTAA CCAACTCTAC with an annealing temperature of 52 ° C). A total of 24 CpGs was covered by the amplicon. For analysis, all high mass, duplicate, and silent peaks were

excluded from the analysis retaining 14 CpGs, which were averaged and used for further analysis.

gDNA extracted from murine adipose tissue F1 ($n \geq 3$, per treatment group) was bisulfite converted using the EZ DNA Methylation kit (Zymo Research, Freiburg, Germany) and subjected to MassARRAY analysis. Genome coordinates of the human *MEST* promoter were lifted over to the mouse genome assembly mm10 and corresponding primer pairs on the forward strand were designed (*Mest* forward primer: aggaagagagAGGAGGTTTGTGTTTTTAATG, reverse: cagtaatacgactcactatagggagaaggctCACCCACTT CTTTTCTACC, annealing temperature: 60 °C, amplicon coordinates: chr6: 30,737,347-30,737,692).

Gene expression analysis

Gene expression analysis in samples of the LINA cohort was performed as described earlier [31] and in more detail in the supplementary material. Briefly, intron-spanning primers were designed, and UPL probes were selected by the Universal Probe Library Assay Design Center. After a preamplification step qPCRs were conducted on 96.96 Dynamic Array (Fluidigm, San Francisco, CA, USA). Gene expression values were determined with *glycerinaldehyd-3-phosphat-dehydrogenase (GAPD)* and *glucuronidase beta (GUSB)* as reference genes and normalized to the lowest measured value. The following primer pairs were used for *MEST* (primer-for 5′- atcgtggaagcgcttttg, -rev 5′-gaccagatcgattctgcttgta, UPL50) and the reference genes *GAPD* and *GUSB* (primer-for 5′-gctctctgctcctcctgttc, -rev 5′-acgaccaaatccgttgactc, UPL 60; -for 5′-cgccctgcctatctgt attc, -rev 5′-tccccacagggagtgtgtag, UPL 57, respectively).

Mest expression in murine fat tissue was assessed by qPCR. Expression values were determined by applying the 2-ΔΔCT method and normalized to *Gapdh and UBC (–for 5′-gtctgctgtgtgaggactgc, rev 5′- cctccagggtga tggtctta UPL 77).*

Furthermore, gene expression of *peroxisome proliferator-activated receptor gamma (PPARG), sterol regulatory element-binding factor 1 (SREBF1), lipoprotein lipase (LPL), leptin (LEP), fatty acid synthase (FASN), mesoderm specific transcript (MEST), estrogen receptor alpha (ESR1),* and

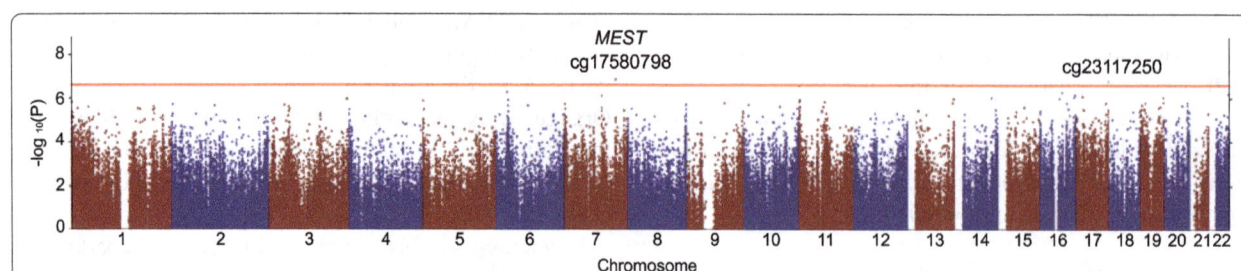

Fig. 1 Epigenome wide analysis and *MEST* methylation assessment. Manhattan-Plot from 450 K array comparing children prenatally exposed to high vs. low BPA. Shown are significant CpGs observed in cord blood that passed threshold for Bonferroni correction (red threshold line, $p < 2.37E-7$)

insulin receptor substrate 2 (*IRS2*) was assessed by qPCR of human in vitro derived adipocytes.

All used primer pairs are listed in Additional file 1: Table S1. All primers were designed as intron spanning assays to assure specificity.

Statistical analyses

To test the equal distribution of parameters in the analyzed sub-cohort and the entire LINA cohort, the chi-squared test was performed. LINA study data were evaluated by STATISTICA for Windows, Version 12 (Statsoft Inc., USA). 450 k data were analyzed and processed using the R packages minfi and qqman (R version 3.3.1, R Foundation for Statistical Computing).

BPA concentrations and DNA methylation levels were log transformed for further statistical analyses. To assess longitudinal associations of gene expression and weight development, a generalized estimating equation (GEE) model was applied. Mediator models for the connection of prenatal BPA exposure with the methylation status and children's BMI z scores were analyzed using the PROCESS macro v2.16.3 in IBM SPSS Statistics version 22 (IBM Corps., USA) [34]. All models were adjusted for the gender of the child, smoking during pregnancy, parental school education, solid food introduction, gestational week at delivery, number of household members, and early delivery (< 37 weeks of gestation). Weight-related confounders were chosen according to a literature review.

Experimental data sets from murine and in vitro studies were processed and analyzed in GraphPad PRISM 7.02 for windows (GraphPad Software, Inc.). All p values ≤ 0.05 were considered to be significant.

Results

General study characteristics

Our analyzed sub-cohort was comprised of the 408 children for whom data on prenatal BPA exposure and the cord blood methylation status were available. General characteristics of the study participants (gender, birth weight, gestational week at delivery, smoking during pregnancy, parental school education, household members, breastfeeding, and introduction to solid food) of the sub-cohort ($n = 408$) were not different from the total LINA cohort ($n = 629$) as shown in Table 1. Median urinary BPA concentrations at pregnancy were 12.7 ng/mg creatinine. Low BPA exposure was defined as < 7.6 ng/mg creatinine ($< 25\%$; 1st or lower quartile) and high BPA exposure as > 15.9 ng/mg creatinine ($> 75\%$, 4th or upper quartile). BMI z scores at year 1 ranged from $- 3.5$ to 2.9 with a median of $- 0.2$, BMI z scores at year 6 ranged from $- 2.2$ to 4.2 with a median of 0.0.

Table 1 General study population characteristics

	Entire LINA cohort n (%), $n = 629^{a}$	Analyzed sub-cohort n (%), $n = 408$	χ^2 test[b]
Gender of the child			0.966
Female	302(48.0)	197(48.3)	
Male	327(52.0)	211(51.7)	
Birth weight			0.941
≤ 3000 g	123(19.6)	68(16.7)	
$> 3000–3500$ g	242(38.5)	157(38.5)	
$> 3500–4000$ g	192(30.6)	129(31.6)	
> 4000 g	71(11.3)	54(13.2)	
Gestational week at delivery			0.834
< 37 weeks	25(4.0)	10(2.5)	
37–40 weeks	389(62.0)	255(62.5)	
> 40 weeks	214(34.0)	143(35.0)	
Smoking during pregnancy			0.833
Never	534(84.9)	358(87.7)	
Occasionally	47(7.4)	23(5.6)	
Daily	48(7.6)	27(6.6)	
Parental school education[c]			0.969
Low	16(2.5)	8(2.0)	
Intermediate	144(22.9)	96(23.5)	
High	469(74.6)	304(74.5)	
Household members			0.932
2	33(5.2)	20(4.9)	
3	365(58.0)	257(63.0)	
> 4	203(32.3)	129(31.6)	
Breastfeeding exclusive			0.968
1–3 months	112(17.8)	69(16.9)	
1–6 months	190(30.2)	121(29.7)	
1–12 months	254(40.4)	172(42.2)	
Introduction to solid food			0.897
1–3 months	23(3.7)	11(2.7)	
4–6 months	251(39.9)	156(38.2)	
7–12 months	305(48.5)	205(50.2)	
Urinary BPA concentration during pregnancy			0.263[d]
Median [ng/mg creatinine]	12.7	12.7	
IQR[e] [ng/mg creatinine]	7.5–16.0	7.6–15.9	
BMI z score at year 1	$n = 564$	$n = 366$	
Median	$- 0.24$	$- 0.16$	
IQR	$- 0.90–0.35$	$- 0.79-0.43$	
BMI z score at year 6	$n = 303$	$n = 192$	
Median	$- 0.02$	0.05	
IQR	$- 0.67-0.50$	$- 0.51-0.54$	

[a]n may be different from 629 due to missing data
[b]Calculated using the chi-squared test for cross relationship
[c]Low = 8 years of schooling ('Hauptschulabschluss'); intermediate = 10 years of schooling ('Mittlere Reife'); high = 12 years of schooling or more ('(Fach-)hochschulreife')
[d]p-value derived by Student's t test between group means
[e]IQR: inter quartile range (25th to 75th percentile)

Prenatal BPA exposure and cord blood DNA methylation of MEST

As there is growing evidence that epigenetic mechanisms such as DNA methylation changes can contribute to prenatal programming of diseases, the potential impact of BPA on children's DNA-methylation pattern was assessed. Using bisulfite converted gDNA from cord blood, genome-wide changes in DNA methylation were evaluated by applying Illumina Infinium HumanMethylation450 BeadChip arrays. Differentially methylated CpG sites were computed using a regression model for high (fourth quartile) versus low (first quartile) prenatal BPA exposure. Two CpGs passed the threshold for Bonferroni correction (Fig. 1a and Table 2), including a hypomethylated CpG (cg17580798) in the *MEST* promoter (chr7:130132199, $p = 1.35E-07$) and cg23117250 (chr17: 80649886, intronic, $p = 1.55E-07$) that is located in an intron of *RAB40B*. *RAB40B* encodes for a poorly characterized protein proposed to be involved in vesicle transport [35] and cancer progression [36].

Thus, we focused further analyses on cg17580798 since *MEST*, as a member of the alpha/beta hydrolase superfamily, is reported to control the initial phase of early adipose tissue expansion by regulating adipocyte size [37]. Although cg17580798 is located in the first intron of *MEST*, ENCODE histone modification data suggest that it is a promoter region. That indeed this region is potentially transcriptionally regulating is supported by its overlap with a DNase I hypersensitivity cluster.

MEST promoter methylation around cg17580798 was validated by MassARRAY (see Additional file 2: Figure S1). The MassARRAY amplicon included 24 CpG sites of which 14 CpG sites passed quality control and were averaged as "total promoter methylation." BPA exposure was associated with total promoter methylation (adj.MR: 0.88, 95% CI (0. 80, 0.97), $p = 0.010$), as well as methylation of the CpG corresponding to cg17580798 only (adj.MR: 0.90, 95% CI (0. 82, 0.99), $p = 0.033$). The methylation difference between low and high BPA exposure was 2.6 and 2.3%, respectively.

BPA associates with MEST promoter methylation and MEST expression in cord blood

MEST expression was measured in 408 cord blood samples of the LINA cohort. Complete information of *MEST* methylation status, *MEST* expression and prenatal BPA

exposure was available for 361 children. High prenatal BPA exposure (> 75%, upper quartile (UQ)) was associated with a decrease in *MEST* promoter methylation at birth as determined by MassARRAY (Fig. 2a). Further, this *MEST* promoter hypomethylation was associated with an increase in *MEST* RNA expression, which was not observed in lowly exposed children (Fig. 2b). There was no direct effect of prenatal BPA exposure on cord blood *MEST* expression. However, applying a mediation model using PROCESS in SPSS, prenatal BPA exposure was linked indirectly to *MEST* expression by *MEST* promoter methylation (ab = 0. 47, 95% CI (0.07, 1.24); Fig. 2c and Additional file 1: Table S2) at time of birth. Furthermore, *MEST* expression at birth was positively correlated with BMI z scores (adj.MR: 1.13, 95% CI (1.02, 1.26), $p = 0.024$).

BPA increases risk for childhood overweight development via MEST methylation

In addition, we were interested whether the changes in *MEST* promoter methylation that were associated with BPA exposure have relevance for the later weight development of the child. Therefore, we applied a mediator analysis, adjusted for weight-related confounders, to assess the impact of prenatal BPA exposure on children's BMI z scores at year 1, which might be mediated by neonatal *MEST* promoter methylation. Indeed the mediation analysis indicates that the effect of prenatal BPA exposure on BMI z scores is mediated by *MEST* promoter methylation in cord blood (ab = 0.29, 95% CI (0.03, 1.09), Fig. 3a and Additional file 1: Table S3). Furthermore, the impact of cord blood *MEST* promoter methylation on BMI z scores at year 6 was mediated by the BMI z scores at year 1 (ab = − 0.18, 95% CI (− 0. 51, − 0.06), Fig. 3b and Additional file 1: Table S4).

MEST expression is associated with longitudinal weight development

The longitudinal impact of altered *MEST* expression at birth due to prenatal BPA exposure was calculated using a generalized estimating equation (GEE) model including BMI z scores and *MEST* expression at birth and year 6 as well as weight related confounders. We found that a longitudinally higher *MEST* expression at birth and year 6 was positively correlated with longitudinal weight development at birth and year 6 (adj.RR: 1.03, 95% CI (1.00, 1.07), $p = 0.021$).

Table 2 Epigenome-wide association study (EWAS) comparing children prenatally exposed to high vs. low BPA. Shown are significant CpGs observed in cord blood that passed Bonferroni correction

CpG	Chromosome	Position	Region	Host gene	p value [a]	Δ β[b]
cg17580798	7	130,132,199	Promoter	*MEST*	1.35E-07	−1.8%
cg23117250	17	80,649,886	Intron	*RAB40B*	1.55E-07	−2.0%

[a]p values are derived from a regression model with prenatal vitamin D level, prenatal benzene exposure, maternal smoking, maternal stress, and cord blood cell composition as confounding parameters
[b]Methylation differences are shown as Δ methylation values (β)

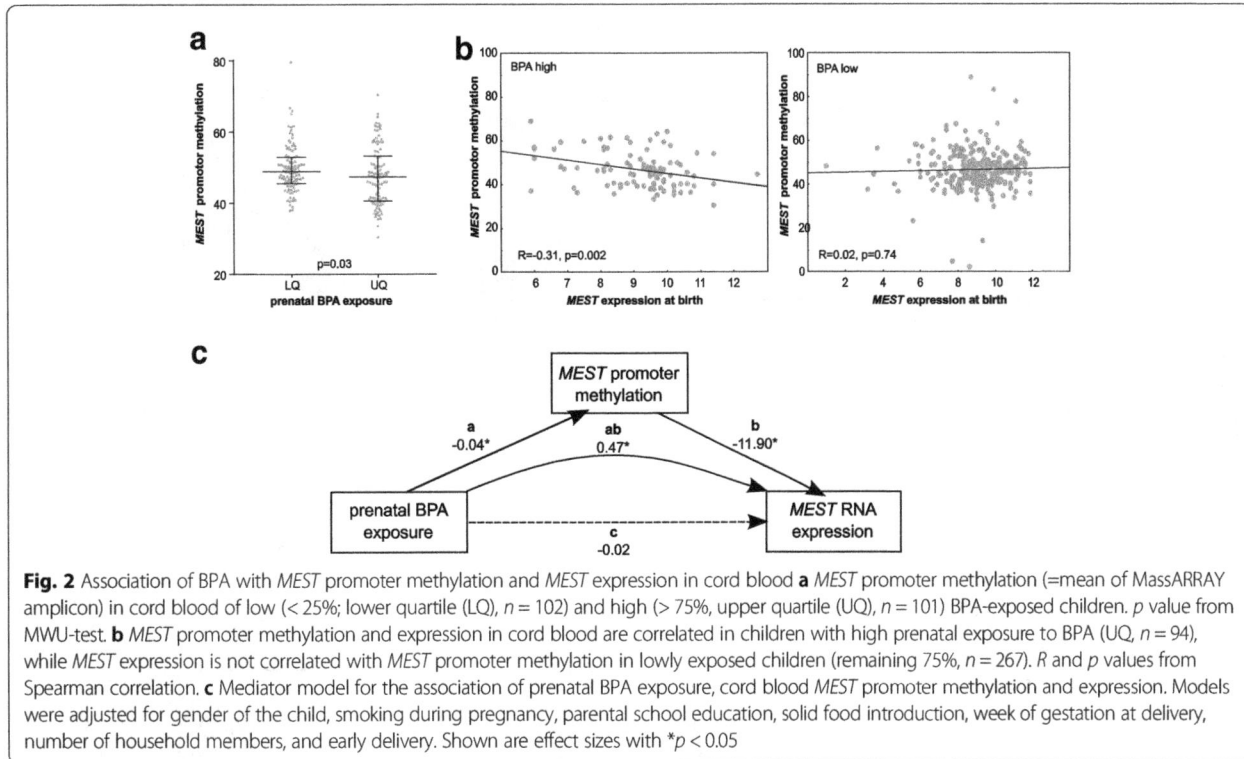

Fig. 2 Association of BPA with *MEST* promoter methylation and *MEST* expression in cord blood **a** *MEST* promoter methylation (=mean of MassARRAY amplicon) in cord blood of low (< 25%; lower quartile (LQ), $n = 102$) and high (> 75%, upper quartile (UQ), $n = 101$) BPA-exposed children. p value from MWU-test. **b** *MEST* promoter methylation and expression in cord blood are correlated in children with high prenatal exposure to BPA (UQ, $n = 94$), while *MEST* expression is not correlated with *MEST* promoter methylation in lowly exposed children (remaining 75%, $n = 267$). R and p values from Spearman correlation. **c** Mediator model for the association of prenatal BPA exposure, cord blood *MEST* promoter methylation and expression. Models were adjusted for gender of the child, smoking during pregnancy, parental school education, solid food introduction, week of gestation at delivery, number of household members, and early delivery. Shown are effect sizes with *$p < 0.05$

In vivo mouse model: impact of prenatal BPA exposure on weight development

To validate our findings from the LINA cohort and add further information on *Mest* methylation and expression in fat tissue, we applied a mouse model under standardized

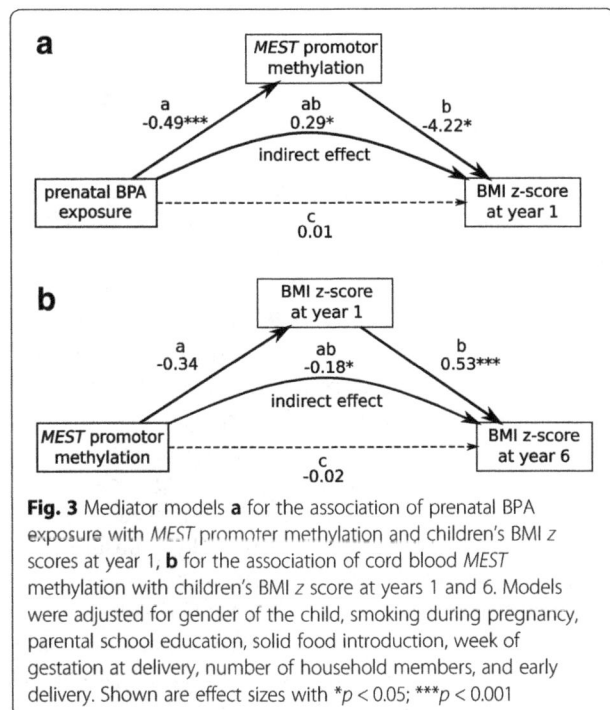

Fig. 3 Mediator models **a** for the association of prenatal BPA exposure with *MEST* promoter methylation and children's BMI z scores at year 1, **b** for the association of cord blood *MEST* methylation with children's BMI z score at years 1 and 6. Models were adjusted for gender of the child, smoking during pregnancy, parental school education, solid food introduction, week of gestation at delivery, number of household members, and early delivery. Shown are effect sizes with *$p < 0.05$; ***$p < 0.001$

conditions. Mice offspring of BPA-exposed mothers were followed up until 10 weeks after delivery. Weight was assessed twice a week, beginning 1 week after delivery, and compared to unexposed control animals (Fig. 4a). Prenatally BPA exposed mice had a significantly higher weight over the entire observation period compared to unexposed control mice ($p = 0.004$, p value derived by ANOVA) with a mean difference of 0.85 g (week 2) to 3.04 g (weeks 3, 8, and 9). There was no gender difference in BPA-dependent weight development (Additional file 3: Figure S2). Furthermore, lean mass and fat mass were assessed at 10 weeks, with BPA-exposed mice showing a 53% higher fat mass than control mice ($p = 0.013$, Fig. 4b). *Mest* methylation and expression was assessed at 10 weeks in fat tissue samples. *Mest* methylation was reduced by 7% in BPA exposed mice ($p < 0.001$, Fig. 4c) with a corresponding increase in *Mest* expression by 2.1-fold in BPA exposed mice ($p = 0.022$, Fig. 4d).

In vitro model: impact of BPA exposure on adipocyte differentiation

Differentiation of human MSC to adipocytes was monitored in real time using the impedance-based xCELLigence System. 10 or 50 μM BPA were applied during the entire differentiation period and compared to a solvent control (EtOH, 0.05%). BPA caused a dose-dependent decrease in cell index values after the differentiation initiation period compared to unexposed controls (Fig. 5a). Significance was reached from day 3 on for 50 μM and

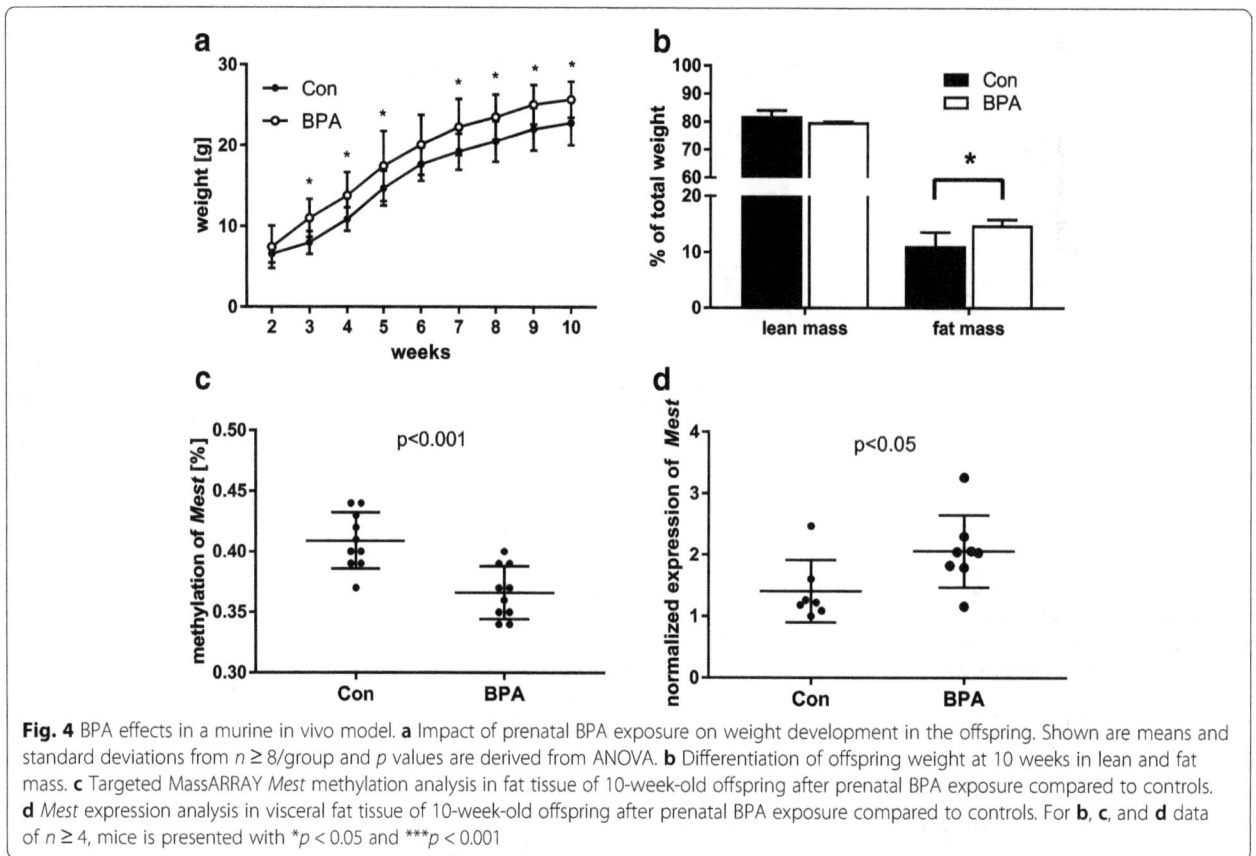

Fig. 4 BPA effects in a murine in vivo model. **a** Impact of prenatal BPA exposure on weight development in the offspring. Shown are means and standard deviations from $n \geq 8$/group and p values are derived from ANOVA. **b** Differentiation of offspring weight at 10 weeks in lean and fat mass. **c** Targeted MassARRAY *Mest* methylation analysis in fat tissue of 10-week-old offspring after prenatal BPA exposure compared to controls. **d** *Mest* expression analysis in visceral fat tissue of 10-week-old offspring after prenatal BPA exposure compared to controls. For **b**, **c**, and **d** data of $n \geq 4$, mice is presented with *$p < 0.05$ and ***$p < 0.001$

from day 5 on for 10 μM BPA until the end of the observational period. Oil Red O staining of lipid droplets showed significantly more droplets for 50 μM BPA ($p < 0.001$; Fig. 5b, c) but not for 10 μM BPA compared to unexposed control cells.

mRNA analysis of adipocyte-specific genes after 17 days of differentiation in the presence of 50 μM BPA revealed a significant upregulation of *PPARγ* (2.2 ± 1.15-fold, $p = 0.005$), its target gene *LPL* (4.4 ± 2.6-fold, $p = 0.029$); *SREBF1* (1.8 ± 0.4-fold, $p = 0.005$), its target gene *IRS2* (1.9 ± 0.6-fold, $p = 0.015$; Fig. 2b), and *ESR1* (8.4 ± 3.8-fold, $p = 0.006$). For 10 μM BPA, a significant increase in gene expression was detected for *LPL* (1.9 ± 0.3-fold, $p = 0.002$), *SREBF1* (1.5 ± 0.1-fold, $p < 0.001$) and *FASN* (1.9 ± 0.7-fold, $p = 0.046$, Fig. 5d).

MEST methylation and expression was measured in differentiated adipocytes as shown in Fig. 5e, f. *MEST* promoter methylation (total and cg17580798) was decreased by 28% after exposure to 50 μM BPA compared to the control. In accordance, *MEST* expression was significantly increased in adipocytes exposed to 50 μM BPA (1.6 ± 0.4-fold, $p = 0.027$, Fig. 5e, f).

Our in vitro results are not influenced by any cytotoxic effects of BPA, as can be seen from the performed MTT assay (Additional file 4: Figure S3). There was no change in cell viability up to 50 μM BPA, although cells exposed

to 100 μM BPA showed a slight but significantly lower cell viability after 48 h ($p = 0.027$).

Discussion

Our study provides first evidence that prenatal BPA exposure causes epigenetic changes in the *MEST* promoter potentially contributing to overweight development in children with longitudinal effects until the age of 6 years (Additional file 5: Figure S4). Results from our experimental models support these epidemiological findings: prenatally BPA exposed mice showed hypo-methylation of the *MEST* promoter region and developed a significantly higher body weight compared to controls. Furthermore, a stimulating impact of BPA on adipocyte differentiation from human MSC was observed. Although these experimental data have to be interpreted with caution, since the applied exposure concentrations were quite different compared to the real human exposure situation, there is some evidence for an involvement of *MEST* in BPA-induced adipogenesis.

Results from this study may provide a first mechanistic explanation how prenatal BPA potentially exposure contributes to overweight development in the children. We identified two differentially methylated CpG sites in cord blood in association to prenatal BPA exposure, among them one hypo-methylated CpG in the *MEST* promoter. *MEST* is a paternally imprinted gene that encodes a

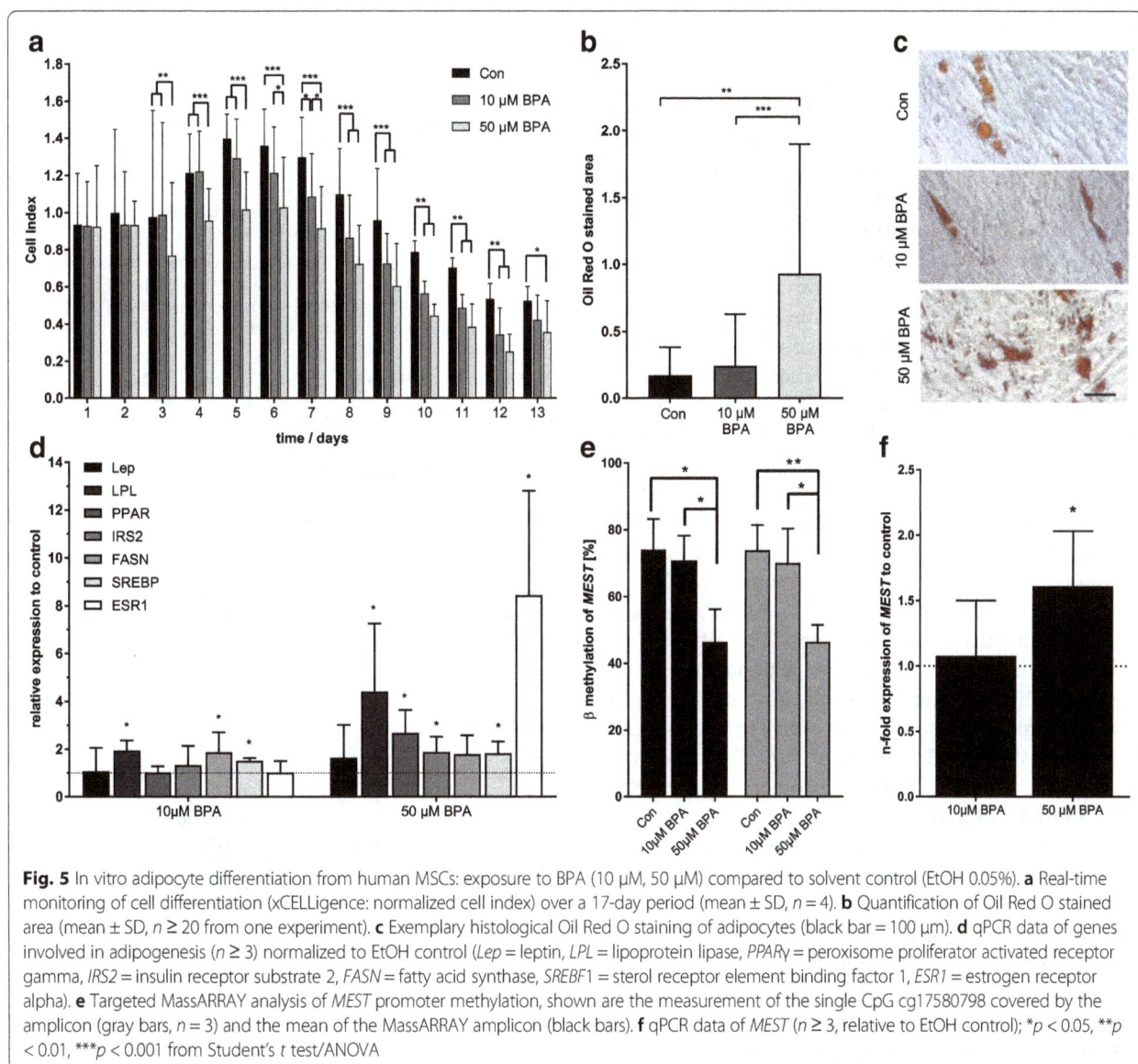

Fig. 5 In vitro adipocyte differentiation from human MSCs: exposure to BPA (10 μM, 50 μM) compared to solvent control (EtOH 0.05%). **a** Real-time monitoring of cell differentiation (xCELLigence: normalized cell index) over a 17-day period (mean ± SD, $n = 4$). **b** Quantification of Oil Red O stained area (mean ± SD, $n ≥ 20$ from one experiment). **c** Exemplary histological Oil Red O staining of adipocytes (black bar = 100 μm). **d** qPCR data of genes involved in adipogenesis ($n ≥ 3$) normalized to EtOH control (*Lep* = leptin, *LPL* = lipoprotein lipase, *PPAR*γ = peroxisome proliferator activated receptor gamma, *IRS2* = insulin receptor substrate 2, *FASN* = fatty acid synthase, *SREBF*1 = sterol receptor element binding factor 1, *ESR1* = estrogen receptor alpha). **e** Targeted MassARRAY analysis of *MEST* promoter methylation, shown are the measurement of the single CpG cg17580798 covered by the amplicon (gray bars, $n = 3$) and the mean of the MassARRAY amplicon (black bars). **f** qPCR data of *MEST* ($n ≥ 3$, relative to EtOH control); *$p < 0.05$, **$p < 0.01$, ***$p < 0.001$ from Student's *t* test/ANOVA

member of the α/β hydrolase fold family, and its expression has been described to be associated with obesity [38–40], adipocyte size [37], and preadipocyte proliferation [41] in mouse and human studies. *MEST* knock-out mice showed reduced body weight and less obesity. *Mest* expression has been associated with variable obesity in mice and is attenuated by a positive energy balance [42]. High *Mest* expression was found in high-gainers even at only 1 week of high fat diet and may therefore be able to foreshadow food metabolism capacity in mice [43–45].

Recently, a link between prenatal BPA exposure and an epigenetic modification in the imprinted *Mest* gene was observed in a murine study. Trapphoff et al. reported hypomethylation of the *Mest* promoter due to BPA exposure in murine oocytes [46]. Perinatal BPA exposure interferes with DNA methyltransferase 3a/3b (DNMT3A/DNMT3B)

expression in mice, specifically affecting the de novo methylation of imprinted genes [47], which might be a contributing factor to the observed hypo-methylation. In this study, we show for the first time that also in humans prenatal BPA exposure is related to DNA methylation changes in the *MEST* promoter. It was already suggested that *MEST* methylation levels are associated with obesity risk in humans [48, 49]. Thus, our observed hypo-methylation in the *MEST* promoter may link prenatal BPA exposure to the overweight development in the offspring. In line with this hypothesis, we showed that *MEST* expression was associated with BMI increase on a longitudinal scale.

Although the observed methylation difference in the *MEST* promoter between BPA high and low exposed children in cord blood samples was only 1%, we nevertheless believe that this very small difference in the methylation status could be of biological relevance. *MEST* is expressed in mesenchymal tissue and also in MSCs, which are the source of adipose tissue, but not in blood cells. Since cord blood contains a sizeable number of MSCs, we suppose that the observed BPA-related hypo-methylation in the cord blood samples of our study relates to an expansion in the cord blood MSC fraction and *MEST* activation. Unfortunately, we were not able to test this hypothesis within our LINA study due to limited cell availability. However, data from an earlier study may support the idea that changes in specific cell populations in response to environmental exposure might be the cause of small DNA methylation differences observed in whole blood samples and, moreover, might be also of biological relevance if this particular cell population is involved in pathophysiology [30].

Since we were not able to isolate and test MSCs from our study participants, we applied an in vitro model to analyze the impact of BPA on MSCs. In adipocytes differentiated from BPA-exposed human MSCs, we showed a hypo-methylation of the *MEST* promoter region and an enhanced *MEST* expression. Although the applied BPA concentrations in this experimental model were much higher compared to the real exposure situation in humans, these data nevertheless may support the hypothesis that BPA induces *MEST* activation in human MSCs, which further corroborates a role of *MEST* in BPA-induced adipogenesis.

A limitation of this study is the missing information about maternal weight before and during pregnancy as a potential confounding factor. Further, BPA concentrations were measured in spot urine samples. BPA concentrations vary widely throughout the day and spot urine BPA concentrations only reflect exposure of the last 4–6 h [7]. Moreover, we cannot exclude the possibility of BPA contaminations introduced by tubing or reaction tubes during the storage and analytical procedure as pointed out to be critical by recent publications [50, 51]. However, samples were all stored in the same tubes and were analyzed at the same time, suggesting rather a systematic overestimation of the BPA concentration than a random contamination effect. The strength of our study is the combination of epidemiological data with in vivo and in vitro experimental models. For the first time, we performed a genome-wide DNA-methylation analysis in the cord blood of prenatally BPA-exposed children and found an epigenetic link between BPA exposure and overweight development.

Conclusion

In conclusion, our study demonstrates that prenatal BPA exposure seems to be a contributing factor in the development of an early overweight phenotype by implicating epigenetic changes in the obesity-related gene *MEST*.

Additional files

Additional file 1: Table S1. Primer for gene expression analysis. **Table S2.** Mediator model for the association of prenatal BPA exposure with cord blood *MEST* DNA methylation and expression (according to Fig. 1c). **Table S3.** Mediator model for the association of prenatal BPA exposure with cord blood *MEST* DNA methylation and children's BMI z scores at year 1 (according to Fig. 3a). **Table S4.** Mediator model for the association of cord blood *MEST* DNA methylation and children's BMI z scores at years 1 and 6 (according to Fig. 3b). (DOCX 45 kb)

Additional file 2: Figure S1. Shown are the location of the *MEST* gene on chromosome 7 (upper part), the 450 K array CpG in the *MEST* promoter (middle part) and the region covered by the MassARRAY amplicon within the promoter region (CpG sites are depicted in red). (PDF 32 kb)

Additional file 3: Figure S2. BPA effect on weight development assessed in a murine in vivo model stratified for gender. Shown are means and standard deviation from $n \geq 8$ mice/group for all, female and male mice separately. p values are derived from ANOVA. (TIFF 1362 kb)

Additional file 4: Figure S3. MTT assay: MTT test for cell viability after exposure to BPA and the solvent control EtOH (0.05%), normalized to unexposed control, Student's t test *$p < 0.05$, mean ± SD, $n = 3$. (JPEG 105 kb)

Additional file 5: Figure S4. Summary scheme: results overview and hypothesis indicating the influence of prenatal BPA exposure on *MEST* methylation and expression that is associated with adipocyte differentiation and overweight development in infant offspring. (PNG 19 kb)

Abbreviations

95% CI: 95% confidence interval; BMI: Body mass index; BPA: Bisphenol A; Con: Control; DNMT: DNA methyltransferase; EDC: Endocrine-disrupting chemicals; *ESR1*: Estrogen receptor alpha; EtOH: Ethanol; *FASN*: Fatty acid synthase; *GAPDH*: Glycerinaldehyd-3-phosphat-dehydrogenase; gDNA: Genomic DNA; GEE: Generalized estimating equation; *GUSB*: Glucuronidase beta; *IRS2*: Insulin receptor substrate 2; *LEP*: Leptin; *LPL*: Lipoprotein lipase; *MEST*: Mesoderm specific transcript; MR: Mean ratio; MSC: Mesenchymal stem cells; MWU: Mann-Whitney U test; *PPARγ*: Peroxisome proliferator-activated receptor gamma; RR: Risk ratio; *SREBF1*: Sterol regulatory element-binding factor 1; UGT: UDP-glucuronosyltransferase; WHO: World Health Organization

Acknowledgements

We thank all LINA families for participation in the study, Anne Hain and Brigitte Winkler for technical support, and Melanie Bänsch for her excellent study organization assistance.

The LINA study was financed via Helmholtz institutional funding (Helmholtz Centre for Environmental Research–UFZ). The work of Ralph Feltens was completely and of Dirk Wissenbach partially funded by the Saxon excellence initiative LIFE. Tobias Bauer was supported by a grant from the German Ministry for Research and Education (BMBF) program PANC-STRAT (01ZX1305A). Martin von Bergen acknowledges funding by DFG CRC 1052.

Funding

The LINA study was financed via Helmholtz institutional funding (Helmholtz Centre for Environmental Research–UFZ). The work of Ralph Feltens was completely and of Dirk Wissenbach partially funded by the Saxon excellence initiative LIFE. Tobias Bauer was supported by a grant from the German Ministry for Research and Education (BMBF) program PANC-STRAT (01ZX1305A). Martin von Bergen acknowledges funding by DFG CRC 1052. Saskia Trump was supported by the Helmholtz cross program activity on Personalized Medicine (iMed).

Authors' contributions

BL, KJ, LT, KL, and AK performed and/or coordinated the experimental work. LT, KG, BL, TB, NI, MS, MBH, and RE performed the epigenetic analysis. DW, RF, and MvB conducted the BPA measurement in LINA. SJ, AS, and TP planned and performed the mouse experiments. SR, MB, and IL collected the data and provided the proband material. KJ, BL, LT, ST, TP, and IL prepared the initial manuscript and figures. IL, RE, KJ, ST, GS, WK, and MvB provided project leadership. All authors contributed to the final manuscript. All authors read and approved the final manuscript.

Competing interests

The authors declare that they have no competing interests.

Author details

[1]Department of Environmental Immunology, Helmholtz Centre for Environmental Research (UFZ), Leipzig, Germany. [2]Department of Dermatology, Venerology and Allergology, Leipzig University Medical Center, Leipzig, Germany. [3]Department Molecular Systems Biology, Helmholtz Centre for Environmental Research (UFZ), Leipzig, Germany. [4]Institute of Forensic Medicine, University Hospital Jena, Jena, Germany. [5]Core Unit for Molecular Tumor Diagnostics (CMTD), National Center for Tumor Diseases (NCT) Dresden, 01307 Dresden, Germany. [6]German Cancer Consortium (DKTK), Dresden, Germany. [7]German Cancer Research Center (DKFZ), 69120 Heidelberg, Germany. [8]German Cancer Research Center (DKFZ), Division of Theoretical Bioinformatics, Heidelberg, Germany. [9]German Cancer Research Center (DKFZ), Genomics and Proteomics Core Facility, Heidelberg, Germany. [10]Medical Faculty, Rudolf-Schönheimer-Institute of Biochemistry, University of Leipzig, Leipzig, Germany. [11]Children's Hospital, Municipal Hospital "St. Georg", Leipzig, Germany. [12]LIFE-Leipzig Research Centre for Civilization Diseases, University of Leipzig, Leipzig, Germany. [13]Hospital for Children and Adolescents-Centre for Pediatric Research, University of Leipzig, Leipzig, Germany. [14]Faculty of Biosciences, Pharmacy and Psychology, Institute of Biochemistry, University of Leipzig, Leipzig, Germany. [15]Institute of Agriculture and Nutritional Sciences, Martin Luther University Halle-Wittenberg, Halle (Saale), Germany. [16]Competence Cluster for Nutrition and Cardiovascular Health (nutriCARD), Halle-Jena Leipzig, Germany. [17]German Cancer Research Center (DKFZ), Heidelberg Center for Personalized Oncology, DKFZ-HIPO, Heidelberg, Germany. [18]Berlin Institute of Health and Charité-Universitätsmedizin Berlin, Center for Digital Health, Berlin, Germany. [19]Health Data Science Unit, Heidelberg University Hospital, Heidelberg, Germany. [20]Unit for Molecular Epidemiology, Berlin Institute of Health (BIH) and Charitè - Universitätsmedizin Berlin, Berlin, Germany.

References

1. Prusinski L, Al-Hendy A, Yang Q. Developmental exposure to endocrine disrupting chemicals alters the epigenome: identification of reprogrammed targets. Gynecol Obstet Res. 2016;3(1):1–6.
2. Gore AC, Heindel JJ, Zoeller RT. Endocrine disruption for endocrinologists (and others). Endocrinology. 2006;147(6 Suppl):S1–3.
3. Vandenberg LN, Hauser R, Marcus M, Olea N, Welshons WV. Human exposure to bisphenol A (BPA). Reprod Toxicol. 2007;24(2):139–77.
4. Calafat AM, Ye XY, Wong LY, Reidy JA, Needham LL. Exposure of the US population to bisphenol a and 4-tertiary-octylphenol: 2003-2004. Environ Health Perspect. 2008;116(1):39–44.
5. Janesick A, Blumberg B. Obesogens, stem cells and the developmental programming of obesity. Int J Androl. 2012;35(3):437–48.
6. Ross MG, Desai M. Developmental programming of offspring obesity, adipogenesis, and appetite. Clin Obstet Gynecol. 2013;56(3):529–36.
7. Volkel W, Colnot T, Csanady GA, Filser JG, Dekant W. Metabolism and kinetics of bisphenol a in humans at low doses following oral administration. Chem Res Toxicol. 2002;15(10):1281–7.
8. Oppeneer SJ, Robien K. Bisphenol a exposure and associations with obesity among adults: a critical review. Public Health Nutr. 2015;18(10):1847–63.
9. Inoue H, Tsuruta A, Kudo S, Ishii T, Fukushima Y, Iwano H, Yokota H, Kato S. Bisphenol a glucuronidation and excretion in liver of pregnant and nonpregnant female rats. Drug Metab Dispos. 2005;33(1):55–9.
10. Strassburg CP, Strassburg A, Kneip S, Barut A, Tukey RH, Rodeck B, Manns MP. Developmental aspects of human hepatic drug glucuronidation in young children and adults. Gut. 2002;50(2):259–65.
11. Burchell B, Coughtrie M, Jackson M, Harding D, Fournelgigleux S, Leakey J, Hume R. Development of human-liver Udp-glucuronosyltransferases. Dev Pharmacol Ther. 1989;13(2–4):70–7.
12. Pacifici GM, Franchi M, Giuliani L, Rane A. Development of the glucuronyltransferase and sulphotransferase towards 2-naphthol in human fetus. Dev Pharmacol Ther. 1989;14(2):108–14.
13. Valvi D, Casas M, Mendez M, Ballesteros-Gomez A, Luque N, Rubio S, Sunyer J, Vrijheid M. Prenatal bisphenol a urine concentrations and early rapid growth and overweight risk in the offspring. Epidemiology. 2013;24(6):791–9.
14. Braun JM, Lanphear BP, Calafat AM, Deria S, Khoury J, Howe CJ, Venners SA. Early-life bisphenol a exposure and child body mass index: a prospective cohort study. Environ Health Perspect. 2014;122(11):1239–45.
15. Harley KG, Aguilar Schall R, Chevrier J, Tyler K, Aguirre H, Bradman A, Holland N, Lustig R, Calafat AM, Eskenazi B. Prenatal and postnatal bisphenol a exposure and body mass index in childhood in the CHAMACOS cohort. Environ Health Perspect. 2013;121(4):514–20.
16. Weinhouse C, Sartor MA, Faulk C, Anderson OS, Sant KE, Harris C, Dolinoy DC. Epigenome-wide DNA methylation analysis implicates neuronal and inflammatory signaling pathways in adult murine hepatic tumorigenesis following perinatal exposure to bisphenol a. Environ Mol Mutagen. 2016;57(6):435–46.
17. Cheong A, Zhang X, Cheung YY, Tang WY, Chen J, Ye SH, Medvedovic M, Leung YK, Prins GS, Ho SM. DNA methylome changes by estradiol benzoate and bisphenol a links early-life environmental exposures to prostate cancer risk. Epigenetics. 2016;11(9):674–89.
18. Faulk C, Kim JH, Anderson OS, Nahar MS, Jones TR, Sartor MA, Dolinoy DC. Detection of differential DNA methylation in repetitive DNA of mice and humans perinatally exposed to bisphenol a. Epigenetics. 2016;11(7):489–500.
19. Herberth G, Herzog T, Hinz D, Roder S, Schilde M, Sack U, Diez U, Borte M, Lehmann I. Renovation activities during pregnancy induce a Th2 shift in fetal but not in maternal immune system. Int J Hyg Environ Health. 2013;216(3):309–16.
20. Weisse K, Winkler S, Hirche F, Herberth G, Hinz D, Bauer M, Roder S, Rolle-Kampczyk U, von Bergen M, Olek S, et al. Maternal and newborn vitamin D status and its impact on food allergy development in the German LINA cohort study. Allergy. 2013;68(2):220–8.
21. Hinz D, Simon JC, Maier-Simon C, Milkova L, Roder S, Sack U, Borte M, Lehmann I, Herberth G. Reduced maternal regulatory T cell numbers and increased T helper type 2 cytokine production are associated with elevated levels of immunoglobulin E in cord blood. Clin Exp Allergy. 2010;40(3):419–26.
22. de Onis M, Martorell R, Garza C, Lartey A, Reference WMG. WHO child growth standards based on length/height, weight and age. Acta Paediatr. 2006;95:76–85.
23. Feltens R, Roeder S, Otto W, Borte M, Lehmann I. Evaluation of population and individual variances of urinary phthalate metabolites in terms of epidemiological studies. J Chromatogr Sep Tech. 2015;6(6):290.
24. Remane D, Grunwald S, Hoeke H, Mueller A, Roeder S, von Bergen M, Wissenbach DK. Validation of a multi-analyte HPLC-DAD method for determination of uric acid, creatinine, homovanillic acid, niacinamide, hippuric acid, indole-3-acetic acid and 2-methylhippuric acid in human urine. J Chromatogr B. 2015;998:40–4.
25. Aryee MJ, Jaffe AE, Corrada-Bravo H, Ladd-Acosta C, Feinberg AP, Hansen KD, Irizarry RA. Minfi: a flexible and comprehensive bioconductor package for the analysis of Infinium DNA methylation microarrays. Bioinformatics. 2014;30(10):1363–9.
26. Du P, Zhang X, Huang CC, Jafari N, Kibbe WA, Hou L, Lin SM. Comparison of beta-value and M-value methods for quantifying methylation levels by microarray analysis. BMC Bioinf. 2010;11:587.
27. Gervin K, Page CM, Aass HC, Jansen MA, Fjeldstad HE, Andreassen BK, Duijts L, van Meurs JB, van Zelm MC, Jaddoe VW, et al. Cell type specific DNA methylation in cord blood: a 450K-reference data set and cell count-based validation of estimated cell type composition. Epigenetics. 2016;11(9):690–8.
28. Gervin K, Hansen KD. FlowSorted.CordBloodNorway.450k: Illumina HumanMethylation data on sorted cord blood cell populations. R package version 1.4.0. 2017. https://bitbucket.com/kasperdanielhansen/Illumina_CordBlood.

29. Junge KM, Bauer T, Geissler S, Hirche F, Thurmann L, Bauer M, Trump S, Bieg M, Weichenhan D, Gu L, et al. Increased vitamin D levels at birth and in early infancy increase offspring allergy risk-evidence for involvement of epigenetic mechanisms. J Allergy Clin Immunol. 2016;137(2):610–3.

30. Bauer M, Fink B, Thurmann L, Eszlinger M, Herberth G, Lehmann I. Tobacco smoking differently influences cell types of the innate and adaptive immune system-indications from CpG site methylation. Clin Epigenetics. 2016;7:83.

31. Bauer T, Trump S, Ishaque N, Thurmann L, Gu L, Bauer M, Bieg M, Gu Z, Weichenhan D, Mallm JP, et al. Environment-induced epigenetic reprogramming in genomic regulatory elements in smoking mothers and their children. Mol Syst Biol. 2016;12(3):861.

32. Trump S, Bieg M, Gu Z, Thürmann L, Bauer T, Bauer M, Ishaque N, Röder S, Gu L, Herberth G, Lawerenz C, Borte M, Schlesner M, Plass C, Diessl N, Eszlinger M, Mücke O, Elvers HD, Wissenbach DK, von Bergen M, Herrmann C, Weichenhan D, Wright RJ, Lehmann I, Eils R. Prenatal maternal stress and wheeze in children: novel insights into epigenetic regulation. Sci Rep. 2016; 6:28616.

33. Du P, Zhang XA, Huang CC, Jafari N, Kibbe WA, Hou LF, Lin SM. Comparison of Beta-value and M-value methods for quantifying methylation levels by microarray analysis. BMC Bioinf. 2010;11.

34. Hayes AF: Introduction to mediation, moderation, and conditional process analysis: a regression-based approach. 2013.

35. Rodriguez-Gabin AG, Almazan G, Larocca JN. Vesicle transport in oligodendrocytes: probable role of Rab40c protein. J Neurosci Res. 2004;76(6):758–70.

36. Li Y, Jia Q, Wang Y, Li F, Jia Z, Wan Y. Rab40b upregulation correlates with the prognosis of gastric cancer by promoting migration, invasion, and metastasis. Med Oncol (Northwood, London England). 2015;32(4):126.

37. Takahashi M, Kamei Y, Ezaki O. Mest/Peg1 imprinted gene enlarges adipocytes and is a marker of adipocyte size. Am J Physiol Endocrinol Metab. 2005;288(1):E117–24.

38. Kamei Y, Suganami T, Kohda T, Ishino F, Yasuda K, Miura S, Ezaki O, Ogawa Y. Peg1/Mest in obese adipose tissue is expressed from the paternal allele in an isoform-specific manner. FEBS Lett. 2007;581(1):91–6.

39. Soubry A, Murphy SK, Wang F, Huang Z, Vidal AC, Fuemmeler BF, Kurtzberg J, Murtha A, Jirtle RL, Schildkraut JM, et al. Newborns of obese parents have altered DNA methylation patterns at imprinted genes. Int J Obes. 2015;39(4): 650–7.

40. Karbiener M, Glantschnig C, Pisani DF, Laurencikiene J, Dahlman I, Herzig S, Amri EZ, Scheideler M. Mesoderm-specific transcript (MEST) is a negative regulator of human adipocyte differentiation. Int J Obes (Lond). 2015;39(12): 1733–41.

41. Kadeta Y, Kawakami T, Suzuki S, Sato M. Involvment of Mesoderm-specific Transcript in Cell Growth of 3T3-L1 Preadipocytes. J Health Sci. 2009;55(5): 814-9.

42. Nikonova L, Koza RA, Mendoza T, Chao PM, Curley JP, Kozak LP. Mesoderm-specific transcript is associated with fat mass expansion in response to a positive energy balance. FASEB J. 2008;22(11):3925–37.

43. Koza RA, Nikonova L, Hogan J, Rim JS, Mendoza T, Faulk C, Skaf J, Kozak LP. Changes in gene expression foreshadow diet-induced obesity in genetically identical mice. PLoS Genet. 2006;2(5):e81.

44. Voigt A, Agnew K, van Schothorst EM, Keijer J, Klaus S. Short-term, high fat feeding-induced changes in white adipose tissue gene expression are highly predictive for long-term changes. Mol Nutr Food Res. 2013;57(8): 1423–34.

45. Jura M, Jaroslawska J, Chu DT, Kozak LP. Mest and Sfrp5 are biomarkers for healthy adipose tissue. Biochimie. 2016;124:124–33.

46. Trapphoff T, Heiligentag M, El Hajj N, Haaf T, Eichenlaub-Ritter U. Chronic exposure to a low concentration of bisphenol a during follicle culture affects the epigenetic status of germinal vesicles and metaphase II oocytes. Fertil Steril. 2013;100(6):1758-+.

47. Kaneda M, Okano M, Hata K, Sado T, Tsujimoto N, Li E, Sasaki H. Essential role for de novo DNA methyltransferase Dnmt3a in paternal and maternal imprinting. Nature. 2004;429(6994):900–3.

48. El Hajj N, Pliushch G, Schneider E, Dittrich M, Muller T, Korenkov M, Aretz M, Zechner U, Lehnen H, Haaf T. Metabolic programming of MEST DNA methylation by intrauterine exposure to gestational diabetes mellitus. Diabetes. 2013;62(4):1320–8.

49. Carless MA, Kulkarni H, Kos MZ, Charlesworth J, Peralta JM, Goring HH, Curran JE, Almasy L, Dyer TD, Comuzzie AG, et al. Genetic effects on DNA methylation and its potential relevance for obesity in Mexican Americans. PLoS One. 2013;8(9):e73950.

50. Teeguarden J, Hanson-Drury S, Fisher JW, Doerge DR. Are typical human serum BPA concentrations measurable and sufficient to be estrogenic in the general population? Food Chem Toxicol. 2013;62:949–63.

51. Teeguarden JG, Hanson-Drury S. A systematic review of bisphenol a "low dose" studies in the context of human exposure: a case for establishing standards for reporting "low-dose" effects of chemicals. Food Chem Toxicol. 2013;62:935–48.

12

Self-reported prenatal tobacco smoke exposure, *AXL* gene-body methylation, and childhood asthma phenotypes

Lu Gao[1], Xiaochen Liu[1], Joshua Millstein[1], Kimberly D. Siegmund[1], Louis Dubeau[1], Rachel L. Maguire[2], Junfeng (Jim) Zhang[3], Bernard F. Fuemmeler[4], Scott H. Kollins[5], Cathrine Hoyo[2], Susan K. Murphy[6] and Carrie V. Breton[1*]

Abstract

Background: Epigenetic modifications, including DNA methylation, act as one potential mechanism underlying the detrimental effects associated with prenatal tobacco smoke (PTS) exposure. Methylation in a gene called *AXL* was previously reported to differ in response to PTS.

Methods: We investigated the association between PTS and epigenetic changes in *AXL* and how this was related to childhood asthma phenotypes. We tested the association between PTS and DNA methylation at multiple CpG loci of *AXL* at birth using Pyrosequencing in two separate study populations, the Children's Health Study (CHS, n = 799) and the Newborn Epigenetic Study (NEST, n = 592). Plasma cotinine concentration was used to validate findings with self-reported smoking status. The inter-relationships among *AXL* mRNA and miR-199a1 expression, PTS, and *AXL* methylation were examined. Lastly, we evaluated the joint effects of *AXL* methylation and PTS on the risk of asthma and related symptoms at age 10 years old.

Results: PTS was associated with higher methylation level in the *AXL* gene body in both CHS and NEST subjects. In the pooled analysis, exposed subjects had a 0.51% higher methylation level in this region compared to unexposed subjects (95% CI 0.29, 0.74; $p < 0.0001$). PTS was also associated with 21.2% lower expression of miR-199a1 (95% CI $-37.9, -0.1$; $p = 0.05$), a microRNA known to regulate *AXL* expression. Furthermore, the combination of higher *AXL* methylation and PTS exposure at birth increased the risk of recent episodes of bronchitic symptoms in childhood.

Conclusions: PTS was associated with methylation level of *AXL* and the combination altered the risk of childhood bronchitic symptoms.

Keywords: Methylation, Epigenetics, Smoke

Background

Tobacco smoking during pregnancy has been linked to several perinatal complications and child health problems [1]. Previous studies have associated prenatal tobacco smoke (PTS) exposure with low birth weight [2], preterm delivery [3], increased asthmatic symptoms, and reduced pulmonary function in childhood [4, 5], as well as cancer in adult life [6]. One hypothesized mechanism for the adverse health effects of PTS on offspring is through epigenetic modifications such as DNA methylation and microRNA expression [7–9]. Alterations in the epigenome established in utero may last across the child's life course to affect disease phenotypes much later and may influence gene expression at various developmental stages. A deeper understanding of the complexities underlying epigenetic responses to PTS, and how these epigenetic changes may affect the health and behavior of offspring, is still lacking.

We previously reported that DNA methylation in the promoter region of *AXL*, a receptor tyrosine kinase of

* Correspondence: breton@usc.edu
[1]Department of Preventive Medicine, USC Keck School of Medicine, 2001 N. Soto Street, Los Angeles, CA 90032, USA
Full list of author information is available at the end of the article

the TAM (*TYRO3*, *AXL*, and *MERTK*) family, was susceptible to maternal smoking during pregnancy [10, 11]. *AXL* was originally discovered in cancer cells and has been shown to regulate various functions including cell survival and growth, clearance of apoptotic cells, and natural killer cell differentiation [12–14]. More recently, studies have shown that *AXL* and its major ligand growth-arrest-specific 6 (*GAS6*) also play an anti-inflammation role by limiting the production of Toll-like receptor (TLR)-induced proinflammatory cytokines [15]. Childhood asthma is the most common chronic disease among children and largely involves airway inflammation [16, 17]. *GAS6* showed higher expression in subjects with severe asthma during exacerbation [18]. However, few studies have addressed the epigenetic regulation of *AXL* in the pathogenesis of childhood asthma [19]. The role that PTS may play in modifying these processes is similarly unknown.

Our previous research in the Children's Health Study (CHS) demonstrated that PTS exposure was associated with increased *AXL* DNA methylation in childhood of one CpG locus located in an Sp1/Sp3 transcription factor binding region, at which the methylation level was reported to correlate with gene expression of *AXL* [10, 20]. In addition to regulation by CpG methylation in its promoter directly, *AXL* expression is also negatively regulated by microRNA 199a1 (miR-199a1) [21]. Based on the above evidence, we sought to investigate the effects of PTS exposure on *AXL* methylation, mRNA expression, and miR-199a1 expression in the offspring earlier in life, at the time of birth. We further hypothesized that *AXL* methylation would be associated with later childhood asthma and related symptoms through innate immune pathways involved in the pathogenesis of asthma.

In this study, we first tested the association between PTS exposure and DNA methylation at multiple CpG loci across the regulatory regions of *AXL* using Pyrosequencing in two separate study populations, the Children's Health Study (CHS) [22] and the Newborn Epigenetic Study (NEST) [23]. In NEST, plasma cotinine concentration was also used to validate our findings using self-reported PTS. We then evaluated the inter-relationships among *AXL* mRNA and miR-199a1 expression, PTS exposure, and *AXL* CpG methylation. Lastly, for functional follow-up of our findings, we evaluated the joint effects of *AXL* methylation and PTS exposure by testing their interaction on the risk of asthma and related symptoms at the age of 10 years in the CHS.

Methods
Study population
This study was primarily conducted in subsets of participants of the Children's Health Study (CHS), a longitudinal study of respiratory health of children in southern California [22, 24–26]. Any subjects with reported chest surgery, chest injury, or cystic fibrosis were excluded from the study population. Based on our ability to link CHS subjects with California birth records and to obtain a newborn bloodspot, a subset of 799 children was selected for an epigenetic study in which DNA methylation at multiple CpG loci on *AXL* was assessed using Pyrosequencing. The sample selected was enriched with subjects exposed to PTS.

Participant's health, personal, parental, socio-demographic characteristics, and medical history were obtained from parent-completed questionnaires at study enrollment and were updated annually throughout the study. Children were considered to have a history of asthma if there was a yes answer the question "Has a doctor ever diagnosed this child as having asthma?" History of wheezing was defined by a yes answer to the question "Has your child's chest ever sounded wheezy or whistling?" and the same question was asked to evaluate wheezing in the previous 12 months. Bronchitic symptoms during the previous 12 months was defined based on the parent's report of a daily cough for 3 months in a row, congestion or phlegm other than when accompanied by a cold or bronchitis.

A subset of 592 Newborn Epigenetic Study (NEST) subjects was also evaluated for the association between PTS exposure and *AXL* methylation. NEST is a prospective study of women and their children [23]. It was designed to identify exposures during pregnancy and early life associated with stable epigenetic alterations in infants that may alter chronic disease susceptibility later in life. Women were recruited from prenatal clinics serving Duke University Hospital and Durham Regional Hospital Obstetrics facilities in Durham, North Carolina and were eligible if they were aged 18 years and older, pregnant, and spoke English or Spanish. Participating women were either consented and interviewed in-person or were given the questionnaire to self-administer and mail back to the study office. Smokers were preferentially enrolled to the extent possible, identified through medical records. The NEST subjects are still under active follow-up and are too young to be assessed for asthma and related symptoms in childhood.

Prenatal tobacco smoke exposure assessment
In CHS participants, a child was considered to be exposed to PTS if the parent completing the questionnaire answered yes to the question "Did this child's biologic mother smoke while she was pregnant with this child?" and unexposed if the answer was no. NEST participants were considered to be exposed to PTS if the mother reported having ever smoked 100 cigarettes or more in her lifetime and smoking at any time during the pregnancy. NEST subjects were classified as unexposed if the mother reported never having smoked 100 cigarettes or

more in her lifetime, or if the mother reported currently not smoking and not smoking anytime in the year before she knew she was pregnant.

Cotinine collection and assay procedures in NEST

Maternal tobacco smoking in NEST was also evaluated by measuring cotinine concentration in maternal plasma samples taken during pregnancy at the time of initial recruitment into the study. Plasma blood samples were collected from women during pregnancy. Assays were completed at the Exposure Biology and Chemistry Lab at Duke University. Cotinine was measured using a high-performance liquid chromatography with tandem mass spectrometric detection (HPLC-MS-MS) method, a highly sensitive assay designed to measure levels of environmental smoke exposure with a limit of detection of 0.05 ng/ml [27–29] and a reproducibility > 94% [27–29]. Details of cotinine assay procedures were described elsewhere [30].

DNA methylation

For CHS subjects, DNA methylation was measured in newborn bloodspots (NBS) that were obtained as part of the routine California Newborn Screening Program from the California Department of Public Health Genetic Disease Screening Program. The NBS were stored by the state of California at − 20 °C. A single complete newborn bloodspot for each requested participant was mailed to us and then stored in our lab at − 80 °C upon receipt. DNA was extracted from whole blood cells using the QiaAmp DNA blood kit (Qiagen Inc., Valencia, CA) and stored at − 80 °C. For NEST subjects, genomic DNA from buffy coat specimens was extracted from umbilical cord blood using Puregene Reagents (Qiagen, Valencia, CA). Laboratory personnel performed DNA methylation analysis by Pyrosequencing (PSQ) [31] and were blinded to study subject information.

Six regions across *AXL* were selected for PSQ, each containing one to three CpGs (Fig. 1). PCR primers were designed by EpigenDx Inc. (http://www.epigendx.com) to cover the loci of interest and the specificity of the primer sequences was confirmed using in silico PCR. Five hundred nanograms of genomic DNA extracted from NEST and CHS samples (randomized together) was bisulfite treated using the EZ DNA Methylation Kit™ (Zymo Research, Irvine, CA, USA) and was purified according to the manufacturer's protocol. Methylation assays (assays ADS6525-FS, ADS8094-FS2, ADS6528-FS, ADS8097-FS, and ADS6570-FS) were performed by EpigenDx Inc. using the PSQ96HS system (Pyrosequencing, Qiagen) according to standard procedures as described in previous work [32, 33]. Two percent of the samples were measured in duplicate to evaluate reproducibility. The methylation level was determined using QCpG software (Pyrosequencing, Qiagen) and was reported as percent of DNA methylation at each CpG locus. Each experiment included cytosines not part of a CpG dinucleotide as internal controls to evaluate incomplete bisulfite conversion of the input DNA. A series of unmethylated and methylated DNA samples were included as controls in each assay. Furthermore, PCR bias testing was performed by mixing unmethylated control DNA with in vitro methylated DNA at different ratios (0, 5, 10, 25, 50, 75, and 100%), followed by bisulfite modification, PCR, and Pyrosequencing analysis. Standard curves for pre-specified ratios against the measured methylation levels were then produced for each assay to check PCR bias and were shown in Additional file 1: Figure S1.

miRNA and mRNA expression in NEST

All measurements of miR-199a1 and *AXL* mRNA expression were conducted in duplicate in cord blood samples from 235 participants in the NEST cohort. Total

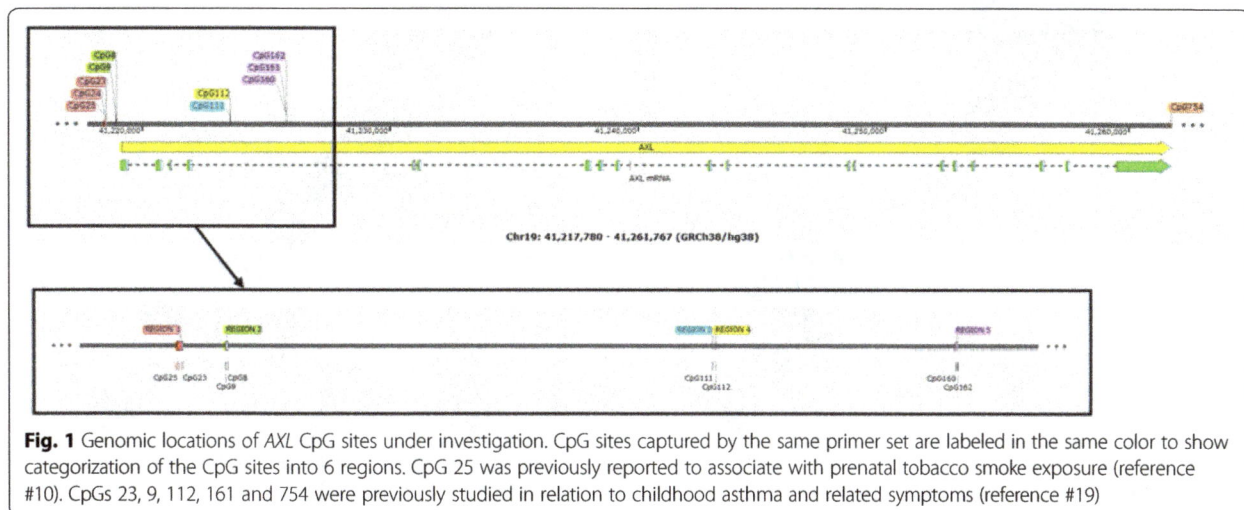

Fig. 1 Genomic locations of *AXL* CpG sites under investigation. CpG sites captured by the same primer set are labeled in the same color to show categorization of the CpG sites into 6 regions. CpG 25 was previously reported to associate with prenatal tobacco smoke exposure (reference #10). CpGs 23, 9, 112, 161 and 754 were previously studied in relation to childhood asthma and related symptoms (reference #19)

mRNA was isolated from stored PAXgene tubes of cord blood using the PAXgene blood miRNA isolation kit (Qiagen, Valencia, CA). Expression of miR-199a1 was quantified using Origene's qStar miRNA detection system (Origene, Rockville, MD) with qStar primer pairs specifically designed for the target (miR-199a1 transcript #HP300226) and its corresponding copy number standard (#HK300226). Plasmid DNA containing a cloned fragment of the target gene was used as the qPCR copy number standard. By utilizing this qPCR standard for the miRNA and employing the standard curve qPCR method, we calculated the absolute copy number of miR-199a1 in each sample. To evaluate reproducibility, 10% repeats were included. Additional details of mRNA expression measurements are described in the Additional file 1: Supplemental methods.

Statistical methods

We first conducted descriptive analyses to examine the distribution of CpG methylation, miR-199a1 and *AXL* mRNA expression, and the population characteristics of both CHS and NEST study participants.

Spearman correlations between methylation levels at CpG sites under investigation were evaluated (Fig. 2). Except for CpG 111 and CpG 112, the methylation levels at CpG sites captured by the same primer set were generally highly correlated, so we averaged their methylation values. In total, six regions across *AXL* were defined (Fig. 1): region 1 was the average of CpG 23-25; region 2 was CpG 8-9; region 3 was CpG 111; region 4 was CpG 112; region 5 was CpG 160-162; and region 6 was CpG 754.

To estimate the main effects of PTS exposure on *AXL* methylation, we first fitted linear regression models using the dichotomized PTS from self-reported questionnaire as described above, and adjusted for child's sex, ethnicity (of child in CHS and of mother in NEST), gestational age, maternal age at delivery, and parental education level. Separate analyses for CHS and NEST were conducted first. Then, a pooled analysis was also conducted, but only included Hispanic, non-Hispanic white, and black subjects due to the different ethnic distribution of these two populations, leaving 1294 subjects for analysis (725 CHS subjects and 569 NEST subjects). All potential covariates were chosen for inclusion based on a priori hypotheses. DNA methylation plate number, parity, and *AXL* genetic polymorphisms did not change the effect estimates by more than 10% and were removed from final models.

In addition to main effects of PTS, we also stratified the analyses by child's sex and ethnicity and tested for interaction by adding the corresponding interaction terms into the models described above. Additionally, to evaluate the association between maternal plasma cotinine concentration and *AXL* methylation in the NEST population, we first categorized cotinine level as non-smoker (0–1 ng/ml), passive smoker (1–10 ng/ml), and active smoker (> 10 ng/ml), and fitted linear regression models with *AXL* methylation [34, 35]. To further explore the nonlinearity of this relationship, we also fitted a linear regression model of log10-transformed cotinine and *AXL* methylation with the two-component linear piecewise spline with a break at 10 ng/ml peak exposure:

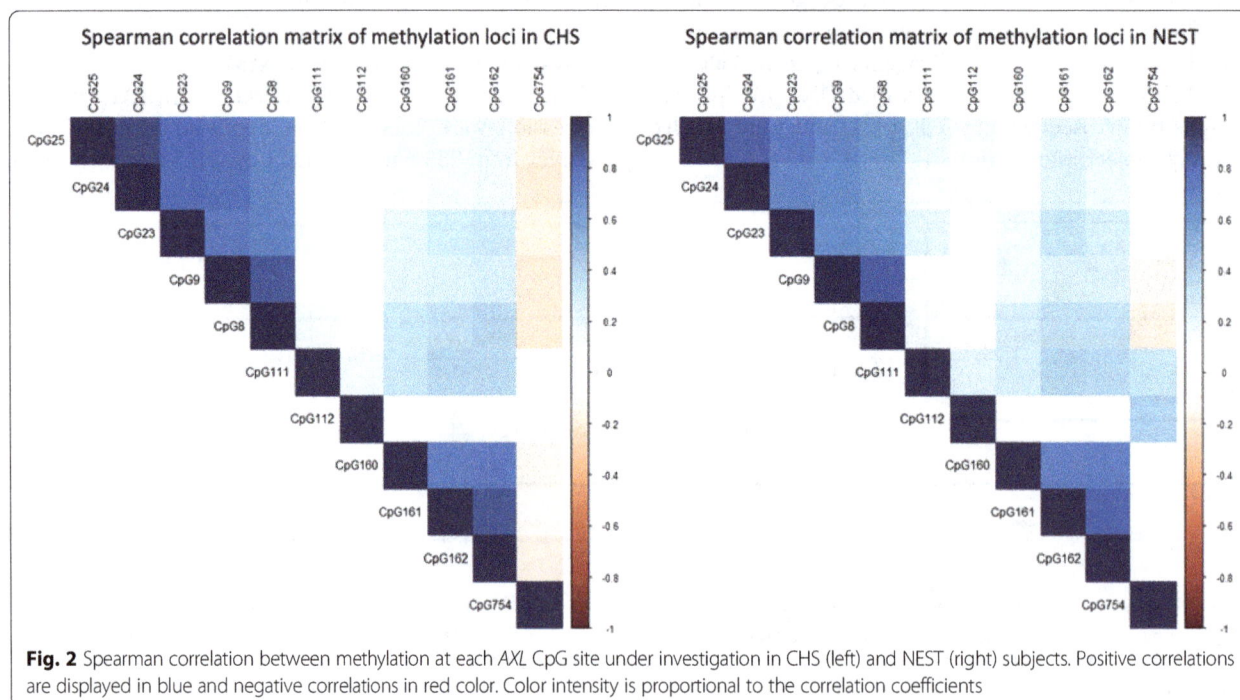

Fig. 2 Spearman correlation between methylation at each *AXL* CpG site under investigation in CHS (left) and NEST (right) subjects. Positive correlations are displayed in blue and negative correlations in red color. Color intensity is proportional to the correlation coefficients

$$\text{Methylation} = \alpha + \beta_1 \times \text{cotinine} + \beta_2$$
$$\times (\text{cotinine}-10)^+ + \text{covariates} + \varepsilon.$$

where $(\text{cotinine} - 10)^+$ takes on a value of 0 when cotinine level is smaller than 10 ng/ml. These models were adjusted for the same covariates as in models using self-reported PTS as well as maternal BMI during pregnancy.

We also evaluated the association between PTS and the expression levels of *AXL* mRNA and miR-199a1 in the NEST population by fitting individual linear regression models. The models were adjusted for child's sex, maternal ethnicity, gestational age, maternal age at delivery, maternal education level, maternal BMI during pregnancy, and miR-199a1 assay number (for miR-199a1 models). Similar models were fitted to assess the association between *AXL* methylation and the expression of *AXL* mRNA and miR-199a1.

Lastly, to evaluate the joint effects of *AXL* methylation and maternal smoking on childhood asthma and related symptoms at age 10 years in CHS subjects, we fitted logistic regression models. An interaction term between methylation and PTS was included, adjusted for child's sex, ethnicity, and city of residence at study entry. Wald tests were used to compute interaction p values.

Statistical analyses were performed using SAS (Statistical Analysis System) version 9.4 (SAS Institute, Cary, NC) and R version 3.3.1 software.

Results

The population characteristics of the CHS and NEST study subjects are described in Table 1. Children's sex was evenly distributed in both populations, while the distribution of ethnicity differed between the two by design. Of the 799 CHS participants, 39% of them were Hispanic white, 49% were non-Hispanic white, and 12% were a mixture of Asian, black, and others; whereas in the 592 NEST participants, there were a much higher proportion of subjects born to black mothers (51%). Both studies were enriched for participants exposed to PTS, and a higher proportion of exposed subjects were observed in NEST (51%) than CHS (27%). With the

Table 1 Demographic characteristics of CHS and NEST subjects

	CHS (N = 799)	NEST (N = 592)	Pooled analysis (N = 1294)[a]
	n (%)	n (%)	n (%)
Sex			
Male	366 (45.8%)	311 (52.5%)	632 (48.8%)
Female	433 (54.2%)	281 (47.5%)	662 (51.2%)
Ethnicity[b]			
Asian	29 (3.6%)	–	–
Black	23 (2.9%)	299 (50.5%)	322 (24.9%)
Hispanic	308 (38.6%)	58 (9.8%)	366 (28.3%)
Non-Hispanic white	394 (49.3%)	212 (35.8%)	606 (46.8%)
Other	45 (5.6%)	23 (3.9%)	–
Highest parental education level[c]			
Less than 12th grade	102 (12.8%)	126 (21.3%)	222 (17.2%)
Completed grade 12	153 (19.2%)	162 (27.4%)	298 (23.0%)
Some college or tech school	352 (44.1%)	159 (26.9%)	483 (37.3%)
Completed 4 years of college or higher	175 (21.9%)	142 (24.0%)	208 (16.1%)
Maternal smoking during pregnancy	217 (27.2%)	303 (51.2%)	500 (38.6%)
Ever MD-diagnosed asthma[d]	141 (17.7%)	–	–
Ever wheezing[d]	284 (35.5%)	–	–
Wheezing in the previous 12 months[d]	145 (18.2%)	–	–
Bronchitic symptoms in the previous 12 months[d]	118 (14.8%)	–	–
Gestational age (weeks), mean ± SD	39.6 ± 2.0	38.6 ± 2.2	39.2 ± 2.1
Maternal age at delivery (years), mean ± SD	27.8 ± 5.9	27.7 ± 5.8	27.7 ± 5.8

Percent number do not always add up to 100% due to missing data
[a]Pooled analysis only included black, Hispanic and non-Hispanic white subjects
[b]Ethnicity of child in CHS and of mother in NEST
[c]Highest education level of either parent in CHS and of mother in NEST
[d]Assessed at mean age 9.96 years (SD 0.37)

current sample, 18% of CHS subjects had a history of physician-diagnosed asthma by age 10 years, and more subjects had experienced wheezing symptoms. Less than 20% of CHS subjects had wheezing or bronchitic symptoms in the previous 12 months.

The distribution of *AXL* methylation in each region under investigation was similar across NEST and CHS subjects (Additional file 1: Table S1). Region 4 was highly methylated with a mean value of 84% (SD = 3.1%) in CHS, and 83% (SD = 5.3%) in NEST. Regions 1, 3, and 6 were moderately methylated with mean values ranging from 37 to 58%. CpG loci in regions 2 and 5 were mostly unmethylated, with mean values ranging from 4 to 13%. miR-199a1 expression level was heavily right-skewed with a median of 184,098 copies/µg RNA (IQR = 258,974 copies/µg RNA) (Additional file 1: Table S1). mRNA expression in cord blood was relatively low and right-skewed (median = 3503 copies/µg cDNA, IQR = 1965 copies/µg cDNA). Cotinine values were also right-skewed, with a median of 1.0 ng/ml (IQR = 28 ng/ml).

Main effects of PTS

We evaluated the association between self-reported PTS exposure and *AXL* methylation in both CHS and NEST populations (Table 2). In CHS, methylation level in region 5 at birth was significantly higher in participants exposed to PTS compared to unexposed participants (β = 0.56; 95% CI 0.31, 0.82; p < 0.0001). We found a similar association at this region in NEST (β = 0.35; 95% CI − 0.03, 0.73; p = 0.07) and in the pooled analysis (β = 0.51; 95% CI 0.29, 0.74; p < 0.0001). In addition, participants exposed to PTS had a 0.58% higher methylation in region 3 compared to the unexposed in CHS subjects, but this association was not replicated in NEST. No associations were observed between PTS and methylation in the other regions. Results for the individual CpG sites in each region were also presented in Additional file 1: Table S2 and were quite consistent with the regional averages. We also tested whether these associations varied by child's sex or ethnicity, but found no significant differences (results not shown).

We further evaluated the association between maternal smoking and *AXL* methylation in NEST subjects using plasma cotinine concentration categorized as non-smoker (0–1 ng/ml), passive smoker (1–10 ng/ml), and active smoker (> 10 ng/ml) (Additional file 1: Table S3). Methylation levels in regions 1, 3, 4, and 5 were positively associated with cotinine level, but none of the effect estimates reached statistical significance, possibly due to a small sample size. To further explore the nonlinear dose-response relationship of cotinine and methylation, we used a piecewise linear regression model with a break at 10 ng/ml and found that methylation levels in regions 1 (p = 0.0001), 2 (p = 0.001), and 6 (p = 0.002) were significantly associated with cotinine level (Additional file 1: Figure S3).

Association between miR-199a1 and AXL mRNA with PTS and AXL methylation

We measured the expression of both *AXL* mRNA and miR-199a1, a microRNA known to regulate *AXL* gene expression, and tested their associations with PTS and *AXL* methylation (Additional file 1: Table S4 and Table S5). We found that *AXL* mRNA was expressed at low levels in cord blood, which is consistent with the relatively low expression in whole blood compared to other tissues using data from the Genotype-Tissue expression (GTEx) project (Additional file 1: Figure S3). In our population, *AXL* mRNA was not associated with self-reported PTS, cotinine concentration, or *AXL* methylation, but was marginally and negatively associated with methylation in region 4 (p = 0.07) and miR-199a1 levels (p = 0.10) (Additional file 1: Table S4).

However, miR-199a1 was associated with methylation and PTS. A 1% higher level of methylation in region 4 was significantly associated with a 2.1% increase in miR-199a1 expression level (95% CI 0.7, 3.5; p = 0.05) (Additional file 1: Table S5). Subjects with PTS exposure had a 21.2% lower miR-199a1 expression level compared to unexposed subjects (95% CI − 37.9, − 0.1; p = 0.05). A similar association was observed using plasma cotinine level, for which a 10% increase in cotinine concentration

Table 2 Association between PTS exposure and *AXL* DNA methylation at birth in CHS and NEST subjects (adjusted for child's sex, ethnicity (of child in CHS and of mother in NEST), gestational age, maternal age at delivery, and parental education level)

	CHS (N = 799)		NEST (N = 592)		Pooled analysis (N = 1294)[a]	
	β (95% CI)	P value	β (95% CI)	P value	β (95% CI)	P value
Region 1	− 0.49 (− 1.56, 0.58)	0.37	0.11 (− 1.16, 1.37)	0.87	− 0.30 (− 1.11, 0.51)	0.47
Region 2	0.01 (− 0.57, 0.59)	0.97	0.59 (− 0.23, 1.42)	0.16	0.23 (− 0.25, 0.72)	0.34
Region 3	0.58 (− 0.06, 1.22)	0.08	− 0.22 (− 1.48, 1.04)	0.73	0.24 (− 0.40, 0.88)	0.47
Region 4	− 0.12 (− 0.67, 0.43)	0.67	0.55 (− 0.45, 1.54)	0.28	0.14 (− 0.41, 0.69)	0.61
Region 5	0.56 (0.31, 0.82)	1.72E−05	0.35 (− 0.03, 0.73)	0.07	0.51 (0.29, 0.74)	7.89E−06
Region 6	0.46 (− 0.16, 1.09)	0.14	− 0.53 (− 1.88, 0.81)	0.44	− 0.10 (− 0.78, 0.57)	0.77

Estimates are showing percent changes in methylation
[a]Pooled analysis only included black, Hispanic, and non-Hispanic white subjects

was significantly associated with a 0.8% lower miR-199a1 level (95% CI -1.3, -0.2; $p = 0.01$).

Interaction between PTS and AXL methylation on asthma and related symptoms

Given the previous findings that PTS was associated with increased risk of childhood asthma and related symptoms, and our observed associations between PTS and methylation in *AXL*, we next sought to test whether they might jointly interact to alter susceptibility to childhood asthma and related symptoms (Table 3). The association between methylation in region 5 and the risk of recent bronchitic symptoms at the age of 10 years significantly differed for subjects with and without PTS exposure (p-interaction = 0.01). Higher methylation level in region 5 at birth was associated with higher risk of bronchitic symptoms (OR = 2.26 per 2SD change in methylation; 95% CI 1.09, 4.72; $p = 0.03$) in children who were exposed to PTS, but not in unexposed children (OR = 0.76 per 2SD change in methylation; 95% CI 0.45, 1.29; $p = 0.31$). No significant interaction with PTS was observed for methylation in other regions on the risk of asthma and related symptoms (Table 3 and Additional file 1: Table S6).

Discussion

We assessed the association between maternal smoking during pregnancy, epigenetic regulation of *AXL* and bronchitic symptoms in childhood. Consistent associations between self-reported PTS and higher *AXL* methylation in one region were observed in both CHS and NEST, despite different underlying population characteristics. Both self-reported PTS and plasma cotinine levels were associated with the expression of miR-199a1, a microRNA known to regulate *AXL* expression. Furthermore, we found synergistic effects between PTS and *AXL* methylation at birth on the risk of bronchitic symptoms 10 years later in childhood.

AXL methylation in the gene body (region 5) was significantly associated with self-reported PTS in CHS and the results were replicated in NEST. Results were unaffected by differences in ethnic distributions or by the use of newborn bloodspots versus cord blood in two populations. However, we previously reported PTS was associated with *AXL* methylation level at CpG 25 in region 1 in a separate subset of CHS subjects [10, 11] but could not replicate this association in the current study. Discrepancies between these findings may be due to a number of factors including differences in cell type and timing of exposure. For example, *AXL* methylation was assessed in buccal cells in the previous papers but in newborn bloodspots in this paper; differences may therefore be due to differences in tissue and cell type [36]. More importantly, *AXL* methylation was measured in childhood in previous studies, but was assessed at birth in this paper, which is a more relevant time window with respect to in utero smoke exposure. Given the dynamic and time-specific nature of DNA methylation, the previously observed changes in region 1 may reflect not only exposure from PTS, but also a summary of other postnatal and childhood exposures such as air pollution, diet, exercise, and environmental tobacco smoke exposure.

Because self-reported PTS may introduce measurement error, we also tested the effects of plasma cotinine level, which is currently regarded as the best biomarker of smoke inhalation in active smokers and in non-smokers exposed to environmental tobacco smoke [37]. We explored both the linear (results not shown) and non-linear relationship of maternal plasma cotinine level and *AXL* methylation in each region. The results were supportive of our findings using self-reported PTS, with the same direction of associations for region 5, and might suggest a non-linear dose-response relationship, though power was limited.

In addition to DNA methylation, both PTS and cotinine level were negatively associated with miR-199a1 expression in this study. Given the generally low expression of *AXL* in cord blood, we were not able to convincingly relate PTS to *AXL* mRNA level. Nonetheless, miR-199a1 expression was marginally associated with lower *AXL* mRNA expression, which is consistent with the previously reported role of miR-199a1 to negatively regulate *AXL* expression in cancer

Table 3 Interaction between *AXL* DNA methylation at birth and PTS exposure in relation to risk of bronchitic symptoms at age 10 years in CHS subjects ($N = 799$) (adjusted for child's sex, ethnicity, and city of residence at study entry. Odds ratios are scaled to per 2SD change in methylation)

	Unexposed to PTS		Exposed to PTS		Interaction *P* value
	OR (95% CI)	*P* value	OR (95% CI)	*P* value	
Region 1	0.96 (0.59, 1.57)	0.87	1.52 (0.72, 3.20)	0.28	0.46
Region 2	1.21 (0.75, 1.96)	0.43	1.85 (0.87, 3.96)	0.11	0.53
Region 3	1.10 (0.69, 1.76)	0.68	1.35 (0.64, 2.82)	0.43	0.64
Region 4	0.93 (0.58, 1.47)	0.74	0.85 (0.40, 1.81)	0.67	0.90
Region 5	0.76 (0.45, 1.29)	0.31	2.26 (1.09, 4.72)	0.03	0.01
Region 6	0.91 (0.59, 1.40)	0.67	0.99 (0.46, 2.17)	0.99	0.62

cell lines [21]. Taken together, these findings illustrate the effects of PTS on multiple aspects of *AXL* regulation (Fig. 3), including methylation at multiple loci, microRNA expression, and potentially mRNA expression.

PTS has been associated with impaired growth in fetal brain, lung, and kidney and infant morbidity and mortality [38–40], lifelong decreases in pulmonary function, and increased risk of childhood asthma [41, 42]. Epigenetic programming may be involved in the consequences of PTS on offspring health outcomes. PTS is now clearly linked to alterations in newborn DNA methylation patterns in multiple tissues, which may persist into childhood and even adolescence and are further linked to adverse fetal and childhood health outcomes [9, 43–46]. Given *AXL*'s key role in innate immune inflammation and lung homeostasis pathways [13–15, 47], it stands to reason that a systemic alteration to *AXL* regulation during fetal development by an exposure such as tobacco smoke might negatively impact function of all tissues and cells in which *AXL* has an active role.

We aimed to investigate this hypothesis—of altered *AXL* programming increasing downstream vulnerability—by investigating whether *AXL* methylation at birth was related to childhood respiratory health. To do so, we tested the interaction between PTS and *AXL* methylation on the risk of childhood asthma and related phenotypes. Methylation in region 5, which showed the strongest association with PTS, was associated with increased risk for recent episodes of bronchitic symptoms only in subjects exposed to PTS. No interactions were observed for asthma or wheezing outcomes. Bronchitic symptoms are suggestive of chronic symptoms that may follow an illness or acute exacerbation of asthma, or chronic inflammation in the airway. The observed

synergistic effects of PTS exposure and *AXL* methylation for higher risk of bronchitic symptoms still held after adjusting for asthma status (results not shown). Interaction between smoke exposure and gene methylation has also been reported to alter the risk of other respiratory diseases [48]. Therefore, one would postulate that PTS exposure may enhance the influence of *AXL* methylation on innate immune pathways and further modify the risk of developing inflammatory phenotypes.

The current study has several strengths. The assessment of methylation pattern occurred in a relevant exposure time window. The prenatal period is highly sensitive to environmental factors and particularly susceptible to epigenetic alterations due to rapid cell division and epigenetic remodeling [49]. Thus, alterations in methylation status at birth may serve as a biomarker for direct consequences of environmental toxicants. We also examined the association between PTS and *AXL* DNA methylation in two separate populations of subjects and were able to replicate the significant findings despite differences in population demographics. Additionally, plasma cotinine concentration was used to validate results with self-report of maternal smoking. Lastly, we related DNA methylation levels at birth to childhood respiratory symptoms 10 years later, removing the possibility of reverse causation.

Several limitations should also be noted. First, our observed effect estimates in DNA methylation associated with PTS are small. However, most studies on DNA methylation changes in newborns in relation to maternal smoking during pregnancy, including meta-analysis of several large cohorts, all identified changes with small magnitudes as low as or less than 0.5% [9, 50–52]. A previous study defined the mean methylation change in response to PTS for both hyper- and hypomethylation as 2% [51]. Furthermore, we previously published a review and summarized that most environmental exposure studies have reported changes in DNA methylation from 2 to 10%, highlighting possible reasons for such small effects and the call for focusing on small magnitude alterations [53]. Second, although we evaluated the effects of PTS on multiple aspects of *AXL* epigenetic modifications, we were not able to test the circulating protein level of *AXL* to functionally interpret the changes in epigenetic marks. Future animal studies may elucidate this by measuring *AXL* protein level in relation to smoke exposure and determining whether this correlates with *AXL* methylation and mRNA levels. Third, PTS was only classified as a dichotomous variable in the analysis, raising the possibility that we may miss finer resolutions in exposure assessment, such as trimester-specific smoking effects. We were also unable to test whether the DNA methylation changes observed at birth persisted into childhood, as the CHS does not have childhood blood

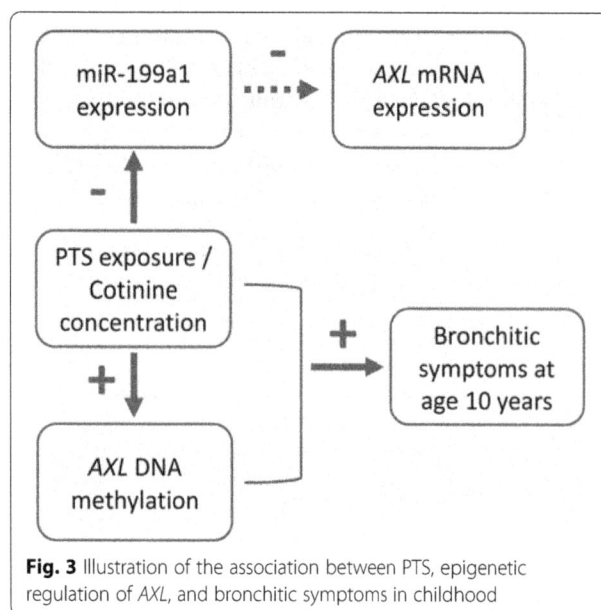

Fig. 3 Illustration of the association between PTS, epigenetic regulation of *AXL*, and bronchitic symptoms in childhood

samples. Besides, asthma and related symptoms in childhood were self-reported in questionnaire and may introduce misclassification bias, however, a previous CHS study has independently verified self-reported physician diagnosed-asthma through a review of medical records and found that the information was highly reliable [54]. Lastly, although we made every effort to control for potential confounders, the possibility of residual confounding by some unknown factors associated with *AXL* DNA methylation levels and PTS cannot be ruled out, for instance, cell type compositions in blood and diet. Future studies may address these issues by inferring cell type compositions from Pyrosequencing methylation data of large numbers of genes.

Conclusions

In conclusion, prenatal tobacco smoke exposure was associated with the regulation of *AXL*, a receptor tyrosine kinase of the TAM family that plays an important role in suppressing Toll-like receptor-induced inflammation. Moreover, *AXL* methylation and tobacco smoke exposure during fetal development may act synergistically to modify the risk of bronchitic symptoms in childhood.

Abbreviations

BMI: Body mass index; CHS: Children's Health Study; CI: Confidence interval; CpG: Cytosine-guanine dinucleotide sites; GTEx: Genotype-Tissue expression; IQR: Interquartile range; miR: Micro RNA; NBS: Newborn bloodspots; NEST: Newborn Epigenetic Study; OR: Odds ratio; PCR: Polymerase chain reaction; PSQ: Pyrosequencing; PTS: Prenatal tobacco smoke; SD: Standard deviation

Acknowledgements

We would like to express our sincere gratitude to Steve Graham and Robin Cooley at the California Biobank Program and Genetic Disease Screening Program within the California Department of Public Health for their assistance and advice regarding newborn bloodspots. The biospecimens and/or data used in this study were obtained from the California Biobank Program, (SIS request number(s) 479)" Section 6555(b), 17 CCR. The California Department of Public Health is not responsible for the results or conclusions drawn by the authors of this publication.

Funding

This research was supported by NIEHS grants 4R01ES022216, K01ES017801, P30ES007048, and P01ES022831, USEPA grant RD-83543701, and NIH grant K24DA023464.

Authors' contributions

CB conceived and designed the study. RM, SKM, and CH aided in the design of the study and provided data for NEST. JZ, BF, and SK provided cotinine measurements in NEST. CB, JM, KS, and LD supervised the project. LG and XL analyzed the data and wrote the manuscript. All authors edited and approved the manuscript.

Author details

[1]Department of Preventive Medicine, USC Keck School of Medicine, 2001 N. Soto Street, Los Angeles, CA 90032, USA. [2]Department of Biological Sciences, Center for Human Health and the Environment, North Carolina State University, Raleigh, NC 27695, USA. [3]Nicholas School of the Environment and Duke Global Health Institute, Duke University, Durham, NC 27701, USA. [4]Department of Health Behavior and Policy, Massey Cancer Center, Virginia Commonwealth University, Richmond, VA 23219, USA. [5]Department of Psychiatry and Behavioral Sciences, Duke University Medical Center, Durham, NC 27705, USA. [6]Division of Reproductive Sciences, Department of Obstetrics and Gynecology, Duke University School of Medicine, Durham, NC 27708, USA.

References

1. Finkelstein JB. Surgeon General's report heralds turning tide against tobacco, smoking. J Natl Cancer Inst. 2006;98:1360–2.
2. Aagaard-Tillery KM, Porter TF, Lane RH, Varner MW, Lacoursiere DY. In utero tobacco exposure is associated with modified effects of maternal factors on fetal growth. Am J Obstet Gynecol. 2008;198(66):e61–6.
3. Shah NR, Bracken MB. A systematic review and meta-analysis of prospective studies on the association between maternal cigarette smoking and preterm delivery. Am J Obstet Gynecol. 2000;182:465–72.
4. Carlsen KH, Lodrup Carlsen KC. Parental smoking and childhood asthma: clinical implications. Treat Respir Med. 2005;4:337–46.
5. Lodrup Carlsen KC, Carlsen KH. Effects of maternal and early tobacco exposure on the development of asthma and airway hyperreactivity. Curr Opin Allergy Clin Immunol. 2001;1:139–43.
6. Doherty SP, Grabowski J, Hoffman C, Ng SP, Zelikoff JT. Early life insult from cigarette smoke may be predictive of chronic diseases later in life. Biomarkers. 2009;14(Suppl 1):97–101.
7. Suter MA, Anders AM, Aagaard KM. Maternal smoking as a model for environmental epigenetic changes affecting birthweight and fetal programming. Mol Hum Reprod. 2013;19:1–6.
8. Maccani MA, Avissar-Whiting M, Banister CE, McGonnigal B, Padbury JF, Marsit CJ. Maternal cigarette smoking during pregnancy is associated with downregulation of miR-16, miR-21, and miR-146a in the placenta. Epigenetics. 2010;5:583–9.
9. Joubert BR, Felix JF, Yousefi P, Bakulski KM, Just AC, Breton C, et al. DNA methylation in newborns and maternal smoking in pregnancy: genome-wide consortium meta-analysis. Am J Hum Genet. 2016;98:680–96.
10. Breton CV, Byun HM, Wenten M, Pan F, Yang A, Gilliland FD. Prenatal tobacco smoke exposure affects global and gene-specific DNA methylation. Am J Respir Crit Care Med. 2009;180:462–7.
11. Breton CV, Salam MT, Gilliland FD. Heritability and role for the environment in DNA methylation in AXL receptor tyrosine kinase. Epigenetics. 2011;6:895–8.
12. Axelrod H, Pienta KJ. Axl as a mediator of cellular growth and survival. Oncotarget. 2014;5:8818–52.
13. Park IK, Giovenzana C, Hughes TL, Yu J, Trotta R, Caligiuri MA. The Axl/Gas6 pathway is required for optimal cytokine signaling during human natural killer cell development. Blood. 2009;113:2470–7.
14. Seitz HM, Camenisch TD, Lemke G, Earp HS, Matsushima GK. Macrophages and dendritic cells use different Axl/Mertk/Tyro3 receptors in clearance of apoptotic cells. J Immunol. 2007;178:5635–42.
15. Rothlin CV, Ghosh S, Zuniga EI, Oldstone MB, Lemke G. TAM receptors are pleiotropic inhibitors of the innate immune response. Cell. 2007;131:1124–36.
16. Moorman JE, Rudd RA, Johnson CA, King M, Minor P, Bailey C, et al. National surveillance for asthma--United States, 1980-2004. MMWR Surveill Summ. 2007;56:1–54.
17. Bousquet J, Jeffery PK, Busse WW, Johnson M, Vignola AM. Asthma. From bronchoconstriction to airways inflammation and remodeling. Am J Respir Crit Care Med. 2000;161:1720–45.
18. Aoki T, Matsumoto Y, Hirata K, Ochiai K, Okada M, Ichikawa K, et al. Expression profiling of genes related to asthma exacerbations. Clin Exp Allergy. 2009;39:213–21.
19. Gao L, Millstein J, Siegmund KD, Dubeau L, Maguire R, Gilliland FD, et al. Epigenetic regulation of AXL and risk of childhood asthma symptoms. Clin Epigenetics. 2017;9:121.

20. Mudduluru G, Allgayer H. The human receptor tyrosine kinase Axl gene—promoter characterization and regulation of constitutive expression by Sp1, Sp3 and CpG methylation. Biosci Rep. 2008;28:161–76.

21. Mudduluru G, Ceppi P, Kumarswamy R, Scagliotti GV, Papotti M, Allgayer H. Regulation of Axl receptor tyrosine kinase expression by miR-34a and miR-199a/b in solid cancer. Oncogene. 2011;30:2888–99.

22. Gauderman WJ, Gilliland GF, Vora H, Avol E, Stram D, McConnell R, et al. Association between air pollution and lung function growth in southern California children: results from a second cohort. Am J Respir Crit Care Med. 2002;166:76–84.

23. Hoyo C, Murtha AP, Schildkraut JM, Forman MR, Calingaert B, Demark-Wahnefried W, et al. Folic acid supplementation before and during pregnancy in the Newborn Epigenetics STudy (NEST). BMC Public Health. 2011;11:46.

24. Peters JM, Avol E, Gauderman WJ, Linn WS, Navidi W, London SJ, et al. A study of twelve Southern California communities with differing levels and types of air pollution. II Effects on pulmonary function. Am J Respir Crit Care Med. 1999;159:768–75.

25. Peters JM, Avol E, Navidi W, London SJ, Gauderman WJ, Lurmann F, et al. A study of twelve Southern California communities with differing levels and types of air pollution. I Prevalence of respiratory morbidity. Am J Respir Crit Care Med. 1999;159:760–7.

26. Berhane K, Chang CC, McConnell R, Gauderman WJ, Avol E, Rapapport E, et al. Association of Changes in air quality with bronchitic symptoms in children in California, 1993-2012. Jama. 2016;315:1491–501.

27. Dempsey DA, Meyers MJ, Oh SS, Nguyen EA, Fuentes-Afflick E, Wu AH, et al. Determination of tobacco smoke exposure by plasma cotinine levels in infants and children attending urban public hospital clinics. Arch Pediatr Adolesc Med. 2012;166:851–6.

28. Bernert JT, Jacob P 3rd, Holiday DB, Benowitz NL, Sosnoff CS, Doig MV, et al. Interlaboratory comparability of serum cotinine measurements at smoker and nonsmoker concentration levels: a round-robin study. Nicotine Tob Res. 2009;11:1458–66.

29. Jacob P 3rd, Yu L, Duan M, Ramos L, Yturralde O, Benowitz NL. Determination of the nicotine metabolites cotinine and trans-3'-hydroxycotinine in biologic fluids of smokers and non-smokers using liquid chromatography-tandem mass spectrometry: biomarkers for tobacco smoke exposure and for phenotyping cytochrome P450 2A6 activity. J Chromatogr B Analyt Technol Biomed Life Sci. 2011;879:267–76.

30. Schechter JC, Fuemmeler BF, Hoyo C, Murphy SK, Zhang JJ, Kollins SH. Impact of smoking ban on passive smoke exposure in pregnant non-smokers in the southeastern United States. Int J Environ Res Public Health. 2018;15:83-98.

31. Delaney C, Garg SK, Yung R. Analysis of DNA methylation by pyrosequencing. Methods Mol Biol. 2015;1343:249–64.

32. Tost J, Dunker J, Gut IG. Analysis and quantification of multiple methylation variable positions in CpG islands by Pyrosequencing. Biotechniques. 2003;35:152–6.

33. Brakensiek K, Wingen LU, Langer F, Kreipe H, Lehmann U. Quantitative high-resolution CpG island mapping with pyrosequencing reveals disease-specific methylation patterns of the CDKN2B gene in myelodysplastic syndrome and myeloid leukemia. Clin Chem. 2007;53:17–23.

34. Homa DM, Neff LJ, King BA, Caraballo RS, Bunnell RE, Babb SD, et al. Vital signs: disparities in nonsmokers' exposure to secondhand smoke—United States, 1999-2012. MMWR Morb Mortal Wkly Rep. 2015;64:103–8.

35. Hukkanen J, Jacob P 3rd, Benowitz NL. Metabolism and disposition kinetics of nicotine. Pharmacol Rev. 2005;57:79–115.

36. Lokk K, Modhukur V, Rajashekar B, Martens K, Magi R, Kolde R, et al. DNA methylome profiling of human tissues identifies global and tissue-specific methylation patterns. Genome Biol. 2014;15:r54.

37. Office On Smoking And Health (US). Publications and Reports of Surgeon General. In The Health Consequences of Involuntary Exposure to Tobacco Smoke: A Report of Surgeon General. Atlanta: Centers for Disease Control and Prevention (US); 2006.

38. Anblagan D, Jones NW, Costigan C, Parker AJ, Allcock K, Aleong R, et al. Maternal smoking during pregnancy and fetal organ growth: a magnetic resonance imaging study. PLoS One. 2013;8:e67223.

39. Chen MF, Kimizuka G, Wang NS. Human fetal lung changes associated with maternal smoking during pregnancy. Pediatr Pulmonol. 1987;3:51–8.

40. Dietz PM, England LJ, Shapiro-Mendoza CK, Tong VT, Farr SL, Callaghan WM. Infant morbidity and mortality attributable to prenatal smoking in the U.S. Am J Prev Med. 2010;39:45–52.

41. Burke H, Leonardi-Bee J, Hashim A, Pine-Abata H, Chen Y, Cook DG, et al. Prenatal and passive smoke exposure and incidence of asthma and wheeze: systematic review and meta-analysis. Pediatrics. 2012;129:735–44.

42. Hollams EM, de Klerk NH, Holt PG, Sly PD. Persistent effects of maternal smoking during pregnancy on lung function and asthma in adolescents. Am J Respir Crit Care Med. 2014;189:401–7.

43. Shorey-Kendrick LE, McEvoy CT, Ferguson B, Burchard J, Park BS, Gao L, et al. Vitamin C prevents offspring DNA methylation changes associated with maternal smoking in pregnancy. Am J Respir Crit Care Med. 2017;196:745–55.

44. Lee KW, Richmond R, Hu P, French L, Shin J, Bourdon C, et al. Prenatal exposure to maternal cigarette smoking and DNA methylation: epigenome-wide association in a discovery sample of adolescents and replication in an independent cohort at birth through 17 years of age. Environ Health Perspect. 2015;123:193–9.

45. Suter M, Ma J, Harris A, Patterson L, Brown KA, Shope C, et al. Maternal tobacco use modestly alters correlated epigenome-wide placental DNA methylation and gene expression. Epigenetics. 2011;6:1284–94.

46. Haley KJ, Lasky-Su J, Manoli SE, Smith LA, Shahsafaei A, Weiss ST, et al. RUNX transcription factors: association with pediatric asthma and modulated by maternal smoking. Am J Physiol Lung Cell Mol Physiol. 2011;301:L693–701.

47. Fujimori T, Grabiec AM, Kaur M, Bell TJ, Fujino N, Cook PC, et al. The Axl receptor tyrosine kinase is a discriminator of macrophage function in the inflamed lung. Mucosal Immunol. 2015;8:1021–30.

48. Sood A, Petersen H, Blanchette CM, Meek P, Picchi MA, Belinsky SA, et al. Wood smoke exposure and gene promoter methylation are associated with increased risk for COPD in smokers. Am J Respir Crit Care Med. 2010;182:1098–104.

49. Foley DL, Craig JM, Morley R, Olsson CA, Dwyer T, Smith K, et al. Prospects for epigenetic epidemiology. Am J Epidemiol. 2009;169:389–400.

50. Joubert BR, Haberg SE, Nilsen RM, Wang X, Vollset SE, Murphy SK, et al. 450K epigenome-wide scan identifies differential DNA methylation in newborns related to maternal smoking during pregnancy. Environ Health Perspect. 2012;120:1425–31.

51. Markunas CA, Xu Z, Harlid S, Wade PA, Lie RT, Taylor JA, et al. Identification of DNA methylation changes in newborns related to maternal smoking during pregnancy. Environ Health Perspect. 2014;122:1147–53.

52. Miyake K, Kawaguchi A, Miura R, Kobayashi S, Tran NQV, Kobayashi S, et al. Association between DNA methylation in cord blood and maternal smoking: the Hokkaido study on environment and Children's Health. Sci Rep. 2018;8:5654.

53. Breton CV, Marsit CJ, Faustman E, Nadeau K, Goodrich JM, Dolinoy DC, et al. Small-magnitude effect sizes in epigenetic end points are important in children's environmental health studies: the children's environmental health and disease prevention research center's epigenetics working group. Environ Health Perspect. 2017;125:511–26.

54. Salam MT, Gauderman WJ, McConnell R, Lin PC, Gilliland FD. Transforming growth factor- 1 C-509T polymorphism, oxidant stress, and early-onset childhood asthma. Am J Respir Crit Care Med. 2007;176:1192–9.

13

Postnatal relative adrenal insufficiency results in methylation of the glucocorticoid receptor gene in preterm infants: a retrospective cohort study

Masato Kantake[1]* , Natsuki Ohkawa[1], Tomohiro Iwasaki[2], Naho Ikeda[1], Atsuko Awaji[1], Nobutomo Saito[1], Hiromichi Shoji[2] and Toshiaki Shimizu[2]

Abstract

Background: To investigate the relationship between early-life stress and glucocorticoid receptor (GR) gene methylation, which may result in long-lasting neurodevelopmental impairment, we performed a longitudinal analysis of the methylation ratio within the GR gene promoter 1F region using next-generation sequencing in preterm infants.

Cell-free DNA was extracted from the frozen serum of 19 preterm birth infants at birth and at 1 and 2 months after birth. All were admitted to the neonatal intensive care unit of Juntendo University Shizuoka Hospital between August 2014 and May 2016 and suffered from chronic lung disease (CLD).

Through bisulfite amplicon sequencing using an Illumina Miseq system and Bismark-0.15.0 software, we identified the rate of cytosine methylation.

Results: Patients' sex and body weight standard deviation were extracted as the associated independent variables at birth. Sex, glucocorticoid administration for treating CLD, and postnatal invasive procedures (surgical operation and blood sampling) were extracted as the associated independent variables at 1 month. Methylation rates increased significantly between postnatal 1 and 2 months at 9 of the 39 CpG sites. Postnatal glucocorticoid administration to treat circulatory collapse was the most-associated independent variable with a positive regression coefficient for a change in methylation rate at these nine CpG sites. It also influenced the methylation ratio at 22 of the 39 CpG sites at 2 months of age. The standard deviation (SD) score at birth was extracted as an independent variable, with a negative regression coefficient at 9 of the 22 CpG sites together with glucocorticoid administration.

Conclusions: The results of this study indicate that a prenatal environment that results in intrauterine growth restriction and postnatal relative adrenal insufficiency requiring glucocorticoid administration leads to GR gene methylation. That, in turn, may result in neurodevelopmental disabilities.

Keywords: Adrenal insufficiency, Chronic lung disease, Circulatory collapse, Epigenetics, Glucocorticoid administration, Glucocorticoid receptor gene, Intrauterine growth restriction, HPA axis, Methylation, NR3C1

* Correspondence: kantake@juntendo.ac.jp
[1]Neonatal Medical Center, Juntendo University Shizuoka Hospital, 1192 Nagaoka, Izunokuni, Shizuoka 410-2295, Japan
Full list of author information is available at the end of the article

Background

The improved survival of babies at early gestational ages (GAs) is considered a success of modern neonatology. In the current post-steroid and post-surfactant era of neonatology, extremely preterm babies who survive have non-negligible rates of neurological disabilities such as cerebral palsy, mental deficits, sensorineural impairment, and cognitive dysfunction ranging from mild to severe [1, 2]. Infants born with a birth weight < 10th percentile or small for gestational age (SGA) [3, 4] and infants with chronic lung disease (CLD) characterized by prolonged inflammation of lung tissue are at increased risk for neonatal mortality, and preterm infants suffer from both short- and long-term morbidities [5, 6].

The most commonly implicated mechanism of these long-term effects is the dysregulation of the hypothalamus–pituitary–adrenal (HPA) axis. Indeed, dysregulation of this axis has been noted in extremely low birth weight and very low birth weight (VLBW) survivors across their lifespan [7, 8]. An impaired HPA axis is an important risk factor for inflammatory disease, somatic fatigue, pain disorders, and psychiatric conditions such as depression and post-traumatic stress disorder [9, 10]. Activity of the HPA axis is regulated by the hypothalamic glucocorticoid receptor (GR) encoded by the nuclear receptor subfamily 3 group C member 1 (NR3C1) gene, which mediates a negative feedback loop [11].

Promoter DNA methylation is a well-established epigenetic regulator of gene expression. Prenatal stressors, such as maternal depression and anxiety and maternal exposure to stressors, are associated with GR gene methylation [12, 13]. Similarly, adults who retrospectively report a history of childhood maltreatment, early parental death, and childhood trauma show associations with GR gene methylation [14–16]. These links have also been demonstrated in postmortem brains from adult suicides [17] as well as from patients who suffer from depression or bipolar disorder [18]. In our previous study, we showed that a postnatal environment that includes the need for acute care and prolonged physical separation under neonatal intensive care affects epigenetic programming of GR expression through methylation of the NR3C1 promoter in premature infants, which might result in glucocorticoid resistance later in life [19]. These studies were performed by using several tissues, such as placenta [12], cord blood [13], peripheral blood [14, 19], saliva [15, 16, 18], and brain [17].

Several important regions are known to exist in the 39 CpG sites analyzed in the present study [20]. Among them, CpG 30–32 are the most important regions known to be binding sites for nerve growth factor inducible protein A (NGFI-A), which has emerged as a central regulator of early inflammatory and immune processes and potentiates GR 1-F promoter activity. The

methylation rate in this region is influenced by an adverse environment during early life [17]. The high methylation status in this region is also known to result in low GR mRNA expression in an animal model in vitro [21]. CpG 35 has been reported to be associated with maternal stress, a low level of prenatal care, and childhood maltreatment. CpG 36 has been associated with maternal psychopathology during pregnancy. CpG 37 methylation has been associated with both early-life stress and maternal psychopathology. CpG 39 methylation has been associated with childhood maltreatment and prenatal stress. However, CpG site-specific methylation findings for CpG 1–29 are scarce.

Recently, Giarraputo et al. showed that the GR gene methylation in infants in neonatal intensive care unit (NICU) is correlated with high medical risk which is defined by many medical variables (Neonatal Therapeutic Intervention Scoring System (NTISS)) [22].

To investigate the relationship between the early-life environment and GR gene (NR3C1) methylation status, which may take part in long-lasting neurodevelopmental impairment, we performed a longitudinal analysis of methylation ratios within the GR gene promoter 1F region using next-generation sequencing in preterm infants with CLD. In this study, we used cell-free DNA which is thought to be derived from proliferating/apoptotic lymphocytes from the participant's peripheral blood [23].

Methods

This study was approved by the Juntendo University Ethics Committee and conducted according to the principles of the Declaration of Helsinki. Nineteen infants admitted to the NICU of Juntendo University Shizuoka Hospital between August 2014 and May 2016 were enrolled in this study after written informed consent had been obtained. All serum samples were routinely collected at birth and at 1 and 2 months after birth and stored at − 80 °C until analysis. The criterion for CLD was the need for additional oxygen after the age of 28 days. Cell-free DNA was extracted from 100 μL frozen serum using a DNA Extractor SP Kit according to the manufacturer's instructions (Wako Pure Chemical Industries, Ltd. Osaka, Japan), and bisulfite-treated DNA was obtained using an EZ DNA Methylation Direct Kit (Zymo Research Corp., Irvine, CA, USA). A 5-μL aliquot of the resulting 10-μL bisulfite-treated genomic DNA solution was subjected to polymerase chain reaction analysis to amplify the GR promoter 1F region, as previously described [19]. The amplicons were purified using a gel-based clean up, and ViewaBlue Stain KANTO (Kanto Chemical Co., Inc. Tokyo, Japan) was used for DNA staining. The purified amplicons were subjected to a NEBNext Ultra II Library Preparation Kit for Illumina (New England Biolabs Japan, Inc., Tokyo,

Japan) including dual indexing. These libraries were multiplexed and sequenced on an Illumina MiSeq system (Illumina Inc., San Diego, CA, USA). The reads were aligned to an in silico converted reference using Bowtie2-2.2.1, and variant calling was used to identify the percentage of methylated cytosines using Bismark-0.15.0. [24]. We analyzed the epigenetic changes in the GR promoter 1F region (containing 39 CpG sites ranging from − 3466 to − 3189 bp upstream of the ATG start site).

Statistical analysis

We performed Wilcoxon's signed-rank test to evaluate longitudinal differences between birth and at 1 and 2 months after birth. A stepwise multiple regression analysis was performed to investigate the relationships of methylation ratio at birth, 1 month, and 2 months with the amount of increase during months 1–2 at each CpG site as dependent variables and pre- and postnatal parameters in preterm infants as independent variables. To perform this analysis, several nominal variables were converted into categorical variables by grouping the values into two categories. The adjusted coefficient of determination $(R)^2$ is the fraction of information of the dependent variable that is explained by the independent variables. A two-tailed p value < 0.05 was considered statistically significant. All of the statistical analyses were performed using SPSS v24.0 (IBM Corp., Armonk, NY, USA) software.

Results

The abbreviations in the present study are listed and described at the end of the main text and in Table 1.

Participant characteristics

Nineteen participants completed the analysis, and their characteristics are shown in Table 1. The GAs and birth weights of the infants ranged from 24 weeks + 3 days to 28 weeks + 2 days and from 316 to 1226 g, respectively. All infants received mechanical ventilation. Four were below − 2 SD of birth weight. Seven infants underwent an operation to close the patent ductus arteriosus (PDA). Twelve infants received antenatal steroid (AS) administration and 11 received postnatal steroid administration. Of these 11 infants, 9 were treated for circulatory collapse and 2 were treated for CLD. Fourteen infants received an opioid for sedation.

Relationship between prenatal parameters and GR gene methylation at birth

We examined the associations between the methylation ratios at the 39 CpG sites in the GR 1F promoter and GA at birth (weeks), body weight SD scores at birth calculated by the Japanese standard, AS administration (mg), and sex. Methylation rates in the GR 1F region were generally low at birth. At 3 of the 39 CpG sites analyzed, only sex (male = 1, female = 0) was correlated with the methylation ratio (CpG 12: $p = 0.046$, regression coefficient, − 0.463; CpG 19: $p = 0.027$, regression coefficient, 0.505; CpG 27: $p = 0.030$, regression coefficient, − 0.497). At 4 of the 39 CpG sites analyzed, only SD scores were correlated with the methylation ratios (CpG 7: $p = 0.048$, regression coefficient, − 0.460; CpG 25: $p = 0.040$, regression coefficient, − 0.475; CpG 36: $p = 0.047$, regression coefficient, − 0.461; CpG 38: $p = 0.002$, regression coefficient, − 0.675). The methylation ratio at CpG 24 was associated only with AS administration ($p = 0.025$, regression coefficient, − 0.512) (Fig. 3).

Relationship between prenatal and postnatal (0–1 month) parameters and GR gene methylation at 1 month

We analyzed the relationships of methylation rates at 1 month with prenatal and postnatal (0–1 month)

Table 1 Patient characteristics

	Range	Number	Mean, SE		Range	Number	Mean, SE
Sex		$M = 12$		AS	0–24	13	12, 2.43
		$F = 7$					
GA	24w3d–28w2d		27w2d, 2d	Gc circ	0–17.4	8	1.44, 0.91
BW	402–1226		825, 54.7	Gc CLD	0–38	3	2.32, 2.0
SD	− 3.95–0.17		− 1.36, 0.31	Opi	0–7	13	3.37, 0.58
dSD	− 2.3–0.97		− 0.61, 0.15	Bf	0.1–7.6	19	4.39, 0.48
Mv	1–60	19	32.4, 5.15	In	0–1.6	15	0.48, 0.10
Hc	30–84	19	57.4, 4.45	PDA		7	

M male, *F* female, *GA* gestational age, *BW* birth weight (g), *SD* standard deviation of body weight, *dSD* change in SD scores between 0 and 2 months, *Mv* duration of mechanical ventilation with intra-tracheal intubation between 0 and 2 months after birth (days), *Hc* heel cut procedure for blood examination between 0 and 2 months after birth (times), *AS* antenatal steroid administration (mg), *Gc circ* glucocorticoid administration between 0 and 2 months after birth as a treatment for circulatory collapse (mg/kg prednisolone), *Gc CLD* glucocorticoid administration between 0 and 2 months after birth as a treatment for or prevention of CLD (mg/kg prednisolone), *Opi* opioid administration between 0 and 2 months after birth (mg fentanyl), *Bf* breast fed volume between 0 and 1 month after birth (mL/kg) (kg was calculated by birthweight + bodyweight at 2 months/2), *In* indomethacin administration for PDA closure (mg/kg), *PDA* underwent surgery to close a patent ductus arteriosus between 0 and 2 months after birth parameters (sex, GA, SD, AS, Hc, Bf, Gc circ, Gc CLD, Opi, dSD, In, and PDA) at the 39 CpG sites. The results are shown in Fig. 3. Briefly, postnatal parameters such as glucocorticoid administration for CLD, surgical operation, or heel-cut blood sampling were extracted as independent variables with positive regression coefficients in CpG 5, 8, 14, 25, 32, 33, 34, 35, and 38, except that sex in CpG 19 had a negative regression coefficient.

Longitudinal changes in methylation status

Methylation rates between birth and postnatal 1 month were stable at all of the 39 CpG sites examined. By contrast, methylation rates significantly increased from postnatal 1 to 2 months at 9 of the 39 CpG sites (CpG 3: $p = 0.043$; CpG 4: $p = 0.047$; CpG 5: $p = 0.031$; CpG 11: $p = 0.014$; CpG 15: $p = 0.038$; CpG 18: $p = 0.047$; CpG 19: $p = 0.005$; CpG 23: $p = 0.0025$; CpG 27: $p = 0.03$) (Fig. 1).

Relationships of the change in methylation ratio during months 1 and 2 with prenatal and postnatal parameters between birth and 2 months of age

We analyzed the relationship between changes in the methylation rates at CpG 3, 4, 5, 11, 15, 18, 19, 23, and 27, when significant increases in methylation rates were observed during months 1–2 after birth, and the prenatal and postnatal environments at 0–2 months of age. The independent variables analyzed at 0–2 months were sex, GA, SD, AS, days of mechanical ventilation (Mv), number of heel-cut (Hc) procedures, breast milk intake (mL/kg) (breast-fed [Bf] baby), amount of glucocorticoid administered (mg/kg prednisolone) for treatment of circulatory collapse (Gc circ), and CLD (Gc CLD), amount of opioid (Opi) administered (times 0.1 mL fentanyl), change in body weight SD scores (dSD), amount of indomethacin (In) administered (mg/kg), and experience of receiving surgery to close a patent ductus arteriosus (PDA) (yes = 1, no = 0).

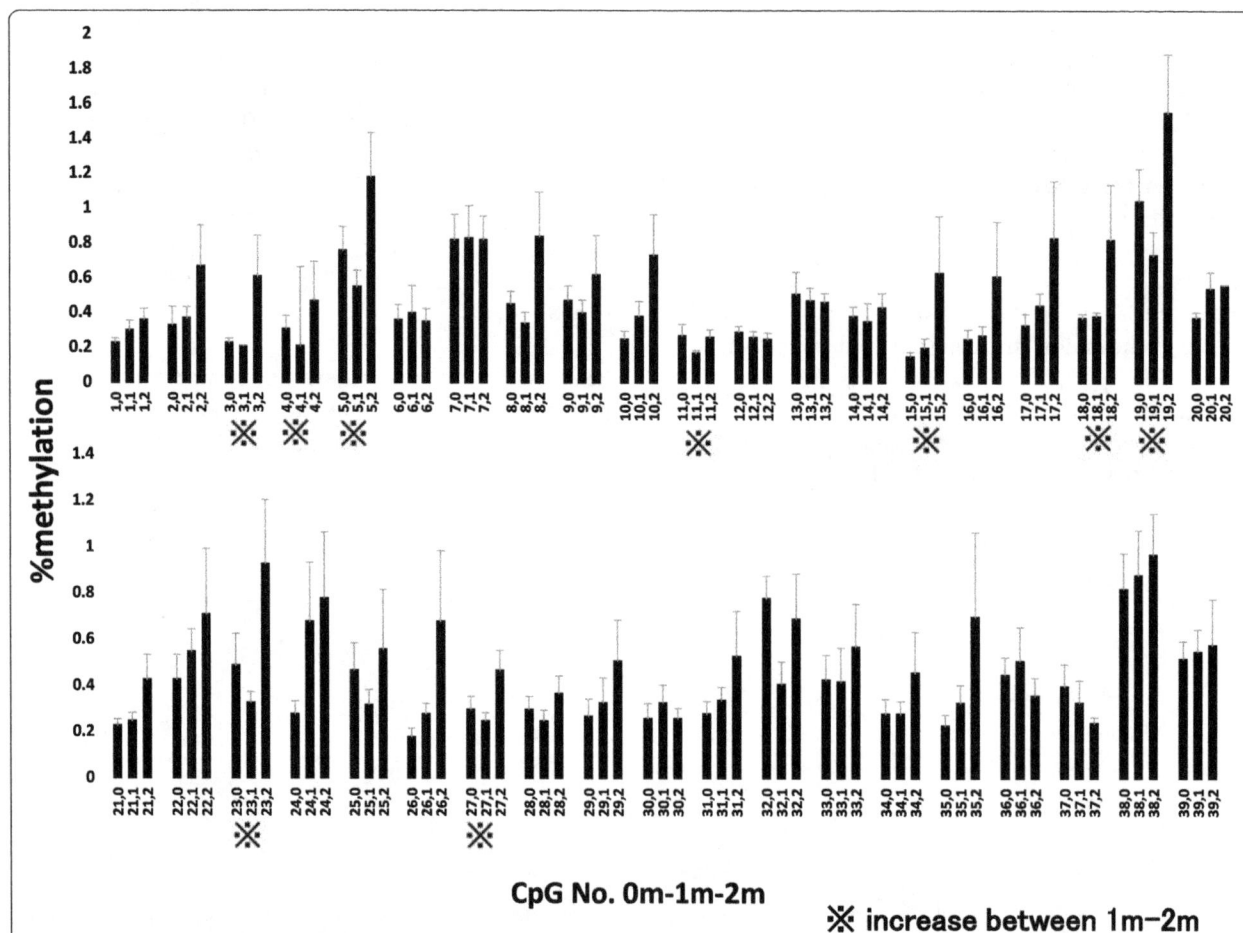

Fig. 1 Longitudinal analysis of glucocorticoid receptor (GR) 1F promoter methylation. Methylation ratios at birth and at 1 and 2 months after birth in the 39 CpG sites analyzed are shown. The left, center, and right triplet bars indicate the methylation rates at birth, 1 month, and 2 months, respectively, with standard error bars. The asterisks under the CpG numbers indicate the methylation rates at CpG sites that significantly increased at between 1 and 2 months after birth

At seven of the nine CpG sites, Gc circ was solely extracted as an efficient independent variable with a positive regression coefficient. CpG 3 (Gc circ [regression coefficient, 0.885, overall $p < 0.001$, adjusted $R^2 = 0.771$]); CpG 4 (Gc circ [regression coefficient, 0.871, overall $p < 0.001$, adjusted $R^2 = 0.744$]); CpG 5 (Gc circ [regression coefficient, 0.687, overall $p = 0.001$, adjusted $R^2 = 0.440$]); CpG 15 (Gc circ [regression coefficient, 0.895, overall $p < 0.001$, adjusted $R^2 = 0.790$]); CpG 18 (Gc circ [regression coefficient, 0.926, overall $p < 0.001$, adjusted $R^2 = 0.848$]); CpG 19 (Gc circ [regression coefficient, 0.689, overall $p = 0.001$, adjusted $R^2 = 0.444$]); and CpG 23 (Gc circ [regression coefficient, 0.800, overall $p < 0.001$, adjusted $R^2 = 0.619$]). None of the eight parameters examined was extracted as an efficient independent variable at the remaining two CpG sites (CpG 11 and CpG 27).

Relationship between methylation rate at postnatal 2 months and prenatal and postnatal parameters

Next, we analyzed the relationship between methylation rates at 2 months after birth and prenatal and postnatal parameters, e.g., sex, GA, SD, AS, Hc, Bf, Gc circ, Gc CLD, Opi dSD, In, and PDA at all of the 39 CpG sites. The results are shown in Table 2. Briefly, some independent variables were extracted from 24 of the 39 CpG sites examined. Gc circ was extracted as an independent variable at 22 CpG sites with a positive regression coefficient. The volume of breast milk consumed was extracted as the sole independent variable at the remaining two CpG sites, with a negative regression coefficient (CpG 11 and CpG 36). SD scores at birth were simultaneously extracted as independent variables at 7 of 22 sites at which Gc circ was extracted, with a negative regression coefficient. AS administration was extracted as an independent variable at 3 of the 22 sites, with a negative regression coefficient. Glucocorticoid administration to treat CLD was extracted as an independent variable at CpG 2 with a negative regression coefficient and at CpG 8 with a positive regression coefficient. Figure 2 is a heat map of the methylation status focused on the effect of three major independent variables (Gc circ, AS, and SD).

Table 2 The relationships between methylation status at 2 months and pre- and postnatal environments

CpG no.	2	3	4	5	8	9	10	11
Gc circ	0.568	0.877	0.968	0.754	0.715	0.855	0.66	
SD	− 0.547						− 0.352	
Gc CLD	− 0.365				0.327			
AS	− 0.193				− 0.298	− 0.254		
Bf								− 0.492
Adjusted R^2	0.922	0.774	0.933	0.544	0.752	0.858	0.724	0.198
Overall p	※	※	※	※	※	※	※	0.032
CpG no.	12	15	16	17	18	19	23	24
Gc circ	0.802	0.789	0.837	0.755	0.887	0.842	0.894	0.639
SD		− 0.255	− 0.234	− 0.285				− 0.364
Gc CLD								
Bf								
Adjusted R^2	0.623	0.838	0.909	0.811	0.89	0.691	0.788	0.702
Overall p	※	※	※	※	※	※	※	※
CpG no.	25	26	31	32	33	34	36	39
Gc circ	0.81	0.865	0.908	0.877	0.892	0.902		0.827
SD	− 0.246							
Gc CLD								
AS								
Bf							− 0.506	
Adjusted R^2	0.869	0.734	0.814	0.756	0.784	0.803	0.213	0.665
Overall p	※	※	※	※	※	※	0.027	※

Regression coefficients of independent variables are shown. A blank means not extracted as independent variables

Gc circ glucocorticoid administration for circulatory collapse, *SD* SD score of birth weight, *Gc CLD* glucocorticoid administration for CLD, *AS* antenatal glucocorticoid administration, *Bf* amount of human milk

※ $p < 0.001$

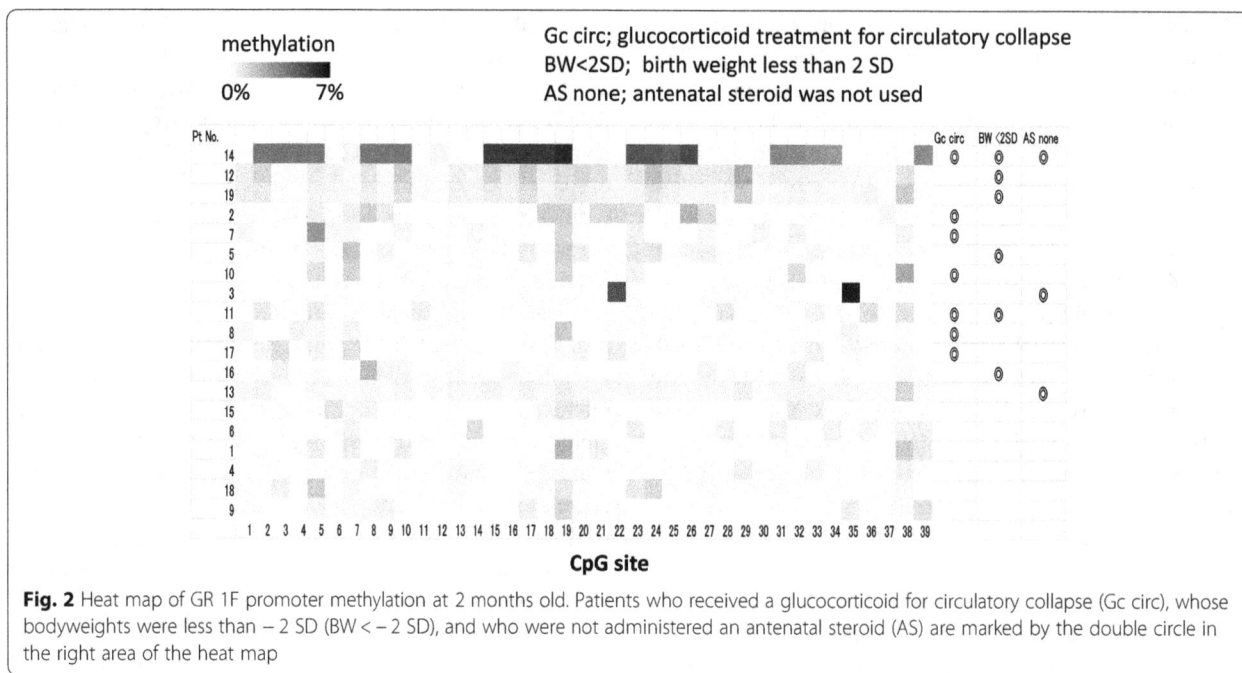

Fig. 2 Heat map of GR 1F promoter methylation at 2 months old. Patients who received a glucocorticoid for circulatory collapse (Gc circ), whose bodyweights were less than − 2 SD (BW < − 2 SD), and who were not administered an antenatal steroid (AS) are marked by the double circle in the right area of the heat map

Discussion

This is the first longitudinal report to demonstrate that prenatal and postnatal environments induce gene methylation. The results of this study show that postnatal Gc circ had positive and strong effects on GR gene methylation at 1–2 months of age, which may result in neurodevelopmental disability in later life due to dysfunction in the HPA axis. Simultaneously, prenatal factors such as SD scores at birth and antenatal glucocorticoid administration had moderate negative effects on GR gene methylation.

In the present study, glucocorticoid administration at 0–1 month influenced GR gene methylation at 1 month (Fig. 3). Our criteria for using glucocorticoid for CLD are as follows: mean airway pressure of mechanical ventilation > 10 mmHg and FiO_2 > 0.4, which indicate a severe lung condition due to relative adrenal insufficiency.

CpG	1	2	3	4	5	6	7	8	9	10	11	12	13	14	15	16	17	18	19	20	21	22	23	24	25	26	27	28	29	30	31	32	33	34	35	36	37	38	39
Sex												-0.5							0.5								-0.5												
SD							**-0.5**																		**-0.5**											**-0.5**		**-0.7**	
0m ↑							p=0.048					p=0.046							p=0.027						p=0.04		p=0.03									p=0.047		p=0.027	
Sex																			-0.5																				
Gc CLD					1			0.6																	0.59							0.8	1		0.7				
Ope														0.6																				0.5					
Hc																																						0.5	
1m ↑					p=0.01			p=0.007						p=0.005					p=0.018						p=0.008							※	※	p=0.031	p=0.001			p=0.045	
SD		**-0.5**								**-0.4**					**-0.3**	**-0.2**	**-0.3**							**-0.4**	**-0.2**														
Gc CLD		-0.4						0.3																															
Gc circ		0.57	0.9	1	1			0.7	0.9	0.7		0.8			0.79	0.84	0.76	0.9	0.84				0.9	0.64	0.81	0.9					0.9	0.9	0.9	0.9					0.8
AS		-0.9						-0.3	-0.3																														
Bf											-0.5																									-0.5			
2m ↑		※	※	※	※			※	※	※	p=0.032	※			※	※	※	※	※				※	※	※	※					※	※	※	※		p=0.027			※

Fig. 3 Extracted independent variables in the 39 CpG sites at birth (0 m), 1 month (1 m), and 2 months (2 m). Regression coefficients of the SD scores are bolded and those of glucocorticoid administration are underlined

Neonatal hypotension is commonly seen in premature neonates, and its incidence is inversely related to GA at delivery. Hypotension in preterm infants is predominantly due to either abnormal peripheral vasoregulation or myocardial dysfunction. Another etiology of hypotension in this population is physiological factors, including the presence of relative adrenal insufficiency secondary to an immature HPA axis [25]. Ng et al. showed an increase in plasma adrenocorticotrophic hormone with the use of inotropes and volume expanders in VLBW infants with hypotension [26]. In addition, low serum cortisol levels were also found in these patients [27]. These findings suggest that the adrenal cortex may be the primary site of dysfunction in this patient population, and not the hypothalamus or pituitary gland. Overall, these findings imply a normal response of the pituitary gland to hypotension, but the adrenal glands are transiently unable to maintain cortisol secretion during the immediate postnatal period. Hydrocortisone is the recommended treatment for hypotensive neonates if volume resuscitation with isotonic saline and dopamine treatment (10 µg/kg/min) are unsuccessful [28]. Our strategy to treat neonatal hypotension, which is defined as a mean blood pressure lower than the neonate's GA, is described above. We also confirmed the effects of glucocorticoids by improvements in blood pressure and urine output soon after administration. We conclude that the hypotension observed in our study population resulted from relative adrenal insufficiency.

Postnatal steroids are widely used to manage preterm infants with CLD. Several reports have indicated that infants with CLD may develop adrenal insufficiency during the first 1–2 weeks of life [26, 29]. All of the infants in this study developed CLD, implying that they may have had some degree of adrenal insufficiency.

Taken together, these findings led us to hypothesize that severe adrenal insufficiency followed by both CLD and circulatory collapse results in GR gene methylation. Adrenal insufficiency during the early stage of life results in upregulation of the HPA axis later in life to respond adequately to stress.

Antenatal glucocorticoid administration had a moderate negative effect on GR gene methylation. In contrast, postnatal glucocorticoid administration for CLD and circulatory collapse had a positive effect on GR gene methylation. Thus, glucocorticoid demand due to relative adrenal insufficiency, not glucocorticoid administration itself, may result in GR gene methylation.

SD scores at birth were related to GR gene methylation at birth and at 2 months of age. Notably, the CpG sites affected at 2 months by SD (CpG 10, 15, 16, 17, 24, and 25) were different from those affected at birth by SD (CpG 7, 25, 36, and 38), except CpG 25. All of the SD effects at birth had disappeared by 1 month, even those in

CpG 25. In addition, SD was always affected together with postnatal glucocorticoid administration only at 2 months. Thus, it is possible that the long-lasting influence of low SD (e.g., intrauterine growth restriction) on GR gene methylation is indirect.

Permanent changes in gene expression have been observed in multiple genes as a consequence of SGA. Dysregulation of the epigenome may explain changes that are propagated from parent to daughter cells in SGA offspring throughout life [30]. The results of this study suggest that dysregulation of several genes induced by intrauterine growth restriction may increase susceptibility to circumstances after birth, particularly relative adrenal insufficiency, leading to GR gene methylation, which in turn results in neurodevelopmental disabilities. Stressful postnatal procedures, such as the Hc procedure or Ope, were correlated with significant positive regression coefficients at three CpG sites at 1 month. Taken together, these findings suggest that relative adrenal insufficiency, which leads to severe CLD and circulatory collapse and the inability to respond to a stressful postnatal environment in the NICU, may result in GR gene methylation at 2 months after birth.

In this study, well-known CpG sites, which are methylated by early-life stress directly, such as CpG 30–32, CpG 35–37, and CpG 39, were affected at 2 months almost only by Gc circ. In contrast, CpG 1–29, which are not well-known as sites methylated by early-life stress, were affected by Gc circ and low SD. CpG 1–29 may be methylated by both the intrauterine and the postnatal environment. Figure 2 shows that CpG 30–39 and CpG 1–29 are widely methylated, which may result in a change in three-dimensional DNA structure.

It should be noted that the volume of mothers' milk fed to infants during the first 2 months after birth had a weak but significant negative effect on GR methylation (CpG 11 and 36). Maternal breastfeeding has been emphasized as an influential factor in early childhood development [31]. However, empirical evidence for the effects of breastfeeding on children's cognitive development has been conflicting. A comprehensive review by the Agency for Healthcare Research and Quality summarized 400 articles and found that breastfeeding had few or small effects on children's cognitive ability [32]. This study may provide new insights into the effects of breastfeeding.

Because epigenetic modifications occur in a tissue-specific manner, it remains unclear whether DNA methylation measured in blood reflects DNA methylation patterns in other tissues including the brain. We used cell-free DNA, which is thought to be derived from proliferating/apoptotic lymphocytes in the participant's peripheral blood [23].

Although research conducted on the effects of early-life stress on methylation of the alternate GR promoter

1F in blood, brain, saliva, and placenta produced similar results [12–19, 33], it should be noted that the correlation of methylation between blood and brain is still controversial. Watson et al. showed that only 7.9% of CpG sites were statistically significant, showing a large correlation between blood and brain tissue [34]. Tylee et al. reviewed seven studies comparing patterns of DNA methylation between the blood and brain and suggested that CpG island methylation levels are generally highly correlated ($r = 0.90$) between them [35].

This study has some limitations. First, cell type and tissue-specific diversity of methylation of the GR gene are noted problems. This study did not include a control for variations in cell type. Second, the participants were homogeneous in race, limiting generalizability of the findings. Another limitation is the lack of information about endogenous glucocorticoid secretion. Further investigations including a longitudinal follow-up study and cell type-specific investigation will enhance our understanding of the relationships between early-life experiences and long-lasting neurodevelopmental disability.

Conclusions

This study revealed that adverse pre- and postnatal environments, such as intrauterine growth restriction and postnatal relative adrenal insufficiency, increased glucocorticoid receptor gene methylation. This, in turn, may result in neurodevelopmental disabilities.

Abbreviations

CLD: Chronic lung disease; GR: Glucocorticoid receptor; HPA: Hypothalamus–pituitary–adrenal gland; SGA: Small for gestational age

Specific abbreviations in the patients' background and perinatal factors

AS: Antenatal steroid administration (mg); Bf: Breast fed volume between 0 and 1 month after birth (mL/kg) (kg was calculated by birthweight + bodyweight at 2 months/2); BW: Birth weight (g); dSD: Change of SD scores between 0 and 2 months; F: Female; GA: Gestational age; Gc circ: Glucocorticoid administration between 0 and 2 months after birth for treatment of circulatory collapse (mg/kg prednisolone); Gc CLD: Glucocorticoid administration between 0 and 2 months after birth for treatment or prevention of CLD (mg/kg prednisolone); Hc: Heel cut procedure for blood examination between 0 and 2 months after birth (times); In: Indomethacin administration for PDA closure (mg/kg); M: Male; Mv: Duration of mechanical ventilation with intra-tracheal intubation between 0 and 2 months after birth (days); Opi: Opioid administration between 0 and 2 months after birth (mg fentanyl); PDA: Experience of receiving surgery to close a patent ductus arteriosus between 0 and 2 month after birth; SD: Standard deviation score of body weight

Acknowledgements

Thank you to Drs. Ryo Matoba and Noriko Ito for the technical assistance. Thank you also to Drs. Koichi Sato and Hajime Orita for their contribution in Shizuoka Medical Research Center for Disaster.

Funding

This study was supported by Ministry of Education, Culture, Sports, Science and Technology (MEXT)-Supported Program for the Strategic Research Foundation at Private Universities, 2015–2019, Japan.

Authors' contributions

MK conceptualized and designed the study, drafted the initial manuscript, and approved the final manuscript as submitted. NO, TI, AA, and NS designed the data collection instruments, coordinated and supervised the data collection, and approved the final manuscript as submitted. NI, HS, and TS carried out the statistical analysis, reviewed and revised the manuscript, and approved the final manuscript as submitted.

Author details

[1]Neonatal Medical Center, Juntendo University Shizuoka Hospital, 1192 Nagaoka, Izunokuni, Shizuoka 410-2295, Japan. [2]Division of Pediatrics, Juntendo University School of Medicine, 3-1-3, Hongo, Bunkyo 113-8421, Japan.

References

1. Marlow N, Wolke D, Bracewell MA, Samara M, EPICure Study Group. Neurologic and developmental disability at six years of age after extremely preterm birth. N Engl J Med. 2005;352:9–19.
2. Larroque B, Ancel PY, Marret S, Marchand L, André M, Arnaud C, EPIPAGE Study Group, et al. Neurodevelopmental disabilities and special care of 5-year-old children born before 33 weeks of gestation (the EPIPAGE study): a longitudinal cohort study. Lancet. 2008;371:813–20.
3. Guellec I, Lapillonne A, Renolleau S, Charlaluk ML, Roze JC, Marret S, et al. Neurologic outcomes at school age in very preterm infants born with severe or mild growth restriction. Pediatrics. 2011;127:e883–91.
4. von Ehrenstein OS, Mikolajczyk RT, Zhang J. Timing and trajectories of fetal growth related to cognitive development in childhood. Am J Epidemiol. 2009;170:1388–95.
5. Anderson PJ, Doyle LW. Neurodevelopmental outcome of bronchopulmonary dysplasia. Semin Perinatol. 2006;30:227–32.
6. Short EJ, Klein NK, Lewis BA, Fulton S, Eisengart S, Kercsmar C, et al. Cognitive and academic consequences of bronchopulmonary dysplasia and very low birth weight: 8-year-old outcomes. Pediatrics. 2003;112:e359.
7. Waxman JA, Lieshout RJ, Boyle MH, Saigal S, Schmidt LA. Linking extremely low birth weight and internalizing behaviors in adult survivors: influences of neuroendocrine dysregulation. Dev Psychobiol. 2015;57:486–96.
8. Kaseva N, Wehkalampi K, Pyhälä R, Moltch-anova E, Feldt K, Pesonen AK, et al. Blunted hypothalamic-pituitary-adrenal axis and insulin response to psycosocial stress in young adults born preterm at very low birth weight. Clin Endocrinol. 2014;80:101–6.
9. Heim C, Binder EB. Current research trends in early life stress and depression: review of human studies on sensitive periods, gene-environment interaction, and epigenetics. Exp Neurol. 2012;233:102–11.
10. Buitelaar JK. The role of the HPA-axis in understanding psychopathology: cause, consequence, mediator, or moderator? Eur Child Adoles Psy. 2013;22:387–9.
11. Jacobson L. Hypothalamic-pituitary-adrenocortical axis regulation. Endocrin Metab Clin. 2005;34:271–92.
12. Conradt E, Lester BM, Appleton AA, Armstrong DA, Marsit CJ. The roles of DNA methylation of NR3C1 and 11beta-HSD2 and exposure to maternal mood disorder in utero on newborn neurobehavior. Epigenetics. 2013;8:1321–9.
13. Oberlander TF, Weinberg J, Papsdorf M, Grunau R, Misri S, Devlin AM. Prenatal exposure to maternal depression, neonatal methylation of human glucocorticoid receptor gene (NR3C1) and infant cortisol stress responses. Epigenetics. 2008;3:97–106.
14. Perroud N, Paoloni-Giacobino A, Prada P, Olié E, Salzmann A, Nicastro R, et al. Increased methylation of glucocorticoid receptor gene (NR3C1) in adults with a history of childhood maltreatment: a link with the severity and type of trauma. Transl Psychiatry. 2011;1:e59.
15. Tyrka AR, Parade SH, Eslinger NM, Marsit CJ, Lesseur C, Seifer R. Methylation of exons 1D, 1F, and 1H of the glucocorticoid receptor gene promoter and exposure to adversity in preschool-aged children. Dev Psychopathol. 2015; 27:577–85.
16. Parade SH, Ridout KK, Seifer R, Armstrong DA, Marsit CJ, McWilliams MA, et al. Methylation of the glucocorticoid receptor gene promoter in preschoolers: links with internalizing behavior problems. Child Dev. 2016;87:86–97.
17. McGowan PO, Sasaki A, D'Alessio AC, Dymov S, Labonté B, Szyf M, et al. Epigenetic regulation of the glucocorticoid receptor in human brain associates with childhood abuse. Nat Neurosci. 2009;12:342–8.

18. Melas PA, Wei Y, Wong CC, Sjöholm LK, Åberg E, Mill J, et al. Genetic and epigenetic associations of MAOA and NR3C1 with depression and childhood adversities. Int J Neuropsychopharmacol. 2013;16:1513–28.

19. Kantake M, Yoshitake H, Ishikawa H, Araki Y, Shimizu T. Postnatal epigenetic modification of glucocorticoid receptor gene in preterm infants: a prospective cohort study. BMJ Open. 2014;4:e005318.

20. Palma-Gudiel H, Córdova-Palomera A, Leza JC, Fananás L. Glucocorticoid receptor gene (NR3C1) methylation processes as mediators of early adversity in stress-related disorders causality: a critical review. Neurosci Biobehav Rev. 2015;55:520–35.

21. Weaver ICG, D'Alessio AC, Brown SE, Hellstrom IC, Dymov S, Sharma S, Szyf M, Meaney MJ. The transcription factor nerve growth factor-inducible protein a mediates epigenetic programming: altering epigenetic marks by immediate-early genes. J Neurosci. 2007;27:1756–68.

22. Giarraputo J, DeLoach J, Padbury J, Uzun A, Marsit C, Hawes K, Lester B. Medical morbidities and DNA methylation of NR3C1 in preterm infants. Ped Res. 2017;81:68–74.

23. Tuaeva NO, Abramova ZI, Sofronov VV. The origin of elevated levels of circulating DNA in blood plasma of premature neonates. Ann N Y Acad Sci. 2008;1137:27–30.

24. Masser DR, Berg AS, Freeman WM. Focused, high accuracy 5-methylcytosine quantitation with base resolution by benchtop next-generation sequencing. Epigenetics Chromatin. 2013;6:33.

25. Seri I. Management of hypotension and low systemic blood flow in very low birth weight neonate during the first postnatal week. J Perinatol. 2006; 26(Suppl 1):S8–S13.

26. Ng PC, Lee CH, Lam CW, Ma KC, Chan IH, Wong E, et al. Early pituitary-adrenal response and respiratory outcomes in preterm infants. Arch Dis Child Fetal Neonatal Ed. 2004;89:F127–30.

27. Helbock HJ, Insoft RM, Conte FA. Glucocorticoid-responsive hypotension in extremely low birth weight newborns. Pediatrics. 1993;92:715–6.

28. Johnson PJ. Hydrocortisone for treatment of hypotension in the newborn. Neonatal Netw. 2015;34:46–50.

29. Watterberg KL, Scott SM. Evidence of early adrenal insufficiency in babies who develop bronchopulmonary dysplasia. Pediatrics. 1995;95:120–5.

30. Einstein F, Thompson RF, Bhagat TD, Fazzari MJ, Verma A, Barzilai N, et al. Cytosine methylation dysregulation in neonates following intrauterine growth restriction. PLoS One. 2010;5:8887.

31. Kramer MS, Aboud F, Mironova E, Vanilovich I, Platt RW, Matush L, et al. Breastfeeding and child cognitive development: new evidence from a large randomized trial. Arch Gen Psychiatry. 2008;65:578–84.

32. Ip S, Chung M, Raman G, Chew P, Magula N, DeVine D, et al. Breastfeeding and maternal and infant health outcome in developed countries. Evid Rep Technol Assess (Full Rep). 2007;153:1–186.

33. Radtke KM, Schauer M, Gunter HM, Ruf-Leuschner M, Sill J, Meyer A, et al. Epigenetic modifications of the glucocorticoid receptor gene are associated with the vulnerability to psychopathology in childhood maltreatment. Transl Psychiatry. 2015;5:e571.

34. Walton E, Hass J, Liu J, Roffman L, Bernardoni F, Roessner V, et al. Correspondence of DNA Methylation Between blood and Brain Tissue and Its Application to Schizophrenia Research. Schizophrenia Bulletin. 2016;42: 406–14.

35. Tylee DS, Kawaguchi DM, Glatt SJ. On the Outside, Looking In: A Review and Evaluation of the Comparability of Blood and Brain "-omes". Am J Med Genet Part B. 2013;162B:595–603.

14

Epigenome-wide association study of total serum immunoglobulin E in children: a life course approach

Cheng Peng[1]*[iD], Andres Cardenas[2], Sheryl L. Rifas-Shiman[2], Marie-France Hivert[2,3], Diane R. Gold[1,4], Thomas A. Platts-Mills[5], Xihong Lin[6], Emily Oken[2], Andrea A. Baccarelli[7], Augusto A. Litonjua[1] and Dawn L. DeMeo[1]

Abstract

Background: IgE-mediated sensitization may be epigenetically programmed in utero, but early childhood environment may further alter complex traits and disease phenotypes through epigenetic plasticity. However, the epigenomic footprint underpinning IgE-mediated type-I hypersensitivity has not been well-understood, especially under a longitudinal early-childhood life-course framework.

Methods: We used epigenome-wide DNA methylation (IlluminaHumanMethylation450 BeadChip) in cord blood and mid-childhood peripheral blood to investigate pre- and post-natal methylation marks associated with mid-childhood (age 6.7–10.2) total serum IgE levels in 217 mother-child pairs in Project Viva—a prospective longitudinal pre-birth cohort in eastern Massachusetts, USA. We identified methylation sites associated with IgE using covariate-adjusted robust linear regressions.

Results: Nineteen methylation marks in cord blood were associated with IgE in mid-childhood (FDR < 0.05) in genes implicated in cell signaling, growth, and development. Among these, two methylation sites (*C7orf50*, *ZAR1*) remained robust after the adjustment for the change in DNA methylation from birth to mid-childhood (FDR < 0.05). An analysis of the change in methylation between cord blood and mid-childhood DNA (Δ-DNAm) identified 395 methylation marks in 272 genes associated with mid-childhood IgE (FDR < 0.05), with multiple sites located within *ACOT7* (4 sites), *EPX* (5 sites), *EVL* (3 sites), *KSR1* (4 sites), *ZFPM1* (3 sites), and *ZNF862* (3 sites). Several of these methylation loci were previously associated with asthma (*ADAM19*, *EPX*, *IL4*, *IL5RA*, and *PRG2*).

Conclusion: This study identified fetally programmed and mid-childhood methylation signals associated with mid-childhood IgE. Epigenetic priming during fetal development and early childhood likely plays an important role in IgE-mediated type-I hypersensitivity.

Keywords: Epigenome-wide association studies, Total serum IgE, Life course analysis

Background

Immunoglobulin E (IgE)—a central mediator for type I hypersensitivity—contributes to the pathogenesis of a wide range of childhood-onset allergic diseases, including asthma, allergic rhinitis, atopic dermatitis, and food allergy [1–4]. IgE-mediated allergic sensitization has its roots very early in life and is likely impacted by the in utero environment [5, 6]. The manifestation of IgE-mediated responses often involves childhood re-exposures to antigens in sensitized individuals, with subsequent IgE-dependent release of inflammatory mediators that give rise to allergic symptoms [3, 4].

To date, the most commonly used therapies for IgE-mediated allergic responses in children focus on acute and chronic symptom relief [7]; no treatment targets the natural history of allergy pathogenesis across the life course. Understanding the molecular origins and mechanisms of IgE-mediated allergic responses, and the plasticity of the associated molecular markers,

* Correspondence: recpe@channing.harvard.edu
[1]Channing Division of Network Medicine and the Division of Pulmonary and Critical Care Medicine, Department of Medicine, Brigham and Women's Hospital, Harvard Medical School, 181 Longwood Avenue, 4th Floor, Boston, MA 02115, USA
Full list of author information is available at the end of the article

would inform more effective screening, prevention, and treatment strategies.

Epigenetic regulatory elements, such as DNA methylation marks, undergo dynamic reprogramming during embryogenesis [8, 9]. The establishment of the human methylome during fetal development coincides with early immune development relevant to IgE-mediated allergic sensitization and makes DNA methylation in cord blood a potential early molecular marker of IgE-mediated disease onset. DNA methylation patterns may vary after birth to reflect the complex interplay between genetics, development and maturation, and environmental exposures. Therefore, plasticity of DNA methylation from birth may portend the development and progression of diseases that were driven by both genetic endowment and the environment, such as IgE-mediated allergic phenotypes during childhood.

Previous studies have reported differential DNA methylation in peripheral blood associated with total serum IgE measures [10–13]. However, these studies were either cross-sectional or case-control studies; the lack of prospective nature of these studies impedes the identification of epigenetic marks that predict development of allergy. Further, most of these studies were conducted in later childhood and adulthood. Since IgE-mediated allergic responses may have a fetal origin, these studies may not capture alterations during critical developmental windows, e. g., the period of fetal immune development during which IgE-dependent predisposition may originate.

To better understand the molecular origins and progression of IgE-mediated responses, we sought to conceptualize the association between epigenome-wide differential methylation in DNA from blood cells and serum IgE measures using a life course framework [14] (Fig. 1). Specifically, we used methylation data from DNA from blood cells at two distinct time points—birth and mid-childhood (mean age = 7.8 years)—to quantify and dissect the influence of prenatal and childhood factors on IgE. We hypothesize that (1) epigenetic marks in cord blood DNA reflecting the prenatal environment serve as early markers of IgE-mediated allergic response susceptibility in childhood, (2) some epigenetic marks established at birth may be associated with IgE levels in childhood independent of factors operating postnatally, and (3) childhood environmental influences—captured by changes in DNA methylation levels between cord blood and mid-childhood peripheral blood—reflect the progression and manifestation of IgE-mediated allergic responses.

Methods

Study population

Our study population is drawn from Project Viva—a prospective longitudinal pre-birth cohort from Massachusetts,

USA. All participants were recruited at their initial obstetric visit at Atrius Harvard Vanguard Medical Associates from 1999 to 2002. Eligible participants were those with single gestation, gestational age < 22 weeks at enrollment, able to answer questions in English, and intended to stay in the study region before delivery. A detailed cohort profile has been published previously [13]. At enrollment, mothers provided information on age at enrollment, smoking habits (never smoker/former smoker/smoked during pregnancy), education level, and familial atopy history of asthma, eczema, or hay fever. We collected date of birth and sex from hospital records and calculated gestational age at birth as previously described [13]. Trained research assistants conducted in-person research visits with mother-child pairs in the hospital following delivery, in early childhood (mean age = 3.3 years), and mid-childhood (mean age = 7.8 years). Mothers reported child race/ethnicity in early childhood.

Of the original 2128 mother-child pairs in the cohort, 616 children had mid-childhood plasma total IgE measures. Among those, 242 children had cord blood DNA methylation measurements at birth, 68 had peripheral blood DNA methylation measurement at early childhood, and 411 had peripheral blood DNA methylation measurements at mid-childhood. Two hundred and seventeen children had DNA methylation measurements at both birth and mid-childhood, while 56 had DNA methylation measurements at all three time points (at birth, early childhood, and mid-childhood) (Fig. 2).

DNA methylation measures

Trained personnel collected blood samples at birth (umbilical cord blood) and early and mid-childhood (peripheral blood). DNA was extracted using the Qiagen Puregene Kit (Valencia, CA) and bisulfite converted using the EZ DNA Methylation-Gold Kit (Zymo Research, Irvine, CA). Samples were allocated to chips and plates using a two-stage randomization algorithm and analyzed with Infinium HumanMethylation450 BeadChip (Illumina, San Diego, CA), which includes ~ 485,000 CpG sites at a single nucleotide resolution. In the quality control step, we removed technical replicates, samples with low quality, genotype mismatch, and sex mismatch. At the probe level, low-quality probes with detection P values > 0.05, probes on sex chromosomes, SNP-associated probes, non-CpG probes, and non-specific and previously identified cross-reactive probes were excluded [15]. We further removed probes within 10 base pairs of a known SNP (UCSC Human Feb. 2009 [GRCh37/hg19] Assembly) with a minor allele frequency (MAF) ≥ 1%. After the quality control, a total of 343,208 probes were included for subsequent analysis. We used the normal-exponential out-of-band ("noob") method for background correction and dye bias

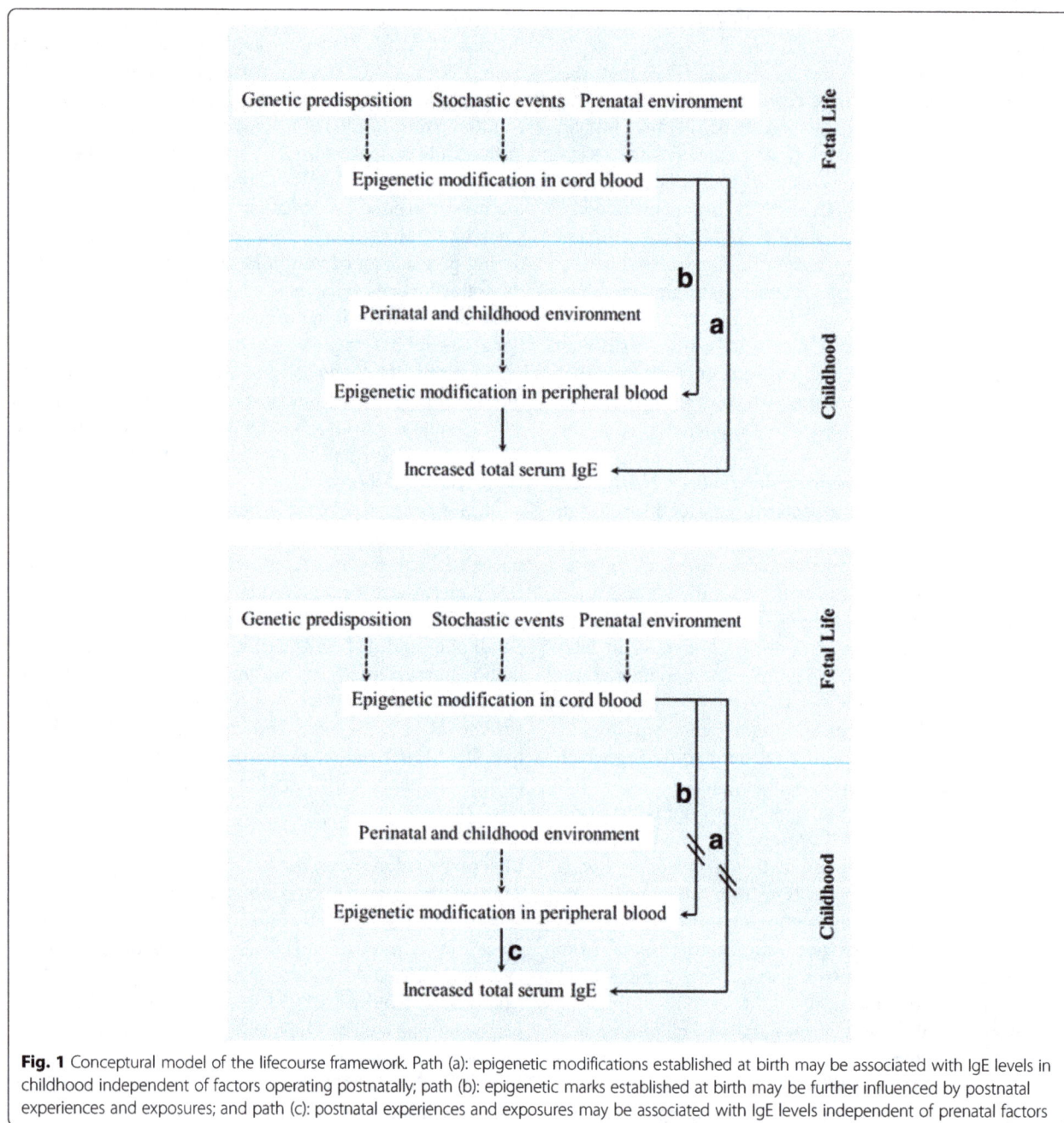

Fig. 1 Conceptual model of the lifecourse framework. Path (a): epigenetic modifications established at birth may be associated with IgE levels in childhood independent of factors operating postnatally; path (b): epigenetic marks established at birth may be further influenced by postnatal experiences and exposures; and path (c): postnatal experiences and exposures may be associated with IgE levels independent of prenatal factors

adjustment [16] and normalized our sample with Beta Mixture Quantile Dilation (BMIQ) [17]. To control for technical variability across sample plates, we applied Combat [18]. We report the percent of methylation for each CpG sites as β values, calculated as the signal intensity of methylated cytosines over the signal intensity of methylated and un-methylated cytosines at the 5C position [β value = M/(M + U)]. In order to control for cell-type heterogeneity, we applied ReFACTor—a reference-free method based on principle component analysis (PCA) with low rank approximation [19]. We chose this method

because ReFACTor components correlate well with measured eosinophil and neutrophil counts [19]. Eosinophils and neutrophils are central effector immune cells that often associate with allergic outcomes. By adequately adjusting for eosinophil and neutrophil counts, we aimed to reduce the influence of changes in eosinophil and neutrophil cellular composition. We computed the first five ReFACTor components in cord blood and the first five ReFACTor components in mid-childhood peripheral blood, and used them in subsequent analysis for the adjustment of cell type composition.

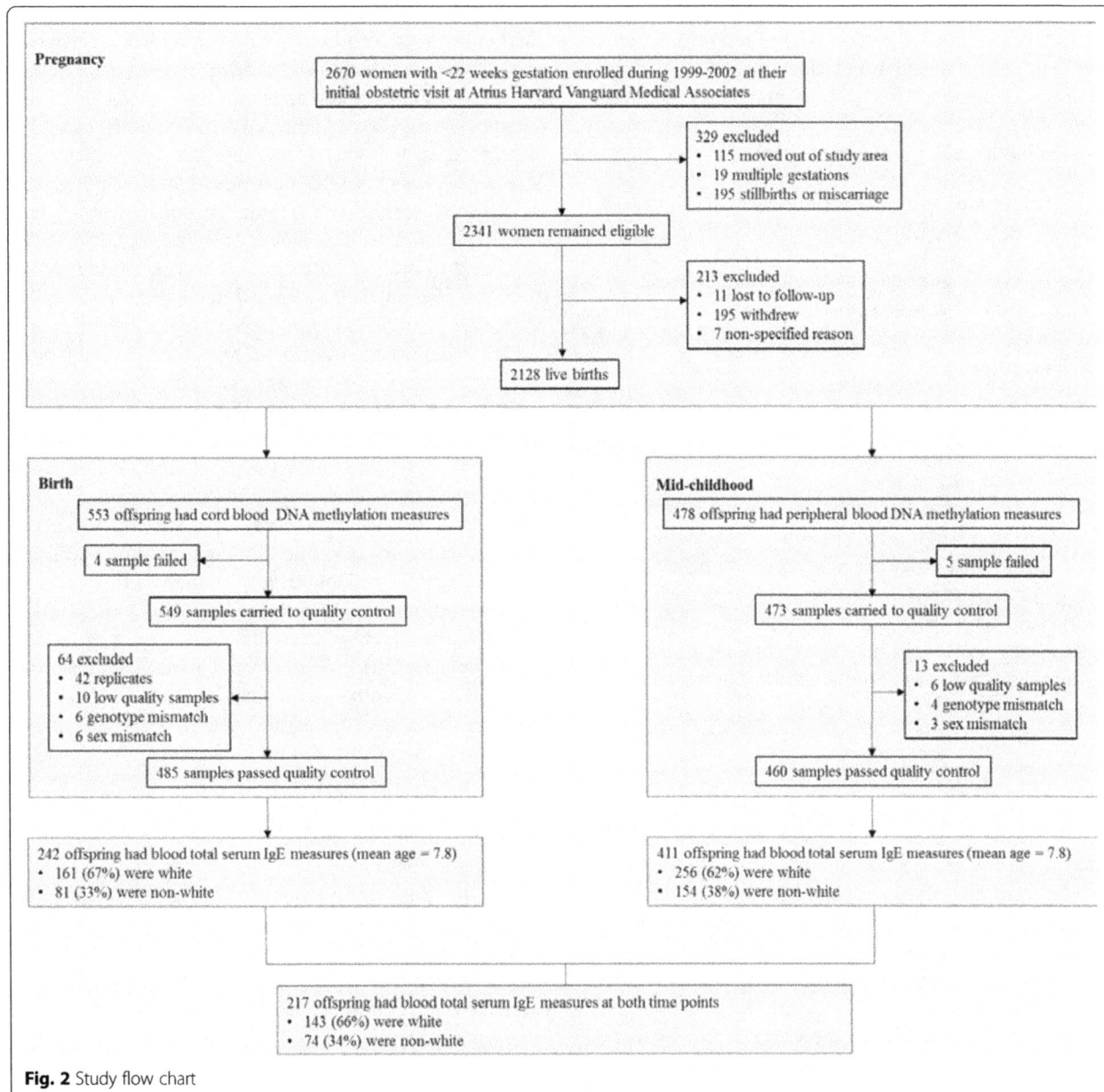

Fig. 2 Study flow chart

Total serum IgE measures

Total serum IgE concentrations were measured in mid-childhood blood using ImmunoCAP (Phadia, Uppsala, Sweden)—a widely used in vitro sandwich immunoassay to quantitatively measure circulating IgE in serum samples.

Statistical analyses

Cord blood DNA methylation and childhood total serum IgE

We evaluated the association of DNA methylation at each individual CpG site in cord blood with total serum IgE measured in mid-childhood using robust linear regression. To remove the influence of extreme methylation outliers, we restricted the methylation values between [25th percentile – 3*IQR] and [75th percentile + 3*IQR], where IQR represents interquantile range. Total serum IgE was natural log-transformed, and model estimates are expressed as the change in the log total serum IgE per 1% increase in methylation values. Regression models were adjusted for the following covariates selected a priori: maternal [age at enrollment (continuous), smoking status (never, former, or during pregnancy), college graduate (yes/no), maternal atopy history (yes/no)], child [sex (female/male), race/ethnicity (white/black/others), gestational age at birth (continuous), age at blood drawn (continuous)], and the first five ReFACTor components computed from cord blood to capture cellular heterogeneity [19]. A methylation site was considered to be epigenome-wide significant if it reached the false discovery rate (FDR)-corrected p value of less than 0.05 based on the method of Benjamini and Hochberg [20]. Additional methylation signals, which were marginally significant (FDR < 0.1), are included in the supplement. The main regression model took the general form:

$$\log(\text{IgE}) = \alpha_0 + \alpha_1 \text{CpG}_{-\text{cbi}} + \alpha_2 X_2 + \ldots + \alpha_p X_p + \varepsilon (\text{Model } 1)$$

where α_0 to the intercept for the population mean, $\alpha_2 X_2 \ldots \alpha_p X_p$ to the covariates we selected a priori, $\alpha_1 \text{CpG}_{-\text{cbi}}$ correspond to ith methylation site in cord blood; ε is the model error term.

Life course analysis

Under the "developmental origins of health and disease" (DOHaD) framework [21], epigenetic endowment from the in utero environment may set the health trajectory of a developing fetus. Hence, some epigenetic marks established at birth may act independently of factors operating after birth and associate with mid-childhood serum IgE. To identify CpG sites that are differentially methylated at birth and not further modified postnatally in our cohort, we considered the following model:

$$\log(\text{IgE}) = \beta_0 + \beta_1 \text{CpG}_{-\text{cbi}} + \beta_2 \Delta \text{CpG}_i + \beta_3 X_3 + \ldots + \beta_p X_p + \eta (\text{Model } 2)$$

where β_0 is the intercept for the population mean, $\beta_3 X_3 \ldots \beta_p X_p$ to the baseline covariates we selected a priori, $\beta_1 \text{CpG}_{-\text{cbi}}$ to the ith methylation site in cord blood measured at birth/baseline, and $\beta_2 \Delta \text{CpG}_i$ corresponds to the difference in DNA methylation at the ith CpG site between cord blood and peripheral blood ($\text{CpG}_{-\text{midchildhoodi}} - \text{CpG}_{-\text{cbi}}$) measured in mid-childhood; η is the model error term.

If we frame this model in the context of a mediation analysis, the term $\text{CpG}_{-\text{cbi}}$ is the direct effect of cord blood methylation on IgE independently of postnatal change in methylation levels. We considered a methylation site to be "early programmed" if $\text{CpG}_{-\text{cbi}}$ reached epigenome-wide significance; a methylation site to capture postnatal environment and experiences if ΔCpG_i reached epigenome-wide significance; and a methylation site to be associated with both prenatal ($\text{CpG}_{-\text{cbi}}$) and postnatal exposure (ΔCpG_i) if both terms remained epigenome-wide significant.

Sensitivity analysis

As a sensitivity analysis, we additionally adjusted for current asthma status at mid-childhood (yes/no) to examine whether the adjustment for asthma would influence our results. We additionally adjusted for asthma status in mid-childhood because (1) children with asthma may have

higher total serum IgE levels compared to non-asthmatic children and (2) children maybe on asthma medication upon diagnosis, which leads to lowered serum IgE levels; for both reasons, asthma status maybe a predictor of our outcome—total serum IgE levels. On the other hand, we did not adjust for other atopic diseases (food allergy and eczema) because both of those variables showed high degree of concordance with asthma (chi-square test p values were both 0.0003). Including highly correlated variables may result in multi-collinearity and decrease model stability. Hence, we only adjust for asthma, a prevalence atopic phenotype in mid-childhood in our dataset (prevalence = 21.7%). We further stratified our analysis by child race/ethnicity (white, non-white) and sex to investigate whether the observed associations were consistent across population strata. We adjusted for white blood cell proportions estimated from blood reference panel [22, 23] and compared the effect estimates with the PCA-based ReFACTor method. We restricted the cord blood analysis to the 217 mother-child pairs who had DNA methylation measures at birth and mid-childhood to examine whether the discrepancy we observe between the cord blood analysis and the life course analysis were driven by a shift in participants' characteristics. We conducted a concurrent analysis among the 210 mother-child pairs who had DNA methylation measures only during mid-childhood and compared results with the postnatal term in the life course analysis. Further, we plotted DNA methylation levels of our top associations at three different time points—birth, early childhood, and mid-childhood ($N = 56$)—to graphically illustrate the change in methylation over time. We also plotted the range of epigenome-wide significant methylation sites identified from the cord blood analysis and the life course analysis.

To investigate the genetic control of methylation for associated CpG sites, we leveraged information from a large-scale genome-wide DNA methylation quantitative trait loci (QTL) analysis of 1000 mother-child pairs to examine whether the differentially methylated sites identified were partly driven by genetic variation (http://www.mqtldb.org/) [24]. The genetic influences on DNA methylation were studied across five different time points in blood in this reference library: maternal [pregnancy, middle-age]; child [at birth, childhood, adolescence]. We focused our mQTL comparisons on the *cis* position (i.e., a genetic variant within ± 500Kb of a methylation locus) measured from cord blood and peripheral blood in childhood. We only considered SNPs with MAF ≥ 5%.

Results

Participants' characteristics

Two-hundred and forty-two children had information on cord blood DNA methylation measurements and mid-childhood total serum IgE measurements (Table 1). Participants included in the current analysis did not differ substantially from the overall Project Viva study population who had serum IgE measures (Additional file 1: Table S1). Ten percent of mothers smoked during pregnancy, and 22% were former smokers (self-reported). Thirty-seven percent of mothers had a history of atopy (which includes asthma, eczema, and hay fever). One hundred and sixty-one children (67%) were white and 117 (48%) were female. Mean ± SD age at blood draw at mid-childhood was 7.8 ± 0.7 years. Total serum IgE levels showed a right-skewed distribution, with a mean ± SD of 146.4 ± 310.2 kU/L. Of the 217 children pairs who had information for both cord blood and mid-childhood DNA methylation measurements, maternal and childhood characteristics did not differ substantially from those who only had DNA methylation measured in cord blood (Table 1).

Cord blood DNA methylation and mid-childhood IgE association

Our epigenome-wide association identified 67 methylated CpG sites (representing 58 annotated genes) in cord blood associated with mid-childhood total serum IgE (FDR < 0.1) (Additional file 1: Table S2; Additional file 2: Figure S1; Fig. 3). These associations include multiple genes that have been implicated in immuno-regulation (*AOAH*, *ALOX5*, *DHX58*, and *STAM2*). Methylation loci associated with obesity (*AEBP2*), calcium signaling (*CAPNS1*), insulin signaling (*INSR*, *PTPRN2*, *RPTOR*) and vasodilation (*VASP*) also appeared to be epigenome-wide significant (Additional file 1: Table S2). With an FDR threshold of less than 0.05, 19 differentially methylated CpG sites located at 18 annotated loci in cord blood showed epigenome-wide significance (Table 2), most of which were involved in cell signaling, growth, and development. We observed minimal inflation in the epigenome-wide association analysis accounting for the first five ReFACTor components (Additional file 2: Figure S2).

Life course analysis
Prenatal influences
We identified 98 differentially methylated CpG sites (located at 82 annotated genes) associated with mid-childhood total serum IgE levels (Additional file 1: Table

Table 1 Descriptive characteristics of study participants in Project Viva with information on DNA methylation and mid-childhood IgE

Participant characteristics	Cord blood DNA methylation data (N = 242)	Mid-childhood DNA methylation data (N = 411)	DNA methylation data at both time points (N = 217)
Maternal characteristics			
Age (years), mean ± SD	32.0 (5.6)	32.3 (5.5)	32.3 (5.4)
Smoking status, N (%)			
Smoked during pregnancy	24 (10%)	41 (10%)	20 (9%)
Former smoker	53 (22%)	83 (20%)	49 (23%)
Never smoker	165 (68%)	287 (70%)	148 (68%)
College graduate, N (%)			
Yes	158 (65%)	271 (66%)*	144 (66%)
No	84 (35%)	138 (34%)	73 (34%)
Atopy history			
Yes	90 (37%)	163 (40%)*	80 (37%)
No	152 (63%)	246 (60%)	137 (63%)
Child characteristics			
Gestational age (weeks), mean ± SD	39.7 (1.6)	39.6 (1.6)	39.7 (1.6)
Age at blood drawn (years), mean ± SD	7.8 (0.7)†	7.8 (0.7)†	7.8 (0.7)
Sex, N (%)			
Female	117 (48%)	201 (49%)	105 (48%)
Male	125 (52%)	210 (51%)	112 (52%)
Race/ethnicity, N (%)			
White	161 (67%)	256 (62%)†	143 (66%)
Black	42 (17%)	77 (19%)	39 (18%)
Other	39 (16%)	77 (19%)	35 (16%)
Total serum IgE level in mid-childhood, (kU/L)	146.4 (310.2)	152.1 (286.2)	142.5 (311.0)

*Number of missing = 2
†Number of missings = 1

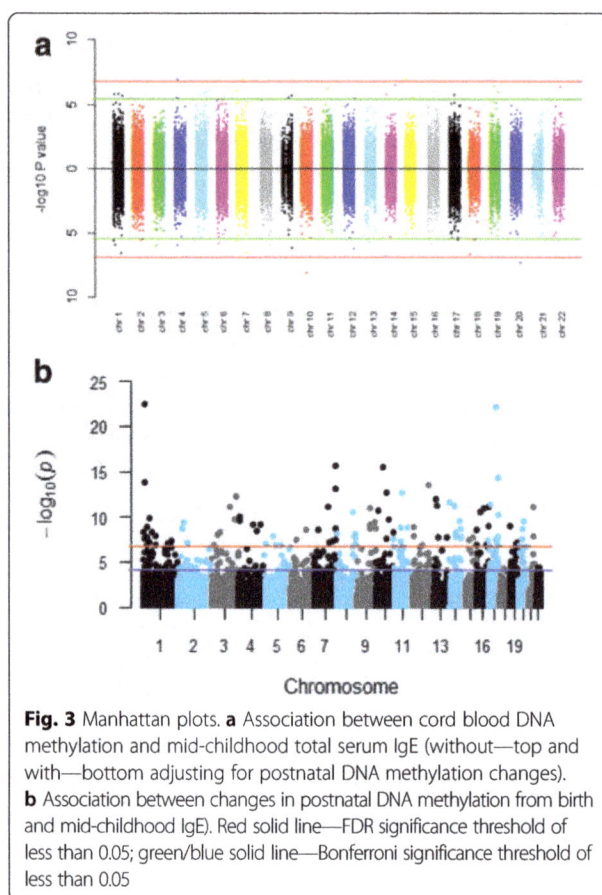

Fig. 3 Manhattan plots. **a** Association between cord blood DNA methylation and mid-childhood total serum IgE (without—top and with—bottom adjusting for postnatal DNA methylation changes). **b** Association between changes in postnatal DNA methylation from birth and mid-childhood IgE). Red solid line—FDR significance threshold of less than 0.05; green/blue solid line—Bonferroni significance threshold of less than 0.05

S3; Additional file 2: Figure S1; Fig. 3), after adjustment for postnatal DNA methylation; 13 methylation sites overlapped with the previous analysis (i.e., showed epigenome-wide significance with and without the adjustment for postnatal DNA methylation changes). The 13 methylation sites are in proximity to/within *ATP10A*, *C22orf45*, *C7orf50*, *DDO*, *INSR*, *KCNIP4*, *LOC100128076*, *MPP2*, *STAM2*, *TGIF1*, *TRIM27*, *XKR6*, and *ZAR1*, respectively (Additional file 1: Table S3). When we further restrict our analysis to an FDR threshold of less than 0.05, we identified 16 differentially methylated CpG sites (FDR < 0.05) located at 15 annotated genes in cord blood associated with mid-childhood total serum IgE levels (Table 3).

Postnatal influences (Δ-DNAm)
We performed an analysis of the change in methylation between cord blood and mid-childhood DNA (Δ-DNAm) and identified 395 differentially methylated sites in 272 independent loci (FDR < 0.05) in blood associated with mid-childhood serum IgE (Additional file 1: Table S4). Table 3 presents the top 20 differentially methylated sites ranked by association *p* value. *ZFPM1*, *ACOT7*, and *MDN1* have been previously associated with total serum

IgE measurements in school-aged children from an independent cohort [12]. Figure 4 shows the regional plot for *ACOT7*—among the FDR-significant CpG sites identified, three of them were located within / close to CpG island of the gene body. Many of the methylation sites we identified have been associated with asthma including *ADAM19*, *EPX*, *IL4*, *IL5RA*, and *PRG2* (Table 4).

Prenatal and postnatal influences
Twenty-two methylation sites showed epigenome-wide significance (FDR < 0.10) for both cord blood and Δ-DNAm (from birth to mid-childhood): including three mitochondrial-related genes associated with the oxidative stress pathway, namely *CS*, *SLC25A26*, and *TOMM34*. With an FDR threshold of less than 0.05, we identified seven differentially methylation sites for both cord blood and Δ-DNAm (Table 3), which include *ASCC1*, *OR4K1*, *FAM20B*, *KCNH2*, *PVT1*, *ARHGAP17*, and *AGPAT1*. In Additional file 1: Table S10, we presented summary statistics of the seven FDR-significant methylation site (FDR < 0.05). We observed higher methylation values in mid-childhood peripheral compared to cord blood among all seven methylation studied (i.e., a positive value for ΔCpG_i). Signs of effect estimates were in the same direction for the prenatal and the postnatal terms.

Sensitivity analysis
Our associations were robust to adjustment for current asthma status, and we observed consistent associations within non-whites and whites, and boys and girls (Additional file 1: Table S5; Additional file 1: Table S6). Further, adjusting for estimated cell proportions from blood, a reference panel did not alter estimates of our top associations identified from the primary analysis (Additional file 1: Table S7; Additional file 2: Figure S5). We observed less genomic inflation with the ReFACTor method (Additional file 2: Figures S2 and S5). Restricting the cord blood analysis to the 217 mother-child pairs who had DNA methylation measures at birth and mid-childhood also did not seem to influence our effect estimates (Additional file 1: Table S8). Among the 210 mother-child pairs who only had DNA methylation measures in mid-childhood, we observed similar effect estimates when we compared the concurrent analysis with the postnatal term of the life course analysis (Additional file 1: Table S11). Our longitudinal plots showed more changes in DNA methylation levels in the first 3 years of life (Additional file 2: Figure S3a; b; c). Even though top hits identified from the epigenome-wide association studies tend to be at the extremes of methylation (either hyper- or hypo-methylated), we still observed a number of methylation sites with greater range of methylation values (Additional file 2: Figure S4).

Among the differentially methylated CpG sites identified in the life course analysis, most of them were not

Table 2 Association between cord blood DNA methylation and mid-childhood IgE (FDR threshold < 0.05). Results are expressed as the change in log(IgE) concentration per 1% increase in cord blood methylation value

CpG	CHR	MAPINFO	Gene	Estimate	P value	FDR
cg06226630	4	48,493,420	ZAR1	− 0.40	1.15E−07	0.013
cg03307893	15	26,108,683	ATP10A	− 0.76	1.20E−07	0.013
cg13322072	7	98,784,083	KPNA7	− 0.11	1.23E−07	0.013
cg16797808	14	99,948,289	SETD3;CCNK	− 0.90	3.18E−07	0.023
cg09535168	19	19,431,582	MAU2	− 1.44	3.91E−07	0.023
cg04122974	22	39,916,495	ATF4	− 3.02	4.46E−07	0.023
cg01527777	11	71,956,145	PHOX2A	− 0.24	6.06E−07	0.027
cg24575275	7	1,094,737	C7orf50	− 0.29	9.23E−07	0.032
cg14920426	5	176,924,420	PDLIM7	− 1.00	1.01E−06	0.032
cg05399209	19	46,010,836	VASP	− 1.33	1.03E−06	0.032
cg09507928	5	140,027,484	IK;NDUFA2	− 2.03	1.46E−06	0.040
cg24114890	14	23,834,349	EFS	− 0.76	1.65E−06	0.040
cg05063806	1	36,772,417	C1orf113	− 1.26	1.79E−06	0.040
cg14167858	1	120,199,593	–	0.10	1.83E−06	0.040
cg02228675	17	40,259,724	DHX58	− 0.27	1.90E−06	0.040
cg14607755	9	139,962,279	C9orf140	− 0.49	2.25E−06	0.044
cg24630419	1	217,311,608	ESRRG	− 0.41	2.49E−06	0.046
cg27212903	15	92,708,880	SLCO3A1	0.97	2.91E−06	0.048
cg14605590	9	94,900,583	LOC100128076	− 0.16	2.93E−06	0.048

Model adjusted for maternal [age at enrollment (continuous), smoking status (smoking during pregnancy/former/never), college graduate (yes/no), maternal atopy history (yes/no)], children [child's sex (female/male), race/ethnicity (white/black/other), gestational age (continuous), age at blood drawn (continuous)], and the cell-type proxys using the first five ReFACTor components estimated from cord blood

Corresponding model: $\log(IgE) = a_0 + a_1 CpG_{-cbi} + a_2 X_2 + \ldots + a_p X_p + \varepsilon$

associated with known genetic variants in the *cis*-position (i.e., ± 500Kb) (Additional file 1: Table S9). We identified four methylation loci with *cis*-mQTL including cg19549714 (*TGIF1*) (childhood peripheral blood), cg18879389 (*TFF2*) (cord blood and childhood peripheral blood), and cg24576940 (*KCNH2*) (cord blood and childhood peripheral blood).

Discussion

To our knowledge, this study is the first epigenome-wide association study to conceptualize IgE-mediated allergic response under an early-childhood life-course framework using longitudinal methylation measured from birth to mid-childhood. Our data show that differential methylation patterns in cord blood are associated with total serum IgE levels in children. A number of associated cord blood methylation signals remained epigenome-wide significant after the adjustment for the change in methylation between cord blood and mid-childhood DNA (Δ-DNAm). Further, change in methylation pattern from cord blood to mid-childhood DNA (Δ-DNAm) may also be associated with total serum IgE levels—independently or in combination with prenatal methylation marks.

It is now recognized that allergic sensitization may occur as early as in utero [5, 6]. Factors such as genetic

predisposition [25, 26], parental atopic status [27–29], and aspects of the intrauterine environment [30–33] including exposures to allergens in amniotic fluid [6] may impact the development of fetal immune responses and Th2 immune responses postnatally. We identified multiple differentially methylated immuno-regulatory loci in cord blood associated with total serum IgE measured in mid-childhood. For example, *AOAH* gene products—released by neutrophils and macrophages—help to neutralize and inactivate bacterial lipopolysaccharides (LPS); *ALOX5* encodes for a lipoxygenase that facilitates leukotriene synthesis—an important inflammatory mediator for allergic reaction; and *DHX58* is involved in antiviral signaling, while *STAM2* responds to cytokine stimulation in the JAK kinase signaling pathway.

In addition to the findings of these immune-regulatory genes, many other top associations have been implicated in obesity (*AEBP2*) (FDR < 0.10), calcium signaling (*CAPNS1*), insulin signaling (*INSR, PTPRN2, RPTOR*), and vasodilation (*VASP*). Abnormal insulin signaling often couples with obesity and increases the risk of asthma and other childhood allergic disorders [34–38], while calcium signaling has a long standing role in hyperpolarization of airway smooth muscle cells—activation of voltage-gated calcium channels may induce airway hyper-responsiveness—a

Table 3 Life course analysis—contribution of fetal and postnatal influences (FDR threshold < 0.05). For the prenatal analysis, results are expressed as the change in log(IgE) concentration per 1% increase in cord blood methylation value. While for the postnatal analysis, results are expressed as the change in log(IgE) concentration per 1% increase in Δ-DNAm methylation value

CpG	CHR	MAPINFO	Gene	Prenatal influences			Postnatal influences (Δ-DNAm)		
				Estimate	P value	FDR	Estimate	P value	FDR
Life course analysis—prenatal influences									
cg25854298	10	73,936,754	ASCC1	− 0.36	8.02E−09	0.003	− 0.40	1.80E−13	6.28E−09
cg16416603	20	57,593,014	TUBB1	0.58	5.17E−08	0.008	0.28	1.32E−04	8.24E−02
cg11848324	14	20,403,845	OR4K1	0.57	1.48E−07	0.016	0.44	3.35E−06	5.26E−03
cg19549714	18	3,447,713	TGIF1	− 2.00	2.40E−07	0.017	− 0.10	4.45E−01	9.71E−01
cg23933289	1	178,998,656	FAM20B	− 0.18	2.66E−07	0.017	− 0.17	8.01E-08	2.54E−04
cg24576940	7	150,648,283	KCNH2	− 1.54	3.31E−07	0.017	− 1.66	2.95E−08	1.10E−04
cg13443997	9	139,743,586	PHPT1	− 3.39	7.11E−07	0.028	− 1.83	1.50E−03	3.32E−01
cg19954205	12	122,211,282	TMEM120B	− 1.20	7.20E−07	0.028	− 0.55	1.72E−02	7.37E−01
cg01782059	1	44,715,942	ERI3	− 0.96	1.25E−06	0.033	− 0.60	4.04E−04	1.69E−01
cg02133716	8	128,981,622	PVT1	− 0.45	1.25E−06	0.033	− 0.54	2.63E−11	3.31E−07
cg06226630	4	48,493,420	ZAR1	− 0.39	1.24E−06	0.033	− 0.02	5.24E−01	9.76E−01
cg20675173	3	43,795,541	–	− 1.22	1.03E−06	0.033	− 0.72	1.11E−03	2.91E−01
cg08067346	16	25,011,481	ARHGAP17	− 0.24	1.44E−06	0.035	− 0.30	2.18E−11	2.85E−07
cg09597192	6	32,141,591	AGPAT1	− 0.31	1.78E−06	0.040	− 0.28	3.70E−06	5.67E−03
cg16096766	13	52,419,714	FLJ37307	− 0.36	2.30E−06	0.048	− 0.19	2.48E−04	1.23E−01
cg00026222	1	2,144,244	–	− 1.02	2.63E−06	0.049	− 0.29	9.59E−02	9.09E−01
cg24575275	7	1,094,737	C7orf50	− 0.31	2.49E−06	0.049	− 0.02	5.23E−01	9.76E−01
Life course analysis—postnatal influences (top 20 methylation sites)									
cg11699125	1	6,341,327	ACOT7	− 0.10	3.29E−02	5.88E−01	− 0.25	2.81E−23	7.95E−18
cg02970679	17	56,269,818	EPX	− 0.17	9.50E−04	2.86E−01	− 0.25	5.06E−23	7.95E−18
cg24491618	7	150,649,807	KCNH2	− 0.12	1.23E−03	3.05E−01	− 0.19	2.12E−16	2.22E−11
cg01614759	10	45,495,435	C10orf25	− 0.17	2.17E−03	3.46E−01	− 0.28	2.97E−16	2.33E−11
cg13054523	17	81,055,722	–	− 0.30	9.45E−05	1.53E−01	−0.43	4.23E−15	2.66E−10
cg21220721	1	6,341,230	ACOT7	0.01	7.03E−01	9.51E−01	− 0.11	1.30E−14	6.81E−10
cg10065736	12	117,440,120	FBXW8	− 0.10	2.28E−02	5.53E−01	− 0.18	2.73E−14	1.23E−09
cg06558622	7	149,543,177	ZNF862	− 0.29	3.37E−05	1.02E−01	− 0.41	8.05E−14	3.16E−09
cg25854298	10	73,936,754	ASCC1	− 0.36	8.02E−09	2.52E−03	− 0.40	1.80E−13	6.28E−09
cg05300717	11	65,546,210	DKFZp761E198	0.0002	9.93E−01	9.99E−01	− 0.33	2.11E−13	6.63E−09
cg09596645	3	181,897,670	–	− 0.15	2.74E−03	3.67E−01	− 0.25	5.56E−13	1.59E−08
cg19928703	13	30,143,971	SLC7A1	− 0.19	3.05E−03	3.75E−01	− 0.31	1.06E−12	2.78E−08
cg18368116	14	21,436,271	–	− 0.13	2.02E−02	5.40E−01	− 0.27	1.91E−12	4.62E−08
cg20885063	17	17,939,419	ATPAF2	− 0.16	1.85E−04	1.90E−01	− 0.23	4.05E−12	9.09E−08
cg08077807	14	62,001,072	PRKCH	− 0.53	7.33E−04	2.63E−01	− 0.76	4.45E−12	9.11E−08
cg07908654	13	41,631,052	–	− 0.20	3.94E−06	5.14E−02	− 0.26	4.64E−12	9.11E−08
cg08940169	16	88,540,241	ZFPM1	− 0.05	1.56E−01	7.57E−01	− 0.18	6.34E−12	1.17E−07
cg18879389	21	43,771,120	TFF2	− 0.16	6.64E−04	2.58E−01	− 0.28	6.73E−12	1.17E−07
cg20263733	3	130,616,293	ATP2C1	− 0.25	4.25E−03	3.99E−01	− 0.50	7.45E−12	1.23E−07
cg02985445	7	97,908,505	–	− 0.08	3.50E−02	5.94E−01	− 0.18	8.09E−12	1.27E−07
Life course analysis—prenatal and postnatal influences									
cg25854298	10	73,936,754	ASCC1	− 0.36	8.02E−09	0.003	− 0.40	1.80E−13	6.28E−09
cg11848324	14	20,403,845	OR4K1	0.57	1.48E−07	0.016	0.44	3.35E−06	0.005

Table 3 Life course analysis—contribution of fetal and postnatal influences (FDR threshold < 0.05). For the prenatal analysis, results are expressed as the change in log(IgE) concentration per 1% increase in cord blood methylation value. While for the postnatal analysis, results are expressed as the change in log(IgE) concentration per 1% increase in Δ-DNAm methylation value *(Continued)*

CpG	CHR	MAPINFO	Gene	Prenatal influences			Postnatal influences (Δ-DNAm)		
				Estimate	P value	FDR	Estimate	P value	FDR
cg23933289	1	178,998,656	FAM20B	− 0.18	2.66E−07	0.017	− 0.17	8.01E−08	2.54E−04
cg24576940	7	150,648,283	KCNH2	− 1.54	3.31E−07	0.017	− 1.66	2.95E−08	1.10 E−04
cg02133716	8	128,981,622	PVT1	− 0.45	1.25E−06	0.033	− 0.54	2.63E−11	3.31E−07
cg08067346	16	25,011,481	ARHGAP17	− 0.24	1.44E−06	0.035	− 0.30	2.18E−11	2.85E−07
cg09597192	6	32,141,591	AGPAT1	− 0.31	1.78E−06	0.040	− 0.28	3.70E−06	0.006

Model adjusted for maternal [age at enrollment (continuous), smoking status (smoking during pregnancy/former/never), college graduate (yes/no), maternal atopy history (yes/no)], children [child's sex (female/male), race (white/black/other), gestational age (continuous), age at blood drawn (continuous)], and the cell-type proxys using the first five ReFACTor components estimated from cord blood

Corresponding model: log(IgE) = $\beta_0 + \beta_1 CpG_{cbl} + \beta_2 \Delta CpG_i + \beta_3 X_3 + \ldots + \beta_p X_p + \eta$

Life course analysis—prenatal influence: association between cord blood methylation and mid-childhood IgE independent of postnatal changes in DNA methylation, which correspond to $\beta_1 CpG_{cbl}$

Life course analysis—postnatal influence: association between changes in postnatal DNA methylation from birth and mid-childhood IgE independent of baseline/cord blood DNA methylation, which correspond to ΔCpG_i

fundamental property of asthma [39]. Although those genes may not be directly involved in immuno-regulation, alterations in these pathways during embryonic development may increase disease susceptibility and make the fetus more prone to the development of IgE-mediated allergic responses later in life.

Leveraging the longitudinal study design of our pre-birth cohort, we aimed to identify differentially methylated sites at birth that are associated with later allergic response and that may or may not be modified postnatally using changes in the epigenome from birth to childhood. We identified 98 differentially methylated CpG sites in cord blood associated with mid-childhood total serum IgE levels, which were independent of changes in DNA methylation postnatally. Thirteen of these methylation sites overlapped with the cord blood analysis where we did not adjust for methylation changes after birth. The fact that methylation levels remained epigenome-wide significant lends support to the DOHaD hypothesis, reinforcing that embryonic development is a vulnerable period with high degree of epigenetic plasticity, and exposures occurring during this period of time may embed epigenetically and could have an effect that persists for decades in life independent of postnatal/childhood influences.

Exposures during early childhood play critical roles in IgE-mediated disease onset and manifestation. We demonstrated that changes in DNA methylation levels from baseline (cord blood) until mid-childhood—potentially an "archive" [40] of the childhood environment—were associated with total serum IgE measures in school-aged children. Specifically, we identified multiple methylation loci in genes previously associated with asthma (*ADAM19*, *EPX*, *IL4*, *IL5RA*, and *PRG2*) from genome-wide and epigenome-wide association studies [10–12, 26]. Many of those methylation sites have been

previously reported in independent large adult cohorts (*EPX*, *IL4*, *IL5RA*, and *PRG2*) [10, 11]. IL4 and IL5RA are well-characterized cytokines responsible for Th2 cell differentiation and effector function, ADAM19 is involved in airway and vasculature remodeling, and PRG2 and EPX are both eosinophil-related proteins that play key roles in eosinophil-related airway inflammation. PRG2 is a major protein component of the crystalline core of the eosinophil granule and is involved in epithelial cell damage, mast cell degranulation, and macrophage and neutrophil activation. EPX is a key peroxidase enzyme in the eosinophil granules, which helps to generate potent oxidizing agents directly implicated in oxidative damage processes. It is not surprising that we identified those well-established IgE-related methylation signals in the postnatal analysis—as children are exposed to a more diverse environment after birth including increased allergen exposures. Hence, we were able to identify a large number of signals related to allergic symptoms and disease manifestation. Moreover, most of these genes identified in the postnatal analysis did not overlap with the baseline signals, which suggests that the fetal environment may not necessarily be associated with disease manifestation; rather, it may help to direct the development of fetal immunity and alters disease susceptibility. Future research is warranted to explore whether the identified methylation marks are on the causal pathway linking in utero and early-life risk factors (i.e., living in rural versus urban areas, having siblings or not, attending daycare or not, antibiotic use, pets at home) and higher total serum IgE levels.

We observed that seven methylation sites showed epigenome-wide significance at both baseline and postnatally (Δ-DNAm). Among these *KCNH2* encodes for a voltage-gated K⁺ channel, *PVT1* is a candidate oncogene and *ARHGAP17* encodes for a GTPase-activating

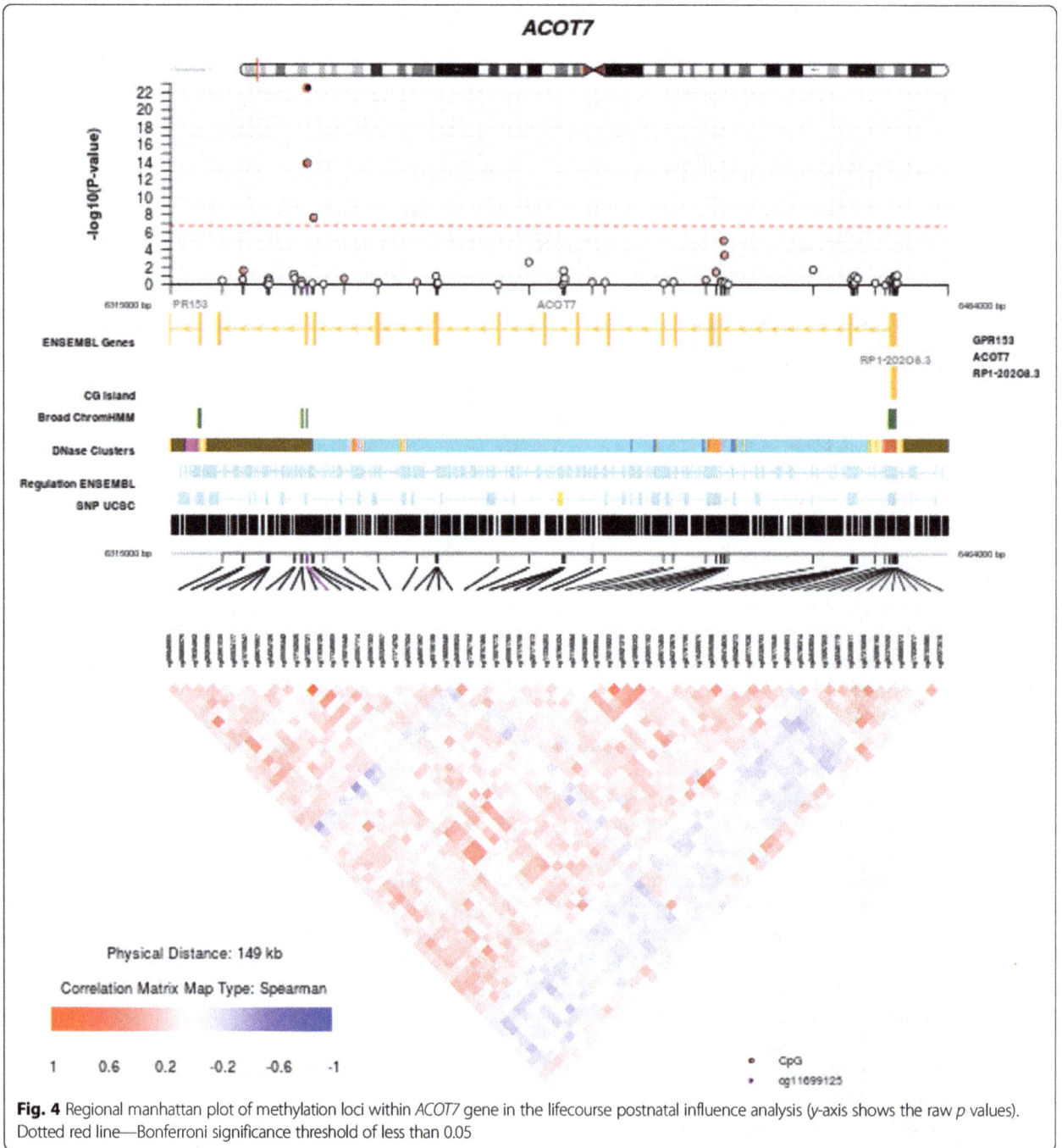

Fig. 4 Regional manhattan plot of methylation loci within *ACOT7* gene in the lifecourse postnatal influence analysis (*y*-axis shows the raw *p* values). Dotted red line—Bonferroni significance threshold of less than 0.05

protein, which participates in the Ca²⁺ dependent regulation of exocytosis. With an FDR threshold less than 0.10, we identified 22 methylation sites (15 additional); several of these genes have been implicated in mitochondrial function (*TOMM34*, *CS*, *SLC25A26*). Mitochondria are critical cellular components that reflect and intensify oxidative stress [41]. Epigenetic alterations in nuclear-encoded mitochondrial genes at both time windows suggest that intrauterine and postnatal cellular oxidative stress may be associated with higher total serum IgE in mid-childhood. A handful of observational studies and clinical trials have shown that maternal antioxidant intake was associated with reduced allergic symptoms in children [33, 42–47], and antioxidant intake during pregnancy and early in life may potentially serves as a first-line preventive regimen to avert childhood allergy.

Since DNA methylation was measured at birth and early and mid-childhood, it would be interesting to explore how methylation patterns change in children who

Table 4 Life course analysis— contribution of fetal and postnatal influences (FDR threshold < 0.05)—asthma pathway. For the prenatal analysis, results are expressed as the change in log(IgE) concentration per 1% increase in cord blood methylation value. While for the postnatal analysis, results are expressed as the change in log(IgE) concentration per 1% increase in Δ-DNAm methylation value

CpG	CHR	MAPINFO	Gene	Prenatal influences			Postnatal influences		
				Estimate	P value	FDR	Estimate	P value	FDR
Life course analysis—postnatal influences (asthma pathway)									
cg26787239	5	132,008,525	IL4	− 0.12	9.00E−02	6.91E−01	− 0.18	1.94E−05	0.020
cg01310029	3	3,152,374	IL5RA	− 0.09	7.48E−02	6.73E−01	− 0.18	3.55E−06	0.005
cg02970679	17	56,269,818	EPX	− 0.17	9.50E−04	2.86E−01	− 0.25	5.06E−23	7.95E−18
cg25173129	17	56,269,410	EPX	− 0.16	5.73E−03	4.22E−01	− 0.22	2.59E−08	9.80E−05
cg27469152	17	56,282,313	EPX	− 0.10	5.02E−02	6.32E−01	− 0.19	2.59E−07	6.53E−04
cg18421167	17	56,276,490	EPX	− 0.09	2.38E−01	8.07E−01	− 0.25	1.83E−06	0.003
cg08105265	17	56,274,480	EPX	− 0.04	6.46E−01	9.40E−01	− 0.22	1.55E−05	0.017
cg12819873	11	57,157,632	PRG2	− 0.12	8.55E−03	4.60E−01	− 0.23	1.21E−09	9.05E−06
cg15700636	11	57,156,050	PRG2	− 0.08	3.19E−02	5.85E−01	− 0.18	4.13E−08	1.46E−04
cg08295410	5	156,990,663	ADAM19	− 0.31	4.79E−03	4.09E−01	− 0.40	2.70E−05	0.026

Model adjusted for maternal [age at enrollment (continuous), smoking status (smoking during pregnancy/former/never), college graduate (yes/no), maternal atopy history (yes/no)], children [child's sex (female/male), race (white/black/other), gestational age (continuous), age at blood drawn (continuous)], and the cell-type proxys using the first five ReFACTor components estimated from cord blood

Corresponding model: $\log(IgE) = \beta_0 + \beta_1 CpG_{\_cbi} + \beta_2 \Delta CpGi + \beta_3 X_3 + \ldots + \beta_p X_p + \eta$

Life course analysis—prenatal influence: association between cord blood methylation and mid-childhood IgE independent of postnatal changes in DNA methylation, which correspond to $\beta_1 CpG_{\_cbi}$;

Life course analysis—postnatal influence: association between changes in postnatal DNA methylation from birth and mid-childhood IgE independent of baseline/cord blood DNA methylation, which correspond to ΔCpG_i

have persistent atopy versus those who transition to a nonatopic state. We computed a two-by-two table of atopic sensitization at early and mid-childhood. We found that 76% of children were sensitized at both time points; only 5% of children ($N = 15$) are no longer atopic by age 8. Such small sample size would make any statistical inference unreliable. It is widely accepted that there is an age-dependent allergic march during childhood [48–50], beginning with food allergy and atopic dermatitis (infancy to early-childhood), followed by asthma and rhinitis (early/mid-childhood to teen) [48–50]. Since we have methylation measurements at birth and early and mid-childhood, the ideal phenotype to study would be food allergy [51, 52]. However, food allergy was only measured at mid-childhood in Project Viva. A transition from early to mid-childhood may not be the right time window to capture subjects no longer categorized as having atopy or asthma phenotypes. Future research is needed to identify differential methylation patterns associated with transient and persistent subtypes at appropriate developmental windows.

Our study has a number of strengths including the longitudinal nature of our analyses that enabled us to conceptualize IgE-mediated disease etiology under an early-childhood life-course framework. We identified some distinct and some overlapping methylation marks at birth and postnatally that potentially reflect IgE-mediated disease sensitization, progression, and manifestation. Most of these methylation sites identified in the life course analysis

were not associated with known genetic variants in the *cis*-position (i.e., ± 500Kb), and thus were likely to be related to endogenous or exogenous exposures. Our results were robust to the adjustment for batch, cell proportions, and maternal atopy history. Although we did not have external replication for our current analysis, many of our top findings have been previously reported in independent cohorts (with comparable effect estimates and direction of effect) [11, 12], suggesting that the observed associations were robust signals and are not cohort specific.

Our study has several limitations. First, we measured DNA methylation from heterogeneous blood cells at birth and in mid-childhood. Different cell types often exhibits distinct DNA methylation patterns, and if the change in relative cell abundance also correlates with total serum IgE measures in mid-childhood, then our observed associations may potentially be confounded by cellular heterogeneity. Although we adjusted for the first five PCs of ReFACTor— a stringent way to control for cell heterogeneity—we cannot rule out the possibility of residual confounding. Future analysis with relevant purified cell types might help elucidate the immune roots for the observed associations. Second, we do not have genetic information on mother-child pairs. Hence, it is difficult to disentangle the influence of genetics and the environment. Even though we studied the genetic control of selected methylation loci using mQTL information from an independent cohort with relatively large sample size ($N = 1000$) [24], obtaining genetic information from our own population will further elucidate whether the identified methylation marks reflect genetic predisposition, the impact of the intrauterine, postnatal and childhood environments, or an interaction of the two.

Conclusion

In summary, leveraging the epigenetic plasticity from the prenatal period till childhood, our work identified differentially methylated patterns—in cord blood, as well as in changes in methylation levels from cord blood to mid-childhood DNA—associated with mid-childhood IgE. Several cord blood methylation marks associated with IgE that were independently of postnatal change in methylation levels. Further, change in methylation pattern from cord blood to mid-childhood DNA were associated with IgE—independently or in combination with cord blood methylation marks. Our study provides evidence for the epigenetic regulatory mechanism of IgE-mediated diseases and offers a scientific basis to promote early prevention of IgE-mediated diseases.

Additional files

Additional file 1: Table S1. Descriptive characteristics of study participants in Project Viva. **Table S2.** Association between cord blood DNA methylation and mid-childhood IgE (FDR threshold < 0.10). **Table S3.** Life course analysis—contribution of fetal influences (FDR threshold < 0.10). **Table S4.** Life course analysis—contribution of postnatal influences (FDR threshold < 0.10). **Table S5.** Stratified analysis of methylation sites identified in the cord blood DNA methylation and mid-childhood IgE analysis. **Table S6.** Stratified analysis of methylation sites identified in the life course analysis. **Table S7.** Association between cord blood DNA methylation and mid-childhood IgE (FDR threshold < 0.05)—we estimated cell proportions using blood reference panels for cord blood. Results are expressed as the change in log(IgE) concentration per 1% increase in cord blood methylation value. **Table S8.** Association between cord blood DNA methylation and mid-childhood IgE (FDR threshold < 0.05) among the 217 children who had DNA methylation measurements both at birth and in mid-childhood. **Table S9.** Genetic influences on DNA methylation of selected top hits—results from mQTL from an independent cohort. **Table S10.** Summary statistics of selected methylation sites and their sign of associations for the prenatal and postnatal influences. **Table S11.** Association between mid-childhood peripheral blood DNA methylation and mid-childhood IgE (FDR threshold < 0.05) among the 210 children who had DNA methylation measurements both at mid-childhood only (top 20 methylation sites). (PDF 2172 kb)

Additional file 2: Figure S1. Scatter plot (cord blood DNA methylation and mid-childhood total serum IgE). Scatter plot (life course analysis: prenatal influence—top 6 methylation sites). Scatter plot (life course analysis: postnatal influences—top 6 methylation sites). Scatter plot (life course analysis: postnatal influences (asthma pathway)—top 6 methylation sites). Scatter plot (life course analysis—contribution of prenatal and postnatal influences—top 6 methylation sites). **Figure S2.** QQ plots. **Figure S3a.** Trend of top hits (reflect life course analysis—prenatal influence) (N = 56). **Figure S3b.** Trend of top hits (reflect life course analysis—prenatal and postnatal influence) (N = 56). **Figure S3c.** Trend of top hits (reflect life course analysis—postnatal influence) (N = 56). **Figure S4.** Distribution of the range of epigenome-wide significant methylation sites identified from the cord blood analysis and the life course analysis. **Figure S5.** QQ plot of cord blood analysis using blood reference panel to adjust for cellular heterogeneity. (PDF 330 kb)

Abbreviations

CpG: Cytosine-guanine dinucleotide sequence; FDR: False discovery rate; IgE: Immunoglobulin E; IQR: Interquantile range; kb: Kilo-bases; MAF: Minor allele frequency; QTL: Quantitative trait locus; ReFACTor: Reference free adjustment for cell-type composition; SD: Standard deviation; SNP: Single nucleotide polymorphism

Acknowledgements

The authors would like to thank all the Project Viva participants.

Funding

This study is supported by grants from the National Institutes of Health (R01 HL 111108, R01 NR013945, P01 HL 105339, P01 HL 114501, P01 132825, K24 HD069408, R01 HD034568, R01 AI102960).

Authors' contributions

CP, DLD, and AAL contributed to the study concept and design; CP, DLD, AAL, AAB, EO, DRG, TAP, MFH, and SLR helped in the acquisition of data. CP, DLD, AAL, XL, AC, and SLR performed the analysis and interpretation of data. CP, DLD, and AAL drafted the manuscript. CP, AC, SLR, MFH, DRG, TAP, XL, EO, AAB, AAL, and DLD approved the final manuscript draft. All authors read and approved the final manuscript.

Competing interests

The authors have declared that they have no conflict of interest.

Author details

[1]Channing Division of Network Medicine and the Division of Pulmonary and Critical Care Medicine, Department of Medicine, Brigham and Women's Hospital, Harvard Medical School, 181 Longwood Avenue, 4th Floor, Boston, MA 02115, USA. [2]Division of Chronic Disease Research Across the Lifecourse, Department of Population Medicine, Harvard Medical School and Harvard Pilgrim Health Care Institute, Boston, MA, USA. [3]Diabetes Unit, Massachusetts General Hospital, Boston, MA, USA. [4]Department of Environmental Health, Harvard T. H. Chan School of Public Health, Boston, MA, USA. [5]Division of Allergy and Clinical Immunology, University of Virginia School of Medicine, Charlottesville, VA, USA. [6]Department of Biostatistics, Harvard T. H. Chan School of Public Health, Boston, MA, USA. [7]Department of Environmental Health Sciences, Columbia University Mailman School of Public Health, New York, NY, USA.

References

1. Galli SJ, Tsai M, Piliponsky AM. The development of allergic inflammation. Nature. 2008;454(7203):445–54.
2. Kay AB. Allergy and allergic diseases. First of two parts. N Engl J Med. 2001; 344(1):30–7.
3. Gould HJ, Sutton BJ. IgE in allergy and asthma today. Nat Rev Immunol. 2008;8(3):205–17.
4. Galli SJ, Tsai M. IgE and mast cells in allergic disease. Nat Med. 2012;18(5): 693–704.
5. Warner JO. The early life origins of asthma and related allergic disorders. Arch Dis Child. 2004;89(2):97–102.
6. Warner JA, Warner JO. Early life events in allergic sensitisation. Br Med Bull. 2000;56(4):883–93.

7. Holgate ST, Polosa R. Treatment strategies for allergy and asthma. Nat Rev Immunol. 2008;8(3):218–30.

8. Feil R, Fraga MF. Epigenetics and the environment: emerging patterns and implications. Nat Rev Genet. 2012;13(2):97–109.

9. Reik W. Stability and flexibility of epigenetic gene regulation in mammalian development. Nature. 2007;447(7143):425–32.

10. Liang L, Willis-Owen SA, Laprise C, Wong KC, Davies GA, Hudson TJ, et al. An epigenome-wide association study of total serum immunoglobulin E concentration. Nature. 2015;520(7549):670–4.

11. Ek WE, Ahsan M, Rask-Andersen M, Liang L, Moffatt MF, Gyllensten U, et al. Epigenome-wide DNA methylation study of IgE concentration in relation to self-reported allergies. Epigenomics. 2017;9(4):407–418. https://doi.org/10.2217/epi-2016-0158. Epub 2017 Mar 21.

12. Chen W, Wang T, Pino-Yanes M, Forno E, Liang L, Yan Q, et al. An epigenome-wide association study of total serum IgE in Hispanic children. J Allergy Clin Immunol. 2017;140(2):571–577. https://doi.org/10.1016/j.jaci.2016.11.030. Epub 2017 Jan 6.

13. Everson TM, Lyons G, Zhang H, Soto-Ramirez N, Lockett GA, Patil VK, et al. DNA methylation loci associated with atopy and high serum IgE: a genome-wide application of recursive random Forest feature selection. Genome Med. 2015;7:89.

14. Ben-Shlomo Y, Kuh D. A life course approach to chronic disease epidemiology: conceptual models, empirical challenges and interdisciplinary perspectives. Int J Epidemiol. 2002;31(2):285–93.

15. Chen YA, Lemire M, Choufani S, Butcher DT, Grafodatskaya D, Zanke BW, et al. Discovery of cross-reactive probes and polymorphic CpGs in the Illumina Infinium HumanMethylation450 microarray. Epigenetics. 2013;8(2):203–9.

16. Triche TJ Jr, Weisenberger DJ, Van Den Berg D, Laird PW, Siegmund KD. Low-level processing of Illumina Infinium DNA Methylation BeadArrays. Nucleic Acids Res. 2013;41(7):e90.

17. Teschendorff AE, Marabita F, Lechner M, Bartlett T, Tegner J, Gomez-Cabrero D, et al. A beta-mixture quantile normalization method for correcting probe design bias in Illumina Infinium 450 k DNA methylation data. Bioinformatics. 2013;29(2):189–96.

18. Johnson WE, Li C, Rabinovic A. Adjusting batch effects in microarray expression data using empirical Bayes methods. Biostatistics. 2007;8(1):118–27.

19. Rahmani E, Zaitlen N, Baran Y, Eng C, Hu D, Galanter J, et al. Sparse PCA corrects for cell type heterogeneity in epigenome-wide association studies. Nat Methods. 2016;13(5):443–5.

20. Benjamini Yoav HY. Controlling the false discovery rate: a practical and powerful approach to multiple testing. J R Stat Soc Ser B Methodol. 1995;57(1):289–300.

21. Barker DJ, Osmond C. Infant mortality, childhood nutrition, and ischaemic heart disease in England and Wales. Lancet. 1986;1(8489):1077–81.

22. Bakulski KM, Feinberg JI, Andrews SV, Yang J, Brown S, L McKenney S, et al. DNA methylation of cord blood cell types: applications for mixed cell birth studies. Epigenetics. 2016;11(5):354–62.

23. Cardenas A, Allard C, Doyon M, Houseman EA, Bakulski KM, Perron P, et al. Validation of a DNA methylation reference panel for the estimation of nucleated cells types in cord blood. Epigenetics. 2016;11(11):773–9.

24. Gaunt TR, Shihab HA, Hemani G, Min JL, Woodward G, Lyttleton O, et al. Systematic identification of genetic influences on methylation across the human life course. Genome Biol. 2016;17:61.

25. Holgate ST, Wenzel S, Postma DS, Weiss ST, Renz H, Sly PD. Asthma. Nat Rev Dis Primers. 2015;1:15025.

26. Cookson W. The alliance of genes and environment in asthma and allergy. Nature. 1999;402(6760 Suppl):B5–11.

27. Litonjua AA, Carey VJ, Burge HA, Weiss ST, Gold DR. Parental history and the risk for childhood asthma. Does mother confer more risk than father? Am J Respir Crit Care Med. 1998;158(1):176–81.

28. Jaakkola JJ, Nafstad P, Magnus P. Environmental tobacco smoke, parental atopy, and childhood asthma. Environ Health Perspect. 2001;109(6):579–82.

29. Oddy WH, Peat JK, de Klerk NH. Maternal asthma, infant feeding, and the risk of asthma in childhood. J Allergy Clin Immunol. 2002;110(1):65–7.

30. Beckhaus AA, Garcia-Marcos L, Forno E, Pacheco-Gonzalez RM, Celedon JC, Castro-Rodriguez JA. Maternal nutrition during pregnancy and risk of asthma, wheeze, and atopic diseases during childhood: a systematic review and meta-analysis. Allergy. 2015;70(12):1588–604.

31. Willers SM, Devereux G, Craig LC, McNeill G, Wijga AH, Abou El-Magd W, et al. Maternal food consumption during pregnancy and asthma, respiratory and atopic symptoms in 5-year-old children. Thorax. 2007;62(9):773–9.

32. Devereux G, Turner SW, Craig LC, McNeill G, Martindale S, Harbour PJ, et al. Low maternal vitamin E intake during pregnancy is associated with asthma in 5-year-old children. Am J Respir Crit Care Med. 2006;174(5):499–507.

33. Devereux G, Litonjua AA, Turner SW, Craig LC, McNeill G, Martindale S, et al. Maternal vitamin D intake during pregnancy and early childhood wheezing. Am J Clin Nutr. 2007;85(3):853–9.

34. Forno E, Han YY, Muzumdar RH, Celedon JC. Insulin resistance, metabolic syndrome, and lung function in US adolescents with and without asthma. J Allergy Clin Immunol. 2015;136(2):304–11. e8.

35. Rastogi D, Bhalani K, Hall CB, Isasi CR. Association of pulmonary function with adiposity and metabolic abnormalities in urban minority adolescents. Ann Am Thorac Soc. 2014;11(5):744–52.

36. Davidson WJ, Mackenzie-Rife KA, Witmans MB, Montgomery MD, Ball GD, Egbogah S, et al. Obesity negatively impacts lung function in children and adolescents. Pediatr Pulmonol. 2014;49(10):1003–10.

37. Rastogi D, Fraser S, Oh J, Huber AM, Schulman Y, Bhagtani RH, et al. Inflammation, metabolic dysregulation, and pulmonary function among obese urban adolescents with asthma. Am J Respir Crit Care Med. 2015;191(2):149–60.

38. Weiss ST. Obesity: insight into the origins of asthma. Nat Immunol. 2005;6(6):537–9.

39. Barnes PJ. Calcium-channel blockers and asthma. Thorax. 1983;38(7):481–5.

40. Heijmans BT, Tobi EW, Stein AD, Putter H, Blauw GJ, Susser ES, et al. Persistent epigenetic differences associated with prenatal exposure to famine in humans. Proc Natl Acad Sci U S A. 2008;105(44):17046–9.

41. Yakes FM, Van Houten B. Mitochondrial DNA damage is more extensive and persists longer than nuclear DNA damage in human cells following oxidative stress. Proc Natl Acad Sci U S A. 1997;94(2):514–9.

42. Litonjua AA, Rifas-Shiman SL, Ly NP, Tantisira KG, Rich-Edwards JW, Camargo CA Jr, et al. Maternal antioxidant intake in pregnancy and wheezing illnesses in children at 2 y of age. Am J Clin Nutr. 2006;84(4):903–11.

43. West CE, Dunstan J, McCarthy S, Metcalfe J, D'Vaz N, Meldrum S, et al. Associations between maternal antioxidant intakes in pregnancy and infant allergic outcomes. Nutrients. 2012;4(11):1747–58.

44. Martindale S, McNeill G, Devereux G, Campbell D, Russell G, Seaton A. Antioxidant intake in pregnancy in relation to wheeze and eczema in the first two years of life. Am J Respir Crit Care Med. 2005;171(2):121–8.

45. Litonjua AA, Carey VJ, Laranjo N, Harshfield BJ, McElrath TF, O'Connor GT, et al. Effect of prenatal supplementation with vitamin D on asthma or recurrent wheezing in offspring by age 3 years: the VDAART randomized clinical trial. JAMA. 2016;315(4):362–70.

46. Chawes BL, Bonnelykke K, Stokholm J, Vissing NH, Bjarnadottir E, Schoos AM, et al. Effect of vitamin D3 supplementation during pregnancy on risk of persistent wheeze in the offspring: a randomized clinical trial. JAMA. 2016;315(4):353–61.

47. Bisgaard H, Stokholm J, Chawes BL, Vissing NH, Bjarnadottir E, Schoos AM, et al. Fish oil-derived fatty acids in pregnancy and wheeze and asthma in offspring. N Engl J Med. 2016;375(26):2530–9.

48. Barnetson RS, Rogers M. Childhood atopic eczema. BMJ. 2002;324(7350):1376–9.

49. Bantz SK, Zhu Z, Zheng T. The atopic march: progression from atopic dermatitis to allergic rhinitis and asthma. J Clin Cell Immunol. 2014;5(2). https://doi.org/10.4172/2155-9899.1000202.

50. Zheng T, Yu J, Oh MH, Zhu Z. The atopic march: progression from atopic dermatitis to allergic rhinitis and asthma. Allergy Asthma Immunol Res. 2011;3(2):67–73.

51. Syed A, Garcia MA, Lyu SC, Bucayu R, Kohli A, Ishida S, et al. Peanut oral immunotherapy results in increased antigen-induced regulatory T-cell function and hypomethylation of forkhead box protein 3 (FOXP3). J Allergy Clin Immunol. 2014;133(2):500–10.

52. Martino D, Dang T, Sexton-Oates A, Prescott S, Tang ML, Dharmage S, et al. Blood DNA methylation biomarkers predict clinical reactivity in food-sensitized infants. J Allergy Clin Immunol. 2015;135(5):1319–28. e1-12.

15

Identification and validation of SRY-box containing gene family member *SOX30* methylation as a prognostic and predictive biomarker in myeloid malignancies

Jing-dong Zhou[1,2†], Yu-xin Wang[3†], Ting-juan Zhang[1,2†], Xi-xi Li[1,2], Yu Gu[1,2], Wei Zhang[1,2], Ji-chun Ma[2,4], Jiang Lin[2,4*] and Jun Qian[1,2*]

Abstract

Background: Methylation-associated *SOX* family genes have been proved to be involved in multiple essential processes during carcinogenesis and act as potential biomarkers for cancer diagnosis, staging, prediction of prognosis, and monitoring of response to therapy. Herein, we revealed *SOX30* methylation and its clinical implication in acute myeloid leukemia (AML) and myelodysplastic syndromes (MDS).

Results: In the discovery stage, we identified that *SOX30* methylation, a frequent event in AML, was negatively associated with *SOX30* expression and correlated with overall survival (OS) and leukemia-free survival (LFS) in cytogenetically normal AML among *SOX* family members from The Cancer Genome Atlas (TCGA) datasets. In the validation stage, we verified that *SOX30* methylation level was significantly higher in AML even in MDS-derived AML compared to controls, whereas *SOX30* hypermethylation was not a frequent event in MDS. *SOX30* methylation was inversely correlated with *SOX30* expression in AML patients. Survival analysis showed that *SOX30* hypermethylation was negatively associated with complete remission (CR), OS, and LFS in AML, where it only affected LFS in MDS. Notably, among MDS/AML paired patients, *SOX30* methylation level was significantly increased in AML stage than in MDS stage. In addition, *SOX30* methylation was found to be significantly decreased in AML achieved CR when compared to diagnosis time and markedly increased in relapsed AML when compared to the CR population.

Conclusions: Our findings revealed that *SOX30* methylation was associated with disease progression in MDS and acted as an independent prognostic and predictive biomarker in AML.

Keywords: *SOX30*, Methylation, Biomarker, MDS, AML

Background

Acute myeloid leukemia (AML) and myelodysplastic syndromes (MDS) are common clonal disorders in myeloid malignancies. AML is etiologically, biologically, and clinically heterogeneous disease characterized by the accumulation of excessive blasts [1], whereas MDS is characterized by ineffective hematopoiesis and has a tendency to evolve into AML [2]. Cytogenetic and molecular analyses can identify recurrent chromosomal aberrations, gene mutations, and abnormal gene expression, which are associated with MDS/AML pathogenesis, response to therapy and prognosis [3, 4]. Despite recent progresses and advancements made in the understanding of disease biology and the personalized and precision treatment regimen, clinical outcome of AML even the MDS-derived AML remains unsatisfactory [1, 2]. Thus, the identification of underlying molecular events which correlated with disease progression and prognosis could make a better understanding of cancer pathogenesis and

* Correspondence: linjiangmail@sina.com; 2651329493@qq.com; qianjun0007@hotmail.com

†Jing-dong Zhou, Yu-xin Wang and Ting-juan Zhang contributed equally to this work.

²The Key Lab of Precision Diagnosis and Treatment of Zhenjiang City, Zhenjiang, Jiangsu, People's Republic of China

¹Department of Hematology, Affiliated People's Hospital of Jiangsu University, 8 Dianli Rd, 212002 Zhenjiang, People's Republic of China

Full list of author information is available at the end of the article

improve treatment outcome by the use of molecular risk-adapted treatment strategies [5].

DNA methylation, a common type of epigenetic DNA modification, plays a crucial role in maintenance of genome integrity, genomic imprinting, transcriptional regulation, and developmental processes [6]. In human cancers, aberrant DNA methylation is known to contribute to various biological processes of cancer development including initiation, promotion, invasion, metastases, and chemotherapy resistance [7]. Clinically, aberrant methylation in cancer-related genes acts as potential biomarkers for diagnosis, staging, prediction of prognosis, and monitoring of response to therapy [7]. As for myeloid malignancies, studies showed that aberrant DNA methylation was a dominant mechanism in MDS progression to AML [8]. For example, our previous investigation revealed that epigenetic dysregulation of *ID4*, which exhibited anti-proliferation and pro-apoptosis effects in leukemia cells, and predicted disease progression and treatment outcome in myeloid malignancies [9].

SOX [sex-determining region Y (SRY) box-containing] genes encode transcription factors belonging to the HMG (High Mobility Group) superfamily [10]. There are, at least, 19 members (*SOX1-15, SOX17, SOX18, SOX21, SOX30*) divided into eight groups (from A to H), based on their HMG sequence identity in humans [10]. The SOX genes have emerged as modulators of canonical Wnt/β-catenin signaling and have been attributed to their properties involving in the regulation of cell differentiation, proliferation, and survival in multiple essential processes during carcinogenesis [11]. Although most *SOX* genes show a property of oncogenes in various cancers, different members of the *SOX* gene family may play distinct roles in different types of cancers including hematological malignancies: some of them show an oncogenic role contributing to cancer development, whereas others act as a tumor suppressor gene to block the growth of cancers [12]. For instance, *SOX4* overexpression resulting from C/EBPα inactivation or cooperating with CREB contributed to the development of AML [13, 14]. Man et al. reported that methylation-dependent *SOX7* was a novel tumor suppressor in AML via a negative modulatory effect on the Wnt/β-catenin pathway [15]. Moreover, *SOX12* exhibited pro-proliferative effect involved in leukemogenesis by regulating the expression of β-catenin and then interfering with TCF/Wnt pathway [16]. Our previous study also showed that reduced *SOX17* expression was associated with adverse prognosis in cytogenetically normal AML (CN-AML) [17].

In this study, we examined the methylation pattern and clinical significance of *SOX30* in AML and MDS. *SOX30* methylation was a novel biomarker associated with prognosis and disease recurrence in AML and correlated with disease evolution in MDS. The results might provide us with novel insights into the mechanisms of MDS/AML leukemogenesis.

Methods

Patients and samples

A total of 196 AML patients (184 de novo AML and 12 MDS-derived AML), 104 MDS patients, and 28 healthy donors were enrolled in the present study approved by the Institutional Ethics Committee of the Affiliated People's Hospital of Jiangsu University. The diagnosis and classification of MDS and AML patients were based on the 2016 World Health Organization (WHO) criteria [18]. The main clinical and laboratory features of AML and MDS patients were presented in Tables 1 and 2. After signing the written informed consents, bone marrow (BM) was collected from all participants at diagnosed time. Moreover, BM from 49 AML patients who achieved complete remission (CR) after induction therapy and 27 relapsed AML patients were also included. BM mononuclear cells (BMMNCs) were separated by density-gradient centrifugation using Lymphocyte Separation Medium (Absin, Shanghai, China) [9].

Treatment regimen

The treatment for MDS patients with lower IPSS scores (Low/Int-1) was symptomatic and supportive treatment with/without thalidomide/lenalidomide or EPO or cyclosporine together with ATG, whereas patients with higher IPSS scores (Int-2/High) received symptomatic and supportive treatment with/without chemotherapy included decitabine or HAG protocol (cytarabine, homoharringtonine, and granulocyte colony stimulating factor) or CAG protocol (cytarabine, aclacinomycin, and granulocyte colony stimulating factor) [19]. AML patients received chemotherapy including induction therapy and subsequent consolidation treatment. For non-M3 patients, induction therapy was daunorubicin/homoharringtonine/mitoxantrone combined with cytarabine. Subsequent consolidation treatment included high-dose cytarabine, mitoxantrone with cytarabine, and homoharringtonine combined with cytarabine. Meanwhile, for M3 patients, induction therapy was oral all-trans retinoic acid (ATRA) together with daunorubicin in combination with cytarabine. Maintenance therapy was oral mercaptopurine, oral methotrexate, and oral ATRA over 2 years [9, 20].

Cytogenetic analysis and gene mutation detection

BM cells were harvested after 1 to 3 days of unstimulated culture in RPMI 1640 medium (BOSTER, Wuhan, China) containing 20% fetal calf serum (ExCell Bio, Shanghai, China). The metaphase cells were banded by trypsin-Giemsa technique and karyotyped according to the recommendations of the International System for

Table 1 Comparison of clinical and laboratory features between *SOX30* hypermethylated and non-hypermethylated AML patients

Patient's features	Total (n = 196)	Non-hypermethylated (n = 96)	Hypermethylated (n = 100)	P value
Sex, male/female	114/82	58/38	56/44	0.564
Median age, years (range)	57 (18–86)	52 (18–83)	59 (18–86)	0.024
Median WBC, × 10^9/L (range)	14.35 (0.3–528.0)	11.35 (0.3–528.0)	15.75 (0.3–249.3)	0.554
Median hemoglobin, g/L (range)	77 (32–147)	75 (34–147)	78 (32–144)	0.536
Median platelets, ×10^9/L (range)	42.5 (3–447)	43 (3–447)	42 (3–399)	0.521
Median BM blasts, % (range)	49.75 (1.0^a–99.0)	49.5 (1.0^a–97.5)	50.5 (5.5^a–99.0)	0.173
FAB classifications				0.005
M0	2	0 (0%)	2 (2%)	
M1	18	11 (11%)	7 (7%)	
M2	83	35 (36%)	48 (48%)	
M3	28	22 (23%)	6 (6%)	
M4	37	17 (18%)	20 (20%)	
M5	20	10 (10%)	10 (10%)	
M6	6	1 (1%)	5 (5%)	
No data	2	0 (0%)	2 (2%)	
Karyotypes				0.020
Normal	95	39 (41%)	56 (56%)	
t(8;21)	14	10 (10%)	4 (4%)	
inv.(16)	2	1 (1%)	1 (1%)	
t(15;17)	27	21 (22%)	6 (6%)	
+8	6	2 (2%)	4 (4%)	
-5/5q-	1	1 (1%)	0 (0%)	
-7/7q-	2	0 (0%)	2 (2%)	
t(9;22)	2	1 (1%)	1 (1%)	
11q23	2	0 (0%)	2 (2%)	
Complex	17	8 (8%)	9 (9%)	
Others	16	8 (8%)	8 (8%)	
No data	12	5 (5%)	7 (7%)	
Gene mutations				
CEBPA (+/−)	23/137	10/68	13/69	0.656
NPM1 (+/−)	17/143	8/70	9/73	> 0.999
FLT3-ITD (+/−)	15/145	5/73	10/72	0.280
C-KIT (+/−)	10/150	6/72	4/78	0.527
N/K-RAS (+/−)	15/145	7/71	8/74	> 0.999
IDH1/2 (+/−)	10/150	2/76	8/74	0.099
DNMT3A (+/−)	8/152	3/75	5/77	0.720
U2AF1 (+/−)	5/155	2/76	3/79	> 0.999
SRSF2 (+/−)	5/155	2/76	3/79	> 0.999
CR (+/−)	75/93	47/41	28/52	0.020

WBC white blood cells, *BM* bone marrow, *FAB* French-American-British classification, *CR* complete remission
^{a}Patients' blasts less than 20% with t(15;17) cytogenetic aberrations

Human Cytogenetic Nomenclature (ISCN). Cytogenetics for AML and MDS patients were analyzed at the new diagnosis time by conventional R-banding method and karyotype risk was classified according to what was reported previously [21]. Mutations in *NPM1*, *C-KIT*, *DNMT3A*, *N/K-RAS*, *U2AF1*, and *SRSF2* were detected

Table 2 Comparison of clinical and laboratory features between *SOX30* hypermethylated and non-hypermethylated MDS patients

Patient's features	Total (n = 104)	Non-hypermethylated (n = 80)	Hypermethylated (n = 24)	P value
Sex (male/female)	61/43	48/32	13/11	0.642
Median age, years (range)	62 (14–86)	63.5 (14–86)	67 (28–86)	0.689
Median WBC, ×10^9/L (range)	2.7 (0.6–82.4)	2.8 (0.6–82.4)	2.5 (1.1–44.4)	0.457
Median hemoglobin, g/L (range)	64 (26–140)	66 (36–140)	56 (26–107)	0.017
Median platelets, ×10^9/L (range)	60 (0–1176)	60 (0–754)	50 (10–1176)	0. 503
Median BM blasts, % (range)	5.0 (0.0–19.0)	5.0 (0.0–19.0)	11.0 (0.0–18.0)	0.006
WHO classifications (2018)				0.020
MDS-SLD	10	9 (11%)	1 (4%)	
MDS-RS	7	6 (8%)	1 (4%)	
MDS-MLD	32	29 (36%)	3 (13%)	
MDS-EB1	20	16 (20%)	4 (17%)	
MDS-EB2	31	18 (23%)	13 (54%)	
MDS with isolated del(5q)	3	1 (1%)	2 (8%)	
MDS-U	1	1 (1%)	0 (0%)	
IPSS scores				0.021
Low	11	9 (11%)	2 (8%)	
Int-1	52	45 (56%)	7 (29%)	
Int-2	22	16 (20%)	6 (25%)	
High	12	5 (6%)	7 (29%)	
No data	7	5 (6%)	2 (8%)	
Gene mutations				
CEBPA (+/−)	3/91	3/71	0/20	> 0.999
IDH1/2 (+/−)	3/91	3/71	0/20	> 0.999
DNMT3A (+/−)	3/91	3/71	0/20	> 0.999
U2AF1 (+/−)	6/88	1/73	5/15	0.001
SRSF2 (+/−)	5/89	4/70	1/19	> 0.999
SF3B1 (+/−)	6/98	4/70	2/18	0.604

WBC white blood cells, *BM* bone marrow, *IPSS* International Prognostic Scoring System

by high-resolution melting analysis (HRMA) as reported previously [22–26], whereas mutations in *FLT3*-ITD and *CEBPA* were detected by DNA sequencing as reported previously [27, 28].

RNA isolation, reverse transcription, and RQ-PCR

Total RNA was isolated by using Trizol reagent and was synthesized into cDNA through reverse transcription as reported previously [9]. The primers used for *SOX30* transcript detection were 5′-TGTCACACTTTTCCAGCCC A-3′ (forward) and 5′-TGAAATCCTGTTGGCGCTC T-3′ (reverse). Real-time quantitative PCR (RQ-PCR) was performed to detect *SOX30* transcript using SYBR Premix Ex Taq II (TaKaRa, Tokyo, Japan). RQ-PCR conditions for *SOX30* transcript level detection were 95 °C for 30 s, followed by 40 cycles at 95 °C for 5 s, 66 °C for 30 s, 72 °C for 30 s, 88 °C for 30 s (collect fluorescence), and finally followed by the melting program at 95 °C for 15 s, 60 °C

for 60 s, 95 °C for 15 s, and 60 °C for 15 s. The housekeeping gene *ABL* detected by RQ-PCR using 2× SYBR Green PCR Mix (Multisciences, Hangzhou, China) was used to calculate the abundance of *SOX30* transcript. Relative *SOX30* transcript level was calculated by $2^{-\Delta\Delta CT}$ methods.

DNA isolation, bisulfite modification, and RQ-MSP

Genomic DNA isolation and modification were performed as reported previously [9]. Real-time quantitative methylation-specific PCR (RQ-MSP) was applied to examine *SOX30* methylation level using AceQ qPCR SYBR Green Master Mix (Vazyme Biotech Co., Piscataway, NJ, USA) with primers reported previously [29]. RQ-MSP conditions for *SOX30* methylation level detection were 95 °C for 5 min, 40 cycles for 10 s at 95 °C, 1 min at 68 °C, 1 min at 72 °C, 80 °C for 30 s (collect fluorescence), and finally followed by the melting program at 95 °C for 15 s, 60 °C for 60 s, 95 °C for 15 s, and 60 °C for 15 s. The gene *ALU* was used to calculate the abundance of *SOX30* methylation level. Relative *SOX30* methylation level was calculated by $2^{-\Delta\Delta CT}$ methods.

BSP

The primers used for *SOX30* methylation density detection were 5′-TTTTTGGGTAGTAGTTATGGAG-3′ (forward) and 5′-AACTTAACCACCCTAAAAACTC-3′ (reverse). Bisulfite sequencing PCR (BSP) was conducted using TaKaRa Taq™ Hot Start Version kit (Tokyo, Japan). BSP conditions for *SOX30* methylation density detection were 10 s at 98 °C, 40 cycles for 10 s at 98 °C, 30 s at 58 °C, 30 s at 72 °C, and followed by a final 7 min at 72 °C. Clone sequencing of BSP products was performed as described previously [9], and five/six independent clones were sequenced (BGI Tech Solutions Co., Shanghai, China).

TCGA databases

SOX gene family methylation (HM450) and mRNA expression (RNA Seq V2 RSEM) data in a cohort of 200 AML patients (NEJM 2013) from The Cancer Genome Atlas (TCGA) [30] were downloaded via cBioPortal (http://www.cbioportal.org) [31, 32].

Bioinformatics analyses

The human disease methylation database DiseaseMeth version 2.0 (http://www.bio-bigdata.com/diseasemeth/analyze.html) was used for differential methylation analysis. The Genomicscape Survival Analysis (http://genomicscape.com/microarray/survival.php) was applied to determine the impact of *SOX30* expression on survival of CN-AML patients.

Statistical analyses

Statistical analyses were conducted using SPSS software version 20.0 and GraphPad Prism 5.0. Mann-Whitney U test was carried to compare the difference of continuous variables between two groups, whereas Pearson chi-square analysis/Fisher exact test was applied to compare the difference of categorical variables between two groups. Correlation analysis was performed by Spearman test. Receiver operating characteristic (ROC) curve and area under the ROC curve (AUC) were carried out to test the performance of *SOX30* methylation level in distinguishing AML patients from controls. CR was obtained after one or two courses of chemotherapy. Overall survival (OS) was measured from diagnosis to last follow-up or death from any cause. Leukemia-free survival (LFS) for MDS was calculated from diagnosis to progression to acute leukemia or the end of follow-up, whereas for AML was calculated from the day that CR was established until either relapse or death without relapse. The prognostic value of *SOX30* methylation for survival (OS and LFS) was

analyzed by Kaplan-Meier analysis and Cox regression analyses (univariate and multivariate analyses). All tests were two sided, and $P < 0.05$ was defined as statistically significant.

Results

Identification of methylation-dependent SOX gene associated with prognosis in AML

For initial selection of prognostic relevant methylation of *SOX* genes, we analyzed 19 members of *SOX* gene family by utilizing TCGA data. Among all *SOX* genes, methylation data was available for *SOX5*, *SOX7*, *SOX8*, *SOX10*, *SOX12*, *SOX15*, *SOX18*, and *SOX30*. To investigate their prognostic value in AML, we divided the patients into two groups by the median methylation level of each gene respectively. In whole-cohort AML patients, we did not observe the prognostic impact of *SOX* genes methylation on OS and LFS besides *SOX30* showed a trend (Additional file 1: Figure S1). However, among CN-AML, OS and LFS were adversely affected by methylation in *SOX10* and *SOX30*, but not in *SOX5*, *SOX7*, *SOX8*, *SOX12*, *SOX15*, and *SOX18* (Fig. 1a).

As is well known, DNA methylation is a major mechanism that regulates gene expression. We next analyzed the association between *SOX* gene methylation and expression in AML patients from TCGA data. Significant negative association was shown in *SOX8*, *SOX18*, and *SOX30*, but not in *SOX5*, *SOX7*, *SOX10*, *SOX12*, and *SOX15* (Fig. 1b). These data suggested methylation in *SOX8*, *SOX18*, and *SOX30* may play a major role in regulating gene expression.

Finally, we used DiseaseMeth version 2.0 (based on TCGA and Gene Expression Omnibus) to identify whether *SOX30* promoter (CpG island) was differentially methylated in AML. According to the analyses, the methylation level of *SOX30* in AML was significantly higher than normal controls ($P < 0.001$, Fig. 1c). In addition, a recent investigation reported *SOX* gene family expression in leukemia and found *SOX30* expression was significantly downregulated in AML [15]. By GenomicScape, patients with lower *SOX30* mRNA level tended to have a shorter OS time than those with higher *SOX30* mRNA level ($P = 0.078$, Fig. 1d). Taken together, we deduced that methylation-dependent *SOX30* played a crucial role in leukemogenesis.

Validation of SOX30 hypermethylation was a frequent event and correlated with prognosis in AML

We designed RQ-MSP and BSP primer sets and assays at the CpG island of *SOX30* gene promoter (Fig. 2a) to validate *SOX30* methylation in AML patients and analyzed its clinical significance. Firstly, *SOX30* methylation was examined by RQ-MSP, and AML patients had a significantly higher *SOX30* methylation level than controls

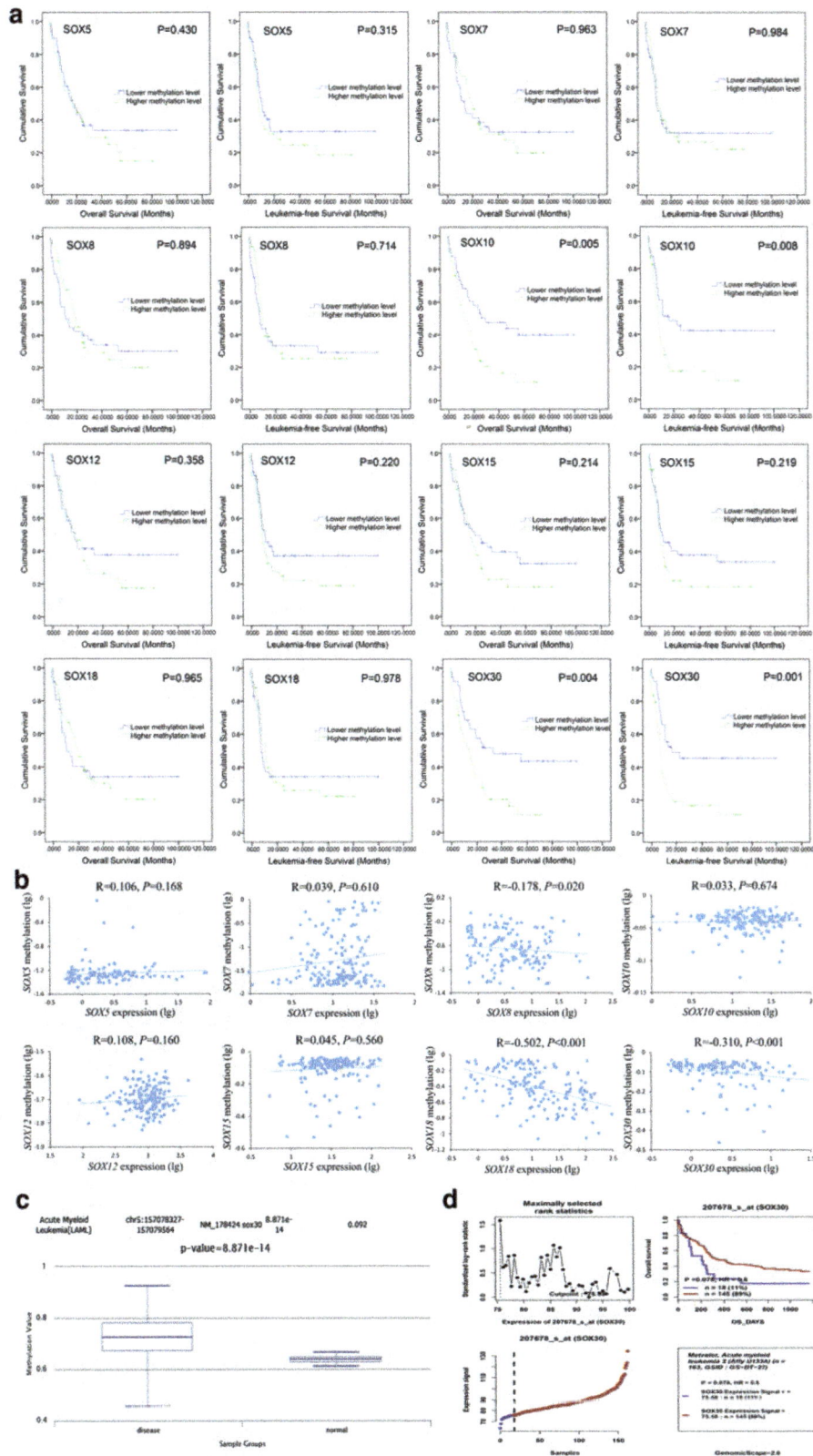

Fig. 1 (See legend on next page.)

(See figure on previous page.)

Fig. 1 Identification of methylation-dependent *SOX* genes associated with prognosis in AML. **a** The prognostic value of *SOX* gene methylation for OS and LFS among CN-AML patients from TCGA databases. *SOX* gene methylation (HM450) data was downloaded via cBioPortal (http://www.cbioportal.org). AML patients were divided into two groups by the median methylation level of each gene respectively. **b** Correlation between *SOX* genes expression and methylation among AML patients from TCGA databases. *SOX* gene methylation (HM450) and mRNA expression (RNA Seq V2 RSEM) data was downloaded via cBioPortal (http://www.cbioportal.org). The correlation analysis was conducted by Spearman test. **c** *SOX30* methylation level in AML patients and controls obtained by bioinformatics analysis. *SOX30* promoter (CpG island) methylation level was obtained through the human disease methylation database DiseaseMeth version 2.0 (http://www.bio-bigdata.com/diseasemeth/analyze.html). **d** The prognostic value of *SOX30* expression for OS among CN-AML patients obtained by bioinformatics analysis. The effect of *SOX30* expression on prognosis was determined by the Genomicscape Survival Analysis (http://genomicscape.com/microarray/survival.php)

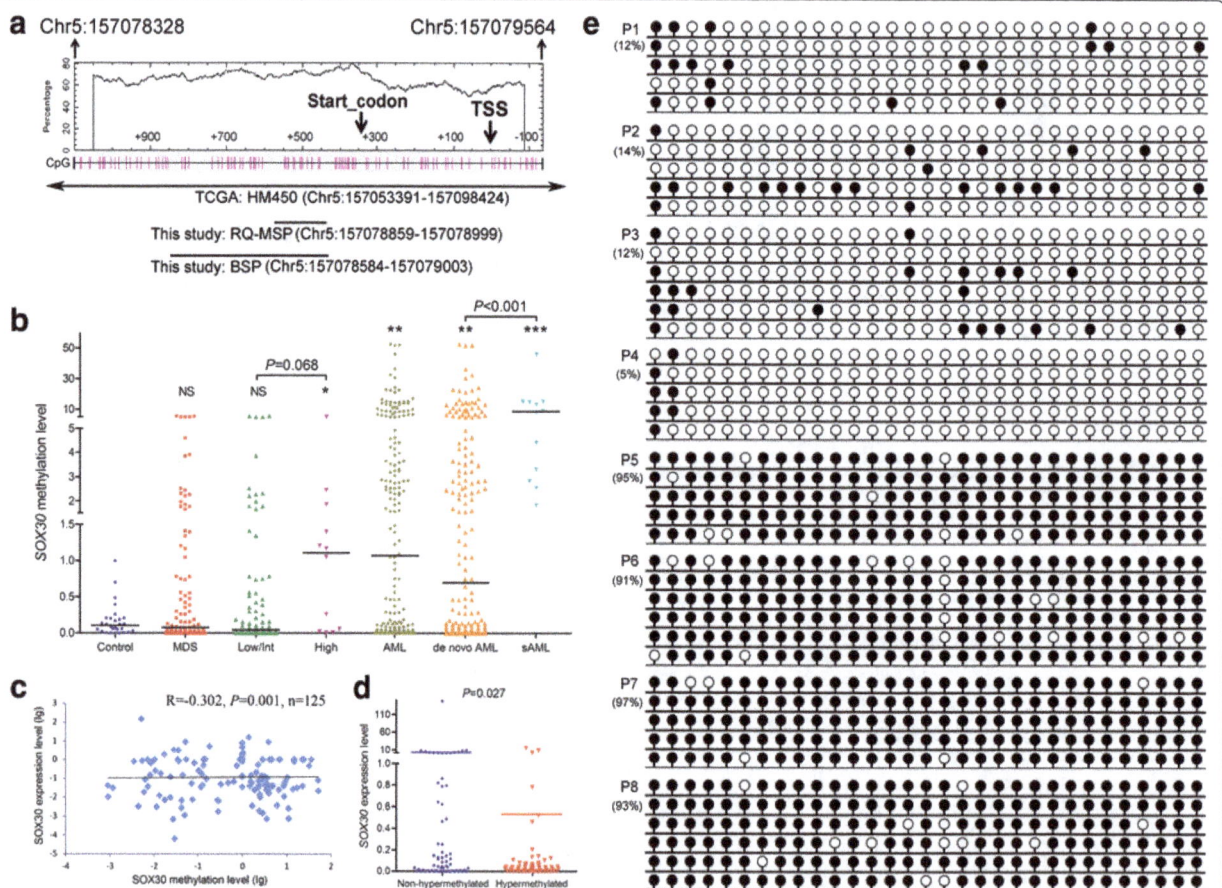

Fig. 2 Validation of *SOX30* methylation in MDS/AML patients. **a** The genomic coordinates (GC) of *SOX30* promoter region CpG island and primer locations. The panel plots the GC content as a percentage of the total. Each vertical bar in the bottom panel represents the presence of a CpG dinucleotide. Black horizontal lines indicate regions amplified by RQ-MSP primer pairs and BSP primer pairs. CpGplot (http://emboss.bioinformatics.nl/cgi-bin/emboss/cpgplot) and Methyl Primer Express v1.0 software were used for creating the figure. TSS: transcription start site; RQ-MSP: real-time quantitative methylation-specific PCR; BSP: bisulfite sequencing PCR. **b** *SOX30* methylation level in controls and MDS/AML patients. *SOX30* methylation level was examined by RQ-MSP. Low/Int and High indicated MDS subtypes based on the classification of IPSS risks. AML included de novo AML and sAML which indicated MDS-derived AML. Each was compared to controls. NS: no significance; *: $P < 0.05$; **: $P < 0.01$; ***: $P < 0.001$. **c** Correlation between *SOX30* methylation level and expression level in AML patients. *SOX30* methylation level and expression level were examined by RQ-MSP and RQ-PCR, respectively. The correlation analysis was conducted by Spearman test. **d** *SOX30* expression level in *SOX30* hypermethylated and non-hypermethylated AML patients. *SOX30* methylation level and expression level were examined by RQ-MSP and RQ-PCR, respectively. **e** *SOX30* methylation density in controls and representative AML patients. *SOX30* methylation density was determined by BSP. P1-P2 indicated two controls selected randomly. P3-P4 represented two AML patients with lower *SOX30* methylation level. P5-P8 showed four AML patients with highest *SOX30* methylation level

(Fig. 2b). Among the tested AML patients with available RNA samples, *SOX30* expression, detected by RQ-PCR, was inversely correlated with *SOX30* methylation ($R = -0.302$, $P = 0.001$, $n = 125$, Fig. 2c). ROC curve analysis showed that *SOX30* methylation may be acted as a potential biomarker for differentiating AML from controls with an AUC of 0.685 (95% CI 0.614–0.756, $P = 0.002$) (Additional file 1: Figure S2). We classified AML patients into two groups (hypermethylated and non-hypermethylated) based on the methylation level (1.024) at the cutoff point by ROC curve analysis (sensitivity = 51%, specificity = 100%, positive predictive value = 100%, negative predictive value = 23%). *SOX30* hypermethylated patients had significantly lower *SOX30* expression level than *SOX30* non-hypermethylated patients ($P = 0.027$, Fig. 2d). Secondly, we performed BSP in eight representative patients (two controls selected randomly, two AML patients with lowest *SOX30* methylation level, and four AML patients with highest *SOX30* methylation level) to validate the RQ-MSP results. As a result, *SOX30* methylation density was heavily correlated with *SOX30* methylation level, and the results of *SOX30* methylation density in representative AML patients were shown in Fig. 2e.

In order to analyze the clinical significance of *SOX30* methylation in AML, we compared the clinical and laboratory features between *SOX30* hypermethylated and *SOX30* non-hypermethylated groups, and results were presented in Table 1. There were no significant differences between two groups among sex, white blood cells, hemoglobin, platelets, and BM blasts. However, *SOX30* hypermethylation was correlated with higher age. Moreover, significant differences were observed between two groups in the distribution of FAB classifications and karyotype. *SOX30* hypermethylation was less frequently occurred in M3/t(15;17) subtypes. Moreover, among gene mutations, there was no significant association of *SOX30* hypermethylation with gene mutations besides *IDH1/2* mutations with a trend.

We next determined the prognostic impact of *SOX30* methylation in AML patients. Follow-up data was available in 175 patients with a survival time ranged from 0.5 to 136 months (median 8 months). Firstly, we observed the association of *SOX30* hypermethylation with CR rate in AML patients. Among whole-cohort AML, *SOX30* hypermethylated patients showed significantly lower CR rate than *SOX30* non-hypermethylated patients (Table 1). In non-M3 AML and CN-AML, patients with *SOX30* hypermethylation tended to have lower CR rate than those with *SOX30* non-hypermethylation [44% (30/68) vs 31% (23/74), $P = 0.121$ and 54% (20/37) vs 33% (15/45), $P = 0.074$]. Secondly, by Kaplan-Meier analysis, *SOX30* hypermethylated patients had significantly shorter OS and LFS than *SOX30* non-hypermethylated patients

(Fig. 3a, b). Significant difference was also observed among non-M3 and CN-AML patients (Fig. 3c–f). In addition, by Cox regression analysis, *SOX30* hypermethylation was an independently adverse prognostic biomarker for OS among whole-cohort AML, non-M3 AML, and CN-AML patients ($P = 0.014$, 0.012, and 0.054, Additional file 1: Table S1-S3).

SOX30 hypermethylation increased the risk of leukemia transformation in MDS

Notably, for AML, *SOX30* methylation level in MDS-derived AML was significantly higher than de novo AML patients (Fig. 2a). Next, we further determined *SOX30* methylation in 12 paired patients during progression from MDS to AML. Expectedly, *SOX30* methylation level was significantly increased in AML stage than in MDS stage among all the paired patients (Fig. 3g).

SOX30 hypermethylation was associated with higher IPSS risks and leukemia-free survival in MDS

We further investigated *SOX30* methylation in a large cohort of MDS patients. *SOX30* methylation level in MDS patients was found similar to controls (Fig. 2a). Nevertheless, *SOX30* methylation in the MDS patients with high IPSS risks were significantly higher than in controls ($P = 0.035$), and also higher than in MDS patients with low/Int IPSS risks ($P = 0.068$) (Fig. 2a). We also used the same cutoff value to define *SOX30* hypermethylation and non-hypermethylation in MDS patients. The comparison of clinical and laboratory features between hypermethylated and non-hypermethylated MDS patients was shown in Table 2. There were no significant differences between two groups among sex, age, white blood cells, and platelets. However, *SOX30* hypermethylation was associated with lower hemoglobin and higher BM blasts. Moreover, significant differences were observed between two groups in the distribution of WHO classifications and IPSS scores. *SOX30* hypermethylation was associated with MDS higher IPSS risks (Int-2/High) and WHO classifications (MDS-EB2). In addition, among gene mutations, we observed the association of *SOX30* hypermethylation with *U2AF1* mutation.

Prognostic impact of *SOX30* methylation in MDS patients was performed in 96 patients with available follow-up data (range 1–113 months, median 19 months). Kaplan-Meier analysis showed that *SOX30* hypermethylated patients had a tendency of shorter OS (Fig. 3h) and significantly shorter LFS (Fig. 3i) than *SOX30* non-hypermethylated patients. However, Cox regression analysis showed that *SOX30* hypermethylation may act as an independently adverse prognostic biomarker for LFS in MDS patients ($P = 0.102$, Additional file 1: Table S4).

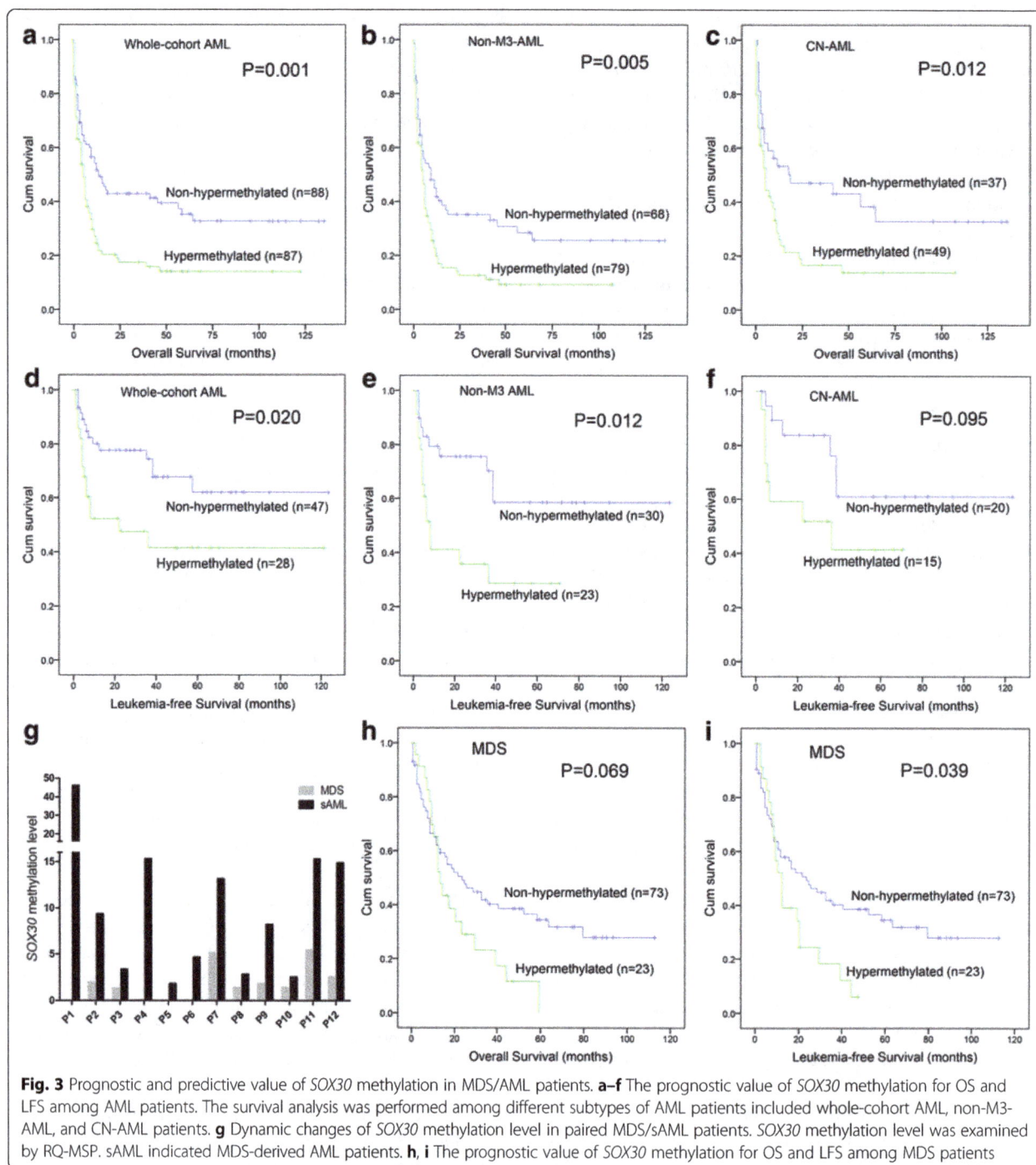

Fig. 3 Prognostic and predictive value of *SOX30* methylation in MDS/AML patients. **a–f** The prognostic value of *SOX30* methylation for OS and LFS among AML patients. The survival analysis was performed among different subtypes of AML patients included whole-cohort AML, non-M3-AML, and CN-AML patients. **g** Dynamic changes of *SOX30* methylation level in paired MDS/sAML patients. *SOX30* methylation level was examined by RQ-MSP. sAML indicated MDS-derived AML patients. **h, i** The prognostic value of *SOX30* methylation for OS and LFS among MDS patients

SOX30 methylation was a predictive biomarker in monitoring disease recurrence in AML

To investigate whether *SOX30* methylation was a potential biomarker in the surveillance of AML, we examined *SOX30* methylation level in different clinical stages of AML patients (49 patients achieved CR and 27 relapsed patients). Significantly, *SOX30* methylation level in CR stage was significantly decreased than in diagnosis time and was markedly increased in relapsed population when compared to CR stage (Fig. 4a). Moreover, the dynamic changes of *SOX30* methylation level in 13 paired patients were also shown in Fig. 4b.

Discussion

SOX30, a member of the *SOX* family, encodes a sequence-specific transcription factor that plays a vital role in gonadal differentiation and development. In species of mouse and human, *SOX30* is considered to be closely

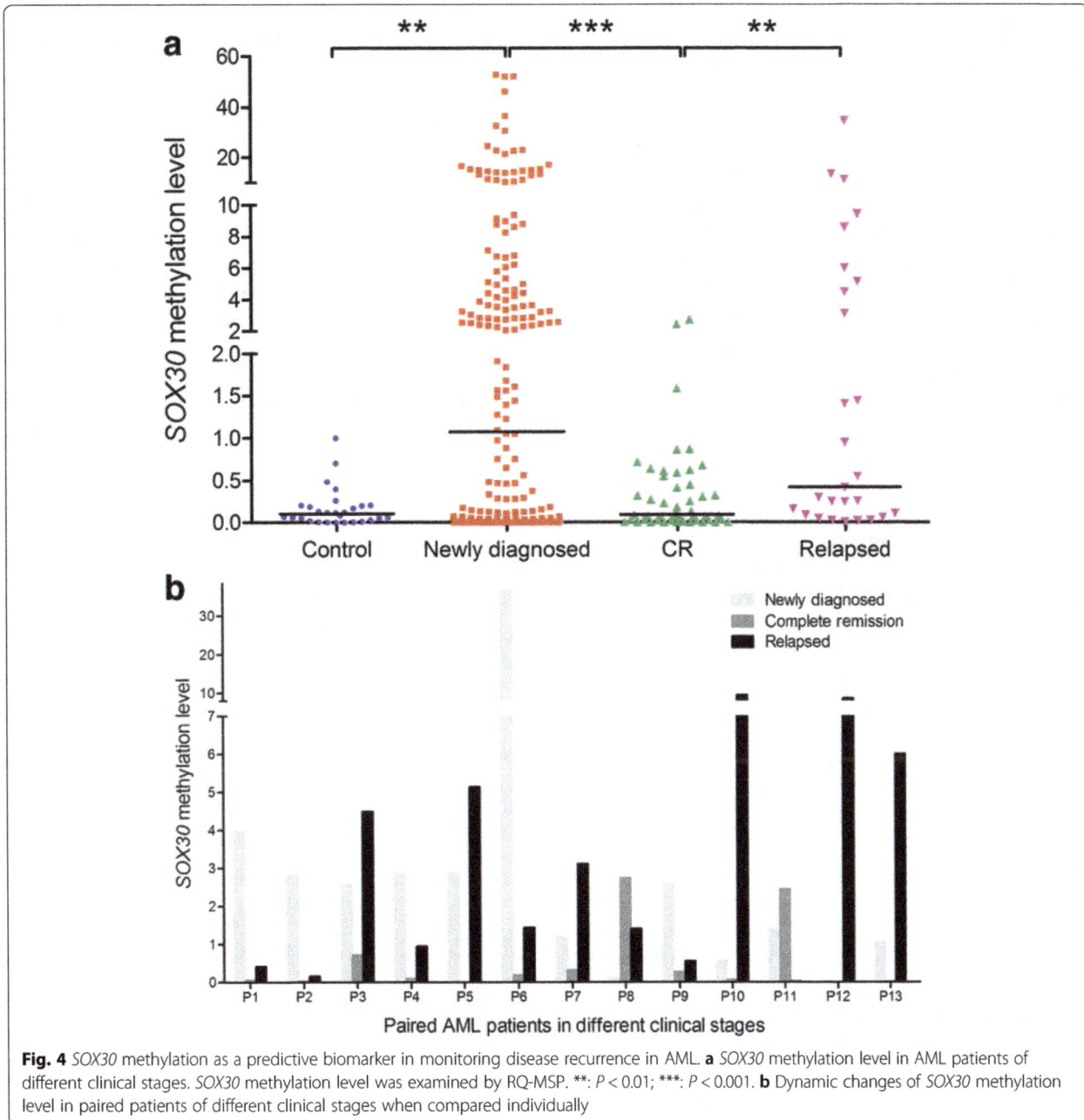

Fig. 4 *SOX30* methylation as a predictive biomarker in monitoring disease recurrence in AML. **a** *SOX30* methylation level in AML patients of different clinical stages. *SOX30* methylation level was examined by RQ-MSP. **: *P* < 0.01; ***: *P* < 0.001. **b** Dynamic changes of *SOX30* methylation level in paired patients of different clinical stages when compared individually

related to spermatogonial differentiation and spermatogenesis [33]. *SOX30* was reported to be highly expressed in male germ cells, human oocytes, or more differentiated cells [34]. Recently, *SOX30* has been validated to be a diagnostic, prognostic, and functional factor in several solid cancers. Han et al. demonstrated that *SOX30* was epigenetically downregulated by promoter methylation and functioned as a novel tumor suppressor partly by transcriptional activating p53 in lung cancer [29]. *SOX30* could also inhibited tumor metastasis through attenuating Wnt signaling via the regulation of β-Catenin in a transcriptional and posttranslational manner in lung cancer

[35]. Furthermore, the expression of *SOX30* was verified to be closely associated with clinical outcomes in lung cancer patients [36]. Also, Guo et al. showed the anti-proliferation effect of *SOX30* overexpression in colon cancer [37]. These results indicated a non-negligible role of *SOX30* that played in the development of cancer.

In this study, we first identified *SOX30* methylation in AML from TCGA datasets and further confirmed that *SOX30* methylation were a frequent event in AML patients. In clinics of AML, *SOX30* methylation was found to be associated with older age and less frequently in FAB-M3/t(15;17), which may be caused by disease entity (less blasts in BM). Notably, *SOX30* methylation seemed to be associated with *IDH1/2* mutations despite that the *P* did not attach statistical significance. As is well known, cancer-associated *IDH* mutations are characterized by neomorphic enzyme activity and resultant 2-hydroxyglutarate production [38] and also contributed to 5-hydroxymethylcytosine depletion in cancer cells [39, 40]. Mutational and epigenetic profiling of a large cohort of AML patients revealed that *IDH1/2*-mutant AMLs displayed global DNA hypermethylation and a specific hypermethylation signature [38]. These indicated that *SOX30* methylation during leukemogenesis may be caused by *IDH1/2* mutations. For MDS, we did not observe the significant association of *SOX30* methylation with *IDH1/2* mutations and older age, which may be caused by limited cases in MDS. However, we found the association of *SOX30* methylation with *U2AF1* mutations. *U2AF1* mutations altered sequence specificity of pre-mRNA binding and splicing and was an important feature of the pathogenesis of MDS and related myeloid neoplasms [41]. Studies showed that *U2AF1* mutations caused differential splicing of hundreds of genes, affecting biological pathways such as DNA methylation (*DNMT3B*) [42]. However, the potential molecular mechanism between *U2AF1* mutation and *SOX30* methylation needs further studies. Importantly, *SOX30* methylation was associated with higher blasts, high-risk MDS, and shorter LFS time. Moreover, *SOX30* methylation showed a higher methylation level in MDS-derived AML compared to de novo AML, and the detection of *SOX30* methylation in 12 paired MDS/sAML patients showed that *SOX30* methylation level was significantly increased in AML stage than in MDS stage. These results suggested *SOX30* methylation might play a crucial role in MDS progression. By gene array technologies, Jiang et al. demonstrated that aberrant DNA methylation, more frequently than chromosome aberrations, was the dominant mechanism for tumor suppressor gene silencing and clonal variation in MDS evolution to AML [8]. However, it was the first time to report *SOX30* methylation in myeloid malignancies, whether *SOX30* functioned as a progression-related driver in MDS needed further studies.

Epigenetic modifications not only played crucial roles in cancer biology but also acted as biomarkers for cancer diagnosis and prognosis especially in blood cancer. Our previous study showed that the long non-coding RNA *H19* overexpression promoted leukemogenesis and predicted unfavorable prognosis in AML [43]. Moreover, besides mutation, dysregulation of *CEBPA* caused by its methylation was also regarded as a prognostic biomarker to guide treatment plan for AML patients [44]. *SOX30* as a prognostic biomarker has been reported in lung cancer [36]. From our study, although *SOX30* methylation was not an independent indicator in MDS, we

revealed that *SOX30* methylation could act as a promising biomarker in AML. Firstly, *SOX30* hypermethylation was associated with lower CR rate, which indicated *SOX30* methylation was associated with chemotherapy response in AML. Secondly, *SOX30* methylation was associated with shorter LFS/OS and acted as independent prognostic factor in AML. Lastly, the dynamic changes of *SOX30* methylation in the surveillance of AML showed it could act as a predictor in monitoring disease recurrence. All these results suggested that determination of the *SOX30* methylation may be useful to predict long-term survival and to guide post-remission therapy in MDS and AML. Interestingly, Božić et al. also used DNA methylation profiles of AML patients from TCGA and identified a CpG site in complement component 1 subcomponent R (C1R) as best suited biomarker to further complement risk assessment in AML [45]. Obviously, prospective studies and integrative analysis are needed before we can routinely use the promising biomarkers for risk stratification and planning therapy in MDS and AML.

Conclusions

Taken together, *SOX30* methylation was associated with disease progression in MDS and acted as an independent prognostic and predictive biomarker in AML.

Abbreviations

AML: Acute myeloid leukemia; ATRA: All-trans retinoic acid; AUC: Area under the ROC curve; BM: Bone marrow; BMMNCs: BM mononuclear cells; BSP: Bisulfite sequencing PCR; CN-AML: Cytogenetically normal AML; CR: Complete remission; GEO: Gene Expression Omnibus; HRMA: High-resolution melting analysis; ISCN: International System for Human Cytogenetic Nomenclature; LFS: Leukemia-free survival; MDS: Myelodysplastic syndromes; OS: Overall survival; ROC: Receiver operating characteristic; RQ-MSP: Real-time quantitative methylation-specific PCR; RQ-PCR: Real-time quantitative PCR; TCGA: The Cancer Genome Atlas

Funding

This work was supported by National Natural Science Foundation of China (81270630), Medical Innovation Team of Jiangsu Province (CXTDB2017002), 333 Project of Jiangsu Province (BRA2016131), Six Talent Peaks Project in Jiangsu Province (2015-WSN-115), Postgraduate Research & Practice Innovation Program of Jiangsu Province (KYCX17_1821, KYCX18_2281), Key Medical Talent Program of Zhenjiang City.

Authors' contributions

JQ, JL and J-d Z conceived and designed the experiments; J-d Z and Y-x W performed the experiments; J-dZ and T-j Z analyzed the data; X-x L, YG and WZ collected the clinical data; J-c M offered technique support; J-d Z wrote the paper. All authors read and approved the final manuscript.

Author details

[1]Department of Hematology, Affiliated People's Hospital of Jiangsu University, 8 Dianli Rd, 212002 Zhenjiang, People's Republic of China. [2]The Key Lab of Precision Diagnosis and Treatment of Zhenjiang City, Zhenjiang, Jiangsu, People's Republic of China. [3]Department of Nephrology and Endocrinology, Traditional Chinese Medicine Hospital of Kunshan City, Kunshan, Jiangsu, People's Republic of China. [4]Laboratory Center, Affiliated People's Hospital of Jiangsu University, 8 Dianli Rd., 212002 Zhenjiang, People's Republic of China.

References

1. Estey E, Döhner H. Acute myeloid leukaemia. Lancet. 2006;368:1894–907.
2. Adès L, Itzykson R, Fenaux P. Myelodysplastic syndromes. Lancet. 2014;383:2239–52.
3. Rowley JD. Chromosomal translocations: revisited yet again. Blood. 2008;112:2183–9.
4. Marcucci G, Haferlach T, Döhner H. Molecular genetics of adult acute myeloid leukemia: prognostic and therapeutic implications. J Clin Oncol. 2011;29:475–86.
5. Chen J, Odenike O, Rowley JD. Leukaemogenesis: more than mutant genes. Nat Rev Cancer. 2010;10:23–36.
6. Wu SC, Zhang Y. Active DNA demethylation: many roads lead to Rome. Nat Rev Mol Cell Biol. 2010;11:607–20.
7. Taby R, Issa JP. Cancer epigenetics. CA Cancer J Clin. 2010;60:376–92.
8. Jiang Y, Dunbar A, Gondek LP, et al. Aberrant DNA methylation is a dominant mechanism in MDS progression to AML. Blood. 2009;113:1315–25.
9. Zhou JD, Zhang TJ, Li XX, Ma JC, Guo H, Wen XM, Zhang W, Yang L, Yan Y, Lin J, Qian J. Epigenetic dysregulation of ID4 predicts disease progression and treatment outcome in myeloid malignancies. J Cell Mol Med. 2017;21:1468–81.
10. Bowles J, Schepers G, Koopman P. Phylogeny of the SOX family of developmental transcription factors based on sequence and structural indicators. Dev Biol. 2000;227:239–55.
11. Kormish JD, Sinner D, Zorn AM. Interactions between SOX factors and Wnt/beta-catenin signaling in development and disease. Dev Dyn. 2010;239:56–68.
12. Dong C, Wilhelm D, Koopman P. Sox genes and cancer. Cytogenet Genome Res. 2004;105:442–7.
13. Sandoval S, Kraus C, Cho EC, Cho M, Bies J, Manara E, Accordi B, Landaw EM, Wolff L, Pigazzi M, Sakamoto KM. Sox4 cooperates with CREB in myeloid transformation. Blood. 2012;120:155–65.
14. Zhang H, Alberich-Jorda M, Amabile G, Yang H, Staber PB, Di Ruscio A, Welner RS, Ebralidze A, Zhang J, Levantini E, Lefebvre V, Valk PJ, Delwel R, Hoogenkamp M, Nerlov C, Cammenga J, Saez B, Scadden DT, Bonifer C, Ye M, Tenen DG. Sox4 is a key oncogenic target in C/EBPα mutant acute myeloid leukemia. Cancer Cell. 2013;24:575–88.
15. Man CH, Fung TK, Wan H, Cher CY, Fan A, Ng N, Ho C, Wan TS, Tanaka T, So CW, Kwong YL, Leung AY. Suppression of SOX7 by DNA methylation and its tumor suppressor function in acute myeloid leukemia. Blood. 2015;125:3928–36.
16. Wan H, Cai J, Chen F, Zhu J, Zhong J, Zhong H. SOX12: a novel potential target for acute myeloid leukaemia. Br J Haematol. 2017;176:421–30.
17. Tang CY, Lin J, Qian W, Yang J, Ma JC, Deng ZQ, Yang L, An C, Wen XM, Zhang YY, Qian J. Low SOX17 expression: prognostic significance in de novo acute myeloid leukemia with normal cytogenetics. Clin Chem Lab Med. 2014;52:1843–50.
18. Arber DA, Orazi A, Hasserjian R, Thiele J, Borowitz MJ, Le Beau MM, Bloomfield CD, Cazzola M, Vardiman JW. The 2016 revision to the World Health Organization classification of myeloid neoplasms and acute leukemia. Blood. 2016;127:2391–405.
19. Zhou JD, Lin J, Zhang TJ, Ma JC, Yang L, Wen XM, Guo H, Yang J, Deng ZQ, Qian J. GPX3 methylation in bone marrow predicts adverse prognosis and leukemia transformation in myelodysplastic syndrome. Cancer Med. 2017;6:267–74.
20. Li Y, Lin J, Yang J, Qian J, Qian W, Yao DM, Deng ZQ, Liu Q, Chen XX, Xie D, An C, Tang CY. Overexpressed let-7a-3 is associated with poor outcome in acute myeloid leukemia. Leuk Res. 2013;37:1642–7.
21. Grimwade D, Hills RK, Moorman AV, Walker H, Chatters S, Goldstone AH, Wheatley K, Harrison CJ, Burnett AK. National Cancer Research Institute Adult Leukaemia Working Group. Refinement of cytogenetic classification in acute myeloid leukemia: determination of prognostic significance of rare recurring chromosomal abnormalities among 5876 younger adult patients treated in the United Kingdom Medical Research Council trials. Blood. 2010;116:354–65.
22. Lin J, Yao DM, Qian J, Chen Q, Qian W, Li Y, Yang J, Wang CZ, Chai HY, Qian Z, Xiao GF, Xu WR. Recurrent DNMT3A R882 muta-tions in Chinese patients with acute myeloid leukemia and myelodysplastic syndrome. PLoS One. 2011;6:e26906.
23. Qian J, Yao DM, Lin J, Qian W, Wang CZ, Chai HY, Yang J, Li Y, Deng ZQ, Ma JC, Chen XX. U2AF1 mutations in Chinese patients with acute myeloid leukemia and myelodysplastic syndrome. PLoS One. 2012;7:e45760.
24. Lin J, Yang J, Wen XM, Yang L, Deng ZQ, Qian Z, Ma JC, Guo H, Zhang YY, Qian W, Qian J. Detection of SRSF2-P95 mutation by high-resolution melting curve analysis and its effect on prognosis in myelodysplastic syndrome. PLoS One. 2014;9:e115693.
25. Yang J, Yao DM, Ma JC, Yang L, Guo H, Wen XM, Xiao GF, Qian Z, Lin J, Qian J. The prognostic implication of SRSF2 mutations in Chinese patients with acute myeloid leukemia. Tumour Biol. 2016;37:10107–14.
26. Lin J, Yao DM, Qian J, Chen Q, Qian W, Li Y, Yang J, Wang CZ, Chai HY, Qian Z, Xiao GF, Xu WR. IDH1 and IDH2 mutation analysis in Chinese patients with acute myeloid leukemia and myelodysplastic syndrome. Ann Hematol. 2012;91:519–25.
27. Wen XM, Lin J, Yang J, Yao DM, Deng ZQ, Tang CY, Xiao GF, Yang L, Ma JC, Hu JB, Qian W, Qian J. Double CEBPA mutations are prognostically favorable in non-APL acute myeloid leukemia patients with wild-type NPM1 and FLT3-ITD. Int J Clin Exp Pathol. 2014;7:6832–40.
28. Wen XM, Hu JB, Yang J, Qian W, Yao DM, Deng ZQ, Zhang YY, Zhu XW, Guo H, Lin J, Qian J. CEBPA methylation and mutation in myelodysplastic syndrome. Med Oncol. 2015;32:192.
29. Han F, Liu W, Jiang X, Shi X, Yin L, Ao L, Cui Z, Li Y, Huang C, Cao J, Liu J. SOX30, a novel epigenetic silenced tumor suppressor, promotes tumor cell apoptosis by transcriptional activating p53 in lung cancer. Oncogene. 2015;34:4391–402.
30. Network CGAR. Genomic and epigenomic landscapes of adult de novo acute myeloid leukemia. N Engl J Med. 2013;368:2059–74.
31. Cerami E, Gao J, Dogrusoz U, Gross BE, Sumer SO, Aksoy BA, Jacobsen A, Byrne CJ, Heuer ML, Larsson E, Antipin Y, Reva B, Goldberg AP, Sander C, Schultz N. The cBio cancer genomics portal: an open platform for exploring multidimensional cancer genomics data. Cancer Discov. 2012;2:401–4.
32. Gao J, Aksoy BA, Dogrusoz U, Dresdner G, Gross B, Sumer SO, Sun Y, Jacobsen A, Sinha R, Larsson E, Cerami E, Sander C, Schultz N. Integrative analysis of complex cancer genomics and clinical profiles using the cBioPortal. Sci Signal. 2013;6:pl1.
33. Osaki E, Nishina Y, Inazawa J, Copeland NG, Gilbert DJ, Jenkins NA, et al. Identification of a novel Sry-related gene and its germ cell-specific expression. Nucleic Acids Res. 1999;27:2503–10.
34. Han F, Wang Z, Wu F, Liu Z, Huang B, Wang D. Characterization, phylogeny, alternative splicing and expression of Sox30 gene. BMC Mol Biol. 2010;11:98.
35. Han F, Liu WB, Shi XY, Yang JT, Zhang X, Li ZM, Jiang X, Yin L, Li JJ, Huang CS, Cao J, Liu JY. SOX30 inhibits tumor metastasis through attenuating Wnt-signaling via transcriptional and posttranslational regulation of β-catenin in lung cancer. EBioMedicine. 2018; https://doi.org/10.1016/j.ebiom.2018.04.026.
36. Han F, Liu W, Xiao H, Dong Y, Sun L, Mao C, Yin L, Jiang X, Ao L, Cui Z, Cao J, Liu J. High expression of SOX30 is associated with favorable survival in human lung adenocarcinoma. Sci Rep. 2015;5:13630.
37. Guo ST, Guo XY, Wang J, Wang CY, Yang RH, Wang FH, Li XY, Hondermarck H, Thorne RF, Wang YF, Jin L, Zhang XD, Jiang CC. MicroRNA-645 is an oncogenic regulator in colon cancer. Oncogene. 2017;6:e335.
38. Figueroa ME, Abdel-Wahab O, Lu C, Ward PS, Patel J, Shih A, Li Y, Bhagwat N, Vasanthakumar A, Fernandez HF, Tallman MS, Sun Z, Wolniak K, Peeters JK, Liu W, Choe SE, Fantin VR, Paietta E, Löwenberg B, Licht JD, Godley LA, Delwel R, Valk PJ, Thompson CB, Levine RL, Melnick A. Leukemic IDH1 and IDH2 mutations result in a hypermethylation phenotype, disrupt TET2 function, and impair hematopoietic differentiation. Cancer Cell. 2010;18:553–67.
39. Kroeze LI, Aslanyan MG, van Rooij A, Koorenhof-Scheele TN, Massop M, Carell T, Boezeman JB, Marie JP, Halkes CJ, de Witte T, Huls G, Suciu S, Wevers RA, van der Reijden BA, Jansen JH. EORTC leukemia group and GIMEMA. Characterization of acute myeloid leukemia based on levels of global hydroxymethylation. Blood. 2014;124:1110–8.
40. Chou NH, Tsai CY, Tu YT, Wang KC, Kang CH, Chang PM, Li GC, Lam HC, Liu SI, Tsai KW. Isocitrate dehydrogenase 2 dysfunction contributes to 5-hydroxymethylcytosine depletion in gastric cancer cells. Anticancer Res. 2016;36:3983–90.
41. Okeyo-Owuor T, White BS, Chatrikhi R, Mohan DR, Kim S, Griffith M, Ding L, Ketkar-Kulkarni S, Hundal J, Laird KM, Kielkopf CL, Ley TJ, Walter MJ, Graubert TA. U2AF1 mutations alter sequence specificity of pre-mRNA binding and splicing. Leukemia. 2015;29:909–17.
42. Ilagan JO, Ramakrishnan A, Hayes B, Murphy ME, Zebari AS, Bradley P, Bradley RK. U2AF1 mutations alter splice site recognition in hematological malignancies. Genome Res. 2015;25:14–26.
43. Zhang TJ, Zhou JD, Zhang W, Lin J, Ma JC, Wen XM, Yuan Q, Li XX, Xu ZJ, Qian J. H19 overexpression promotes leukemogenesis and predicts unfavorable prognosis in acute myeloid leukemia. Clin Epigenetics. 2018;10:47.

16

Epigenome-wide DNA methylation profiling of periprostatic adipose tissue in prostate cancer patients with excess adiposity—a pilot study

Yan Cheng[1,2], Cátia Monteiro[3,4], Andreia Matos[5,6], Jiaying You[1], Avelino Fraga[6,7], Carina Pereira[3,8], Victoria Catalán[9,10], Amaia Rodríguez[9,10], Javier Gómez-Ambrosi[9,10], Gema Frühbeck[9,10,11], Ricardo Ribeiro[3,5,6,12,13]*[†] and Pingzhao Hu[1]*[†] (ID)

Abstract

Background: Periprostatic adipose tissue (PPAT) has been recognized to associate with prostate cancer (PCa) aggressiveness and progression. Here, we sought to investigate whether excess adiposity modulates the methylome of PPAT in PCa patients. DNA methylation profiling was performed in PPAT from obese/overweight (OB/OW, BMI > 25 kg m^{-2}) and normal weight (NW, BMI < 25 kg m^{-2}) PCa patients. Significant differences in methylated CpGs between OB/OW and NW groups were inferred by statistical modeling.

Results: Five thousand five hundred twenty-six differentially methylated CpGs were identified between OB/OW and NW PCa patients with 90.2% hypermethylated. Four hundred eighty-three of these CpGs were found to be located at both promoters and CpG islands, whereas the representing 412 genes were found to be involved in pluripotency of stem cells, fatty acid metabolism, and many other biological processes; 14 of these genes, particularly *FADS1*, *MOGAT1*, and *PCYT2*, with promoter hypermethylation presented with significantly decreased gene expression in matched samples. Additionally, 38 genes were correlated with antigen processing and presentation of endogenous antigen via MHC class I, which might result in fatty acid accumulation in PPAT and tumor immune evasion.

Conclusions: Results showed that the whole epigenome methylation profiles of PPAT were significantly different in OB/OW compared to normal weight PCa patients. The epigenetic variation associated with excess adiposity likely resulted in altered lipid metabolism and immune dysregulation, contributing towards unfavorable PCa microenvironment, thus warranting further validation studies in larger samples.

Keywords: DNA methylation, Periprostatic adipose tissue, Obesity, Prostate cancer, Microenvironment

Background

Prostate cancer (PCa) is one of the most frequent malignancies in men and the second leading cause of cancer-related death in the North America and most western European countries [1, 2]. Epidemiological studies support obesity or excess adiposity as an important environmental risk factor for PCa, being primarily associated with advanced disease and death [3]. Periprostatic adipose tissue (PPAT), a white fat depot surrounding the prostate capsular-like structure, has been recognized to have the potential to exert pro-tumoral endocrine and paracrine influences on prostate cancer cell's biological phenotypes [4]. There is now evidence that obesity and overweight result in excess fat deposit at PPAT [5], altered fatty acid profile [6], migration of tumor cells [7], secretion of a variety of adipokines, such as interleukin-1 beta (IL-1b), osteopontin, leptin, tumor necrosis factor alpha (TNF-a),

---

* Correspondence: ricardo.ribeiro@i3s.up.pt; pingzhao.hu@umanitoba.ca
[†]Equal contributors
[3]Molecular Oncology Group, Portuguese Institute of Oncology, Porto, Portugal
[1]Department of Biochemistry and Medical Genetics & Department of Electrical and Computer Engineering, University of Manitoba, Winnipeg, Canada
Full list of author information is available at the end of the article

and decreased adiponectin, thus contributing to a tumor microenvironment that ultimately facilitates PCa aggressiveness [7, 8].

DNA methylation is a well-known epigenetic mechanism resulting from the interaction between environmental factors and the genome [9]. DNA methylation with variation of CpG sites is associated with tissue-specific gene modulation and involved in phenotype transmission and in the development of diseases [10]. Excess adiposity, as a consequence of environmental factors such as excessive food consumption or inactive lifestyle, has been identified as a regulator of epigenetic modification in adipose tissue. Recent findings from experimental studies suggested that modification of DNA methylation pattern in adipose tissue and adipocytes was related with development of cancer, type 2 diabetes, and cardiovascular diseases through influencing metabolism and inflammation [11–13]. Additionally, several studies reported altered DNA methylation in PCa cells as compared with adjacent benign tissue, and some significantly methylated CpG sites and genes were found to be responsible for the occurrence and progression of PCa [14–16]. Nevertheless, the epigenome-wide DNA methylation profile of PPAT from excess adiposity PCa patients is currently unknown despite its potential mechanistic involvement in obesity association with PCa.

The aim of this study was to perform a epigenetic-wide association study (EWAS) in order to evaluate DNA methylation profile of PPAT obtained from obese/overweight (OB/OW) in comparison with normal weight (NW) PCa patients and identify differentially methylated sites. We also explored the consequential potential biological functions that account for the effect of PPAT from OB/OW subjects in PCa molecular mechanisms.

Methods

Study samples

This study included ten prostate cancer patients from the Portuguese Institute of Oncology, Porto Centre. Inclusion criteria and conditions of this study have been previously reported, including the procedures for PPAT collection, handling, and storage [4]. Briefly, PPAT was collected and immediately processed in the operating room and transported to the laboratory within 2 h in appropriate culture media and temperature conditions, in order to minimize pre-analytical errors. Patients' signed informed consent and research procedures were approved by the institute's ethics committee.

The clinical and pathological characteristics of participants are presented in Table 1. The ten subjects were selected from a larger group of patients undergoing prostate surgery ($n = 51$) [4, 17] that fitted the strict inclusion and exclusion criteria, in order to control for variables that might influence adipose tissue gene

Table 1 Clinicopathological characteristics of PCa patients by BMI category

Character	NW ($n = 5$)	OB/OW ($n = 5$)	P value
Age (years)	65.2 ± 3.8	63.2 ± 2.5	0.67[a]
BMI (kg/m²)	23.0 ± 0.3	29.0 ± 0.9	0.0003[a]
Gleason score			
< 7	2 (40%)	1 (20%)	
≥ 7	3 (60%)	4 (80%)	1.00[b]
Stage			
OCPCa	2 (40%)	2 (40%)	
EPCa	3 (60%)	3 (60%)	1.00[b]
Smoking status			
Yes	1	5	
No	4	0	0.05[b]
PSA (ng/ml)	10.7 ± 2.7	12.1 ± 3.23	0.74[a]

Data are presented as mean ± SD or number (%). Significant difference between OB/OW and NW was evaluated using [a]t test and [b]Fisher's exact test

OB/OW obese/overweight, NW normal weight, BMI body mass index; PSA, prostate specific antigen; PCa, prostate cancer; OCPCa, organ-confined prostate cancer; EPCa, extra-prostatic PCa

expression or methylation (e.g., anti-diabetic or anti-dyslipidemia drugs, stage of disease and PSA, concomitant diseases such as diabetes, other neoplasia or metabolic syndrome). Subjects were matched for age at diagnosis, PSA value, Gleason grade, and stage of disease, which differed in body mass index (BMI). BMI was calculated by dividing weight in kilograms by the squared height in meters and categorized using the WHO (World Health Organization) criteria: normal weight, BMI < 25 kg m^{-2}, overweight, $25 \leq BMI < 30$ kg m^{-2}, and obese, BMI ≥ 30 kg m^{-2}. Obese and overweight were combined into one excess adiposity group ($n = 5$, BMI≥25 kg m^{-2}) versus normal weight group ($n = 5$, BMI < 25 kg m^{-2}). Therefore, the two groups were selected to differ only by BMI, in order to reflect our objective of assessing whether excess adiposity (BMI) influences PPAT methylation profile.

Epigenome-wide DNA methylation analysis

DNA was isolated from PPAT using Puregene hisalt extraction method (Qiagen/Gentra). Briefly, the tissue was minced with scalpels in a sterile petri dish on ice and then transferred to Puregene Cell Kit for overnight Proteinase K digest at 55 °C. A second Proteinase K digest was done the next morning for 5 h. DNA from the digested tissue was purified using Puregene extraction protocol (Qiagen/Gentra). Purified DNA was washed 2× with 70% ethanol and DNA pellet air dried and rehydrated in TE (10 mM Tris-Cl, 1 mM EDTA pH 7.5). Epigenome-wide DNA methylation was analyzed using the Infinium Human Methylation450 (HM450) BeadChip (Illumina, San Diego, CA, USA) in the Center for Applied Genomics (Toronto). This array contains 485,577 probes, which cover 21,231 (99%) RefSeq genes. Briefly, DNA was bisulfite-converted using the EZ DNA methylation kit (Zymo Research, Orange, CA, USA) and then used on the Infinium Assay® followed by the Infinium HD Assay Methylation Protocol (Illumina). The imaging data on the BeadChips was captured by Illumina iScan system.

Data filtering and normalization

Raw methylation level for each probe was represented by methylation β value, which was calculated based on β = intensity of the methylated allele/(intensity of the unmethylated allele + intensity of the methylated allele + 100). M values were the logit transformation of β values based on $M = \log_2 (\beta/(1 - \beta))$, which makes the data more homoscedastic and appropriate for further bioinformatic and statistical analysis.

Methylation values were normalized using the functional normalization algorithm implemented in Minfi R package [18]. Quality control was performed by excluding CpG probes, which are found by Chen et al. to be cross-reactive with areas of the genome not at the site of interest [19], as well as control probes and probes on sex chromosomes. We analyzed a total of 438,458 CpG sites from the PPAT of 5 OB/OW PCa patients and 5 NW PCa patients.

Differential methylation analysis

A statistical linear modeling approach was applied to the detected differentially methylated CpG sites (DMCs) associated with obesity in PPAT using the Bioconductor "limma" package [20]. Hyper- or hypomethylation was determined when methylation levels of CpGs increased or decreased between the OB/OW PCa group and the NW PCa group based on mean different $\beta > 0$ or < 0. False discovery rate (FDR)-corrected P values were determined according to the method of Benjamin and Hochberg's (BH method) multiple testing procedure [21].

Differentially methylated regions (DMRs) were identified using the "Bumphunter" method implemented in the "chAMP" R package with the parameters ($B = 1000$, useWeights = TRUE, minProbes = 10, pickCutoff = TRUE, and other settings with default values) [22].

The proportions of significant hyper- or hypomethylated CpGs were calculated and visualized according to their relation to the nearest genes or to the CpG islands, separately. Gene promoter region was defined as 1500 base pairs (bp) and 200 bp upstream of the transcription start site (TSS) (TSS1500 and TSS200) [23]. Identified genes were selected when more than two significantly hypermethylated CpGs were simultaneously located in the promoter region.

Functions, pathway, and network enrichment analysis

Gene ontology (GO) and KEGG pathway enrichment analyses were performed to explore the biological functions of significantly methylated genes using the online bioinformatic tool Enrichr [24]. Protein-protein interaction (PPI) analysis of all DMC-related genes was performed using NetworkAnalyst according to STRING database [25].

Association analysis between DNA methylation and gene expression

We have previously performed gene expression experiment of the PPAT of the 5 OB/OW PCa patients and the 5 NW PCa patients using the HG-U133 Plus 2.0 Affymetrix GeneChip Array (Affymetrix, Santa Clara, CA, USA) [4]. Differential gene expression (DGE) analysis between the OB/OW PCa patients and the NW PCa patients was re-performed using the Bioconductor "limma" package as previously described [4]. Spearman's rank correlation analysis was performed between the methylation profiles of the hypermethylated CpGs and the gene expression profiles of the genes in PPAT.

Results

Clinical characteristics

Clinical characteristics of PCa patients in this study were stratified according to obesity classification groups and are presented in Table 1. Mean age, PSA level, Gleason sum score, and cancer stage in subjects with PCa were similar (P value > 0.05) between OB/OW and NW groups. As expected, the mean BMI of the OB/OW group was significantly higher than that of the NW subjects (P value < 0.01). All the patients in the OB/OW group are ex-smokers or active smokers, while only one patient in the NW group is a smoker (P value = 0.05).

Epigenome-wide DNA methylation profiling of PPAT

To study the impact of obesity status on DNA methylation profiles and to identify differentially methylated CpG sites in PPAT from OB/OW and NW prostate cancer patients, we conducted epigenome-wide DNA methylation analyses. A flowchart of the data analysis is depicted in Additional file 1: Figure S1. After quality control and filtering, the Infinium array generated methylation data for 438,458 CpG sites, from which 5526 were differentially methylated after FDR control in the PPAT of OB/OW PCa patients compared to NW (adjusted P value < 0.25; Additional file 2: Table S1 and Table 2). The unsupervised hierarchical clustering of DMCs showed differential DNA methylation patterns in PPAT between OB/OW and NW samples (Additional file 3: Figure S2). The majority of DMCs were hypermethylated ($n = 4985$, 90.2%), with 9.8% hypomethylated CpG sites ($n = 541$) in OB/OW versus NW prostate cancer patients (Fig. 1a, b, c).

Table 2 Differentially methylated CpG sites in PPAT between obese/overweight PCa patients and normal weight controls

Probe ID	Chromosome and coordinate (GRCh37)	Nearest gene	Relation to gene region	Relation to CpG island	DNAm β difference (%)	P value	Adjusted P value (< 0.25)
Hypermethylated CpG sites							
cg09476130	chr1:159870086	CCDC19	TSS200	Island	12.1	1.87E−03	0.213
cg21293934	chr18:14748230	ANKRD30B	TSS200	Island	11.2	1.83E−03	0.212
cg16925210	chr2:216946718	PECR	TSS200	Island	11.2	2.44E−03	0.226
cg11625005	chr5:1295737	TERT	TSS1500	Island	11.1	1.38E−03	0.196
cg07039560	chr5:140683681	SLC25A2	TSS200	Island	10.5	2.24E−03	0.222
cg00329447	chr8:145028170	PLEC1	TSS200	Island	10.1	3.41E−03	0.244
cg24463471	chr1:25257978	RUNX3	TSS1500	Island	9.9	3.58E−04	0.155
cg26149485	chr19:2428350	TIMM13	TSS1500	Island	9.7	3.36E−04	0.154
cg05156901	chr22:51016646	CPT1B	TSS200	Island	9.3	3.05E−03	0.238
cg18689454	chr21:45705694	AIRE	TSS200	Island	9.3	7.33E−04	0.174
cg01454592	chr3:49236800	CCDC36	TSS200	Island	9.3	2.89E−03	0.236
cg24041556	chr19:10736059	SLC44A2	TSS200	Island	9.1	2.15E−05	0.110
cg22257574	chr9:135754383	C9orf98	TSS200	Island	9.0	1.97E−05	0.110
cg23005885	chr15:90543450	ZNF710	TSS1500	Island	8.9	6.20E−04	0.169
cg05726756	chr17:46608288	HOXB1	TSS200	Island	8.6	1.67E−03	0.206
cg12782180	chr7:127880932	LEP	TSS1500	Island	8.5	9.78E−04	0.184
cg04675542	chr5:150284416	ZNF300	TSS200	Island	8.4	3.42E−03	0.244
cg10134527	chr6:33283015	TAPBP	TSS1500	Island	8.4	3.19E−03	0.241
cg23387569	chr12:58120011	LOC100130776	TSS200	Island	8.4	3.39E−04	0.155
cg17205324	chr14:23835595	EFS	TSS1500	Island	8.3	1.46E−04	0.133
cg24402300	chr19:55591437	EPS8L1	TSS1500	Island	8.2	2.02E−03	0.216
cg18081258	chr14:21494161	NDRG2	TSS1500	Island	8.2	1.05E−03	0.187
cg00730561	chr10:102279703	SEC31B	TSS200	Island	8.1	4.82E−04	0.162
cg17791651	chr1:38513489	POU3F1	TSS1500	Island	8.0	1.31E−04	0.133
Hypomethylated CpG sites							
cg03462171	chr16:1664488	CRAMP1L	TSS200	Island	− 8.2	2.30E−03	0.223
cg11648730	chr5:92907151	FLJ42709	TSS1500	Island	− 6.4	1.72E−03	0.207
cg04558166	chr1:210001279	C1orf107	TSS200	Island	− 4.0	1.75E−03	0.209
cg25472897	chr8:145560555	SCRT1	TSS1500	Island	− 3.1	1.53E−03	0.201
cg17612948	chr5:110427863	WDR36	TSS200	Island	− 3.0	1.70E−03	0.207
cg21665057	chr3:196295764	WDR53	TSS1500	Island	− 2.4	2.42E−03	0.225
cg12683173	chr7:69063404	AUTS2	TSS1500	Island	− 1.4	3.30E−03	0.242
cg04872557	chr1:76190008	ACADM	TSS200	Island	− 1.0	1.96E−03	0.215

Chromosomal distribution of the DMCs

To further explore the methylation profile, we investigated the chromosome distribution of DMCs. Results showed that hypermethylated CpG sites were located at chromosomes 1, 6, 11, and 17 (proportion > 6%, Fig. 1d) and hypomethylated CpG sites were located at chromosomes 1, 2, 6, 7, and 11 (proportion > 6%, Fig. 1e).

Methylation variations of hypermethylated DMCs and hypomethylated DMCs were found mainly distributed on chromosomes 1, 6, and 11, suggesting that the DNA methylation alterations in these chromosomes were correlated with the body weight changes in prostate patients. Furthermore, we compared the distribution of the DMCs (hyper- and hypomethylated, separately) with the distribution of all evaluated CpG sites based on their relation to nearest gene regions (Fig. 2f, Additional file 4: Table S2) or their relation to CpG islands (Fig. 2g, Additional file 5: Table S3) using χ^2 test. The results showed that hypermethylated CpGs are mainly located at TSS1500 (transcription start sites 1500), IGR (intergenic

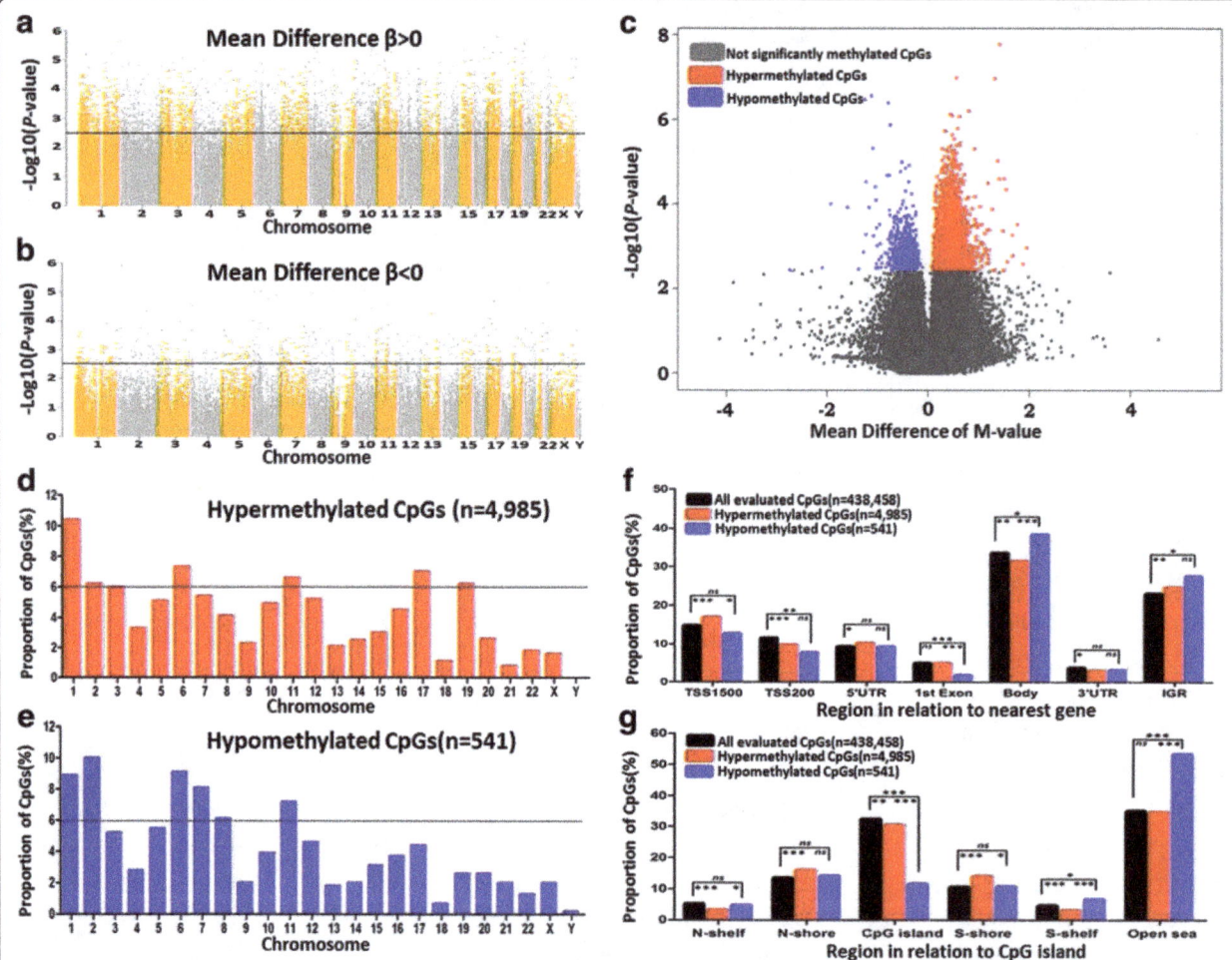

Fig. 1 Epigenetic profiles of differentially methylated CpGs of PPAT between OB/OW and NW groups. Manhattan plots show epigenetic profiles of all increased methylated CpGs (**a**) and all decreased methylated CpGs (**b**). The X-axis shows chromosomes, and the Y-axis is a −log10 (P value). The black line represents the threshold of adjusted P value = 0.25. CpGs above the black line are significantly hyper- or hypomethylated. The volcano plot of DNA methylation (**c**) shows a significant difference in PPAT between the OB/OW and NW groups. Four thousand nine hundred eighty-five hypermethylated CpGs are labeled in red, and 541 hypomethylated CpGs are labeled in green (adjusted P value > 0.25). The proportions of hyper- and hypomethylated CpGs on each chromosome are shown in (**d**) and (**e**). The black line indicates if the proportions of hyper- and hypomethylated CpGs on a chromosome are higher than 6%. The distribution of significant DMCs (hyper- or hypomethylated CpGs) and globe DNA methylation CpGs in locations related to the nearest gene regions and CpG islands are shown in **f** and **g**. Hypermethylated CpGs are mainly located at TSS1500 (transcription start sites 1500), IGR (intergenic region), N-shore (the 2 kb regions upstream of the CpG island boundaries), and S-shore (the 2 kb regions downstream of the CpG island boundaries), and hypomethylated CpGs are mostly located at the gene body and open sea. The difference of the proportion of CpGs among the three CpG groups was calculated based on the χ^2 test (*P < 0.05, **P < 0.01, ***P < 0.001, ns not significant). CpG islands were defined as DNA sequences (500 base windows; excluding most repetitive Alu-elements) with a GC base composition greater than 50% and a CpG observed/expected ratio of more than 0.6. The 2 kb regions immediately upstream (N_Shore) and downstream (S_Shore) of the CpG island boundaries were defined as "CpG island shores," and the 2 kb regions upstream (N_Shelf) and downstream (S_Shelf) of the CpG island shores were referred as "CpG island shelves." Open seas were the regions more than 4 kb from CpG islands

region), N-shore, and S-shore, and hypomethylated CpGs are mostly located at the gene body and open sea.

Functional enrichment analysis of significantly obesity-associated DMCs

To investigate the potential biological relevance of the significant DMCs, we further filtered 483 DMCs (distributed within 413 genes) from a total of 5526 DMCs according to their locations at both the gene promoter and CpG

island (Additional file 6: Table S4). Four hundred seventy-five of the 483 DMCs (representing 404 genes) were hypermethylated. Functional enrichment analysis of the hypermethylated genes showed that these genes were enriched for biological processes, such as pattern specification process, neuron differentiation, neuron fate specification, and negative regulation of phosphate metabolic process (adjusted P value < 0.05, Additional file 7: Table S5), as well as molecular functions, such as

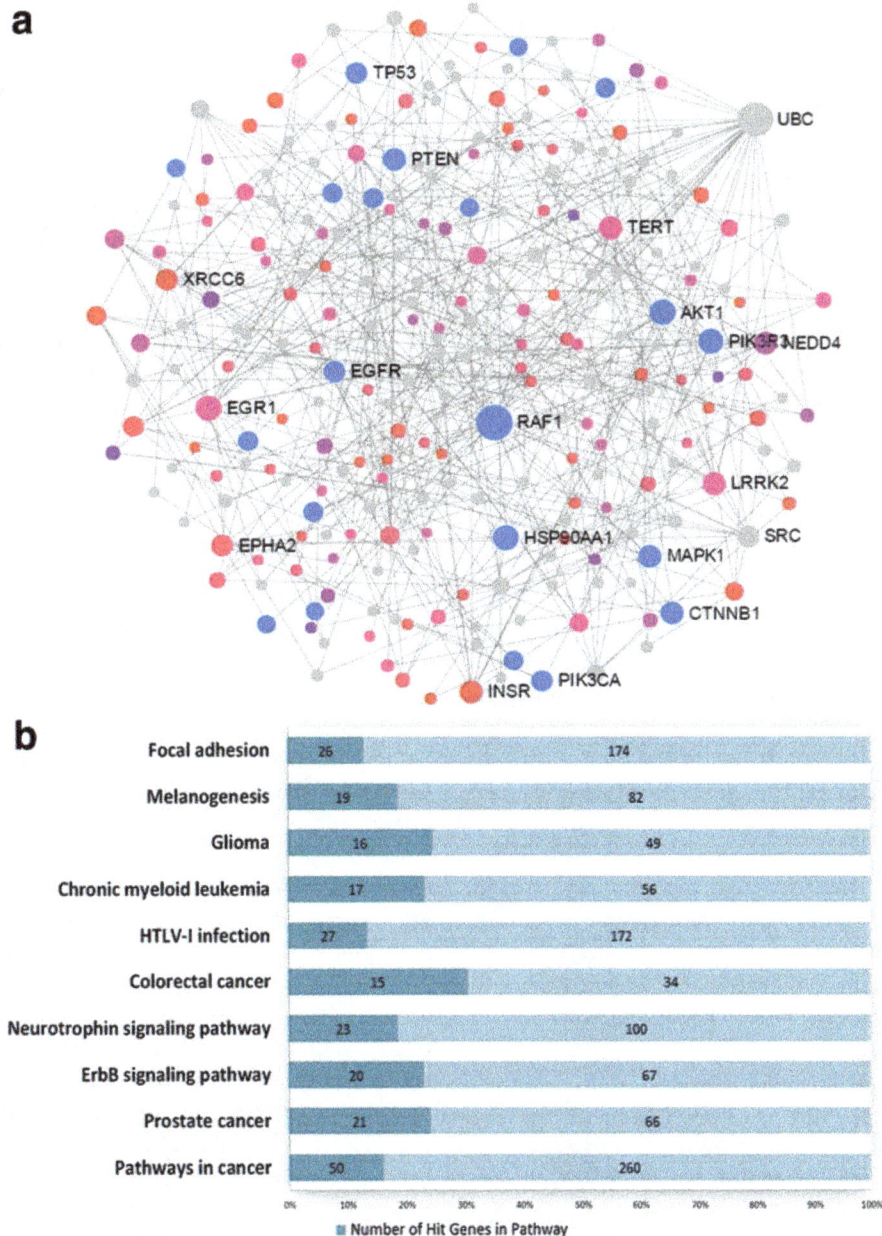

Fig. 2 Protein-protein interaction analysis. **a** A subnetwork composing of 247 nodes and 403 edges was generated using methylated genes. Blue dots represent the genes involved in prostate cancer; red and pink dots represent the seeds (methylated genes) according to the different *P* values; the gray dots represent the proteins which were closely interacted with the seeds, and the circle size represents the node degree. **b** The pathway enrichment analysis shows the subnetwork is mainly enriched in cancer pathways (*P* < 0.0001)

neuropeptide receptor activity and sequence-specific DNA-binding RNA polymerase II transcription factor activity (adjusted *P* value < 0.1, Additional file 8: Table S6). KEGG pathway enrichment analysis showed that hypermethylated genes were involved in signaling pathways regulating pluripotency of stem cells, fatty acid metabolism, basal cell carcinoma, non-alcoholic fatty liver disease (NAFLD), and AMPK signaling pathway (*P* value < 0.05, Additional file 9: Table S7).

We mapped the 404 hypermethylated genes to the STRING database and generated a protein-protein interaction (PPI) network by the NetworkAnalyst. The largest subnetwork was identified to include 247 nodes (genes) and 403 edges (Fig. 2a). In the network, the size of the nodes was based on their degree values and the color of nodes was based on their *P* values. This network contained 118 seed genes from the DMCs, and the enrichment pathway analysis showed that the genes of the subnetwork were mostly involved in the pathways of prostate cancer and other cancers (Fig. 2b, Additional file 10: Table S8, adjusted P value < 0.05). Particularly, the gene *UBC* (ubiquitin C) was found to be a hub connecting with many other nodes in the network, suggesting that the gene may play important biological roles in the PPAT of obese PCa patients.

Selected genes with multiple methylated CpG sites

In order to explore repression of genes by DNA methylation modifications, we selected genes which had multiple hypermethylated CpG sites (the number of methylated CpG sites ≥ 2, in at least one of the sites with a mean difference of β > 3% and an adjusted P value < 0.25) (Additional file 1: Figure S1 and Additional file 11: Table S9). A total of 38 genes with 100 differentially methylated CpG sites were selected, which included *TAPBP, RUNX3, CPT1B, CPT1C, MOGAT3, WNT2,* and *AIRE* (Additional file 11: Table S9). Notably, the promoter region of *TAPBP* (TAP-binding protein) had eight hypermethylated CpG sites in the promoter (Fig. 3a), which were significantly more methylated in the OB/OW than those in the NW groups (Fig. 3b), with a mean difference of β value greater than 5% (Additional file 10: Table S8). Spearman's rank correlation showed strong association ($r^2 = 0.73$–0.97) of the eight hypermethylated CpGs in the *TAPBP* promoter with their methylation levels (Fig. 3c). Pathway analysis of these genes revealed enrichment for fatty acid metabolism, PPAR signaling pathway, glucagon signaling pathway, AMPK signaling pathway, glycerolipid metabolism, basal cell carcinoma, antigen processing and presentation, ECM receptor interaction, and insulin resistance (adjusted P value < 0.25) (Additional file 12: Table S10).

Differential methylated regions analysis

Ten DMRs were identified ($P < 0.01$) in obesity PPAT samples compared to normal weight controls (Table 3). The size of the DMRs varied from 161 to 1287 bp. Noteworthy, four out of the ten DMRs were discovered on chromosome 6. Eight regions were located in genes, and two were in the intergenic region. Four regions were in the gene promoter of *FAM104A, C17orf80, HOXA4A,* and *TAPBP*.

Association analysis between DNA methylation and mRNA expression

Increased DNA methylation of promoter in CpG islands was obviously linked to gene transcriptional silencing [26]. Therefore, we related hypermethylated CpG sites in PPAT with genes showed decreased gene expression level from our previously generated mRNA expression data [4]. DNA methylation of 16 CpG sites, corresponding to 14 genes, was associated with significantly decreased transcripts in OB/OW group (P value < 0.05) (Table 4). The Spearman's

rank correlation analysis showed that eight of the 14 genes have significantly negative association (P value < 0.05) between the methylation profiles and the gene expression profiles of these genes (Table 4). The repression genes were mainly involved in metabolic pathways (Additional file 13: Table S11, adjusted P value < 0.25), such as *MOGAT1* (glycerolipid metabolism), *FADS1* (fatty acid metabolism and biosynthesis of unsaturated fatty acids), and *PCYT2* (glycerophospholipid metabolism). The mRNA expression level of *FADS1* was significantly decreased in the PPAT of obese with prostate cancers in our previous study using qRT-PCR [4]. Besides these, GO enrichment analysis showed that these genes are functionally related to receptor binding (neuropeptide receptor binding, dopamine receptor binding, and insulin receptor binding) and enzyme activity (acid phosphatase activity, metallocarboxypeptidase activity, and acylglycerol *O*-acyltransferase activity) (Additional file 14: Table S12, adjusted P value < 0.25).

Discussion

This pilot study revealed significant differences of DNA methylation profiles between the PPATs from OB/OW versus NW PCa patients. Variations in global DNA methylation demonstrated that excess adiposity played an important role in DNA methylation level of PPAT tissues in prostate cancer patients, which provide an opportunity to explore the effect of obesity on PPAT epigenetic modification and subsequently on prostate cancer. These findings reported for the first time in PPAT depot are in concordance with previous works reporting that excess adiposity and BMI activate DNA methylation in adipose tissue [27–29]. Thus, considering the present understanding of the potential causal relationship between excess adiposity and cancer [30], diabetes [11], and cardiovascular disease [31], our results provide methylated candidate genes, which might foster research on the potential biological mechanisms underlying epigenetic regulation of PPAT by excess adiposity and prostate cancer.

Given that DNA methylation of CpGs located at promoters and islands are associated with gene transcription silencing, we performed a strict filtering of DMCs and explored the biological functions of all promoter hypermethylated genes, aiming to find the critical methylated CpGs in the PPAT between the obese and normal weight PCa patients. Bioinformatic analysis showed that the enriched pathways were mostly involved in metabolic disorders, particularly fatty acid degradation and glycerolipid and choline metabolism. These pathways are known to mediate the pro-tumoral effect of white adipose tissue in tumors, thus contributing to tumorigenesis and metastasis [32, 33], particularly in prostate cancer [5]. Findings from other oncological models highlight excess adiposity-associated impact in methylation

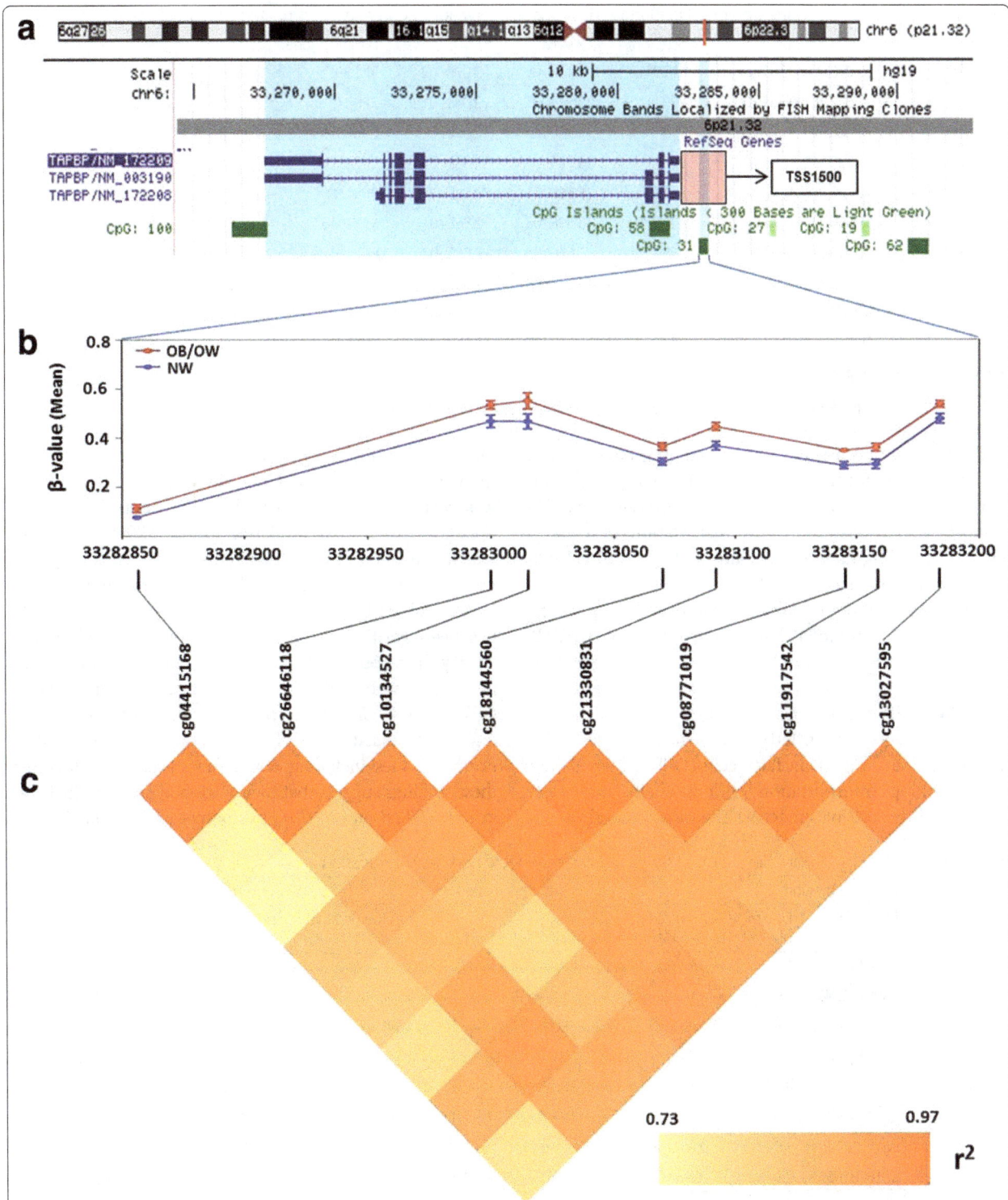

Fig. 3 Visualization and analysis of hypermethylated CpG sites in TAPBP promoter. **a** The chromosome positions of hypermethylated CpG sites show that DMCs are located at chr6 (p21.32), which is in the region of TSS1500 (pink square) of TAPBP and at the location of CpG island 31. **b** Methylation levels of eight CpG sites in PPAT from OB/OW and NW PCa patients have shown a significant difference. **c** Correlation analysis shows strong correlation (Spearman correlation coefficient r^2 0.73~ 0.97) between the eight hypermethylated CpG sites based on the mean β value difference of individual probes

Table 3 Differentially methylated regions (DMR) in PPAT of obese/overweight PCa patients compared to normal weight controls

DMR	Chr	Start–end (bp)	Size (bp)	P value	FDR	Located gene	DMCs*	Relation to CpG island
1	6	30,038,791–30,039,801	1010	5.11E−05	2.07E−02	RNF39	37(0)	Island
2	6	29,648,161–29,649,084	923	1.54E−03	2.08E−01	ZFP57#	22(0)	Open sea
3	17	71,228,123–71,228,832	709	3.10E−03	2.86E−01	FAM104A	4(3)	Island
4	17	71,228,123–71,228,832	709	3.10E−03	2.86E−01	C17orf80	10(8)	Island
5	12	42,720,006–42,720,167	161	5.56E−03	2.86E−01	PPHLN1	4(0)	Island
6	6	31,650,735–31,651,158	423	5.59E−03	2.86E−01	MIR4646#	16(0)	Island
7	7	27,169,674–27,170,961	1287	5.66E−03	2.86E−01	HOXA4	17(11)	Island
8	6	33,282,736–33,283,145	409	5.87E−03	2.86E−01	TAPBP	18(18)	Island
9	20	57,463,763–57,464,129	366	6.74E−03	2.86E−01	GNAS	15(0)	Island
10	16	86,546,938–86,547,322	384	7.03E−03	2.86E−01	FOXF1	4(0)	Shore

#The DMR is located at the intergenic region
Chr chromosome
*The number in the bracket is the quantities of DMCs located at the promoter (TSS200 and TSS1500) regions

markers known to associate with potential effect in the cancer microenvironment (e.g., aromatase, prostaglandin E_2 receptor in breast cancer) [34, 35]. Obesity has also been shown to associate with methylation of cancer-related genes (E-cadherin, p16, and RAR-β(2)) directly in malignant breast cells [36, 37].

Pathway enrichment analysis showed a strong association between promoter hypermethylation of CPT1B, CPT1C, ACADM, and FADS1, with fatty acid metabolism. CPT1B (carnitine palmitoyltransferase 1B) and CPT1C (carnitine palmitoyltransferase 1C) genes encode rate-limiting enzymes in fatty acid degradation and play critical roles in long-chain fatty acid (LCFA) β-oxidation by controlling transportation of long-chain fatty acyl-CoAs from the cytoplasm across the outer mitochondria

membrane [38]. Maple et al. reported that increased methylation of specific CpGs in the CPT1B promoter was correlated with decreased CPT1B transcripts in the skeletal muscle after lipid oversupply in severe obesity, which resulted in obese individual's incapacity to increase fat oxidation, contributing to metabolic inflexibility [39]. Although the biochemical function of CPT1C has been verified to be necessary for the regulation of energy homeostasis in CPT1C knockout mouse brain [40], the study of CPT1C methylation was absent. CPT1B and CPT1C were previously reported to be highly expressed in the muscle, brain, and many other normal tissues including adipocytes [41]. Taken together, these findings suggest that methylation of specific CpG sites in the CPT1B and CPT1C promoters likely result in gene

Table 4 Genes hypermethylated in promoters with significantly decreased gene expression

Gene symbol	DNA methylation			Gene expression			Correlation analysis	
	Probe ID	DNAm β diff. (%)	Adjusted P value (< 0.25)	Probe ID	FC	P value (< 0.05)	Spearman's rank correlation coefficient	P value (< 0.05)
UCN	cg20442078	5.6	0.17	8051061	− 1.12	3.61E−02	− 8.42E−01	2.23E−03
CCHCR1	cg00160818	1.9	0.17	8124868	− 1.14	1.73E−02	− 7.45E−01	9.21E−03
CRB3	cg14782015	4.3	0.20	8025041	− 1.13	1.84E−02	− 7.21E−01	1.21E−02
AGBL4	cg21834207	3.2	0.13	7915971	− 1.17	1.29E−02	− 6.73E−01	1.97E−02
INSL3	cg10174482	4.2	0.13	8035345	− 1.13	4.94E−02	− 6.36E−01	2.72E−02
ANKRD30B	cg21293934	11.2	0.21	8069499	− 1.17	2.24E−02	− 6.08E−01	3.11E−02
FADS1	cg16213375	3.6	0.16	7948612	− 1.8	9.55E−04	− 5.88E−01	4.01E−02
PAPL	cg18481683	2.3	0.24	8028570	− 1.19	1.45E−02	− 5.52E−01	5.21E−02
MOGAT1	cg12678667	4	0.15	8048725	− 1.28	3.87E−02	− 4.67E−01	8.91E−02
PPP1R1B	cg09762778	5	0.12	8006865	− 1.27	4.74E−02	− 4.67E−01	8.91E−02
PRUNE2	cg00390775	4.4	0.15	8161884	− 1.31	1.91E−02	− 3.82E−01	1.39E−01
CIDEA	cg18309817	1.8	0.18	8020211	− 1.32	3.21E−02	− 2.97E−01	2.03E−01
PCYT2	cg19583655	6.2	0.21	8019280	− 1.26	6.38E−04	− 1.88E−01	3.04E−01
SCUBE1	cg07697597	1.7	0.23	8076586	− 1.23	9.03E−03	− 4.24E−02	4.59E−01

FC fold change, *DNAm β diff.* DNAm β difference

expression silencing, thus consequently contributing to fatty acid accumulation in adipocytes by decreasing long-chain fatty acid β-oxidation in the mitochondria (Fig. 4).

LCFA and *ACADM* genes (aliases MCAD, medium-chain acyl-CoA dehydrogenase) coding for metabolic enzymes presented increased methylation in the PPAT of the OB/OW group. *ACADM* is the critical enzyme of the initial step of β-oxidation and controls the medium-chain fatty acid (MCFA) metabolism by catalyzing the

dehydrogenation of medium-chain Acyl-CoA, which is the common middle product of MCFA and LCFA, in the mitochondria. Mutations in *ACADM* cause MCAD deficiency, which resulted in fatty acid oxidation disorder leading to disease or infantile death [42–44]. Greco et al. [45] reported inverse association between *ACADM* transcript abundance with fat content in the human liver. Our findings suggest that the hypermethylated *ACADM* found in the PPAT of OB/OW PCa patients might fail to

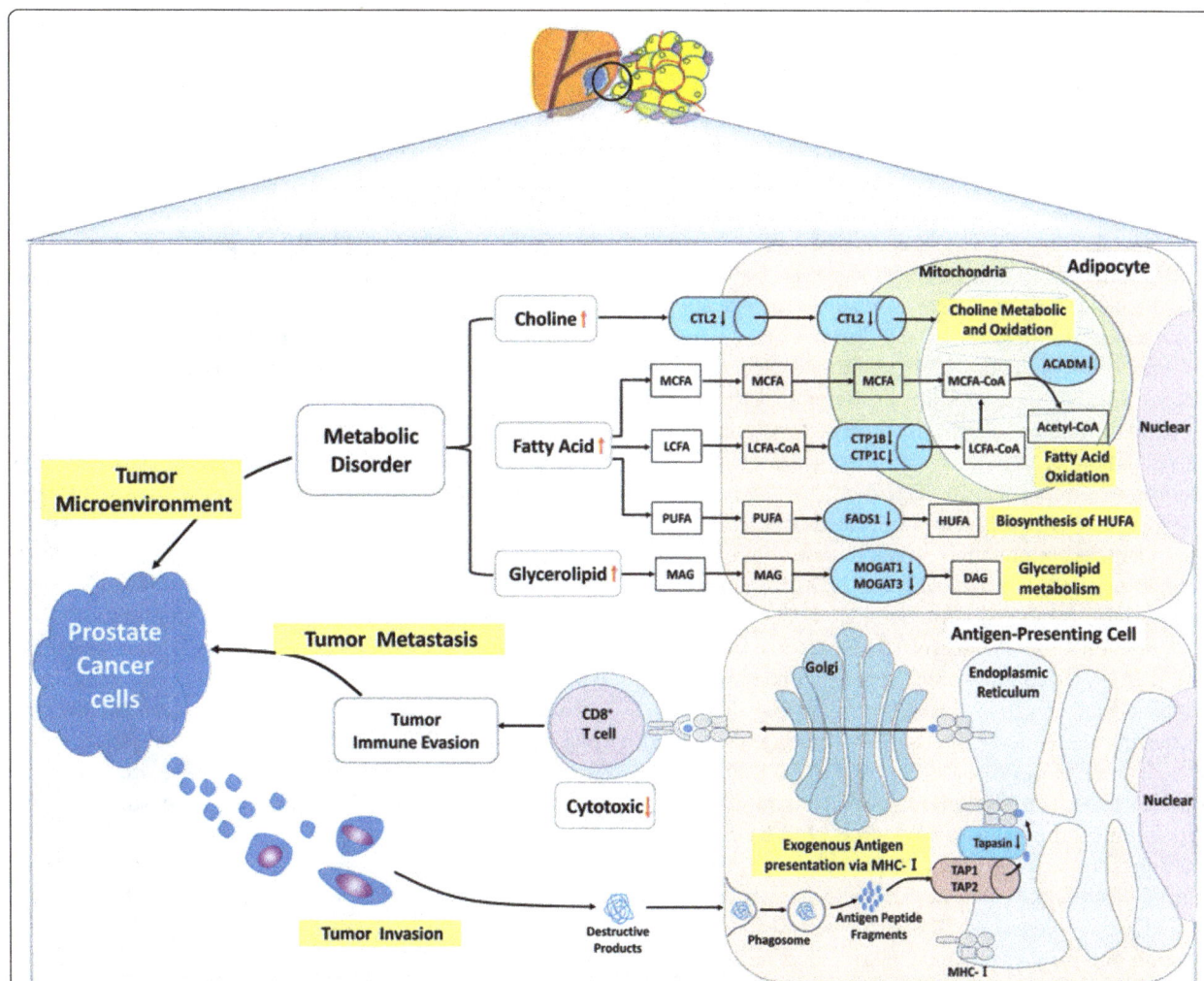

Fig. 4 Proposed mechanisms with differentially methylated genes from PPAT of OB/OW prostate cancer patients. Hypermethylated genes in periprostatic adipose tissue of patients with increased adiposity might contribute towards the modulation of prostate tumor microenvironment. The genes that might be related to tumor microenvironment include choline transporter-like protein 2 (*CTL2*, which was a rate-limiting step of choline metabolism by transporting extracellular choline into cell and mitochondria), carnitine palmitoyltransferase 1B and 1C (*CPT1B* and *CPT1C*, which encode the rate-limiting enzymes of long-chain fatty acid β-oxidation by controlling transportation of long-chain fatty acyl-CoAs from cytoplasm across outer mitochondria membrane), medium-chain-specific acyl-CoA dehydrogenase (*ACADM*, which catalyzes the initial step of medium-chain fatty acid β-oxidation in mitochondria), fatty acid desaturase 1 (*FADS1*, which was correlated with fatty acid metabolism by catalyzing polyunsaturated fatty acid biosynthesis), monoacylglycerol O-acyltransferases 1 and 3 (*MOGAT1* and *MOGAT3*, which catalyze the formation of diacylglycerol by transferring fatty acyl-CoA to 2-monoacylglycerol), which contributes to metabolic disorder in adipose tissue by regulating the metabolism of lipid, choline, and glycerolipid. Another gene with hypermethylated promoter, *TAPBP* (transporter associated with antigen processing (TAP) transport protein), could influence tumor supervision of immune cells in PPAT by altering tumor antigen presentation process from TAP to MHC class I in endoplasmic reticulum and result in tumor metastasis and cancer progression. The black downward arrows represent the promoter hypermethylated genes (in blue containers), and the red arrows represent the possible consequence of these methylated genes. *LCFA* long-chain fatty acid, *MCFA* media-chain fatty acid, *PUFA* polyunsaturated fatty acid, *HUFA* high unsaturated fatty acid, *MAG* monoacylglycerol, *DAG* dionoacylglycerol

generate medium-chain acyl-CoA β-oxidation and result in MCFA and LCFA accumulation in adipose tissue, providing a favorable tumor microenvironment for PCa cell aggressiveness (Fig. 4). Additional functional studies are required to confirm this assumption.

The hypermethylation of the *FADS1* (fatty acid desaturase 1) promoter, whose transcriptional activity was significantly decreased in OB/OW PCa patients in agreement with our previous study [4], has been described as correlated with polyunsaturated fatty acid (PUFA) metabolism by catalyzing the biosynthesis of highly unsaturated fatty acids (HUFA) from the catalysis of dihomo-gamma-linoleic acid (DGLA, 20:3 n-6) and eicosatetraenoic acid (ETA, 20:4 n-3) desaturation, in order to generate arachidonic acid (AA, 20:4 n-6) and eicosapentaenoic acid (EPA, 20:5 n-3) [46]. Genetic variants in the *FADS1* and *FADS2* gene clusters have been associated with altered (n-6) and (n-3) PUFA metabolism [47, 48], whereas metabolic disorder in PUFA exerted effects on PCa by mediating the formation of eicosanoid inflammatory mediators (prostaglandins, leukotrienes, thromboxanes, and lipoxins), angiogenesis, immune cell regulation, and membrane structure and function [49, 50]. These results illustrated that the epigenetic modifications of *FADS1* may play important roles in the regulation of fatty acid metabolic genes on PPAT in response to excess adiposity (Fig. 4).

Besides abnormal fatty acid metabolism, DMC-related genes identified in our study were also correlated with glycerolipid metabolism. *MOGAT1* and *MOGAT3* encode the monoacylglycerol *O*-acyltransferase (MOGAT) and catalyze the formation of diacylglycerol (DAG) from monoacylglycerol (MAG), which is the precursor of phosphatidylcholine, phosphatidylethanolamine, and triacylglycerol (TAG), by transferring fatty acyl-CoA to 2-monoacylglycerol [51]. While human *MGAT1* (aliases for MOGAT1) is involved in intestinal dietary fat absorption and TAG synthesis in the liver, its function in adipose tissue has yet to be elucidated. The expression of *MGAT1* was increased in the liver of diet-induced obese mice with nonalcoholic fatty liver disease (NAFLD), but, interestingly, there was increased DAG accumulation and no inflammatory injury reduction in hepatocytes after *MGAT1* knockdown. Similarly, *MOGAT3* was mostly expressed in the human intestine and liver and maintained a significant DGAT (diacylglycerol *O*-acyltransferase) activity. Although results indicate that the metabolic mechanism of lipid regulation by *MGAT1* and *MOGAT3* was altered, evidence of association between lipid metabolic disorders caused by aberrant expression of MGAT1/MOGAT3 and PCa are lacking. Our data indicate the methylation of *MOGAT1* and *3* genes in PPAT may play important roles in response to excess adiposity by modulating glycerolipid metabolism (Fig. 4).

Choline metabolic disorder might be caused by epigenetic regulation of *SLC44A2* (solute carrier family 44 member 2), which encodes choline transporter-like protein 2 (CTL2) and is mainly expressed on blood plasma and mitochondrial membrane of different organisms and cell types. This transporter is a rate-limiting step in choline metabolism by transporting extracellular choline into cell and mitochondria. Choline is essential for synthesizing membrane phospholipid and neurotransmitter acetylcholine and used as a donor of methyl groups via choline oxidized in mitochondria [52]. The choline transporter has been associated with choline metabolic disorders, thus playing an important role in regulating immune response, inflammation, and oxidation [53, 54]. Concordantly, abnormal choline metabolism emerged as a metabolic hallmark, associated with oncogenesis and tumor progression in prostate cancer and other malignancies [55–57]. The increased uptake of choline by the cancer cell was important to meet the needs of phosphatidylcholine synthesis [58]. We hypothesize that hypermethylated *SLC44A2* in adipocytes might be associated with lower uptake and oxidation of extracellular choline, resulting in choline accumulation in PPAT extracellular media (Fig. 4) and increasing the availability of choline for PCa cell metabolism.

Besides metabolic modifications, altered immune regulation pathways were also enriched in DMC-related genes. *TAPBP* (alias tapasin) encodes a transmembrane glycoprotein, which mediates the interaction between MHC class I molecules and a transport protein TAP (transporter associated with antigen processing), being responsible for antigen processing and presentation. This mechanism occurs via mediating TAP to translocate endo/exogenous antigen peptides from the cytoplasm into the endoplasmic reticulum and deliver the antigen peptides to MHC class I molecules. The cancer cell's survival depends on successful escape to immune surveillance. Loss of MHC class I has been described as a major immune evasion strategy for cancer cells. Downregulation of antigen-presenting MHC class I pathway in tumor cells was a common mechanism for tumor cells escaped from specific immune responses, which can be associated with coordinated silencing of antigen-presenting machinery genes, such as *TAPBP* [59]. Cross-presentation is the ability of certain antigen-presenting cells to take up, process, and present extracellular antigens with MHC class I molecules to CD8[+] T cells. This process is necessary for immunity against most tumors. Recent studies revealed that *TAPBP* is a major target for cancer immune evasion mechanisms and decreased *TAPBP* expression in cancer was associated with reduced CD8[+] T cell-mediated killing of the tumor cells, lowered immune responses, and enhanced tumor metastases via downregulation of antigen presentation the MHC class I pathway [60, 61]. Our results showed that *TAPBP* promoter hypermethylation in the PPAT of obese PCa subjects likely reduced the expression or activity of *TAPBP*, downregulating tumor cell's antigen presentation of immune cells in PPAT, leading to impaired CD8$^+$ T cell activation (Fig. 4). This indicates that methylation of *TAPBP* might be a mechanism by which prostate cancer cells escape the immune surveillance and provide an appropriate microenvironment for tumor aggressiveness, allowing prostatic cancer cells' transfer, spread, and growth. The significant DMR identified with eight DMCs located in the *TAPBP* promoter further supported its role in prostate cancer.

From the PPI analysis, the network which was connected through ubiquitin C is characterized, suggesting *UBC* played a significant biological function with the methylated genes in PPAT between OB/OW and NW patients and somehow was correlated with the methylation. Ubiquitin is much known with the functions including roles in protein degradation, DNA repair, cell cycle regulation, kinase modification, and cell signaling pathways [62]. Recent reports expressed that the ubiquitin-proteasome system was associated with the progression and metastasis of prostate cancers [63, 64]. And long-term silencing of the *UBC* was found to be correlated with DNA methylation at the promoters [65]. Additional studies are needed to clarify whether the protein network for methylated genes impacts prostate cancer and if this difference is associated with ubiquitin C.

Although we present the first report on periprostatic adipose tissue methylation profile in association with excess adiposity measured by BMI, our results should be interpreted in the context of several potential limitations. This study is limited by small sample size, even though representative groups of OB/OW and NW are likely to be selected following the strict inclusion/exclusion criteria and between-group match by clinicopathological and demographic variables. Although we matched patients by clinicopathological characteristics between adiposity groups, tobacco smoking was more frequent among OB/OW compared with NW patients. Actually, albeit we cannot exclude an effect of smoking status on the presumably adiposity-associated findings presented herein, due to a known effect of tobacco on overall DNA methylation, data from previous reports indicate that methylation profiles are tissue-specific [66, 67] and that adiposity-associated DNA methylation occurs independently of tobacco smoking [68, 69]. Future studies will benefit from the confirmation of these results in larger sample sizes, determination of correspondence to matched prostate tumor methylation patterns, investigation of interactome at the interface between tumor and PPAT, and prospective investigations on the value of PPAT epigenetic modifications on cancer recurrence and survival. Future validation and replication are important to establish the accuracy and generalizability of the reported associations.

In summary, we observed differences in PPAT methylation between NW and OB individuals at several loci known to be involved in the metabolism of choline (*SLC44A2*), fatty acids (*CPT1B, CPT1C, ACADM, FADS1*), and glycerolipid (*MOGAT1, MOGAT3*) and in the regulation of exogenous tumor antigen presentation (*TAPBP*). These findings suggest a relationship of adiposity status with the methylation profile, which ultimately modulates tumor microenvironment and may influence PCa behavior.

Conclusions

In this preliminary study, we report DNA methylation changes in PPAT underlying the association between excess adiposity and PCa. Whole epigenome methylation profiling of PPAT of PCa patients revealed significant differences in OB/OW versus normal weight subjects. Epigenetic imprinting in association with excess adiposity expressed the methylated modifications in genes functionally related with lipid metabolism and immune function, which could ultimately contribute to an unfavorable tumor microenvironment and decreased immune surveillance for prostate tumors. This association analyses provided us novel insights into how prostate cancer patients with excess adiposity differ from those of patients with normal weight in epigenome. Findings from this study warrant confirmation in PPAT samples from larger number of patients.

Additional files

Additional file 1: Figure S1. Research flowchart. Whole research flowchart. NW normal weight, OB/OW obese/overweight, BMI body mass index, PPAT periprostatic adipose tissue, QC quality control, DMCs differentially methylated CpG sites, DMRs differentially methylated regions, Limma linear models for microarray and RNA-seq analysis data using *R*, GO gene ontology, KEGG Kyoto Encyclopedia of Genes and Genomes, PPI protein-protein interaction network. (JPEG 128 kb)

Additional file 2: Table S1. Differentially methylated CpG sites in PPAT between obese/overweight PCa patients and normal weight controls. The table shows 5526 DMCs in PPAT between obese/overweight PCa patients and normal weight patients, which were identified by using the "Limma" method. (XLSX 663 kb)

Additional file 3: Figure S2. Heatmap of differentially methylated CpG sites between the PPAT of OB/OW PCa and NW PCa patients. The graphical display of hierarchical clustering for DMCs. The selected CpGs are those with FDR < 0.25 and beta difference between obesity and normal weight group larger than 10%. (JPEG 1797 kb)

Additional file 4: Table S2. Distribution of differentially methylated CpG sites in relation to the nearest gene regions. The table shows the distribution of DMCs according to the relation to the nearest gene regions. (XLSX 11 kb)

Additional file 5: Table S3. Distribution of differentially methylated CpG sites in relation to CpG islands. The table shows the distribution of DMCs according to the relation to CpG islands. (XLSX 13 kb)

Additional file 6: Table S4. Differentially methylated CpG sites located at both gene promoters and CpG islands. This table shows the 483 DMCs which locate at both gene promoters and CpG islands. (XLSX 76 kb)

Additional file 7: Table S5. GO biological process analysis of promoter hypermethylated genes. GO biological process analysis for 404 promoter hypermethylated genes. (XLSX 18 kb)

Additional file 8: Table S6. GO molecular function analysis of promoter hypermethylated genes. GO molecular function analysis for 404 promoter hypermethylated genes. (XLSX 13 kb)

Additional file 9: Table S7. Pathway enrichment analysis of promoter hypermethylated genes. Pathway enrichment analysis for 404 promoter hypermethylated genes. (XLSX 11 kb)

Additional file 10: Table S8. Pathway enrichment analysis of the genes included in PPI networks. Pathway enrichment analysis for methylated genes and related genes included in PPI networks. (XLSX 13 kb)

Additional file 11: Table S9. Selected genes with multiple hypermethylated CpG sites in PPAT with obese/overweight. The table shows the 38 selected genes which have multiple hypermethylated CpG sites. (XLSX 24 kb)

Additional file 12: Table S10. Pathway enrichment analysis of the selected genes with multiple hypermethylated CpG sites. Pathway enrichment analysis for the 38 selected genes which have multiple hypermethylated CpG sites. (XLSX 13 kb)

Additional file 13: Table S11. Pathway enrichment analysis of the overlapping genes. Pathway enrichment analysis for the 14 overlapping genes. (XLSX 13 kb)

Additional file 14: Table S12. GO molecular function analysis of the overlapping genes. GO molecular function analyses for the 14 overlapping genes. (XLSX 13 kb)

Abbreviations

AA: Arachidonic acid; ACADM: Aliases MCAD, medium-chain acyl-CoA dehydrogenase; BH: Benjamin and Hochberg; BMI: Body mass index; CPT1B: Carnitine palmitoyltransferase 1B; CPT1C: Carnitine palmitoyltransferase 1C; CTL2: Choline transporter-like protein 2; DAG: Diacylglycerol; DGAT: Diacylglycerol O-acyltransferase; DGAT2: Diacylglycerol O-acyltransferase 2; DGEs: Differential gene expressions; DGLA: Dihomo-gamma-linoleic acid; DMCs: Differentially methylated CpG sites; DMRs: Differentially methylated regions; EPA: Eicosapentaenoic acid; ER: Endoplasmic reticulum; EWAS: Epigenetic-wide Association Studies; FADS1: Fatty acid desaturase 1; FDR: False discovery rate; GO: Gene ontology; GWAS: Genome-wide Association Studies; HUFA: Highly unsaturated fatty acid; KEGG: Kyoto Encyclopedia of Genes and Genomes; LCFA: Long-chain fatty acids; limma: Linear models for microarray and RNA-seq data; MAG: Monoacylglycerol; MCFA: Medium-chain fatty acid; MGAT1: Aliases for MOGAT1; MHC: Major histocompatibility complex; MOGAT: Monoacylglycerol O-acyltransferase; MOGAT1: Monoacylglycerol O-acyltransferase 1; MOGAT3: Monoacylglycerol O-acyltransferase 3; NAFLD: Nonalcoholic fatty liver disease; PCa: Prostate cancer; PPAT: Periprostatic adipose tissue; PPI: Protein-protein interaction analysis; PSA: Prostate-specific antigen; PUFA: Polyunsaturated fatty acid; QC: Quality control; SLC44A2: Solute carrier family 44 member 2; TAG: Triacylglycerol; TAP: Transporter associated with antigen processing; TAPBP: TAP binding protein; TSS: Transcription start site; TSS1500: 1500 bp upstream of the transcription start site; TSS200: 200 bp upstream of the transcription start site; UBC: Ubiquitin C

Funding

This work was supported in part by the Natural Sciences and Engineering Research Council of Canada, Manitoba Research Health Council, University of Manitoba, and China Scholarship Council.

Authors' contributions

YC designed and implemented the experiments and drafted the manuscripts. JY helped generate the figures. PH supervised and monitored the whole project. RR, CM, AM, CP, VC, JGA, GF, and AR performed the tissue handling and processing, isolated the RNA, and conducted the gene expression experiment. RR, AF, AM, and CM collected the adipose tissue and clinicopathological patient information and edited the manuscript. RR, GF, and PH designed the study and edited the manuscript. All authors read, edited, and approved the final manuscript.

Author details

[1]Department of Biochemistry and Medical Genetics & Department of Electrical and Computer Engineering, University of Manitoba, Winnipeg, Canada. [2]Experimental Center, Northwest University for Nationalities, Lanzhou, People's Republic of China. [3]Molecular Oncology Group, Portuguese Institute of Oncology, Porto, Portugal. [4]Research Department, Portuguese League Against Cancer–North, Porto, Portugal. [5]Laboratory of Genetics and Environmental Health Institute, Faculty of Medicine, University of Lisboa, Lisbon, Portugal. [6]Tumor & Microenvironment Interactions, i3S/INEB, Institute for Research and Innovation in Health, and Institute of Biomedical Engineering, University of Porto, Porto, Portugal. [7]Department of Urology, Centro Hospitalar Universitário do Porto, Porto, Portugal. [8]CINTESIS, Center for Health Technology and Services Research, Faculty of Medicine, e, University of Porto, Porto, Portugal. [9]Metabolic Research Laboratory, Universidad de Navarra, Pamplona, Spain. [10]CIBER Fisiopatología de la Obesidad y Nutricion, Instituto de Salud Carlos III, Madrid, Spain. [11]Department of Endocrinology, Clínica Universidad de Navarra, Pamplona, Spain. [12]Department of Clinical Pathology, Centro Hospitalar e Universitário de Coimbra, Coimbra, Portugal. [13]i3S/INEB, Instituto de Investigação e Inovação em Saúde/Instituto Nacional de Engenharia Biomédica, Universidade do Porto, Tumor & Microenvironment Interactions, Rua Alfredo Allen, 208 4200-135 Porto, Portugal.

References

1. Labbé DP, Zadra G, Ebot EM, Mucci LA, Kantoff PW, Loda M, Brown M. Role of diet in prostate cancer: the epigenetic link. Oncogene. 2014; 34(36):4683–91.
2. Sutcliffe S, Colditz GA. Prostate cancer: is it time to expand the research focus to early-life exposures? Nat Rev Cancer. 2013;13:208–18.
3. Peisch SF, Van Blarigan EL, Chan JM, Stampfer MJ, Kenfield SA. Prostate cancer progression and mortality: a review of diet and lifestyle factors. World J Urol. 2017;35(6):867–74.
4. Ribeiro R, Monteiro C, Catalán V, Hu P, Cunha V, Rodríguez A, Gómez-Ambrosi J, Fraga A, Príncipe P, Lobato C, Lobo F, Morais A, Silva V, Sanches-Magalhães J, Oliveira J, Pina F, Lopes C, Medeiros R, Frühbeck G. Obesity and prostate cancer: gene expression signature of human periprostatic adipose tissue. BMC Med. 2012;10:108.
5. Venkatasubramanian PN, Brendler CB, Plunkett BA, Crawford SE, Fitchev PS, Morgan G, Cornwell ML, McGuire MS, Wyrwicz AM, Doll JA. Periprostatic adipose tissue from obese prostate cancer patients promotes tumor and endothelial cell proliferation: a functional and MR imaging pilot study. Prostate. 2014;74:326–35.
6. Iordanescu G, Brendler C, Crawford SE, Wyrwicz AM, Venkatasubramanian PN, Doll JA. MRS measured fatty acid composition of periprostatic adipose tissue correlates with pathological measures of prostate cancer aggressiveness. J Magn Reson Imaging. 2015;42(3):651–7.
7. Laurent V, Guérard A, Mazerolles C, Le Gonidec S, Toulet A, Nieto L, Zaidi F, Majed B, Garandeau D, Socrier Y, Golzio M, Cadoudal T, Chaoui K, Dray C, Monsarrat B, Schiltz O, Wang YY, Couderc B, Valet P, Malavaud B, Muller C. Periprostatic adipocytes act as a driving force for prostate cancer progression in obesity. Nat Commun. 2016;7:10230.
8. Ribeiro R, Monteiro C, Cunha V, Oliveira MJ, Freitas M, Fraga A, Príncipe P, Lobato C, Lobo F, Morais A, Silva V, Sanches-Magalhães J, Oliveira J, Pina F, Mota-Pinto A, Lopes C, Medeiros R. Human periprostatic adipose tissue promotes prostate cancer aggressiveness in vitro. J Exp Clin Cancer Res. 2012;31:32.
9. Liu L, Li Y, Tollefsbol TO. Gene-environment interactions and epigenetic basis of human diseases. Curr Issues Mol Biol. 2008;10(2):25–36.
10. Tost J. DNA methylation: an introduction to the biology and the disease-associated changes of a promising biomarker. Methods Mol Biol. 2009;507:3–20.
11. Barres R, Zierath J. DNA methylation in metabolic disorders. Am J Clin Nutr. 2011;93:897S–00.
12. Pinnick KE, Karpe F. DNA methylation of genes in adipose tissue. Proc Nutr Soc. 2011;70(1):57–63.
13. Benton MC, Johnstone A, Eccles D, Harmon B, Hayes MT, Lea RA, Griffiths L, Hoffman EP, Stubbs RS, Macartney-Coxson D. An analysis of DNA methylation in human adipose tissue reveals differential modification of obesity genes before and after gastric bypass and weight loss. Genome Biol. 2015;16:8.

14. Wu Y, Davison J, Qu X, Morrissey C, Storer B, Brown L, Vessella R, Nelson P, Fang M. Methylation profiling identified novel differentially methylated markers including OPCML and FLRT2 in prostate cancer. Epigenetics. 2016; 11(4):247–58.

15. Shui IM, Wong CJ, Zhao S, Kolb S, Ebot EM, Geybels MS, Rubicz R, Wright JL, Lin DW, Klotzle B, Bibikova M, Fan JB, Ostrander EA, Feng Z, Stanford JL. Prostate tumor DNA methylation is associated with cigarette smoking and adverse prostate cancer outcomes. Cancer. 2016;122(14):2168–77.

16. Kobayashi Y, Absher D. DNA methylation profiling reveals novel biomarkers and important roles for DNA methyltransferases in prostate cancer. Genome Res. 2011;21(7):1017–27.

17. Fraga A, Ribeiro R, Vizcaíno JR, Coutinho H, Lopes JM, Príncipe P, Lobato C, Lopes C, Medeiros R. Genetic polymorphisms in key hypoxia-regulated downstream molecules and phenotypic correlation in prostate cancer. BMC Urol. 2017;17:12.

18. Aryee MJ, Jaffe AE, Corrada-Bravo H, Ladd-Acosta C, Feinberg AP, Hansen KD, Irizarry RA. Minfi: a flexible and comprehensive Bioconductor package for the analysis of Infinium DNA methylation microarrays. Bioinformatics. 2014;30(10):1363–9.

19. Chen YA, Lemire M, Choufani S, Butcher DT, Grafodatskaya D, Zanke BW, Gallinger S, Hudson TJ, Weksberg R. Discovery of cross-reactive probes and polymorphic CpGs in the Illumina Infinium HumanMethylation450 microarray. Epigenetics. 2013; 11:8(2).

20. Ritchie ME, Phipson B, Wu D, Hu Y, Law CW, Shi W, Smyth GK. Limma powers differential expression analyses for RNA-sequencing and microarray studies. Nucleic Acids Res. 2015;43(7):289–300.

21. Benjamini Y, Hochberg Y. Controlling the false discovery rate: a practical and powerful approach to multiple testing. J R Stat Soc B. 1995;57(1):289–300.

22. Morris TJ, Butcher LM, Feber A, Teschendorff AE, Chakravarthy AR, Wojdacz TK, Beck S. ChAMP: 450k chip analysis methylation pipeline. Bioinformatics. 2014;30(3):428–30.

23. Wang D, Yan L, Hu Q, Sucheston LE, Higgins MJ, Ambrosone CB, Johnson CS, Smiraglia DJ, Liu S. IMA: an R package for high-throughput analysis of Illumina's 450K Infinium methylation data. Bioinformatics. 2012;28(5):729–30.

24. Chen EY, Tan CM, Kou Y, Duan Q, Wang Z, Meirelles GV, Clark NR, Ma'ayan A. Enrichr: interactive and collaborative HTML5 gene list enrichment analysis tool. BMC Bioinformatics. 2013;14:128.

25. Xia J, Gill EE, Hancock REW. NetworkAnalyst for statistical, visual and network-based meta-analysis of gene expression data. Nat Protoc. 2015; 10(6):823–44.

26. Jones PA, Takai D. The role of DNA methylation in mammalian epigenetics. Science. 2001;293(5532):1068–70.

27. Dick KJ, Nelson CP, Tsaprouni L, Sandling JK, Aïssi D, Wahl S, Meduri E, Morange PE, Gagnon F, Grallert H, Waldenberger M, Peters A, Erdmann J, Hengstenberg C, Cambien F, Goodall AH, Ouwehand WH, Schunkert H, Thompson JR, Spector TD, Gieger C, Trégouët DA, Deloukas P, Samani NJ. DNA methylation and body-mass index: a genome-wide analysis. Lancet. 2014;383(9933):1990–8.

28. Rönn T, Volkov P, Gillberg L, Kokosar M, Perfilyev A, Jacobsen AL, Jørgensen SW, Brøns C, Jansson PA, Eriksson KF, Pedersen O, Hansen T, Groop L, Stener-Victorin E, Vaag A, Nilsson E, Ling C. Impact of age, BMI and HbA1c levels on the genome-wide DNA methylation and mRNA expression patterns in human adipose tissue and identification of epigenetic biomarkers in blood. Hum Mol Genet. 2015;24(13):3792–813.

29. Zhang B, Zhou Y, Lin N, Lowdon RF, Hong C, Nagarajan RP, Cheng JB, Li D, Stevens M, Lee HJ, Xing X, Zhou J, Sundaram V, Elliott G, Gu J, Shi T, Gascard P, Sigaroudinia M, Tlsty TD, Kadlecek T, Weiss A, O'Geen H, Farnham PJ, Maire CL, Ligon KL, Madden PA, Tam A, Moore R, Hirst M, Marra MA, Zhang B, Costello JF, Wang T. Functional DNA methylation differences between tissues, cell types, and across individuals discovered using the M&M algorithm. Genome Res. 2013;23(9):1522–40.

30. Dedeurwaerder S, Desmedt C, Calonne E, Singhal SK, Haibe-Kains B, Defrance M, Michiels S, Volkmar M, Deplus R, Luciani J, Lallemand F, Larsimont D, Toussaint J, Haussy S, Rothé F, Rouas G, Metzger O, Majjaj S, Saini K, Putmans P, Hames G, van Baren N, Coulie PG, Piccart M, Sotiriou C, Fuks F. DNA methylation profiling reveals a predominant immune component in breast cancers. EMBO Mol Med. 2011;3(12):726–41.

31. Wang X, Zhu H, Snieder H, Su S, Munn D, Harshfield G, Maria BL, Dong Y, Treiber F, Gutin B, Shi H. Obesity related methylation changes in DNA of peripheral blood leukocytes. BMC Med. 2010;8:87.

32. Booth A, Magnuson A, Fouts J, Foster M. Adipose tissue, obesity and adipokines: role in cancer promotion. Horm Mol Biol Clin Investig. 2015;21(1):57–74.

33. Hefetz-Sela S, Scherer PE. Adipocytes: impact on tumor growth and potential sites for therapeutic intervention. Pharmacol Ther. 2013;138(2):197–210.

34. Zeng XC, Ao X, Yang HF, Zhang GX, Li WH, Liu QL, Tang YL, Xie YC, He WG, Huang YN, Zhang L, Li RJ. Differential expression of stromal aromatase in obese females is regulated by DNA methylation. Mol Med Rep. 2014;10(2):887–90.

35. To SQ, Takagi Y, Miki Y, Suzuki K, Abe E, Yang Y, Sasano H, Simpson ER, Knower KC, Clyne CD. Epigenetic mechanisms regulate the prostaglandin E receptor 2 in breast cancer. J Steroid Biochem Mol Biol. 2012;132:331–8.

36. Tao MH, Marian C, Nie J, Ambrosone C, Krishnan SS, Edge SB, Trevisan M, Shields PG, Freudenheim JL. Body mass and DNA promoter methylation in breast tumors in the Western New York Exposures and Breast Cancer Study. Am J Clin Nutr. 2011;94(3):831–8.

37. Zolochevska O, Shearer J, Ellis J, Fokina V, Shah F, Gimble JM, Figueiredo ML. Human adipose-derived mesenchymal stromal cell pigment epithelium-derived factor cytotherapy modifies genetic and epigenetic profiles of prostate cancer cells. Cytotherapy. 2014;16(3):346–56.

38. Serra D, Mera P, Malandrino MI, Mir JF, Herrero L. Mitochondrial fatty acid oxidation in obesity. Antioxid Redox Signal. 2013;19(3):269–84.

39. Maples JM, Brault JJ, Witczak CA, Park S, Hubal MJ, Weber TM, Houmard JA, Shewchuk BM. Differential epigenetic and transcriptional response of the skeletal muscle carnitine palmitoyltransferase 1B (CPT1B) gene to lipid exposure with obesity. Am J Physiol Endocrinol Metab. 2015;309(4):E345–56.

40. Wolfgang MJ, Kurama T, Dai Y, Suwa A, Asaumi M, Matsumoto S, Cha SH, Shimokawa T, Lane MD. The brain-specific carnitine palmitoyltransferase-1c regulates energy homeostasis. Proc Natl Acad Sci U S A. 2006;103(19):7282–7.

41. van Tienen FHJ, van der Kallen CJH, Lindsey PJ, Wanders RJ, van Greevenbroek MM, Smeets HJM. Preadipocytes of type 2 diabetes subjects display an intrinsic gene expression profile of decreased differentiation capacity. Int J Obes. 2011;35(9):1154–64.

42. Hara K, Tajima G, Okada S, Tsumura M, Kagawa R, Shirao K, Ohno Y, Yasunaga S, Ohtsubo M, Hata I, Sakura N, Shigematsu Y, Takihara Y, Kobayashi M. Significance of ACADM mutations identified through newborn screening of MCAD deficiency in Japan. Mol Genet Metab. 2016;118(1):9–14.

43. Grünert SC, Wehrle A, Villavicencio-Lorini P, Lausch E, Vetter B, Schwab KO, Tucci S, Spiekerkoetter U. Medium-chain acyl-CoA dehydrogenase deficiency associated with a novel splice mutation in the ACADM gene missed by newborn screening. BMC Med Genet. 2015;16(1):56–65.

44. Ji S, Yang R, Lu C, Qiu Z, Yan C, Zhao Z. Differential expression of PPARγ, FASN, and ACADM genes in various adipose tissues and longissimus dorsi muscle from Yanbian yellow cattle and Yan yellow cattle. Asian-Australasian J Anim Sci. 2014;27(1):10–8.

45. Greco D, Kotronen A, Westerbacka J, et al. Gene expression in human NAFLD. 2008:1281–1287. doi:https://doi.org/10.1152/ajpgi.00074.2008.

46. Berquin IM, Edwards IJ, Kridel SJ, Chen YQ. Polyunsaturated fatty acid metabolism in prostate cancer. Cancer Metastasis Rev. 2011;30(3–4):295–309.

47. Lattka E, Illig T, Koletzko B, Heinrich J. Genetic variants of the FADS1 FADS2 gene cluster as related to essential fatty acid metabolism. Curr Opin Lipidol. 2010;21(1):64–9.

48. Glaser C, Heinrich J, Koletzko B. Role of FADS1 and FADS2 polymorphisms in polyunsaturated fatty acid metabolism. Metabolism. 2010;59(7):993–9.

49. Suburu J, Chen YQ. Lipids and prostate cancer. Prostaglandins Other Lipid Mediat. 2012;98(1–2):1–10.

50. Chen YQ, Edwards IJ, Kridel SJ, Thornburg T, Berquin IM. Dietary fat–gene interactions in cancer. Cancer Metastasis Reviews. 2007;26(3–4):535–51.

51. Schweitzer GG, Finck BN. Targeting hepatic glycerolipid synthesis and turnover to treat fatty liver disease. Advances in Hepatology 2014;2014:498369.

52. Glunde K, Bhujwalla ZM, Ronen SM. Choline metabolism in malignant transformation. Nat Rev Cancer. 2011;11(12):835–48.

53. Snider S. Choline transport links phospholipid metabolism and inflammation in macrophages. 2017. http://hdl.handle.net/10393/35715. Accessed 28 July 2017.

54. Traiffort E, O'Regan S, Ruat M. The choline transporter-like family SLC44: properties and roles in human diseases. Mol Asp Med. 2013;34(2–3):646–54.

55. Kouji H, Inazu M, Yamada T, Tajima H, Aoki T, Matsumiya T. Molecular and functional characterization of choline transporter in human colon carcinoma HT-29 cells. Arch Biochem Biophys. 2009;483(1):90–8.

56. Nishiyama R, Nagashima F, Iwao B, Kawai Y, Inoue K, Midori A, Yamanaka T, Uchino H, Inazu M. Identification and functional analysis of choline transporter in tongue cancer: a novel molecular target for tongue cancer therapy. J Pharmacol Sci. 2016;131(2):101–9.

57. Mattie M, Raitano A, Morrison K, Morrison K, An Z, Capo L, Verlinsky A, Leavitt M, Ou J, Nadell R, Aviña H, Guevara C, Malik F, Moser R, Duniho S, Coleman J, Li Y, Pereira DS, Doñate F, Joseph IB, Challita-Eid P, Benjamin D, Stover DR. The discovery and preclinical development of ASG-5ME, an antibody-drug conjugate targeting SLC44A4-positive epithelial tumors including pancreatic and prostate cancer. Mol Cancer Ther. 2016;15(11):2679–87.

58. Sutinen E, Nurmi M, Roivainen A, Varpula M, Tolvanen T, Lehikoinen P, Minn H. Kinetics of [11C]choline uptake in prostate cancer: a PET study. Eur J Nucl Med Mol Imaging. 2004;31(3):317–24.

59. Vlková V, Štěpánek I, Hrušková V, Šenigl F, Mayerová V, Šrámek M, Šímová J, Bieblová J, Indrová M, Hejhal T, Dérian N, Klatzmann D, Six A, Reiniš M. Epigenetic regulations in the IFNγ signalling pathway: IFNγ-mediated MHC class I upregulation on tumour cells is associated with DNA demethylation of antigen-presenting machinery genes. Oncotarget. 2014;5(16):6923–35.

60. Pedersen MH, Hood BL, Beck HC, Conrads TP, Ditzel HJ, Leth-Larsen R. Downregulation of antigen presentation-associated pathway proteins is linked to poor outcome in triple-negative breast cancer patient tumors. Oncoimmunology. 2017;6(5):e1305531.

61. Ylitalo EB, Thysell E, Jernberg E, Lundholm M, Crnalic S, Egevad L, Stattin P, Widmark A, Bergh A, Wikström P. Subgroups of castration-resistant prostate cancer bone metastases defined through an inverse relationship between androgen receptor activity and immune response. Eur Urol. 2017;71(5):776–87.

62. Lucia Radici MB, Rita Crinelli, Mauro Magnani. Ubiquitin C gene: structure, function, and transcriptional regulation. Adv Biosci Biotechnol 2013;4:1057–1062.

63. Song HM, Lee JE, Kim JH. Ubiquitin C-terminal hydrolase-L3 regulates EMT process and cancer metastasis in prostate cell lines. Biochem Biophys Res Commun. 2014;452(3):722–7.

64. Jang MJ, Baek SH, Kim JH. UCH-L1 promotes cancer metastasis in prostate cancer cells through EMT induction. Cancer Lett. 2011;302(2):128–35.

65. Hawkins PG, Santoso S, Adams C, Anest V, Morris KV. Promoter targeted small RNAs induce long-term transcriptional gene silencing in human cells. Nucleic Acids Res. 2009;37(9):2984–95.

66. Wahl S, Drong A, Lehne B, et al. Epigenome-wide association study of body mass index, and the adverse outcomes of adiposity. Nature. 2017;541(7635):81–6.

67. Rahmioglu N, Drong AW, Lockstone H, Tapmeier T, Hellner K, Saare M, Laisk-Podar T, Dew C, Tough E, Nicholson G, Peters M, Morris AP, Lindgren CM, Becker CM, Zondervan KT. Variability of genome-wide DNA methylation and mRNA expression profiles in reproductive and endocrine disease related tissues. Epigenetics. 2017;12(10):897–908.

68. Agha G, Houseman EA, Kelsey KT, Eaton CB, Buka SL, Loucks EB. Adiposity is associated with DNA methylation profile in adipose tissue. Int J Epidemiol. 2015;44(4):1277–87.

69. Turcot V, Tchernof A, Deshaies Y, Pérusse L, Bélisle A, Marceau S, Biron S, Lescelleur O, Biertho L, Vohl MC. LINE-1 methylation in visceral adipose tissue of severely obese individuals is associated with metabolic syndrome status and related phenotypes. Clin Epigenetics. 2012;4(1):10.

17

Histone demethylase JARID1B/KDM5B promotes aggressiveness of non-small cell lung cancer and serves as a good prognostic predictor

Kuang-Tai Kuo[1,2], Wen-Chien Huang[3,4], Oluwaseun Adebayo Bamodu[5,6], Wei-Hwa Lee[7], Chun-Hua Wang[8,9], M. Hsiao[10], Liang-Shun Wang[1*] and Chi-Tai Yeh[5,6*]

Abstract

Background: Lung cancer is the leading cause of cancer death worldwide. Recently, epigenetic dysregulation has been known to promote tumor progression and therefore may be a therapeutic target for anticancer therapy. JARID1B, a member of histone demethylases, has been found to be related to tumorigenesis in certain kinds of cancers. However, its biological roles in non-small cell lung cancer (NSCLC) remain largely unclear.

Methods: We firstly examined the expression of JARID1B in surgical specimens and six NSCLC cell lines. Then, we evaluated the relationship between JARID1B expression and clinicopathologic parameters in 72 NSCLC patients, thereby established its prognostic importance. We subsequently studied the functional roles of JARID1B in tumorigenesis to verify its clinicopathologic significance.

Results: Our results showed that JARID1B was overexpressed in NSCLC cells and JARID1B overexpression was associated with tumor size, lymph node metastasis, advanced stages, and poor overall survival in NSCLC patients. JARID1B overexpression resulted in increased cell proliferation and formation of tumorspheres and correlated positively with the expression of cancer stem cells (CSCs) and epithelial-mesenchymal transition (EMT) markers, while the c-Met signaling pathway was actively involved. It also correlated with the strength of resistance to cisplatin and doxorubicin. On the contrary, downregulation of JARID1B expression by applying shRNA or JARID1B inhibitor PBIT reversed these phenomena.

Conclusions: JARID1B worsens prognosis of NSCLC patients by promotion of tumor aggressiveness through multiple biological facets which were associated with activation of the c-Met signaling, and can be a novel prognostic biomarker and therapeutic target for NSCLC.

Keywords: JARID1B, Lung cancer, Prognosis, Cancer stem cells, c-Met

Background

Lung cancer is one of the most frequently diagnosed malignancies and the leading cause of cancer death worldwide, with an estimated global incidence of 1.82 million and mortality of 1.59 million in 2012 [1]. Non-small cell lung carcinoma (NSCLC) accounts for 85% of all lung cancers, and only few patients are diagnosed with early

disease [2]. Despite the advance of treatment in all aspects, the all-stage 5-year survival of lung cancer remains less than 20% [3]. During the past decade, new chemotherapeutic agents and target therapies have improved survival of lung cancer patients but the effect was not overwhelming, mostly due to development of therapeutic resistance after treatment [4, 5]. Several studies have shown a small subpopulation of tumor cells called cancer stem cells (CSCs) modulate tumor initiation, growth, metastasis, and resistance to anticancer therapy [6, 7]. These CSCs are characterized by enhanced propensity for self-renewal, unrestricted proliferation, de-differentiation, and tumor

---

* Correspondence: wangls72269@yahoo.com.tw; ctyeh@s.tmu.edu.tw
[1]Division of Thoracic Surgery, Department of Surgery, Shuang Ho Hospital, Taipei Medical University, New Taipei City, Taiwan
[5]Department of Medical Research and Education, Shuang Ho Hospital, Taipei Medical University, New Taipei City, Taiwan
Full list of author information is available at the end of the article

propagation. Several somatic stem cell markers including SOX2, KLF4, c-Myc, NANOG, and OCT 3/4 have been applied to identify CSCs, and some additional markers such as ALDH and CD133 have also been proposed for lung cancer stem cells (LCSCs) [8].

The last decade has witnessed increasing implication of enhanced mesenchymal-to-epithelial transition (MET) signaling in the formation, resistance to therapy, and progression of NSCLC [9]. It has also been suggested that MET is required for epithelial growth factor (EGF)-induced cell invasion and motility in EGFR wild-type NSCLC cells, especially as the pharmacological inhibition of c-Met or its siRNA knockdown reduced EGF-induced invasion and motility, indicating that EGFR requires c-Met activity and/or expression to maximize the invasive phenotypes of NSCLC cells [10]. However, the molecular mechanisms of these c-Met activities in NSCLC cells remain unclear, especially its epigenetic underlying molecular mechanism, thus forming a basis for continued exploration of the pharmacologic and molecular targetability, as well as the epigenetic modulation of MET signaling in NSCLC patients.

There is accumulating evidence that besides the genetic mutations, epigenetic changes and chromatin dynamics are actively involved in the initiation and disease progression of several malignancies, including NSCLC [11–14]. However, the underlying mechanisms of epigenetic activities such as histone modification in NSCLC tumorigenesis have largely been underexplored until now. Like other types of histone modification, methylation and demethylation of the lysine residue of the histone protein modulate genetic activities while concurrently serve as a transcription switch of gene expression in both physiological and diseased condition. In the past decade, several studies have demonstrated the oncogenicity of histone demethylases and implicated their dysregulation in tumor formation and progression [15–17].

JARID1B, also known as KDM5B or PLU-1, is one member of the Jumonji, AT-rich interactive domain 1 (JARID1) histone demethylase protein family that possesses H3K4 histone demethylase activity [18, 19]. Our previous studies have shown that JARID1B was associated with tumorigenicity in oral cancer and breast cancer [20, 21]. Recently, it was also reported that an inhibitor of KDM5 family could reduce survival of drug-tolerant cancer cells, including NSCLC cells [22]. This implied the possible link between JARID1B and LCSCs. Nevertheless, the functional and prognostic roles of JARID1B in NSCLC have not been well clarified so far. Meanwhile, the relationship between JARID1B, LCSCs, and c-Met is also obscure. In this study, we evaluated the expression of JARID1B in NSCLC tumor tissues and cell lines, analyzed its clinicopathologic significance in NSCLC patients, and finally investigated its biological roles in NSCLC tumorigenesis.

Methods

Cell lines and culture

The human bronchial epithelial cell line BEAS-2B and NSCLC cell lines, CL1-0, CL1-5, A549, and PC9 were grown in Dulbecco's modified Eagle medium (Gibco®D-MEM, Thermo Fisher Scientific Inc., Waltham, MA, USA), while NSCLC cell lines H441 and H1299 were grown in Gibco®RPMI1640 medium (Thermo Fisher Scientific Inc.). The culture media contain 10% FBS (Gibco, Thermo Fisher Scientific Inc.) supplemented with penicillin (100 U/mL) and streptomycin (100 mg/mL) (Gibco, Thermo Fisher Scientific Inc.). Cells were incubated at 37 °C in a 5% CO_2 humidified atmosphere. Culture media were changed every 72 h and cells passaged at 80% confluence. All cell lines were purchased from ATCC.

Western blot analysis

Normal bronchial epithelial and NSCLC cells were lysed in RIPA lysis buffer; total protein were quantified by BCA protein assay kit (Thermo Fisher Scientific Inc.) and then analyzed by Western blot assay. Primary antibodies used were listed in Additional file 1: Table S1. Secondary antibodies were Alexa Fluor 680-conjugated affinity purified anti-mouse or anti-rabbit IgG (Invitrogen, Thermo Fisher Scientific Inc.) detected using the UVP Imaging.

Immunohistochemical staining and scoring

This study was conducted in a cohort of patients with lung cancer who underwent resection. at Taipei Medical University Shuang-Ho hospital, Taipei, Taiwan, between January 2010 to December 2017. A predesigned data collection format was used to review the patients' medical records for evaluation of clinicopathologic characteristics and survival outcomes. The study was reviewed and approved by the institute review board (IRB:201403007). Clinical samples from NSCLC patients were fixed in 10% formalin, embedded in paraffin, deparaffinized, and then rehydrated. For immunohistochemical (IHC) staining, rehydrated sections were subjected to antigen retrieval and their endogenous peroxidase activity blocked for 30 min in 1% H_2O_2/PBS solution. After blocking, the slides were exposed to JARID1B antibody (1:200), c-Met (1:150), or Vimentin (1:200) at 4 °C overnight, at 4 °C overnight, washed and incubated in biotinylated link universal antiserum for 1 h at room temperature. Slides were then rinsed, and stain was developed using the chromogen, 3, 3-diaminobenzidine hydrochloride. Finally, sections were rinsed with ddH₂O and counterstained with hematoxylin. Slides were observed under microscope, with the selection of five fields of view randomly. Evaluation and quantification of JARID1B, c-Met, or Vimentin expression were done manually by two independent investigators in a blind manner. The percentage of stained area to the selected field was recorded in a 5% interval, ranging from 0 to 100%. The staining intensity was graded into three categories (absent or weak, 1; moderate, 2; strong, 3). Quick score (Q-score) was derived from the product of percentage (P) of tumor cells with characteristic IHC staining (0–100%) and the intensity (I) of IHC staining (1–3) ($Q = P \times I$; maximum = 300). For survival analysis, we used Q-score = 150 as a cutoff value to divide the patients into two groups.

JARID1B-knockdown cell lines

NSCLC H1299 and H441 cells were infected with JARID1B small hairpin RNA (shRNA, Clone ID: TRCN0000329952, target sequence: ATCGCTTGCTTCATCGATATT for shJARID1B-1 and GTGCCTGTTTACCGAACTAAT for shJARID1B-2), or vector (pLKO_TRC005) obtained from the National RNAi Core Facility, Academia Sinica, Taiwan. Treatment with puromycin did selection of positive shJARID1B-1 and shJARID1B-2. Both H1299 and H441 cells were used for phenotypic assays, but only H441 cell lysates were prepared 48 h after transfection and used for Western blot or cytotoxicity assays.

Sulforhodamine B (SRB) cell proliferation assay

The sulforhodamine B (SRB) assay is used for cell density determination, and the principle has been well described [23]. Cells with the amount of 5×10^3 cells/well from H1299 and H441 were seeded into a 96-well plate and allowed to grow and attach in 200 µL serum-free RPMI 1640 for 24 h. After cell attachment, the media were changed to new serum-free RPMI 1640 and incubated for 24, 48, and 72 h, respectively. At the end of incubation, the cells were washed with PBS for three times. Then, 100 µL of SRB (Sigma-Aldrich, St. Louis, MO) solution 0.4% (w/v) in 1% acetic acid was added to each well and incubated at room temperature for 1 h. After staining, unbound dye was removed and bound stain was solubilized with 200 µL/well 10 mM Tris base for 30 min. The absorbance was read on an automated microplate reader (96 well) at 490 nm. Each condition of each cell line was repeated for six times.

Colony formation assay

Five thousand wild-type or JARID1B shRNA H441 cells/ 60-mm dishes were seeded and cultured in complete growth medium with 0.125 µg/mL puromycin (Gibco, Thermo Fisher Scientific Inc.) for 10–12 days. Colonies were then fixed in ice-cold methanol and stained with 0.1% crystal violet solutions, photographed, and visible colonies counted under microscope. The assays were performed in triplicate.

Flow-cytometric analysis of cell cycle progression

Cell cycle progression was analyzed by resuspension of 1×10^6 H441 WT or JARID1B shRNA H441 cells per 1 mL PBS, followed by addition of 0.05 mg/mL propidium iodide (PI) in a 0.1% Triton X-100/0.1% sodium citrate solution. Cells were harvested, washed with cold PBS twice, and fixed in 70% ethanol at – 20 °C overnight. The cells were then centrifuged (1500 rpm, 10 min) and washed twice using phosphate-buffered saline (PBS). Next, the cells were resuspended in 0.5 mL of PBS containing 50 µg/mL RNase A for 1 h at 37 °C. The cells were then loaded with 65 µg/mL PI for 30 min in the dark at 4 °C. The percentage of cells in distinct phases of the cell cycle was measured by flow cytometry (FACSCalibur, BD Biosciences) with excitation set at 488 nm and emission detected at the FL-2 channel (565–610 nm). The assays were performed in triplicate.

Cell migration and invasion assays

NSCLC cells were cultured to 90% confluence in 6-well plates, and then, a scratch was made horizontally through the confluent cells using sterile 10-µL pipette tips. Phosphate-buffered saline (PBS) was used to wash off displaced cells and cellular debris. Five visual fields were randomly selected in each dish for comparison of wound closure. For assessment of cell migration, images were captured under microscope at 0 and 24 h. For invasion assay, matrigel-coated transwell inserts with micropore membranes (BD Biosciences, San Jose, CA, USA) were placed in 24-well plates. 3×10^4 cells were plated in 100 µl of medium containing 1% FBS in the upper chamber, while the lower chamber was filled with 600 µl complete growth medium. Cells were incubated in 5% CO_2 humidified atmosphere at 37 °C for 48 h. The non-invading cells were scraped from the upper chamber of each insert with cotton swab, and invaded cells attached to the lower surface of the insert membrane were incubated in 0.1% crystal violet at 37 °C for 30 min, washed twice with PBS, and viewed under a microscope.

Tumorsphere formation assay

For the analysis of sphere forming ability, H441 NSCLC cells were cultured under serum-deprived conditions and in Ultra-Low Attachment Plates (Corning Incorporated). H441 cells (10^3 cells/mL) were suspended and seeded in the tumorsphere medium containing 20 ng/mL epidermal growth factor, 10 ng/mL basic fibroblast growth factor, 5 µg/mL insulin, 0.4% bovine serum albumin. Approximately 3–5 days of incubation, tumorsphere numbers were counted under a phase-contrast microscope using the × 40 magnification lens. The ability of tumor formation was represented by the average number of spheres obtaining from counts from different views (at least three random fields).

Immunofluorescence staining

H441 sphere cells were seeded on 24-well plates with a coverslip on the bottom of each well. After shJARID1B treatment, cells were washed twice with PBS, fixed with 4% formaldehyde, and probed with primary antibody (JARID1B, and SOX-2) at 4 °C for overnight. Fluorophore-conjugated antibody (Alexa Fluor; Life Technologies) was used to track the in-situ interaction of protein-primary antibody. Double-stranded DNA staining (4′,6-diamidino-2-phenylindole (DAPI); Invitrogen, USA) was used as nuclear staining. The fluorescence signal was captured under confocal microscopy (Nikon, Japan).

Isolation of side-population (SP) cancer cells using fluorescence-activated cell sorting (FACS)

H441 WT or JARID1B shRNA H441 cells in logarithmic growth phase were harvested using trypsin/EDTA and resuspended in pre-warmed appropriate culture media (according to each cell type), at a concentration of 5×10^5 viable cells/mL. Single-cell suspensions were incubated with Hoechst-33342 dye (2.5 μg/mL, Sigma) at 37 °C for 90 min in a water bath and in the dark, with occasional agitation to prevent cell aggregation. Negative control samples were treated with Verapamil (50 μM, Sigma), a wide spectrum ATP-binding cassette (ABC) transporter inhibitor for 15 min, before being incubated with Hoechst-33342. Afterwards, cells were washed with ice-cold PBS, centrifuged at 4 °C, and resuspended in ice-cold PBS with propidium iodide (1 μM), to identify and exclude dead cells. All samples were maintained at 4 °C until flow cytometry acquisition. Hoechst-33342 dye was excited at 355 nm using a UV laser, and its dual wavelengths were detected using 450/50-nm band-pass and 450LP filters (Hoechst-33342 Blue), and 655LP filter (Hoechst-33,342 Red), for the discrimination of side-population cells. At least 10,000 events were acquired in the side-population region. Dead cells were excluded by gating propidium iodide-positive cells on forward vs. side scatter dotplots. Data were acquired using FACSAria™ III sorter (BD Biosciences, Taiwan).

Statistical analysis

All assays were performed in triplicate. Reported data results are expressed as means ± S.E.M. All statistical analyses were performed using GraphPad prism (v.6.0. GraphPad Software Inc., CA, USA). Survival analysis was performed using the Kaplan-Meier plots and log-rank test. The correlation between JARID1B expression and the clinicopathologic parameters was assessed by the χ^2 test and bivariate analysis. For comparisons between two groups, student's t test was used while for more than two groups, one-way ANOVA was used. A p value < 0.05 was considered statistically significant ($*p < 0.05$, $**p < 0.01$, $***p < 0.001$).

Results

JARID1B is overexpressed in NSCLC tissues and cell lines

Nuclear staining of JARID1B was intense, but cytoplasmic staining to some extent was also noted. We demonstrated that while the normal alveoli tissues showed scanty JARID1B staining, JARID1B expression was obviously stronger in the NSCLC tissues (Fig. 1a). To further verify this finding, we comparatively evaluated the expression of JARID1B in paired tumor and adjacent non-tumor tissues by Western blot and observed that JARID1B was overexpressed in the tumor (T) samples as compared to the adjacent non-tumor (NT) samples (Fig. 1b). We subsequently analyzed the expression of JARID1B in six widely used NSCLC cell lines, CL1-0, CL1-5, A549, PC9, H441, and H1299 as well as in the human fibroblast cell line WI-38 plus human alveolar epithelial cell line BEAS-2B. The results showed that JARID1B expression was elevated in almost all the NSCLC cell lines as compared to WI-38 or BEAS-2B. JARID1B expression was stronger in H1299 and H441 cells; modest in CL1-5, A549, and PC9 cells; and mild in CL1-0 cells (Fig. 1c). Notably, the more aggressive CL1-5 cells had stronger JARID1B expression as compared to the non-metastatic CL1-0 cells. These results indicated that JARID1B is overexpressed in human NSCLC tissues and cell lines. To investigate the potential role of other KDM5 family members in NSCLC, we explored the Oncomine database and used The Cancer Genome Atlas (TCGA) database for comparison. We demonstrated that as compared with normal lung tissues from the same individuals, overexpression of KDM5B and KDM5C was found in NSCLC patients while KDM5A was not (Additional file 2: Figure S1).

JARID1B overexpression correlates with advanced disease and poor prognosis

In the first cohort, we analyzed 29 patients of NSCLC with all stages. The representative pictures of each stage were shown in Fig. 2a. The IHC results showed that JARID1B overexpression was positively correlated with advanced tumor stages ($p = 0.001$) (Fig. 2b). Concurrently, a positive correlation was observed between the stage-dependent increase in JARID1B protein expression and enhanced expression of the tyrosine kinase c-Met and the type III intermediate filament protein Vimentin (Fig. 2a), where the former is implicated in cell proliferation, scattering and survival, while the latter is associated with the mesenchymal phenotype. In the second cohort, 72 NSCLC patients with stage I to stage III disease undergoing curative surgery were enrolled for clinical outcome analysis. Our results showed that patients with higher JARID1B expression (Q-score ≥ 150, $n = 53$) had significantly worse overall survival than patients with lower JARID1B expression (Q-score < 150, $n = 19$) ($p = 0.009$) (Fig. 2c). In the JARID1B-high group, 5-year overall survival rate was 17.4% with the median survival of 31.62 months, whereas in the JARID1B-low group, 5-year overall survival rate was 54.8% with the median survival of 50.15 months. As shown in Table 1, a significantly positive correlation

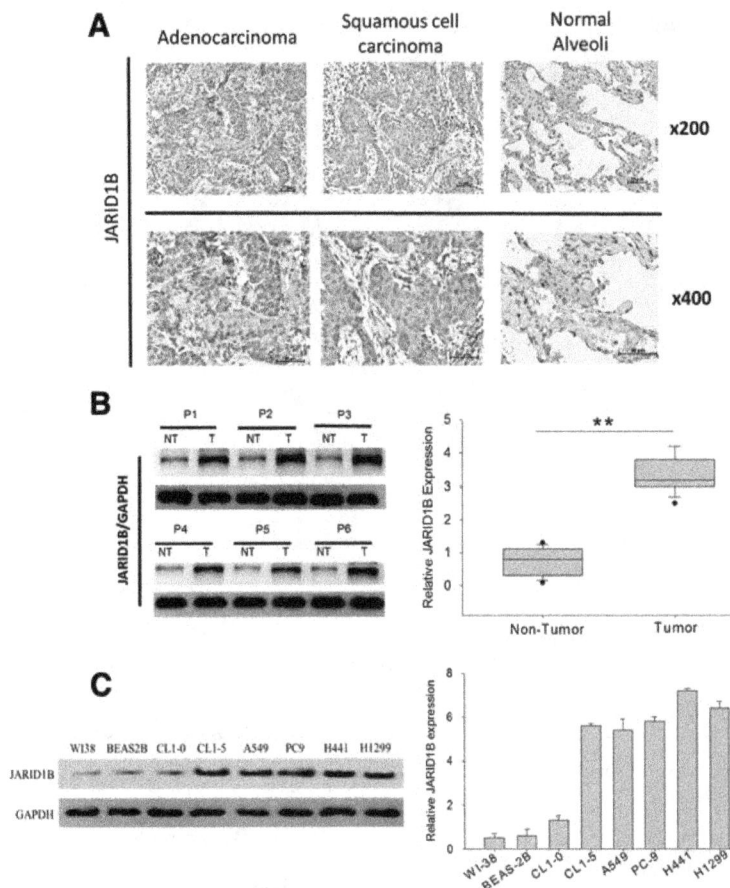

Fig. 1 JARID1B is overexpressed in NSCLC tissues and cell lines. **a** IHC staining of clinical specimens. JARID1B overexpression was demonstrated by strong staining intensity of NSCLC tissues while scanty staining was observed in normal alveoli tissues. **b** Representative Western blot data showed upregulation of JARID1B in most of the NSCLC tumor tissues (T) as compared to the adjacent non-tumor (NT) lung tissues. **c** Western blot showed elevated expression of JARID1B in NSCLC cell lines but very weak expression in the human alveolar epithelial cell line BEAS-2B. The H441 and H1299 cells had stronger JARID1B expression. GAPDH served as the loading control

between JARID1B expression and tumor size ($p = 0.007$, $\chi^2 = 7.25$), lymph node (LN) metastasis ($p = 0.005$, $\chi^2 = 7.827$), and tumor stage ($p = 0.033$, $\chi^2 = 4.527$). No statistically significant correlation between JARID1B expression and patient age ($p = 0.737$, $\chi^2 = 0.112$) or tumor differentiation ($p = 0.382$, $\chi^2 = 0.828$) was observed. These data suggested the potential role of JARID1B as a marker of tumor progression and a useful predictor of clinical outcome in NSCLC.

JARID1B knockdown inhibits NSCLC cell proliferation and colony formation, cell migration, and invasion

The cell line H1299 and H441 which expressed stronger JARID1B were used for knockdown study to determine whether JARID1B is necessary for cell proliferation and invasiveness of NSCLC cells. The JARID1B-knockdown efficiency in the shRNA-transfected H441 cells was verified using Western blot (Fig. 3a). The markers of epithelial-mesenchymal transition (EMT) were evaluated, and we found that the expression of EMT markers was parallel to the expression of JARID1B. The H3K4me3 activity and the expression of p21 and BAK1 were also increased after knocking down JARID1B, indicating not only enzymatic activity of JARID1B but also suppression of JARID1B may increase apoptosis. Consistent with this, result of our cell cycle analysis showed that depletion of JARID1B not only inhibited H441 cell proliferation via enhanced cell death, but also had an uncoupling effect on the NSCLC cell cycle progression as demonstrated by the shJARID1B-induced significant reduction in the population of cells in G0/G1 and S-phases, while increasing the number of cells in G2/M phase, which is indicative of reduced tumor cell growth and DNA replication, coupled with enhanced DNA damage (Additional file 3: Figure S3). Meanwhile, the SRB assay revealed that knockdown of JARID1B reduced cell proliferation remarkably in the H1299 and H441 cells (Fig. 3b). Reduced anchorage-independent growth in soft agar and lesser number of large colonies, as compared to the control groups, were also noted (Fig. 3c). Corresponding to the changes of EMT markers, significant

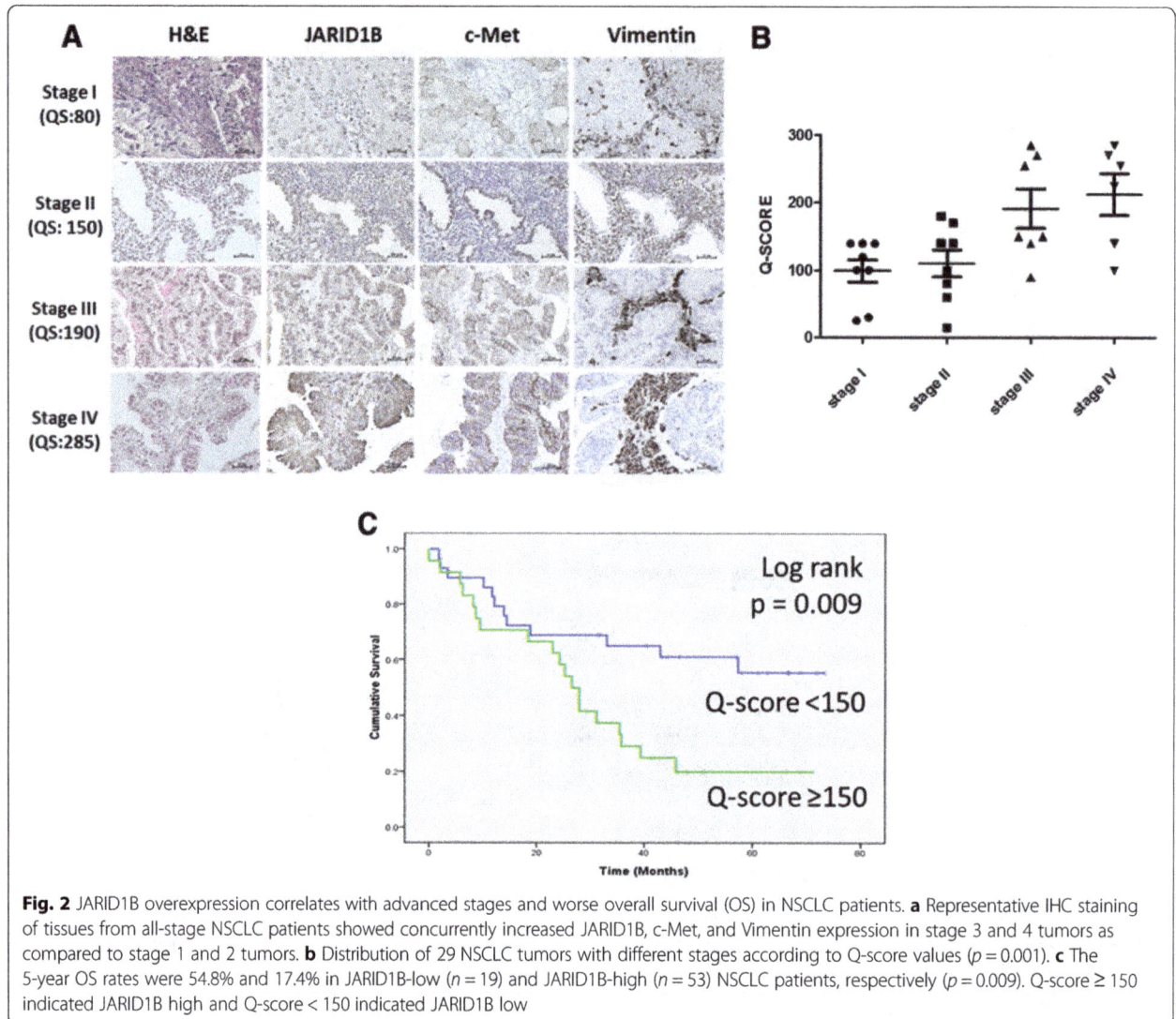

Fig. 2 JARID1B overexpression correlates with advanced stages and worse overall survival (OS) in NSCLC patients. **a** Representative IHC staining of tissues from all-stage NSCLC patients showed concurrently increased JARID1B, c-Met, and Vimentin expression in stage 3 and 4 tumors as compared to stage 1 and 2 tumors. **b** Distribution of 29 NSCLC tumors with different stages according to Q-score values ($p = 0.001$). **c** The 5-year OS rates were 54.8% and 17.4% in JARID1B-low ($n = 19$) and JARID1B-high ($n = 53$) NSCLC patients, respectively ($p = 0.009$). Q-score ≥ 150 indicated JARID1B high and Q-score < 150 indicated JARID1B low

inhibition of cell migration and invasion after 24 h was also observed in the JARID1B-knockdown cells in comparison to the control groups (Fig. 3d). Collectively, these data indicated that endogenous expression of JARID1B is essential for proliferation and formation of invasive phenotype in NSCLC cells, while both apoptosis and EMT phenomenon were important in these processes.

JARID1B expression correlates with activation of the c-Met signaling pathway and facilitates CSC-like phenotype in NSCLC

To validate whether JARID1B expression is related to LCSCs, based on the documented evidence showing that markers such as c-Myc, OCT4, SOX2, KLF4, NANOG, and survivin are useful to define the LCSCs [8, 24], we evaluated the association between the expression of these markers and JARID1B by Western blot, immunofluorescent staining, tumorsphere formation, and flow cytometry side-population (SP) assays. Comparing JARID1B expression in H441

adherent cells and tumorspheres, we observed that JARID1B protein was expressed more in H441 tumorspheres as compared to the adherent cells, and this expression pattern was also noted for LCSC markers such as c-Myc, SOX2, KLF4, CD133, and survivin. Interestingly, c-Met and its downstream proteins including MAPK, STAT3, and FAK were also increased in H441 tumorspheres (Fig. 4a). This highlighted the possible involvement of the c-Met pathway between JARID1B and LCSCs. Additionally, JARID1B knockdown significantly diminished the ability of H441 cells to form tumorspheres, which were the in vitro models of CSCs, and correlated with significant downregulation of c-Myc and c-Met protein expression (Fig. 4b). Thus, the expression of stem cell markers JARID1B and SOX2 in wild-type parental and spheroid H441 cells were analyzed using the dual-color immunofluorescence staining technique. Results showed that the in vitro H441 tumorsphere models displayed significantly higher expression of JARID1B and SOX2, compared with their parental cell counterparts,

Table 1 Correlation between JARID1B expression and clinicopathological parameter in NSCLC patients

Parameters	JARID1B-low expression (n = 19)	JARID1B-high expression (n = 53)	χ^2 value	p value
Age (years)				
≦ 50	8 (42.1%)	20 (37.7%)	0.112	0.737
> 50	11 (57.9%)	33 (62.3%)		
Tumor size				
≦ 2 cm	12 (63.2%)	15 (28.3%)	7.250	*0.007
> 2 cm	7 (36.8%)	38 (71.7%)		
Differentiation				
Poor	6 (31.6%)	23 (43.4%)	0.828	0.382
Moderate	12 (63.2%)	28 (52.8%)		
Well	1 (5.2%)	2 (3.8%)		
LN metastasis				
Negative	16 (84.2%)	25 (47.2%)	7.827	*0.005
Positive	3 (15.8%)	28 (52.8%)		
Stage				
I, II	14 (73.7%)	24 (45.3%)	4.527	*0.033
III	5 (26.3%)	29 (54.7%)		

*Statistically significant values

H441-parental. Nuclear localization of these stem cell markers was also observed in H441 tumorspheres, as demonstrated by their immensely positive co-localization with DAPI staining (Fig. 4c). Furthermore, shRNA knockdown of JARID1B was sufficient to cause a 91.4% reduction in H441 side population (which exhibited higher efflux of DNA-binding dye Hoechst 33342 and were likely to be the LCSCs), an inhibitory effect comparable to what was obtained in verapamil-treated cells (94.3% in control H441 cells, 97.1% in shJARID1B H441 cells) (Fig. 4d). The immunofluorescent staining showed that while JARID1B and SOX2 were strongly co-expressed and co-localized in the nucleus of JARID1B-high H441 cells, their expression was significantly diminished in the JARID1B-knockdown H441 cells (Fig. 4e). Overall, these results documented the relationship between JARID1B and the LCSCs subpopulation and were suggestive of the active role of JARID1B in facilitating the formation of CSCs-like phenotype of NSCLC cells. Additionally, the c-Met signaling pathway was found to play a significant role in this process.

JARID1B expression is associated with chemoresistance
We next evaluated whether JARID1B knockdown increases sensitivity to chemotherapeutic agents by depleting JARID1B expression in H441 cells with two JARID1B shRNAs (Fig. 4f) and measuring cell viability upon treatment of cisplatin and doxorubicin. Knockdown of JARID1B resulted in decreased cell viability as compared to the control vehicle (0.01% DMSO)-treated cells upon

treatment with increasing concentrations of cisplatin and doxorubicin in H441 cells (Fig. 4g, h). These results suggested that JARID1B may contribute to chemoresistance in NSCLC cells.

PBIT suppresses JARID1B expression and inhibits CSCs-like phenotype of NSCLC
PBIT is a potent and specific inhibitor of JARID1B [25] (Fig. 5a), and we herein investigated the role of PBIT in NSCLC and evaluated its ability to suppress the potential and/or CSC phenotype of NSCLC cells. The Western blot assay demonstrated that PBIT significantly downregulates JARID1B protein expression in a dose-dependent manner. Similar to its inhibitory effect on JARID1B, PBIT also resulted in a correlative downregulation of OCT4, SOX2, Vimentin, and c-Met-associated proteins. At the same time, PBIT induced a dose-dependent upregulation of E-cadherin (Fig. 5b). Using the tumorsphere formation assay, we found that shJARID1B caused a significant (72.5%) reduction in the ability to form tumorspheres in NSCLC cells. In addition, 5 μM PBIT not only significantly suppressed tumorsphere formation (57.2%) in control H441 cells, but further potentiated the suppression of tumorsphere formation (95.6%) in shJARID1B H441 cells (Fig. 5c, d). These results suggested that PBIT suppresses JARID1B expression, diminishes EMT phenomenon, and inhibits the LCSCs phenotype, likely through the activation of the c-Met signaling pathway.

Discussion
In the present study, we showed that JARID1B was significantly overexpressed in NSCLC tumor samples and cell lines, and JARID1B overexpression correlated positively with tumor size, lymph node metastasis, advanced tumor stages (Fig. 2b), and poor overall survival in NSCLC patients (Fig. 2c). The overexpression of JARID1B was associated with c-Met and Vimentin protein overexpression and was stage-dependent in nature. We then demonstrated that overexpression of JARID1B promoted cell proliferation, migration and invasion, drug resistance, and CSC-like phenotype of NSCLC cell in vitro. The cell line studies corroborated the clinicopathologic findings well and suggested that JARID1B may facilitate the oncogenic network of events through the epigenetic modulation of epithelial-mesenchymal transition (EMT) regulators including vimentin, snail, and E-cadherin, plus upregulation of a subset of pluripotent transcription factors such as OCT4, SOX2, KLF4, and c-Myc, and finally contribute to aggressiveness and stemness of NSCLC cells. Meanwhile, the c-Met signaling seemed to play a significant role in these processes. These results are consistent with previous studies implicating JARID1B as an oncogene and demonstrating the role of JARID1B to be a marker of disease progression and possible therapeutic target [18, 26–29].

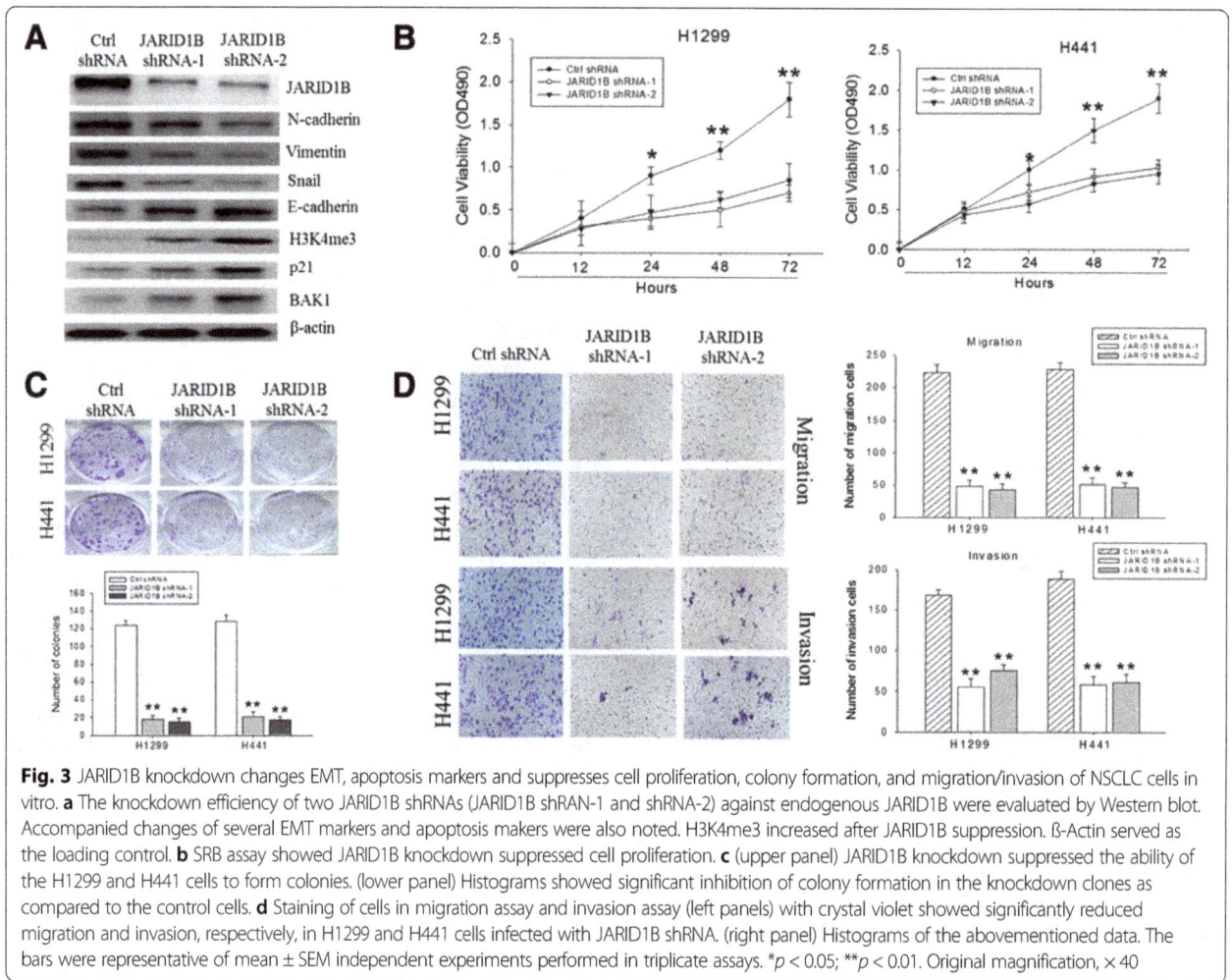

Fig. 3 JARID1B knockdown changes EMT, apoptosis markers and suppresses cell proliferation, colony formation, and migration/invasion of NSCLC cells in vitro. **a** The knockdown efficiency of two JARID1B shRNAs (JARID1B shRAN-1 and shRNA-2) against endogenous JARID1B were evaluated by Western blot. Accompanied changes of several EMT markers and apoptosis makers were also noted. H3K4me3 increased after JARID1B suppression. ß-Actin served as the loading control. **b** SRB assay showed JARID1B knockdown suppressed cell proliferation. **c** (upper panel) JARID1B knockdown suppressed the ability of the H1299 and H441 cells to form colonies. (lower panel) Histograms showed significant inhibition of colony formation in the knockdown clones as compared to the control cells. **d** Staining of cells in migration assay and invasion assay (left panels) with crystal violet showed significantly reduced migration and invasion, respectively, in H1299 and H441 cells infected with JARID1B shRNA. (right panel) Histograms of the abovementioned data. The bars were representative of mean ± SEM independent experiments performed in triplicate assays. *$p < 0.05$; **$p < 0.01$. Original magnification, × 40

There is accumulating evidence showing EMT in the malignant transformation of benign cells, endowment of increased motility, acquisition of an invasive phenotype, and subsequently disease progression [30]. EMT is principally characterized by the repression of the cell adhesion protein, E-cadherin, which inhibits the motility of malignant cells and inversely correlates with the upregulation of mesenchymal markers such as N-cadherin, vimentin, and snail, which are known suppressors of E-cadherin [30]. Consistent with these characteristics, our results indicated that JARID1B knockdown induced a corresponding downregulation of N-cadherin, vimentin, and snail, while conversely upregulated E-cadherin (Fig. 3a). We therefore hypothesized that expression of JARID1B and its alterations in the NSCLC cells are associated with loss of cellular polarity and cell-cell adhesion following diminished E-cadherin levels, detachment of malignant cells, increased cell motility, and finally metastatic dissemination. By demonstrating contrary events after JARID1B suppression, we established a positive correlation between JARID1B overexpression and enhanced NSCLC cell motility

as well as acquisition of the EMT phenotype (Fig. 3d). We also showed that JARID1B knockdown resulted in upregulation of p21 and BAK1, therefore inhibited apoptosis and increased cell proliferation (Fig. 3a–c).

Based on accruing evidence coupling the induction of EMT with the acquisition of CSCs-like phenotype [31], plus the aforementioned results regarding JARID1B and EMT, we assumed that JARID1B could be both a mediator of NSCLC cell invasiveness and a modulator of its CSCs-like phenotype. Our Western blot results showed that overexpression of JARID1B was present in H441 tumorspheres and was associated with upregulation of pluripotency transcription factors (c-Myc, SOX2, KLF4), CSCs-facilitating oncogenic factor (c-Met), and the apoptotic inhibitor survivin (Fig. 4a). We further demonstrated that loss of ability to form tumorspheres, downregulation of c-Met and c-Myc proteins, loss of co-expression and nuclear co-localization of JARID1B with SOX2, as well as the significantly diminished proportion of side population, after knocking down JARID1B (Fig. 4b–e) or applying JARID1B inhibitor PBIT (Fig. 5). Taking together, we speculated that overexpression

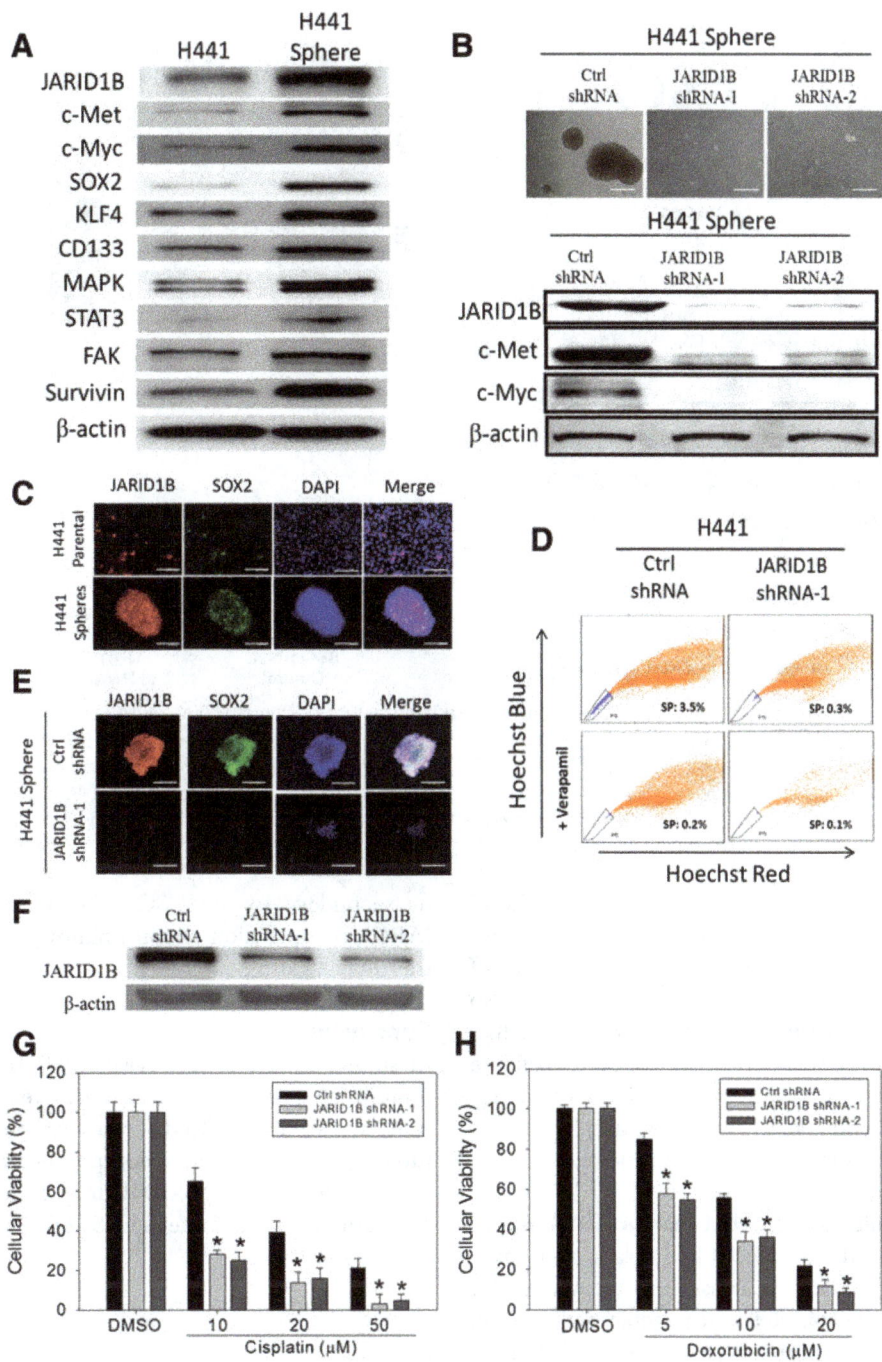

Fig. 4 JARID1B expression activates the c-Met signaling pathway, facilitates CSCs-like phenotype in NSCLC, and JARID1B knockdown increases sensitivity to chemotherapy. **a** The expression of JARID1B, c-Met, c-Myc, SOX2, KLF4, MAPK, STAT3, FAK, survivin in H441, and H441 tumorspheres (spheroids) were shown. β-Actin served as the loading control. **b** Tumorsphere formation assay showed the inhibitory effect of JARID1B knockdown on tumorsphere formation (upper panel) as well as on the expression of c-Met and c-Myc (lower panel). **c** Immunofluorescence staining showing that H441 tumorspheres had greater expression of JARID1B and SOX2, compared with their H441-parental counterparts. **d** Fluorescence-activated cell sorter (FACS) analysis demonstrated the reduction of Hoechst 33342 efflux in shJARID1B cells as compared to the control H441 cells. The percentages indicated the proportion of side population (SP) cells. The gated R5 region (blue) represented the Hoechst stain effluxing SP cells. The SP cell proportion reduced with verapamil treatment. **e** Dual-color immunofluorescence showed the co-expression and co-localization of JARID1B (red) and Sox2 (green). DAPI (blue) is the nuclear marker. Their expression was significantly diminished in the JARID1B-knockdown H441 cells. **f** Western blot for JARID1B in the control H441 cells and in the shJARID1B H441 cells. The control and JARID1B-knockdown cells were treated with increasing concentration of **g** cisplatin or **h** doxorubicin for 24 h. Cell viability was measured by SRB assay. *$p < 0.05$

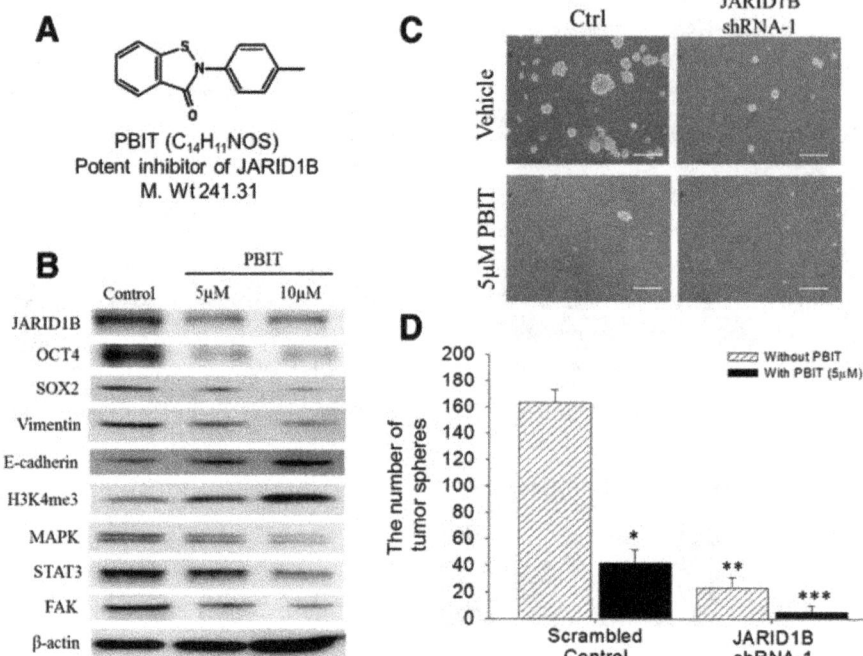

Fig. 5 PBIT suppresses JARID1B expression and inhibits CSCs-like phenotype. **a** The molecular structure of PBIT ($C_{14}H_{11}NOS$), with molecular weight of 241.31 g/mol. **b** Western blot showed the dose-dependent inhibition of expression of JARID1B, Oct4, Sox2, vimentin, MAPK, STAT3, FAK expression, as well as upregulation of E-cadherin and H3K4me3 by PBIT treatment. β-Actin served as the loading control. **c** Tumorsphere formation assay showed the effects of JARID1B knockdown and/or 5 μM PBIT treatment in NSCLC-derived tumorspheres. **d** The histograms of data in **c**. shJARID1B, JARID1B shRNA-silenced; NC, negative control. The bars were representative of mean ± SEM of independent experiments performed in triplicate assays. *$p < 0.05$; **$p < 0.01$; ***$p < 0.001$

of JARID1B promotes NSCLC cell proliferation, cell motility, invasiveness, and tumorsphere formation in vitro, not only allude to a novel role of JARID1B in the modulation of EMT and CSCs-like phenotype in NSCLC cells, but also give a mechanistic insight into the clinical observations that NSCLC patients with stronger JARID1B expression are more prone to have metastasis and significantly shorter overall survival. In addition, pharmacological inhibition of JARID1B effectively suppressed these phenomena caused by JARID1B overexpression.

Our current results also revealed that JARID1B knockdown enhanced cell death induced by cisplatin and doxorubicin in NSCLC cells. We considered the underlying mechanisms to be complicated and possibly multifaceted. As previously reported, histone demethylases could either decrease [32] drug resistance in prostate cancer cells or increase [33, 34] drug resistance in several other cancer cells. As for the role of JARID1B, previous reports were few and most described that JARID1B overexpression increased drug resistance in melanoma in vitro and in vivo [35, 36]. One study including only human subjects suggested that JARID1B is associated with poor prognosis and chemotherapy resistance in epithelial ovarian cancer [37]. On the other hand, it is well known that drug resistance is one typical characteristic of CSCs [38, 39]. Whether our current finding is due to the biological effects of JARID1B itself

or secondary to the CSCs phenotype resulting from JARID1B expression is still unknown and deserves further investigation.

Conclusion

In summary, our study reveals JARID1B-mediated promotion of EMT and CSCs characteristics in NSCLC cells, shows that JARID1B can be a putative marker of tumor progression and poor prognosis in NSCLC patients, and suggests JARID1B may be a good molecular or pharmacological target in NSCLC.

Abbreviations
CSCs: Cancer stem cells; FGFR: Fibroblast growth factor receptor; H&E: Hematoxylin and eosin; JARID1: Jumonji, AT-rich interactive domain 1; LCSCs: Lung cancer stem cells; PDGFR: Platelet-derived growth factor receptors; SRB: Sulforhodamine B; VEGFRs: Vascular endothelial growth factor

Funding
This work was supported by the Ministry of Science and Technology of Taiwan grant to Kuang-Tai Kuo (MOST103-2314-B-038-034-MY2) and grants from Taipei Medical University-Shuang Ho Hospital (106TMU-SHH-22) to Kuang-Tai Kuo and grants from Taipei Medical University—National Taiwan University of Science and Technology Joint Research Program (TMU-NTUST-103-03) to Chi-Tai Yeh. The authors thank the laboratory assistants (Translational
Research Lab, Department of Medical Research and Education, Taipei Medical University-Shuang Ho Hospital) for their technical assistance.

Authors' contributions

KTK and WCH conceived and designed the study. KTK, WCH, and BOA performed the experiments. KTK, WCH, and OAB analyzed the data. KTK and OAB wrote the paper. WHL, CHW, LSW, and CTY provided reagents, materials, and experimental infrastructure. All authors read and approved the definitive version of the manuscript.

Author details

[1]Division of Thoracic Surgery, Department of Surgery, Shuang Ho Hospital, Taipei Medical University, New Taipei City, Taiwan. [2]Division of Thoracic Surgery, Department of Surgery, School of Medicine, College of Medicine, Taipei Medical University, Taipei, Taiwan. [3]Division of Thoracic Surgery, Department of Surgery, MacKay Memorial Hospital, Taipei, Taiwan. [4]MacKay Medical College, Taipei, Taiwan. [5]Department of Medical Research and Education, Shuang Ho Hospital, Taipei Medical University, New Taipei City, Taiwan. [6]Division of Hematology/Oncology, Department of Medicine, Shuang Ho Hospital, Taipei Medical University, New Taipei City, Taiwan. [7]Department of Pathology, Shuang Ho Hospital, Taipei Medical University, New Taipei City, Taiwan. [8]Department of Dermatology, Taipei Tzu Chi Hospital, Buddhist Tzu Chi Medical Foundation, New Taipei City, Taiwan. [9]School of Medicine, Buddhist Tzu Chi University, Hualien, Taiwan. [10]Genomics Research Center, Academia Sinica, Taipei, Taiwan.

References

1. Ferlay J, Soerjomataram I, Dikshit R, Eser S, Mathers C, Rebelo M, et al. Cancer incidence and mortality worldwide: sources, methods and major patterns in GLOBOCAN 2012. Int J Cancer. 2015;136:E359–86.
2. Siegel R, DeSantis C, Virgo K, Stein K, Mariotto A, Smith T, et al. Cancer treatment and survivorship statistics, 2012. CA Cancer J Clin. 2012;62:220–41.
3. Siegel RL, Miller KD, Jemal A. Cancer statistics, 2016. CA Cancer J Clin. 2016;66:7–30.
4. Azzoli CG, Baker S Jr, Temin S, Pao W, Aliff T, Brahmer J, et al. American Society of Clinical Oncology clinical practice guideline update on chemotherapy for stage IV non-small-cell lung cancer. J Clin Oncol. 2009;27:6251–66.
5. Tan DS, Yom SS, Tsao MS, Pass HI, Kelly K, Peled N, et al. The international association for the study of lung cancer consensus statement on optimizing management of EGFR mutation-positive non-small cell lung cancer: status in 2016. J Thorac Oncol. 2016;11:946–63.
6. Singh S, Chellappan S. Lung cancer stem cells: molecular features and therapeutic targets. Mol Asp Med. 2014;39:50–60.
7. MacDonagh L, Gray SG, Breen E, Cuffe S, Finn SP, O'Byrne KJ, et al. Lung cancer stem cells: the root of resistance. Cancer Lett. 2016;372:147–56.
8. Zakaria N, Yusoff NM, Zakaria Z, Lim MN, Baharuddin PJ, Fakiruddin KS, et al. Human non-small cell lung cancer expresses putative cancer stem cell markers and exhibits the transcriptomic profile of multipotent cells. BMC Cancer. 2015;15:84.
9. Breindel JL, Haskins JW, Cowell EP, Zhao M, Nguyen DX, Stern DF. EGF receptor activates MET through MAPK to enhance non-small cell lung carcinoma invasion and brain metastasis. Cancer Res. 2013;73:5053–65.
10. Dulak AM, Gubish CT, Stabile LP, Henry C, Siegfried JM. HGF-independent potentiation of EGFR action by c-Met. Oncogene. 2011;30:3625–35.
11. Dawson MA, Kouzarides T. Cancer epigenetics: from mechanism to therapy. Cell. 2012;150:12–27.
12. Seol HS, Akiyama Y, Shimada S, Lee HJ, Kim TI, Chun SM, et al. Epigenetic silencing of microRNA-373 to epithelial-mesenchymal transition in non-small cell lung cancer through IRAK2 and LAMP1 axes. Cancer Lett. 2014;353:232–41.
13. Mehta A, Dobersch S, Romero-Olmedo AJ, Barreto G. Epigenetics in lung cancer diagnosis and therapy. Cancer Metastasis Rev. 2015;34:229–41.
14. Shi L, Zheng M, Hou J, Zhu B, Wang X. Regulatory roles of epigenetic modulators, modifiers and mediators in lung cancer. Semin Cancer Biol. 2017;42:4–12.
15. Arcipowski KM, Martinez CA, Ntziachristos P. Histone demethylases in physiology and cancer: a tale of two enzymes, JMJD3 and UTX. Curr Opin Genet Dev. 2016;36:59–67.
16. Perrigue PM, Najbauer J, Barciszewski J. Histone demethylase JMJD3 at the intersection of cellular senescence and cancer. Biochim Biophys Acta. 2016;1865:237–44.
17. McGrath J, Trojer P. Targeting histone lysine methylation in cancer. Pharmacol Ther. 2015;150:1–22.
18. Kristensen LH, Nielsen AL, Helgstrand C, Lees M, Cloos P, Kastrup JS, et al. Studies of H3K4me3 demethylation by KDM5B/Jarid1B/PLU1 reveals strong substrate recognition in vitro and identifies 2,4-pyridine-dicarboxylic acid as an in vitro and in cell inhibitor. FEBS J. 2012;279:1905–14.
19. Horton JR, Engstrom A, Zoeller EL, Liu X, Shanks JR, Zhang X, et al. Characterization of a linked Jumonji domain of the KDM5/JARID1 family of histone H3 lysine 4 demethylases. J Biol Chem. 2016;291:2631–46.
20. Lin CS, Lin YC, Adebayo BO, Wu A, Chen JH, Peng YJ, et al. Silencing JARID1B suppresses oncogenicity, stemness and increases radiation sensitivity in human oral carcinoma. Cancer Lett. 2015;368:36–45.
21. Bamodu OA, Huang WC, Lee WH, Wu A, Wang LS, Hsiao M, et al. Aberrant KDM5B expression promotes aggressive breast cancer through MALAT1 overexpression and downregulation of hsa-miR-448. BMC Cancer. 2016;16:160.
22. Vinogradova M, Gehling VS, Gustafson A, Arora S, Tindell CA, Wilson C, et al. An inhibitor of KDM5 demethylases reduces survival of drug-tolerant cancer cells. Nat Chem Biol. 2016;12:531–8.
23. Vichai V, Kirtikara K. Sulforhodamine B colorimetric assay for cytotoxicity screening. Nat Protoc. 2006;1:1112–6.
24. Chen S, Li X, Lu D, Xu Y, Mou W, Wang L, et al. SOX2 regulates apoptosis through MAP4K4-survivin signaling pathway in human lung cancer cells. Carcinogenesis. 2014;35:613–23.
25. Sayegh J, Cao J, Zou MR, Morales A, Blair LP, Norcia M, et al. Identification of small molecule inhibitors of Jumonji AT-rich interactive domain 1B (JARID1B) histone demethylase by a sensitive high throughput screen. J Biol Chem. 2013; 288:9408–17.
26. Yamamoto S, Wu Z, Russnes HG, Takagi S, Peluffo G, Vaske C, et al. JARID1B is a luminal lineage-driving oncogene in breast cancer. Cancer Cell. 2014;25: 762–77.
27. Wang Z, Tang F, Qi G, et al. KDM5B is overexpressed in gastric cancer and is required for gastric cancer cell proliferation and metastasis. Am J Cancer Res. 2014;5:87–100.
28. Cui Z, Song L, Hou Z, Han Y, Hu Y, Wu Y, et al. PLU-1/JARID1B overexpression predicts proliferation properties in head and neck squamous cell carcinoma. Oncol Rep. 2015;33:2454–60.
29. Rasmussen PB, Staller P. The KDM5 family of histone demethylases as targets in oncology drug discovery. Epigenomics. 2014;6:277–86.
30. Kalluri R, Weinberg RA. The basics of epithelial-mesenchymal transition. J Clin Invest. 2009;119:1420–8.
31. Scheel C, Weinberg RA. Cancer stem cells and epithelial-mesenchymal transition: concepts and molecular links. Semin Cancer Biol. 2012;22:396–403.
32. Komura K, Jeong SH, Hinohara K, Qu F, Wang X, Hiraki M, et al. Resistance to docetaxel in prostate cancer is associated with androgen receptor activation and loss of KDM5D expression. Proc Natl Acad Sci U S A. 2016;113:6259–64.
33. Osawa T, Tsuchida R, Muramatsu M, Shimamura T, Wang F, Suehiro J, et al. Inhibition of histone demethylase JMJD1A improves anti-angiogenic therapy and reduces tumor-associated macrophages. Cancer Res. 2013;73:3019–28.
34. Lei ZJ, Wang J, Xiao HL, Guo Y, Wang T, Li Q, et al. Lysine-specific demethylase 1 promotes the stemness and chemoresistance of Lgr5(+) liver cancer initiating cells by suppressing negative regulators of β-catenin signaling. Oncogene. 2015;34:3188–98.
35. Roesch A, Vultur A, Bogeski I, Wang H, Zimmermann KM, Speicher D, et al. Overcoming intrinsic multidrug resistance in melanoma by blocking the mitochondrial respiratory chain of slow-cycling JARID1B(high) cells. Cancer Cell. 2013;23:811–25.
36. Zubrilov I, Sagi-Assif O, Izraely S, Meshel T, Ben-Menahem S, Ginat R, et al. Vemurafenib resistance selects for highly malignant brain and lung-metastasizing melanoma cells. Cancer Lett. 2015;361:86–96.
37. Wang L, Mao Y, Du G, He C, Han S. Overexpression of JARID1B is associated with poor prognosis and chemotherapy resistance in epithelial ovarian cancer. Tumour Biol. 2015;36:2465–72.
38. Carnero A, Garcia-Mayea Y, Mir C, Lorente J, Rubio IT, LLeonart ME. The cancer stem-cell signaling network and resistance to therapy. Cancer Treat Rev. 2016;49:25–36.
39. Zhao J. Cancer stem cells and chemoresistance: the smartest survives the raid. Pharmacol Ther. 2016;160:145–58.

18

Vitamin D and the promoter methylation of its metabolic pathway genes in association with the risk and prognosis of tuberculosis

Min Wang[1,2†], Weimin Kong[3†], Biyu He[1], Zhongqi Li[1], Huan Song[1], Peiyi Shi[1] and Jianming Wang[1,4*] (iD)

Abstract

Background: A variety of abnormalities in vitamin D metabolism have been reported in patients with active tuberculosis. However, intervention trials have produced inconsistent results. We hypothesized that genetic and epigenetic changes in the key genes of the vitamin D metabolic pathway may partly explain the differences between studies.

Methods: We performed a case-control study followed by a prospective cohort study. We recruited 122 patients with pulmonary tuberculosis and 118 healthy controls. The serum 25-hydroxyvitamin D and 1,25-dihydroxyvitamin D levels were measured. The methylation of the promoter regions of key genes in the vitamin D metabolic pathway (CYP24A1, CYP27A1, CYP27B1, CYP2R1, and VDR) was detected using the Illumina MiSeq platform. The specific methylation profiles were examined as epigenetic biomarkers. The sensitivity, specificity, and receiver operating characteristic (ROC) curves were used to estimate the predictive value of the biomarkers.

Results: The baseline serum 25-hydroxyvitamin D and 1,25-dihydroxyvitamin D concentrations in the cases were significantly lower than those in the controls (51.60 ± 27.25 nmol/L vs. 117.50 ± 75.50 nmol/L, $Z = -8.515$, $P < 0.001$; 82.63 ± 51.43 pmol/L vs. 94.02 ± 49.26 pmol/L, $Z = -2.165$, $P = 0.03$). We sequenced 310 CpG sites in five candidate genes. After Bonferroni correction, there were 55 differentially methylated CpG sites between cases and controls; 41.5% were in the CYP27B1 gene, 31.7% were in the CYP24A1 gene, 14.7% were in the VDR gene, and 12.3% were in the CYP27A1 gene. When we designated the CpG sites that remained significant after the Bonferroni correction as the biomarkers, the area under the curve (AUC) for the cumulative methylation was 0.810 (95% CI 0.754–0.866). There was an interaction between CYP27A1 methylation level and 1,25-dihydroxyvitamin D concentration associated with the risk of TB ($OR_{interaction} = 4.11$, 95% CI 1.26–13.36, $P = 0.019$). The serum 1,25-dihydroxyvitamin D concentration at the end of the intensive treatment stage was related to a patient's prognosis ($P = 0.008$). There were 23 CpG sites that were individually related to the treatment outcomes, but the relationships were not significant after the Bonferroni correction.

Conclusion: Both serum vitamin D concentrations and the methylation levels of key genes in the vitamin D metabolic pathway are related to the risk and prognosis of tuberculosis.

Keywords: Tuberculosis, DNA methylation, Vitamin D, Risk, Prognosis

* Correspondence: jmwang@njmu.edu.cn
†Min Wang and Weimin Kong contributed equally to this work.
[1]Department of Epidemiology, School of Public Health, Nanjing Medical University, 101 Longmian Ave, Nanjing 211166, People's Republic of China
[4]Key Laboratory of Infectious Diseases, School of Public Health, Nanjing Medical University, Nanjing, People's Republic of China
Full list of author information is available at the end of the article

Background

Despite the widespread use of the Bacillus Calmette-Guérin (BCG) vaccine, *Mycobacterium tuberculosis* (M.tb) infection and active tuberculosis (TB) remain major public health threats [1, 2]. TB is the ninth leading cause of death worldwide and is the leading cause of death from a single infectious agent, ranking above HIV/AIDS. In 2016, 10.4 million people fell ill with TB and there were an estimated 1.3 million TB deaths among HIV-negative people and an additional 374,000 deaths among HIV-positive people [3].

Factors related to the risk of TB include low socioeconomic status, poor nutrition, traditional/cultural traits, tobacco smoking, contacts with sputum smear-positive index patients, and genetic susceptibility [4–8]. Studies have correlated vitamin D deficiency with susceptibility to TB since 1651 when vitamin deficiency was found to be associated with TB for the first time [9]. Moreover, Stead et al. have shown racial differences in the incidence of TB associated with the levels of 25-hydroxyvitamin D (25(OH)D). Recently, studies have reported that hypovitaminosis D results in lower antimycobacterial immunity [10, 11] and is related to increased risk of TB [12, 13]. In vitro studies have revealed that 1,25-dihydroxyvitamin D ($1,25(OH)_2D$) enhances innate immunity by increasing the expression of antimicrobial peptides, including cathelicidin, and inducing the autophagy of infected cells, thus restricting the intracellular growth of M.tb in macrophages [14]. Some studies have shown that vitamin D supplementation during the intensive phase of antimicrobial treatment can increase sputum negative conversion rates [15, 16]. Vitamin D supplementation has been believed to be beneficial in the treatment of patients with TB in observational studies; however, results from clinical trials have been inconclusive [17]. Confounding factors and reverse causation may partly explain the inconsistencies [18], but individual variations in vitamin D metabolism and related variations in immune responses should not be neglected.

Previous studies have mainly focused on genetic polymorphisms of genes in the vitamin D metabolic pathway. With the development of molecular biology, the role of epigenetic traits in gene expression has received greater attention [19]. DNA methylation, which involves the addition of a methyl group to the cytosine in a CpG dinucleotide, is a key epigenetic trait related to a number of biological processes including genomic imprinting, X-chromosome inactivation, aging, and carcinogenesis [20]. Studies have shown that hypermethylation in the promoter region of the cytochrome P450 gene can silence the gene and affect the vitamin D activity [21], but the role of this hypermethylation in the risk of TB has not been systematically studied. Thus, we performed a molecular epidemiological study in a Chinese population aiming to explore the effect of aberrant DNA methylation in the vitamin D metabolic pathway on serum 25(OH)D and $1,25(OH)_2D$ levels and to determine its relation to the risk and prognosis of pulmonary TB.

Methods

Study design and study population

This study used a mixed case-control and prospective cohort design. We recruited 122 patients with pulmonary TB from Zhenjiang and Lianyungang in the province of Jiangsu in China during 2014 and 2016. TB cases were group-matched (by sex and age) with 118 controls from a pool of individuals who participated in community-based health examination programs. Among these controls, individuals with a history of TB, malignancy, diabetes, and HIV were excluded. This study was approved by the Ethics Committee of Nanjing Medical University. After informed consent was obtained from all participants, questionnaires were used to collect demographic data. Venous blood samples were collected for vitamin D measurement and molecular analyses.

Serum 25(OH)D and $1,25(OH)_2D$ measurement

We measured the serum vitamin D using a 25-hydroxyvitamin D kit and a 1,25-dihydroxyvitamin D EIA (Immunodiagnostic Systems Limited, UK). The intra- and interassay coefficient of variation (CV) were < 9% for 25(OH)D and < 20% for $1,25(OH)_2D$. The minimum detection limits were 12 nmol/L for 25(OH)D and 6 pmol/L for $1,25(OH)_2D$.

Methylation analysis

We selected five key genes (CYP24A1, CYP27A1, CYP27B1, CYP2R1, and VDR) in the vitamin D metabolic pathway and sequenced the CpG islands in the promoter region of the candidate genes using the Illumina MiSeq platform. The DNA was subjected to sodium bisulfite treatment using an EZ DNA Methylation™-GOLD Kit (Zymo Research, Orange, CA, USA) according to the manufacturer's protocols. Primers were designed to amplify the regions of interest from the bisulfite-converted DNA (Table 1).

Multiplex PCR was performed using the optimized primer sets. A 20-µl PCR reaction mixture was prepared for each reaction that included 2 µl of template DNA, 3 mM Mg^{2+}, 0.2 mM dNTP, 0.1 µM of each primer, 1× buffer (Takara, Tokyo, Japan), and 1 U of HotStarTaq polymerase (Takara, Tokyo, Japan). The cycling program was 95 °C for 2 min; 11 cycles of 94 °C for 20 s, 63 °C for 40 s with a decreasing temperature step of 0.5 °C per cycle, and 72 °C for 1 min; 24 cycles of 94 °C for 20 s, 65 °C for 30 s, and 72 °C for 1 min; and 72 °C for 2 min.

PCR amplicons from different panels were quantified and pooled, diluted, and subjected to a second round of amplification using the indexed primers. A 20-µl mixture was prepared for each reaction that included 0.3 µM index primer,

Table 1 Primers designed for multiplex PCR

Gene	Fragment	Forward primer	Reverse primer
CYP24A1	CYP24A1 _1	TAGAGGAGGGYGGAGTGGTTT	CACACCCRATAAACTCCRAACTTC
	CYP24A1 _2	GGAGATAATTTTTAGGAAGTTATGYGAAGTT	CACTTCAATCCAAACTAAAAATATCTAACTC
CYP27A1	CYP27A1 _1	TTGGTTTYGTGGGGGTAGAG	CACCRCRTCCCTCTCCTACAA
	CYP27A1 _2	GGAGGGTYGAGTAAAGGTTAGTTAGAT	AAAACCTATCCCRATATAAAACTTCC
	CYP27A1 _3	ATTTTGGGYGGGGGTGTAG	CCCTCCAAAAATCAAATAACTAACC
	CYP27A1 _4	TTTTYGGATTGATTTYGGAGTTAGT	ACTATACRTTTTCCRTACTATATTACTCTTTCC
	CYP27A1 _5	GGTTGAGATTAGATTTYGTAGATGATG	ACCAACTATACCATCCTACTAAATCCT
CYP27B1	CYP27B1 _1	GGTTGAGATATGATGTTTAGGAGAAG	TCCCTTCCTACCTACAACTCRTATA
	CYP27B1 _2	TTTGGYGTGGGTATAGGTTAAGTTG	CTCACRCAATAAACAATCCRCAAAC
	CYP27B1 _3	GAGTTGTTGYGATAGGAGGGATT	CAACCRACCTCCCACCA
CYP2R1	CYP2R1 _1	TTAATGGGAGTATGGTAGGGTTG	AAAAACCCATCRACCRCCTCTA
	CYP2R1 _2	GGTAGGGAGGGTYGTTAGGTTG	CAAAACTAAATCRCCTCRAAACCTC
	CYP2R1 _3	TGTAGGGGGAGTTTYGTTTTTGT	CAAACACCRAAAAACCTACTATTAACC
	CYP2R1 _4	GGAAAATTAAGGYGTTTTGAGTTTTA	CACACAAAAAACRCCTTTTAAATATCTAC
VDR	VDR _1	GTAGTTATTTATAATTTTAGGTTTTAGGAGGTAG	CTCAACCTAATCCCACAAATTAAAA
	VDR _2	AGGTGATATYGGGTGGGAGTAAT	CCACCTAAACTAACCAAACCAA
	VDR _3	GGTGTTAGTYGGTAGGYGTTTTTTAG	CATAAAACAAAACACRCTTCTACCCT
	VDR _4	TTTYGATTAATATAGGTTGAAGYGGGTA	CCCACAAATCCAATCCTCTC
	VDR _6	GAATTYGGGAGTAGYGGGAAAG	TACTAAACACTATATTAACRAAACATTTCTCC

0.3 μM forward primer, 0.3 mM dNTP, 1× buffer (New England Biolabs, MA, the USA), 1 U of Q5™ DNA polymerase (New England Biolabs), and 1 μL of diluted template. The cycling program was 98 °C for 30 s; 11 cycles of 98 °C for 10 s, 65 °C for 30 s, and 72 °C for 30 s; and 72 °C for 5 min. The PCR products were separated by agarose gel electrophoresis and purified using a QIAquick Gel Extraction Kit (Qiagen, Hilden, Germany). The libraries from the different samples were quantified and pooled together, then sequenced on the Illumina MiSeq platform according to the manufacturer's protocols. Sequencing was performed with 2×300 bp (overall sequencing read length) paired-end runs.

Table 2 General characteristics of cases and controls

Variables	Controls ($n = 118$)	Cases ($n = 122$)	t/χ^2	P
Age (years)				
Mean ± SD	51.97 ± 12.49	50.83 ± 20.04	0.530	0.597
Sex [n(%)]			1.104	0.293
Male	86 (72.9)	96 (78.7)		
Female	32 (27.1)	26 (21.3)		
Marital status [n(%)]				
Unmarried	3 (2.5)	25 (20.5)	18.777	< 0.001
Married	111 (94.1)	94 (77.0)		
Widowed/divorced	4 (3.4)	3 (2.5)		
Smoking [n(%)]			0.329	0.566
Never	72 (61.0)	70 (57.4)		
Ever	46 (39.0)	52 (42.6)		
Drinking [n(%)]			0.351	0.554
Never	83 (70.3)	90 (73.8)		
Ever	35 (29.7)	32 (26.2)		

Table 3 Sequenced sites of selected genes

Gene	Fragment	Start/stop	Size(bp)	Number of CpG sites
CYP24A1	CYP24A1_1	52790591/52790815	224	13
	CYP24A1_2	52790767/52791019	252	28
CYP27A1	CYP27A1_1	219646982/219646721	261	22
	CYP27A1_2	219646810/219646561	249	22
	CYP27A1_3	219646624/219646403	221	18
	CYP27A1_4	219646465/219646204	261	8
	CYP27A1_5	219646286/219646037	249	3
CYP27B1	CYP27B1_1	58160882/58160619	263	16
	CYP27B1_2	58160053/58159785	268	23
	CYP27B1_3	58159890/58159688	202	14
CYP2R1	CYP2R1_1	14913830/14913634	196	14
	CYP2R1_2	14913505/14913273	232	15
	CYP2R1_3	14913339/14913061	278	24
	CYP2R1_4	14913116/14912845	271	15
VDR	VDR_1	48299590/48299323	267	18
	VDR_2	48299412/48299179	233	19
	VDR_3	48299247/48299017	230	13
	VDR_4	48299106/48298885	221	10
	VDR_6	48298733/48298464	269	15

Table 4 Methylation levels of specific sites between cases and controls

Gene	Fragment	Methylation level of controls ($n = 118$)		Methylation level of cases ($n = 122$)	
		Mean ± SD	Median	Mean ± SD	Median
CYP24A1	CYP24A1_1	0.39 ± 0.13	0.374	0.35 ± 0.12	0.335
	CYP24A1_2	0.48 ± 0.08	0.461	0.41 ± 0.07	0.397
CYP27A1	CYP27A1_1	0.87 ± 0.23	0.818	0.75 ± 0.27	0.678
	CYP27A1_2	0.78 ± 0.24	0.716	0.63 ± 0.24	0.557
	CYP27A1_3	0.54 ± 0.20	0.508	0.43 ± 0.18	0.398
	CYP27A1_4	0.72 ± 0.17	0.697	0.63 ± 0.12	0.606
	CYP27A1_5	1.79 ± 0.20	1.804	1.76 ± 0.01	1.784
CYP27B1	CYP27B1_1	3.22 ± 0.56	3.167	2.78 ± 0.56	2.664
	CYP27B1_2	1.56 ± 0.33	1.493	1.40 ± 0.32	1.345
	CYP27B1_3	0.60 ± 0.14	0.578	0.53 ± 0.14	0.499
CYP2R1	CYP2R1_1	0.13 ± 0.01	0.129	0.13 ± 0.01	0.126
	CYP2R1_2	0.15 ± 0.01	0.152	0.15 ± 0.01	0.148
	CYP2R1_3	0.22 ± 0.05	0.223	0.22 ± 0.05	0.213
	CYP2R1_4	0.13 ± 0.02	0.124	0.12 ± 0.01	0.123
VDR	VDR_1	0.94 ± 0.23	0.097	0.02 ± 0.23	0.781
	VDR_2	0.37 ± 0.05	0.362	0.33 ± 0.06	0.313
	VDR_3	0.21 ± 0.10	0.196	0.20 ± 0.10	0.188
	VDR_4	0.13 ± 0.02	0.132	0.12 ± 0.02	0.122
	VDR_6	0.26 ± 0.07	0.270	0.27 ± 0.07	0.263

Table 5 Cumulative methylation levels of multiple CpG sites in each gene between cases and controls using different models

Gene	Model 1				Model 2				Model 3				Model 4			
	Cumulative methylation level		t	P	Cumulative methylation level		t	P	Cumulative methylation level		t	P	Cumulative methylation level		t	P
	Controls ($n = 118$)	Cases ($n = 122$)			Controls ($n = 118$)	Cases ($n = 122$)			Controls ($n = 118$)	Cases ($n = 122$)			Controls ($n = 118$)	Cases ($n = 122$)		
CYP24A1	0.87 ± 0.16	0.76 ± 0.17	5.120	<0.001	0.46 ± 0.08	0.38 ± 0.08	7.929	<0.001	0.46 ± 0.08	0.38 ± 0.08	7.929	<0.001	0.28 ± 0.06	0.23 ± 0.05	7.699	<0.001
CYP27A1	4.70 ± 0.74	4.19 ± 0.68	5.537	<0.001	2.40 ± 0.57	1.96 ± 0.51	6.182	<0.001	2.40 ± 0.57	1.96 ± 0.51	6.182	<0.001	0.59 ± 0.17	0.47 ± 0.16	5.803	<0.001
CYP27B1	5.37 ± 0.97	4.72 ± 0.95	5.271	<0.001	4.95 ± 0.92	4.31 ± 0.90	5.417	<0.001	4.95 ± 0.92	4.31 ± 0.90	5.417	<0.001	3.05 ± 0.61	2.57 ± 0.61	5.998	<0.001
CYP2R1	0.63 ± 0.06	0.61 ± 0.06	2.118	0.035	0.08 ± 0.02	0.07 ± 0.02	2.203	0.029	0.07 ± 0.01	0.06 ± 0.01	6.207	<0.001	–	–	–	–
VDR	1.92 ± 0.32	1.74 ± 0.32	4.203	<0.001	1.12 ± 0.22	0.97 ± 0.23	4.909	<0.001	1.04 ± 0.21	0.88 ± 0.22	5.812	<0.001	0.40 ± 0.07	0.33 ± 0.08	6.237	<0.001

Statistical analysis

Data were entered with EpiData 3.1 software (Denmark) and analyzed using STATA 12.0 (StataCorp, College Station, TX, USA). Student's t test and the chi-square test were used to compare the distributions of demographic variables and risk factors between cases and controls. Univariate and multivariate logistic regression models were used to calculate odds ratios (ORs) and 95% confidence intervals (CIs). We analyzed both individual and cumulative methylation levels of the candidate genes. The sensitivity, specificity, and the area under the receiver operating characteristic (ROC) curve were estimated to assess the diagnostic value of the biomarkers. A Spearman correlation was used to estimate the relationship between serum vitamin D levels and methylation status. A Kaplan-Meier curve was used to analyze the effect of methylation level on initial sputum conversion.

Results

General characteristics of study subjects

In total, 122 TB cases (78.7% males and 21.3% females) and 118 controls (72.9% males and 27.1% females) were involved in the analysis. The average age (± standard deviation, SD) was 50.83 (20.04) years in cases and 51.97 (± 12.49) years in controls. Due to the frequency matching, there was no significant difference in the distribution of age and sex between the two groups. However, the distribution of marital status was significantly different ($P < 0.001$). The proportion of those who had ever smoked in the cases was slightly higher than that in the controls (42.6% vs. 39.0%), while the percentage of those who drank alcohol was slightly lower in the cases than in the controls (26.2% vs. 29.7%), although there was not a significant difference (Table 2). Among the cases, 46 (37.7%) were cured, 61 (50.0%) completed treatment, and 15 (12.3%) failed to be treated. We categorized the cases into two groups: successful (cured or completed treatment) and unsuccessful.

Serum vitamin D concentrations and methylation levels of CpG sites and the risk of TB

The baseline concentrations of serum 25(OH)D and 1,25(OH)$_2$D were 51.60 ± 27.25 nmol/L and 82.63 ± 51.43 pmol/L among cases, respectively, which were significantly lower than those in the controls (25(OH)D 117.50 ± 75.50 nmol/L, $Z = -8.515$, $P < 0.001$; 1,25(OH)$_2$D 94.02 ± 49.26 pmol/L, $Z = -2.165$, $P = 0.03$). The serum level of 1,25(OH)$_2$D declined during the early phase of antituberculosis treatment, while at the end of the intensive treatment stage, it was 70.81 ± 44.50 pmol/L ($Z = -2.606$, $P = 0.009$).

We sequenced 310 CpG sites in the promoter regions of the candidate genes (Table 3). The methylation levels of specific sites between cases and controls are shown in Table 4. The correlations for methylation levels in each region with 1,25(OH)$_2$D concentrations were listed in Additional file 1. After Bonferroni correction, there were 55 differentially methylated CpG sites between cases and controls, 41.5% of which were in the CYP27B1 gene, 31.7% of which were in the CYP24A1 gene, 14.7% of which were in the VDR gene, and 12.3% of which were in the CYP27A1 gene. We calculated the cumulative methylation levels by adding the frequencies for all the CpG sites in each gene region and found that the methylation level of CYP27A1_3 was significantly associated with the level of serum 1,25(OH)$_2$D ($P = 0.045$). To further analyze the cumulative methylation levels by considering multiple CpG sites in each gene, we constructed four models. In model 1, we calculated the cumulative methylation levels by adding the frequencies for all the CpG sites in each gene. In model 2, we calculated the cumulative methylation levels by adding the frequencies for the statistically significant CpG sites in each gene. Model 3 only included hypermethylated CpG sites in the cases and excluded CpG sites with inverse relations between cases and controls. Model 4 only included CpG sites that were statistically significant after the Bonferroni correction.

Model 1

We calculated the cumulative methylation levels by adding the frequencies for all the CpG sites in each gene. The cumulative methylation levels of CYP24A1, CYP27A1, CYP27B1, CYP2R1, and VDR were significantly different between cases and controls ($P < 0.05$, Table 5). The area under the curve (AUC) for each gene is listed in Table 6. The cumulative methylation levels of the CYP27A1 gene showed the highest diagnostic value, with an AUC of

Table 6 Diagnostic values for TB of selected genes using different models

Gene	Model 1			Model 2			Model 3			Model 4		
	AUC	95% CI	P	AUC	95% CI	P	AUC	95% CI	P	AUC	95% CI	P
CYP24A1	0.707	0.641–0.772	< 0.001	0.794	0.737–0.851	< 0.001	0.794	0.737–0.851	< 0.001	0.793	0.736–0.850	< 0.001
CYP27A1	0.739	0.675–0.802	< 0.001	0.760	0.699–0.821	< 0.001	0.760	0.699–0.821	< 0.001	0.747	0.685–0.809	< 0.001
CYP27B1	0.735	0.671–0.799	< 0.001	0.739	0.675–0.803	< 0.001	0.739	0.675–0.803	< 0.001	0.747	0.684–0.810	< 0.001
CYP2R1	0.578	0.506–0.650	0.037	0.611	0.540–0.683	0.003	0.743	0.679–0.806	< 0.001	–	–	–
VDR	0.664	0.596–0.732	< 0.001	0.709	0.644–0.775	< 0.001	0.740	0.677–0.803	< 0.001	0.758	0.696–0.819	< 0.001

AUC area under the curve, *CI* confidence interval

Table 7 Correlation analysis between cumulative methylation levels and 25-hydroxyvitamin D levels

Gene	Model 1		Model 2		Model 3		Model 4	
	r	P	r	P	r	P	r	P
CYP24A1	0.213	< 0.001	0.287	< 0.001	0.287	< 0.001	0.303	< 0.001
CYP27A1	0.294	< 0.001	0.279	< 0.001	0.279	< 0.001	0.227	< 0.001
CYP27B1	0.195	0.002	0.201	0.002	0.201	0.002	0.210	0.001
CYP2R1	0.021	0.742	0.078	0.232	0.231	< 0.001	–	–
VDR	0.177	0.006	0.202	0.002	0.238	< 0.001	0.308	< 0.001

r correlation coefficient

0.739 (95% CI 0.675–0.802), followed by CYP27B1 (AUC 0.735, 95% CI 0.671–0.799). The AUC obtained by combining the cumulative methylation levels of the CpG sites in all genotyped genes was 0.747 (95% CI 0.685–0.809).

Model 2

We calculated the cumulative methylation levels by adding the frequencies for the statistically significant CpG sites in each gene. The cumulative methylation levels of CYP24A1, CYP27A1, CYP27B1, CYP2R1, and VDR remained significantly different between cases and controls ($P < 0.05$). As shown in Table 6, the AUC of each gene was higher than that in model 1. CYP24A1 showed the highest diagnostic value, with an AUC of 0.794 (95% CI 0.737–0.851). The AUC obtained by combining the cumulative methylation levels of the CpG sites in model 2 was 0.805 (95% CI 0.749–0.860).

Model 3

We further excluded CpG sites with inverse relations between cases and controls and only included 164 hypermethylated CpG sites in the cases for analysis. The cumulative methylation levels of CYP24A1, CYP27A1, CYP27B1, CYP2R1, and VDR remained significantly different between cases and controls ($P < 0.001$). The CpG sites of the CYP24A1, CYP27A1, and CYP27B1 genes included in model 3 were the same as those in model 2. For the CYP2R1 and VDR genes, the AUC increased to 0.743 (95% CI 0.679–0.806) and 0.740 (95% CI: 0.677–0.803), respectively (Table 6). The AUC obtained by combining the cumulative methylation levels of all of the aforementioned CpG sites was 0.838 (95% CI 0.789–0.888).

Model 4

We included 55 methylated CpG sites that remained statistically significant after the Bonferroni correction. As shown in Table 5, CYP24A1, CYP27A1, CYP27B1, and VDR had significantly different methylation levels between cases and controls ($P < 0.001$). The AUC obtained by combining the cumulative methylation levels of all the aforementioned CpG sites was 0.810 (95% CI 0.754–0.866).

Interaction between serum vitamin D and methylation levels

As shown in Table 7, the methylation levels of the CYP24A1, CYP27A1, CYP27B1, and VDR genes were significantly associated with the levels of serum 25(OH)D ($P < 0.05$). To explore the interaction between vitamin D and methylation in the risk of TB, we categorized the genes into hyper- and hypomethylated genes based on the ROC curves and divided the serum vitamin D levels into low and high levels based on the median. There was a significant interaction between CYP27A1 methylation levels and $1,25(OH)_2D$ concentrations in model 1 and model 4 and between the methylation levels of VDR and CYP2R1 and $1,25(OH)_2D$ concentrations in model 3 ($P < 0.05$, Table 8). Based on model 4, the OR$_{interaction}$ was 4.11 (95% CI 1.26–13.36, $P = 0.019$) (Table 9).

Treatment outcomes of patients with TB

The baseline serum $1,25(OH)_2D$ concentration was related to the treatment outcome ($Z = -2.655$, $P = 0.008$). Patients with high serum $1,25(OH)_2D$ concentrations had a decreased risk of treatment failure (adjusted relative risk (RR) 0.07, 95% CI 0.01–0.39). As shown in Fig. 1, the sputum

Table 8 Interaction analysis of CpG island methylation levels and 1,25-dihydroxyvitamin D levels in TB risk

Gene	Model 1			Model 2			Model 3			Model 4		
	OR	95% CI	P	OR	95% CI	P	OR	95% CI	P	OR	95% CI	P
VDR	1.99	0.68–5.84	0.209	2.72	0.89–8.30	0.078	3.51	1.11–11.12	0.033	2.45	0.78–7.68	0.125
CYP27B1	2.39	0.69–8.34	0.171	2.60	0.68–10.01	0.164	2.60	0.68–10.01	0.164	2.19	0.67–7.18	0.197
CYP24A1	1.79	0.51–6.29	0.367	2.52	0.75–8.47	0.136	2.52	0.75–8.47	0.136	2.39	0.69–8.29	0.169
CYP2R1	1.19	0.40–3.47	0.756	2.06	0.71–5.98	0.184	4.34	1.30–14.49	0.017	–	–	–
CYP27A1	3.49	1.10–11.08	0.034	2.47	0.77–7.98	0.129	2.47	0.77–7.98	0.129	4.11	1.26–13.36	0.019

Table 9 Crossover analysis of CYP27A1 methylation levels and 1,25-dihydroxyvitamin D levels in the risk of TB

1,25(OH)$_2$D[a]	Cumulative methylation level[b]	Cases	Controls	OR	95% CI
Low	High	23	50	0.30	0.14–0.66
High	High	21	42	0.33	0.15–0.73
Low	Low	52	9	3.78	1.48–9.62
High	Low	26	17	1	

OR$_{interaction}$ = 4.11 (95% CI 1.26–13.36, $P = 0.019$)

[a]Cutoff point of 1,25(OH)$_2$D 86 pmol/L
[b]Cutoff point of cumulative methylation level of CYP27A1 0.48

conversion rate was significantly higher in patients with higher serum 1,25(OH)$_2$D levels ($\chi^2 = 8.85$, $P = 0.003$).

There were 23 CpG sites that were significantly related to the treatment outcomes ($P < 0.05$). The percentage of differentially methylated sites was 14.6% in the CYP24A1 gene, 2.7% in the CYP27A1 gene, 5.7% in the CYP27B1 gene, 5.9% in the CYP2R1 gene, and 10.7% in the VDR gene. However, no CpG sites remained significant after the Bonferroni correction. The cumulative methylation levels were categorized into three groups based on quartile (hypomethylation P$_0$–P$_{25}$; moderate methylation P$_{25}$–P$_{75}$; hypermethylation P$_{75}$–P$_{100}$). No significant relation was found between cumulative methylation level and sputum bacterium conversion (Fig. 2). We conducted crossover analysis and found no evidence of an interaction between CYP27A1 methylation level and 1,25(OH)$_2$D concentration in sputum bacterium conversion (Table 10).

Discussion

Vitamins are being revisited for their role in pathogenicity and for their antimycobacterial properties. Vitamin C and vitamin D have been shown to possess antimycobacterial properties [9]. Previous studies have reported an association between vitamin D and immunity against TB [22, 23]. High levels of vitamin D can decrease the reactivation of latent TB and reduce the severity of active TB [24–27]. Vitamin D deficiency is believed to be a risk factor for the acquisition of TB infection [28, 29]. However, vitamin D supplementation to improve outcomes in TB patients has resulted in contradictory results [30, 31] that may be partly attributable to individual variation in vitamin D metabolic capacity and immunity. Previous studies have suggested that activation or silencing of certain signaling pathways plays a role in TB development [32]. Genetic information is carried not only in DNA sequences but also in epigenetic variations [33, 34]. In this study, we used next-generation sequencing to quantify the methylation levels of five vitamin D metabolic pathway genes and observed a significant association with the risk of TB.

Vitamin D has two main active metabolites: 25(OH)D and 1,25(OH)$_2$D [35]. It binds to the vitamin D receptor on the membrane or cell nucleus to begin its activity in the transcription process [36]. In the present study, we observed that TB patients had significantly lower serum 1,25(OH)$_2$D concentrations than controls and that the concentrations decreased after the initiation of antituberculosis therapy. 1,25(OH)$_2$D is the biologically active form of vitamin D [37] and is associated with treatment outcomes of TB patients. The higher the 1,25(OH)$_2$D concentration, the greater the likelihood of successful treatment and the higher the sputum negative conversion rate. Our findings support the hypothesis that we can assist TB treatment by increasing sunlight radiation

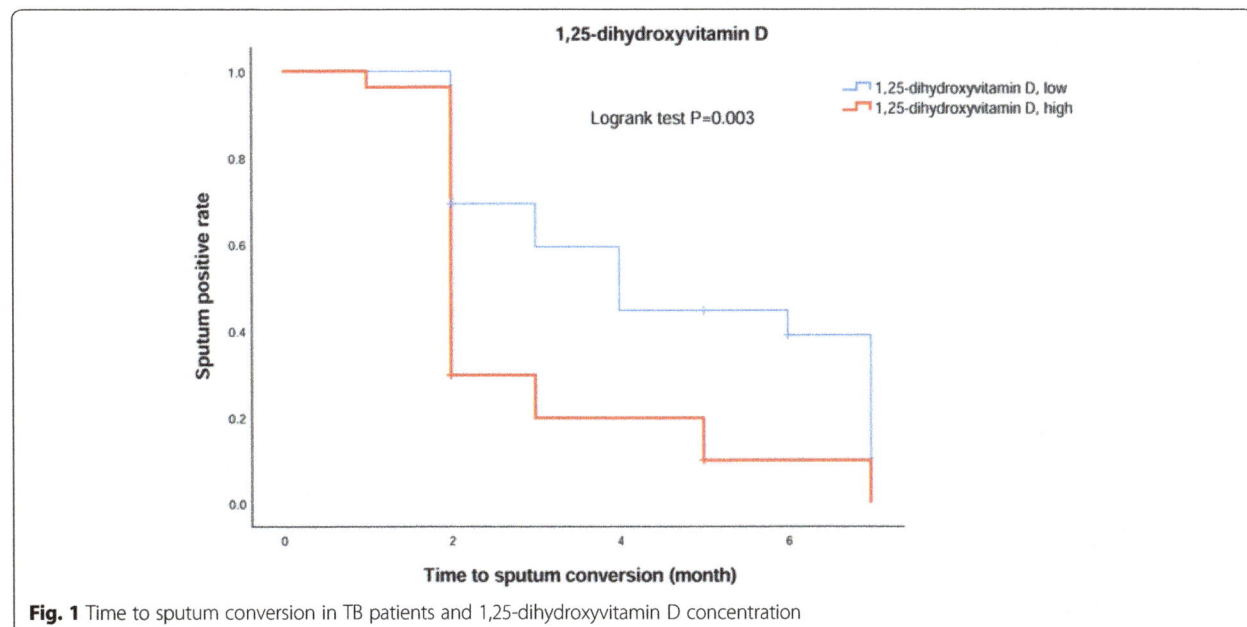

Fig. 1 Time to sputum conversion in TB patients and 1,25-dihydroxyvitamin D concentration

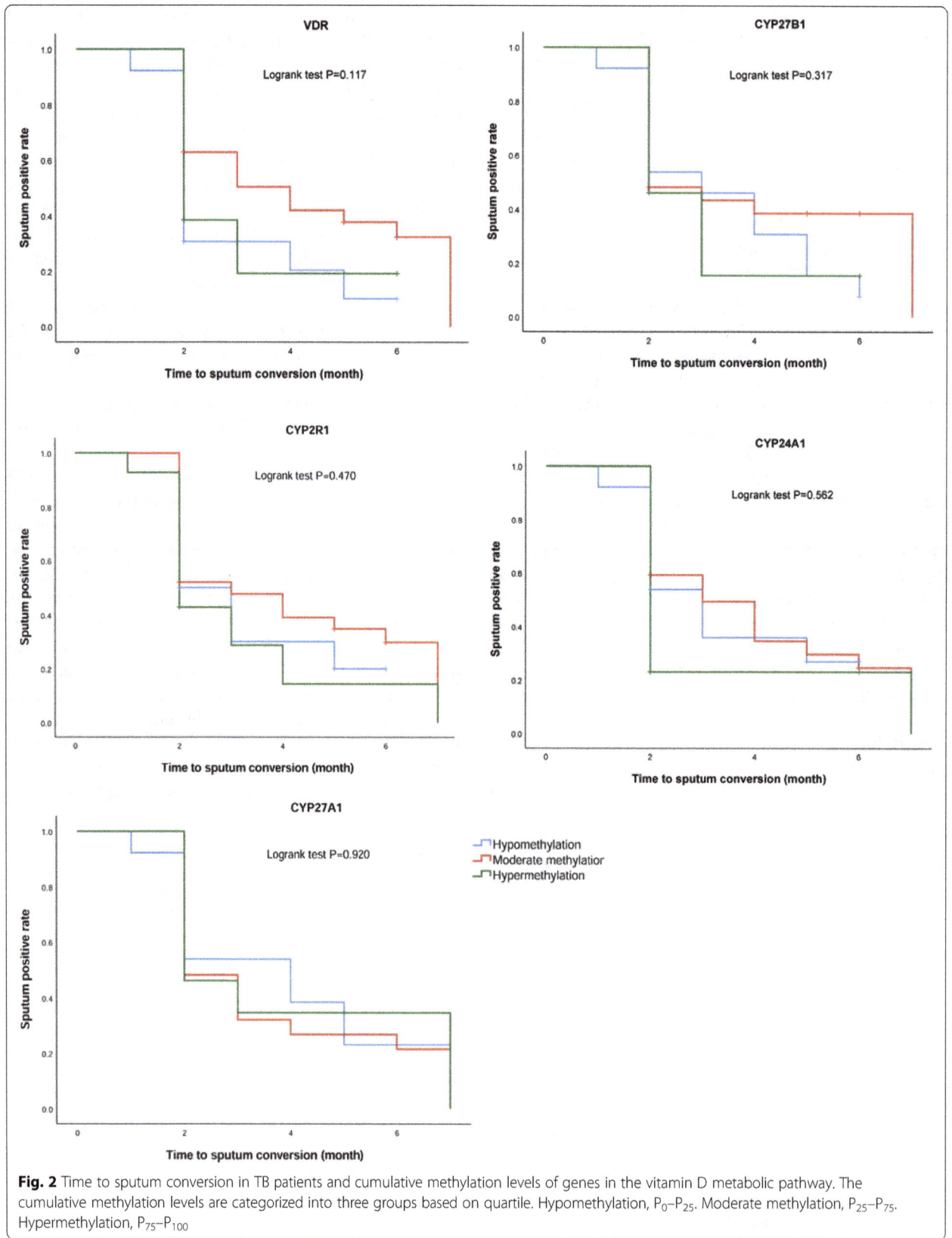

Fig. 2 Time to sputum conversion in TB patients and cumulative methylation levels of genes in the vitamin D metabolic pathway. The cumulative methylation levels are categorized into three groups based on quartile. Hypomethylation, P_0–P_{25}. Moderate methylation, P_{25}–P_{75}. Hypermethylation, P_{75}–P_{100}

Table 10 Crossover analysis of CYP27A1 methylation levels and 1,25-dihydroxyvitamin D levels in the sputum conversion of patients with TB

1,25(OH)$_2$D[a]	Cumulative methylation level[b]	Sputum conversion		OR	95% CI
		Yes	No		
Low	High	9	3	0.27	0.02–3.09
High	High	10	4	0.23	0.02–2.39
Low	Low	11	4	0.25	0.02–2.61
High	Low	11	1	1	

[a]Cutoff point of 1,25(OH)$_2$D 79 pmol/L
[b]Cutoff point of cumulative methylation level of CYP27A1 0.435

and vitamin D intake. In a randomized double-blind placebo-controlled trial among 120 Mongolian children, vitamin D supplementation seemed to prevent the conversion of the tuberculin skin test [38]. However, another report suggested that the time to sputum conversion was not reduced with vitamin D supplementation [17].

VDR is essential for adequate immune function [22]. One study examined the methylation statuses of 17 CpGs in VDR and determined their relation to TB [39]. Our findings showed that hypomethylation of the VDR promoter may be a potential biomarker of TB, but its impact on VDR expression remains to be studied. CYP2R1 is a hepatic microsomal enzyme responsible for the 25-hydroxylation of vitamin D that is highly conserved among species ranging from fish to humans [40, 41]. CYP24A1 encodes 24-hydroxylase, which initiates the metabolism of both 25(OH)D and 1,25(OH)$_2$D [40]. Zhou et al. conducted an intervention trial with vitamin D supplementation in postmenopausal women and reported that the baseline DNA methylation levels of CYP2R1 and CYP24A1 were negatively correlated with the concentrations of active 25(OH)D metabolite after vitamin D supplementation and that subjects with high DNA methylation levels needed higher vitamin D supplementation to reach optimal serum levels [42]. The CYP27A1 gene codes for 27-hydroxylase [43]. The methylation of CYP27A1 has been reported to be associated with the balance of bile acid in nonalcoholic fatty liver disease and in drug metabolism [44]. CYP27B1 catalyzes the de novo production of 1,25(OH)$_2$D from accumulated 25(OH)D; 1,25(OH)$_2$D is delivered to the cells via the vitamin D-binding protein (DBP), which is encoded by GC. The liganded VDR-transcription factor complex binds to vitamin D response elements (VDREs) in cathelicidin antimicrobial peptide (CAMP), activating CAMP expression [45]. The methylation level of CYP27B1 is elevated in primary lymphoma and leukemia cells [46].

There are several limitations in this study. First, we only measured the vitamin D levels at the baseline and at the end of the intensive treatment stage of TB patients; long-term continuous monitoring for the whole course of the disease may provide more information. Second, the regulation of gene transcription is complex, including genetic variation, modulation of the interactions of control factors with the transcriptional machinery, and epigenetic modification. These regulatory pathways do not function independently. Previous studies have reported methylation variation in association with genetic variation across individuals [47]. Genetic and epigenetic mechanisms may interact and together affect biological processes and disease development [48]. In this study, we only measured the methylation of the promoter regions of key genes in the vitamin D metabolic pathway. We noticed that the difference in methylation was subtle between cases and controls, although the P value was significant. Whether this subtle methylation difference could alter vitamin D metabolism and change macrophage M.tb killing capacity is not clear and needs more exploration. Other factors, such as genetic polymorphisms, sunlight exposure, food intake, and drug supplementation, can also affect vitamin D levels and the risk of TB [45]. Third, immune responses downstream of the vitamin D metabolic pathway should also be considered. Vitamin D has no direct antimycobacterial action, but its active metabolite 1,25(OH)$_2$D modulates host responses to M.tb infection [49]. 1,25(OH)$_2$D has been shown to induce antimycobacterial activity in macrophages in vitro, upregulate protective innate host responses, and trigger antimicrobial peptides such as cathelicidin [50]. M.tb entry into the body is mediated by macrophage toll-like receptors, which induce antibacterial autophagy by upregulating and activating VDR and increasing 1a-hydroxylase. Calcitriol activation of VDR induces CAMP gene expression and the subsequent production of cathelicidin, which disrupts the bacterial cell membrane and induces autophagy in monocytes [51]. Exogenous 1,25(OH)$_2$D induces a superoxide burst and enhances phagolysosome fusion in M.tb-infected macrophages [49]. Simultaneously, the T cells secrete IFN-g, which promotes antimicrobial peptide expression, autophagy, phagosomal maturation, and antimicrobial action against M.tb within macrophages [51]. In this study, we did not evaluate the immune responses downstream of the vitamin D metabolic pathway. These immune responses should be considered in future studies.

In conclusion, our results suggest that the methylation levels of the CYP24A1, CYP27A1, CYP27B1, CYP2R1, and VDR genes in the metabolic pathway of vitamin D are related to the risk and prognosis of TB. Investigating the role of abnormal metabolism of vitamin D is important for the prevention and control of TB. Individualized vitamin D intervention based on epigenetic traits of key genes in its metabolic pathway will be valuable for the prevention and control of tuberculosis.

Abbreviations

1,25(OH)₂D: 1,25-dihydroxyvitamin D; 25(OH)D: 25-hydroxyvitamin D; AUC: Area under the curve; BCG: Bacillus Calmette-Guérin; CAMP: Cathelicidin antimicrobial peptide; CI: Confidence interval; CV: Coefficient of variation; DBP: Vitamin D-binding protein; M.tb: *Mycobacterium tuberculosis*; OR: Odds ratio; ROC: Receiver operating characteristic; RR: Relative risk; SD: Standard deviation; TB: Tuberculosis; VDREs: Vitamin D response elements

Acknowledgements

We would like to thank all the participants for their contribution.

Funding

This work was supported by the National Natural Science Foundation of China (81473027, 81673249), the National Key R&D Program of China (2017YFC0907000), the Social Development Project in Jiangsu Province (BE2015694), Scientific Research Innovation Project for Graduate Students in Jiangsu Province (KYCX17_1293), the Six Talent Peaks Project in Jiangsu Province (2014-YY-023), and the Priority Academic Program Development of Jiangsu Higher Education Institutions (PAPD). The funders had no role in the study design, data collection and analysis, decision to publish, or preparation of the manuscript.

Authors' contributions

MW and JW conceived, initiated, and led the study. MW, WK, BH, ZL, HS, PS, and JW analyzed the data with input from all the authors. MW, WK, and JW prepared the manuscript. All authors reviewed and approved the final manuscript.

Author details

[1]Department of Epidemiology, School of Public Health, Nanjing Medical University, 101 Longmian Ave, Nanjing 211166, People's Republic of China. [2]Department of Preventive Health Care, People's Hospital of Suzhou High-tech Zone, Suzhou, People's Republic of China. [3]Department of Nursing, The First People's Hospital of Yancheng City, Yancheng, People's Republic of China. [4]Key Laboratory of Infectious Diseases, School of Public Health, Nanjing Medical University, Nanjing, People's Republic of China.

References

1. Kaushal D, Foreman TW, Gautam US, Alvarez X, Adekambi T, Rangel-Moreno J, Golden NA, Johnson AM, Phillips BL, Ahsan MH, et al. Mucosal vaccination with attenuated Mycobacterium tuberculosis induces strong central memory responses and protects against tuberculosis. Nat Commun. 2015;6:8533.
2. Xu G, Mao X, Wang J, Pan H. Clustering and recent transmission of Mycobacterium tuberculosis in a Chinese population. Infect Drug Resist. 2018;11:323–30.
3. WHO. Global Tuberculosis report 2017. 2017; http://www.who.int/tb/publications/global_report/en/. Accessed 1 Aug 2018.
4. Maro I, Lahey T, MacKenzie T, Mtei L, Bakari M, Matee M, Pallangyo K, von Reyn CF. Low BMI and falling BMI predict HIV-associated tuberculosis: a prospective study in Tanzania. Int J Tuberc Lung Dis. 2010;14(11):1447–53.
5. Rhines AS. The role of sex differences in the prevalence and transmission of tuberculosis. Tuberculosis (Edinb). 2013;93(1):104–7.
6. Melsew YA, Doan TN, Gambhir M, Cheng AC, McBryde E, Trauer JM. Risk factors for infectiousness of patients with tuberculosis: a systematic review and meta-analysis. Epidemiol Infect. 2018;146(3):345–53.
7. Feng Y, Wang F, Pan H, Qiu S, Lu J, Wu L, Wang J, Lu C. Obesity-associated gene FTO rs9939609 polymorphism in relation to the risk of tuberculosis. BMC Infect Dis. 2014;14:592.
8. Lu J, Pan H, Chen Y, Tang S, Feng Y, Qiu S, Zhang S, Wu L, Xu R, Peng X, et al. Genetic polymorphisms of IFNG and IFNGR1 in association with the risk of pulmonary tuberculosis. Gene. 2014;543(1):140–4.
9. Tyagi G, Singh P, Varma-Basil M, Bose M. Role of vitamins B, C, and D in the fight against tuberculosis. Int J Mycobacteriol. 2017;6(4):328–32.
10. Venturini E, Facchini L, Martinez-Alier N, Novelli V, Galli L, de Martino M, Chiappini E. Vitamin D and tuberculosis: a multicenter study in children. BMC Infect Dis. 2014;14:652.
11. Keflie TS, Nolle N, Lambert C, Nohr D, Biesalski HK. Vitamin D deficiencies among tuberculosis patients in Africa: a systematic review. Nutrition. 2015; 31(10):1204–12.
12. Nnoaham KE, Clarke A. Low serum vitamin D levels and tuberculosis: a systematic review and meta-analysis. Int J Epidemiol. 2008;37(1): 113–9.
13. Zeng J, Wu G, Yang W, Gu X, Liang W, Yao Y, Song Y. A serum vitamin D level <25nmol/l pose high tuberculosis risk: a meta-analysis. PLoS One. 2015;10(5):e0126014.
14. Selvaraj P, Harishankar M, Afsal K, Vitamin D. Immuno-modulation and tuberculosis treatment. Can J Physiol Pharmacol. 2015;93(5):377–84.
15. Nursyam EW, Amin Z, Rumende CM. The effect of vitamin D as supplementary treatment in patients with moderately advanced pulmonary tuberculous lesion. Acta Med Indones. 2006;38(1):3–5.
16. Martineau AR, Timms PM, Bothamley GH, Hanifa Y, Islam K, Claxton AP, Packe GE, Moore-Gillon JC, Darmalingam M, Davidson RN, et al. High-dose vitamin D(3) during intensive-phase antimicrobial treatment of pulmonary tuberculosis: a double-blind randomised controlled trial. Lancet. 2011; 377(9761):242–50.
17. Xia J, Shi L, Zhao L, Xu F. Impact of vitamin D supplementation on the outcome of tuberculosis treatment: a systematic review and meta-analysis of randomized controlled trials. Chin Med J. 2014;127(17):3127–34.
18. Scragg R. Limitations of vitamin D supplementation trials: why observational studies will continue to help determine the role of vitamin D in health. J Steroid Biochem Mol Biol. 2018;177:6–9.
19. Manjrekar J. Epigenetic inheritance, prions and evolution. J Genet. 2017; 96(3):445–56.
20. Guastafierro T, Bacalini MG, Marcoccia A, Gentilini D, Pisoni S, Di Blasio AM, Corsi A, Franceschi C, Raimondo D, Spano A, et al. Genome-wide DNA methylation analysis in blood cells from patients with Werner syndrome. Clin Epigenetics. 2017;9:92.
21. Zhu H, Wang X, Shi H, Su S, Harshfield GA, Gutin B, Snieder H, Dong Y. A genome-wide methylation study of severe vitamin D deficiency in African American adolescents. J Pediatr. 2013;162(5):1004–9 e1001.
22. Wahyunitisari MR, Mertaniasih NM, Amin M, Artama WT, Koendhori EB. Vitamin D, cell death pathways, and tuberculosis. Int J Mycobacteriol. 2017; 6(4):349–55.
23. Tessema B, Moges F, Habte D, Hiruy N, Yismaw S, Melkieneh K, Kassie Y, Girma B, Melese M, Suarez PG. Vitamin D deficiency among smear positive pulmonary tuberculosis patients and their tuberculosis negative household contacts in Northwest Ethiopia: a case-control study. Ann Clin Microbiol Antimicrob. 2017;16(1):36.
24. Eklund D, Persson HL, Larsson M, Welin A, Idh J, Paues J, Fransson SG, Stendahl O, Schon T, Lerm M. Vitamin D enhances IL-1beta secretion and restricts growth of Mycobacterium tuberculosis in macrophages from TB patients. Int J Mycobacteriol. 2013;2(1):18–25.
25. Harishankar M, Selvaraj P. Influence of Cdx2 and TaqI gene variants on vitamin D3 modulated intracellular chemokine positive T-cell subsets in pulmonary tuberculosis. Clin Ther. 2017;39(5):946–57.
26. Huang SJ, Wang XH, Liu ZD, Cao WL, Han Y, Ma AG, Xu SF. Vitamin D deficiency and the risk of tuberculosis: a meta-analysis. Drug Des Devel Ther. 2017;11:91–102.
27. Azam F, Shaheen A, Arshad R. Frequency of hypovitaminosis D and its associated risk factors in newly diagnosed pulmonary tuberculosis patients. Pak J Med Sci. 2016;32(2):480–4.
28. Iftikhar R, Kamran SM, Qadir A, Haider E, Bin UH. Vitamin D deficiency in patients with tuberculosis. J Coll Physicians Surg Pak. 2013;23(10):780–3.
29. Talat N, Perry S, Parsonnet J, Dawood G, Hussain R. Vitamin d deficiency and tuberculosis progression. Emerg Infect Dis. 2010;16(5):853–5.
30. Sharma V, Mandavdhare HS, Kumar A, Sharma R, Sachdeva N, Prasad KK, Rana SS. Prevalence and clinical impact of vitamin D deficiency on abdominal tuberculosis. Ther Adv Infect Dis. 2017;4(3):83–6.

31. Choi R, Jeong BH, Koh WJ, Lee SY. Recommendations for optimizing tuberculosis treatment: therapeutic drug monitoring, pharmacogenetics, and nutritional status considerations. Ann Lab Med. 2017;37(2):97–107.

32. Esterhuyse MM, Weiner J 3rd, Caron E, Loxton AG, Iannaccone M, Wagman C, Saikali P, Stanley K, Wolski WE, Mollenkopf HJ, et al. Epigenetics and proteomics join transcriptomics in the quest for tuberculosis biomarkers. MBio. 2015;6(5):e01187–15.

33. He L, Gao L, Shi Z, Li Y, Zhu L, Li S, Zhang P, Zheng G, Ren Q, Li Y, et al. Involvement of cytochrome P450 1A1 and glutathione S-transferase P1 polymorphisms and promoter hypermethylation in the progression of anti-tuberculosis drug-induced liver injury: a case-control study. PLoS One. 2015; 10(3):e0119481.

34. Shnorhavorian M, Schwartz SM, Stansfeld B, Sadler-Riggleman I, Beck D, Skinner MK. Differential DNA methylation regions in adult human sperm following adolescent chemotherapy: potential for epigenetic inheritance. PLoS One. 2017;12(2):e0170085.

35. Zerwekh JE. Blood biomarkers of vitamin D status. Am J Clin Nutr. 2008; 87(4):1087S–91S.

36. Norval M, Coussens AK, Wilkinson RJ, Bornman L, Lucas RM, Wright CY. Vitamin D status and its consequences for health in South Africa. Int J Environ Res Public Health. 2016;13(10):1019.

37. Hussein H, Ibrahim F, Boudou P. Evaluation of a new automated assay for the measurement of circulating 1,25-dihydroxyvitamin D levels in daily practice. Clin Biochem. 2015;48(16–17):1160–2.

38. Verrall AJ, Netea MG, Alisjahbana B, Hill PC, van Crevel R. Early clearance of Mycobacterium tuberculosis: a new frontier in prevention. Immunology. 2014;141(4):506–13.

39. Andraos C, Koorsen G, Knight JC, Bornman L. Vitamin D receptor gene methylation is associated with ethnicity, tuberculosis, and TaqI polymorphism. Hum Immunol. 2011;72(3):262–8.

40. Wang TJ, Zhang F, Richards JB, Kestenbaum B, van Meurs JB, Berry D, Kiel DP, Streeten EA, Ohlsson C, Koller DL, et al. Common genetic determinants of vitamin D insufficiency: a genome-wide association study. Lancet. 2010; 376(9736):180–8.

41. Cheng JB, Levine MA, Bell NH, Mangelsdorf DJ, Russell DW. Genetic evidence that the human CYP2R1 enzyme is a key vitamin D 25-hydroxylase. Proc Natl Acad Sci U S A. 2004;101(20):7711–5.

42. Zhou Y, Zhao LJ, Xu X, Ye A, Travers-Gustafson D, Zhou B, Wang HW, Zhang W, Lee Hamm L, Deng HW, et al. DNA methylation levels of CYP2R1 and CYP24A1 predict vitamin D response variation. J Steroid Biochem Mol Biol. 2014;144:207–14 Pt A.

43. Nie S, Chen G, Cao X, Zhang Y. Cerebrotendinous xanthomatosis: a comprehensive review of pathogenesis, clinical manifestations, diagnosis, and management. Orphanet J Rare Dis. 2014;9:179.

44. Schioth HB, Bostrom A, Murphy SK, Erhart W, Hampe J, Moylan C, Mwinyi J. A targeted analysis reveals relevant shifts in the methylation and transcription of genes responsible for bile acid homeostasis and drug metabolism in non-alcoholic fatty liver disease. BMC Genomics. 2016;17:462.

45. Meyer V, Saccone DS, Tugizimana F, Asani FF, Jeffery TJ, Bornman L. Methylation of the vitamin D receptor (VDR) gene, together with genetic variation, race, and environment influence the signaling efficacy of the toll-like receptor 2/1-VDR pathway. Front Immunol. 2017;8:1048.

46. Wjst M, Heimbeck I, Kutschke D, Pukelsheim K. Epigenetic regulation of vitamin D converting enzymes. J Steroid Biochem Mol Biol. 2010;121(1–2):80–3.

47. Schultz MD, He Y, Whitaker JW, Hariharan M, Mukamel EA, Leung D, Rajagopal N, Nery JR, Urich MA, Chen H, et al. Human body epigenome maps reveal noncanonical DNA methylation variation. Nature. 2015; 523(7559):212–6.

48. Olsson AH, Volkov P, Bacos K, Dayeh T, Hall E, Nilsson EA, Ladenvall C, Ronn T, Ling C. Genome-wide associations between genetic and epigenetic variation influence mRNA expression and insulin secretion in human pancreatic islets. PLoS Genet. 2014;10(11):e1004735.

49. Martineau AR, Honecker FU, Wilkinson RJ, Griffiths CJ. Vitamin D in the treatment of pulmonary tuberculosis. J Steroid Biochem Mol Biol. 2007; 103(3–5):793–8.

50. Wejse C, Gomes VF, Rabna P, Gustafson P, Aaby P, Lisse IM, Andersen PL, Glerup H, Sodemann M. Vitamin D as supplementary treatment for tuberculosis: a double-blind, randomized, placebo-controlled trial. Am J Respir Crit Care Med. 2009;179(9):843–50.

51. Turnbull ER, Drobniewski F. Vitamin D supplementation: a comprehensive review on supplementation for tuberculosis prophylaxis. Expert Rev Respir Med. 2015;9(3):269–75.

19

Association of internal smoking dose with blood DNA methylation in three racial/ethnic populations

Sungshim L. Park[1*], Yesha M. Patel[1], Lenora W. M. Loo[2], Daniel J. Mullen[3], Ite A. Offringa[3], Alika Maunakea[4], Daniel O. Stram[1], Kimberly Siegmund[1], Sharon E. Murphy[5], Maarit Tiirikainen[2] and Loïc Le Marchand[2*]

Abstract

Background: Lung cancer is the leading cause of cancer-related death. While cigarette smoking is the primary cause of this malignancy, risk differs across racial/ethnic groups. For the same number of cigarettes smoked, Native Hawaiians compared to whites are at greater risk and Japanese Americans are at lower risk of developing lung cancer. DNA methylation of specific CpG sites (e.g., in *AHRR* and *F2RL3*) is the most common blood epigenetic modification associated with smoking status. However, the influence of internal smoking dose, measured by urinary nicotine equivalents (NE), on DNA methylation in current smokers has not been investigated, nor has a study evaluated whether for the same smoking dose, circulating leukocyte DNA methylation patterns differ by race.

Methods: We conducted an epigenome-wide association study (EWAS) of NE in 612 smokers from three racial/ethnic groups: whites ($n = 204$), Native Hawaiians ($n = 205$), and Japanese Americans ($n = 203$). Genome-wide DNA methylation profiling of blood leukocyte DNA was measured using the Illumina 450K BeadChip array. Average β value, the ratio of signal from a methylated probe relative to the sum of the methylated and unmethylated probes at that CpG, was the dependent variables in linear regression models adjusting for age, sex, race (for pan-ethnic analysis), and estimated cell-type distribution.

Results: We found that NE was significantly associated with six differentially methylated CpG sites (Bonferroni corrected $p < 1.48 \times 10-7$): four in or near the FOXK2, PBX1, FNDC7, and FUBP3 genes and two in non-annotated genetic regions. Higher levels of NE were associated with increasing methylation beta-valuesin all six sites. For all six CpG sites, the association was only observed in Native Hawaiians, suggesting that the influence of smoking dose on DNA methylation patterns is heterogeneous across race/ethnicity (p interactions $< 8.8 \times 10-8$). We found two additional CpG sites associated with NE in only Native Hawaiians.

Conclusions: In conclusion, internal smoking dose was associated with increased DNA methylation in circulating leukocytes at specific sites in Native Hawaiian smokers but not in white or Japanese American smokers.

Keywords: Smoking, Nicotine equivalents, DNA methylation, Japanese Americans, Native Hawaiians, Whites

Background

Globally, lung cancer is the second most common cancer, after prostate and breast cancer in men and women, respectively. It is also the most common cause of cancer-related death. Approximately 90% of lung cancer cases are ever smokers; however, only 11–24%
of smokers will develop lung cancer in their lifetime [1]. Moreover, for the same quantity smoked, compared to whites, Native Hawaiians have been found to have a ~ 50% higher risk of lung cancer, whereas Japanese Americans have been shown to have a ~ 25% lower risk of disease [2, 3]. The lower risk of lung cancer in Japanese Americans can in part be explained by their slower nicotine metabolism (measured by CYP2A6 activity), which has been shown to influence smoking intensity (measured by biomarkers of internal smoking dose) resulting in a lower exposure to tobacco carcinogens [4, 5]. However, the higher risk of lung cancer in Native Hawaiians is inconsistent with

---

* Correspondence: sungship@usc.edu; Loic@cc.hawaii.edu
[1]Department of Preventive Medicine, Norris Comprehensive Cancer Center, Keck School of Medicine, University of Southern California, 1450 Biggy Street, NRT 1509G, Los Angeles, CA 90033, USA
[2]Epidemiology Program, University of Hawaii Cancer Center, 701 Ilalo Street, Honolulu, HI 96813, USA
Full list of author information is available at the end of the article

their smoking intensity and nicotine metabolism rate, measured by CYP2A6 activity (the ratio of total trans-3′-hydroxycotinine over total cotinine), which is intermediate between that of whites and Japanese Americans. To date, this higher risk in Native Hawaiians is not explained by other known lung cancer risk factors.

DNA methylation of CpG sites is one of the most commonly studied epigenetic modification, and DNA methylation microarrays are the most common method to characterize the epigenome [6] in population studies. Multiple epigenome-wide association studies (EWAS) of smoking status have been conducted using DNA from blood leukocytes [7–19]. The most recent and largest study ($n = 15,907$) comparing current to never smokers found that 2623 CpG sites in 1405 genes were differentially methylated (Bonferroni corrected $p = 1.48 \times 10^{-7}$) [17]. The strongest association was with CpG sites located in the aryl-hydrocarbon receptor repressor (AHRR) gene, coagulation factor II (thrombin) receptor-like 3 (F2RL3) gene, G protein-coupled receptor (GPR15) gene, alkaline phosphatase genes, placental-like (ALPPL2) gene, and in genetic regions in 2q37.1 and 6p21.33 [18]. Hypomethylation of cg05575921 located in intron 3 of AHRR is one of the most frequently replicated findings and may serve as a marker for current smoking status, cumulative amount smoked (smoking pack-years), smoking dose (cigarettes per day [CPD]), and time since quitting [7–16]. However, the literature investigating the influence of self-reported smoking dose (assessed by CPD) or internal dose (assessed by cotinine measurement) is limited to four and three studies, respectively. To our knowledge, no EWAS of nicotine equivalents (NE) has been conducted. NE is a more comprehensive measure of internal smoking dose than other smoking metabolites, such as cotinine, as it is the sum of the major metabolites of nicotine: total cotinine (nmol/mL), total nicotine (nmol/mL), and total trans-3′-hydroxycotinine (3-HC, in nmol/mL), which includes their glucuronides, accounting for ~ 80% of nicotine uptake [20]. Thus, unlike cotinine, NE accounts for the variations in nicotine metabolism across multiethnic populations [5, 21]. Moreover, no study has evaluated whether peripheral blood DNA methylation patterns differ by race/ethnicity for the same NE. Characterization of these differences might be enlightening since racial/ethnic groups have been found to have variations in nicotine uptake per cigarette [5]. The differential impact of smoking dose on the epigenome may in part contribute to the ethnic variations in smoking-related lung cancer risk.

We conducted the first EWAS of NE in three populations with different risks for lung cancer to identify potential mechanisms for the differences in smoking-related disease risks. We hypothesized that an increase in smoking dose will be associated with differential methylation of epigenetic regions in blood leukocyte DNA and that for the same dose, the associations may vary across race/ethnicity. We also evaluated potential biological pathways based on the genes involved in our top associations.

Results

Table 1 presents the characteristics of the 612 Japanese Americans, Native Hawaiians, and white participants enrolled in this study. Native Hawaiians were slightly younger than Japanese Americans and whites (mean age = 57 years versus 62 years, respectively). The distribution of males and females was very similar as an equal number of men and women were targeted for recruitment. Native Hawaiians were heavier (body mass index [BMI] = 29.3 kg/m^2) followed by whites (26.6 kg/m^2) and Japanese Americans (25.5 kg/m^2). Whites reported smoking the most CPD and had the highest NE (CPD = 26.3 and NE = 55.2 nmol/ml), followed by Native Hawaiians (CPD = 21 and NE = 50.3 nmol/ml) and Japanese Americans (CPD = 19 and NE = 35.0 nmol/ml). Lifetime smoking quantity was lowest in Native Hawaiians (42.4 pack-years), which is expected as Native Hawaiians on average were younger at time of urine collection, followed by Japanese Americans (44.7 pack-years) and whites (56.8 pack-years). We found that the cell type by race/ethnicity differed for CD8, T cells, B cells, natural killer cells, and monocytes (p values < 0.005) (Table 1). Also, heterogeneity in the relationship between NE and cell types by race/ethnicity was also detected. Specifically, NE was inversely associated with natural killer cells in Native Hawaiians and Japanese Americans, inversely associated with monocytes in whites, and positively associated with B cells in Native Hawaiians (Additional file 1: Table S1). Among 35 never smokers (11 Japanese Americans, 12 Native Hawaiians, and 12 whites) who were included in only the EWAS of smoking status, the distribution of males and females were ~ 50% in each racial/ethnic group. The Japanese American and Native Hawaiians were older (69 and 67 years of age, respectively) than their current smoking counterparts, whereas the white never smokers were similar in age as their current smoking counterpart (63 years).

Additional file 1: Table S2 presents a list of probes ($n = 55$) that have been found in at least five EWAS of blood leukocytes to be differentially methylated by smoking status (current versus never). This table also presents the parameter estimates and p values from the association tests for these probes with smoking status, NE, and CPD within our study population. Among the ten most frequently replicated (> 10 studies) probes (marked with an asterisk (*)), all ten were also found to be associated with another measure of smoking quantity pack-years, CPD, or cotinine (from at least one EWAS or candidate-probe analyses). In our EWAS of smoking status ($n = 612$ current smokers versus 35 never smokers), after adjustments for age, sex, race/ethnicity, and cell type,

Table 1 Demographic characteristics of study population current smokers at time of biospecimen collection stratified by race/ethnicity

	Japanese Americans	Native Hawaiians	Whites
N	203	205	204
Age (years), mean (SD)	61 (6.95)	57 (12.82)	62 (6.85)
Gender, N (%)			
Males	101 (49.7)	101 (49.3)	101 (49.5)
Females	102 (50.3)	104 (50.7)	103 (50.5)
BMI (kg/m^2), mean (SD)	25.53 (4.71)	29.29 (7.05)	26.61 (5.78)
Pack-years, mean (SD)	44.68 (17.95)	42.44 (24.15)	56.82 (24.53)
CPD, mean (SD)	19.93 (7.45)	21.15 (9.5)	26.32 (11.38)
CYP2A6 activity, mean (SD)	0.85 (1.47)	1.08 (1.14)	1.43 (1.73)
NE (nmol/ml)	34.98 (27.78)	50.26 (41.49)	55.20 (48.86)
Cell types, mean (SD)			
CD8 cells**	0.03 (0.04)	0.05 (0.04)	0.02 (0.03)
CD4T cells	0.16 (0.07)	0.16 (0.06)	0.16 (0.08)
Natural killer cells*	0.06 (0.04)	0.06 (0.04)	0.04 (0.03)
B cells**	0.08 (0.04)	0.08 (0.03)	0.06 (0.03)
Monocytes	0.05 (0.04)	0.05 (0.03)	0.06 (0.04)
Granulocytes*	0.67 (0.12)	0.66 (0.11)	0.69 (0.12)

*P value for trend < 0.005, indicating significant ethnic differences
**P value for trend < 0.0005, indicating significant ethnic differences

24 of the previously 55 replicated probes were associated with smoking status at a Bonferroni significance level ($p = 1.48 \times 10^{-7}$). Among our three most significant hits, cg0591221 and cg21566642 in 2q37.1 ($p = 1.95 \times 10^{-67}$ and 4.4×10^{-67}) and cg05575921 in *AHRR* ($p = 7.99 \times 10^{-67}$), current smoking status was associated with decreasing methylation beta values. For all 24 replicated probes, we found that the associations had greater statistical significance in whites than the other two racial/ethnic groups, despite a similar sample size across the three ethnic populations (e.g., for *AHRR*, cg05575921 $p = 4.3 \times 10^{-31}$ for whites, $p = 2.9 \times 10^{-20}$ for Japanese Americans, and $p = 7.1 \times 10^{-19}$ for Native Hawaiians).

In our pan-ethnic EWAS of smoking dose in smokers, after adjusting for age, sex, race/ethnicity, and cell type, we found that NE was associated with six differentially methylated probes (Bonferroni corrected $p < 1.48 \times 10^{-7}$) (Fig. 1). For all six probes, higher levels of NE were associated with increasing methylated beta-values (Table 2). These six CpG probes were mapped in or near the *FOXK2*, *PBX1*, *FNDC7*, and *FUBP3* genes and two in non-annotated regions. Associations with these six probes also showed statistically significant interactions with race, where the associations were only statistically significant in Native Hawaiians ($p < 1.1 \times 10^{-8}$). These differences indicate that Native Hawaiians may have greater differential DNA methylation patterns in relation to smoking dose, compared to whites and Japanese Americans (p interaction

$< 8.8 \times 10^{-8}$) (Figs. 2 and 3). In ethnic-specific EWAS (Additional file 1: Table S4), higher NE was associated with increasing methylation beta-values of two additional probes, cg00812246 in *BSND* and cg01924952 in 2p25.1 ($p < 1.2 \times 10^{-7}$), in only Native Hawaiians (Table 2). When investigating the association between CPD and DNA methylation, no significant pan-ethnic or ethnic-specific

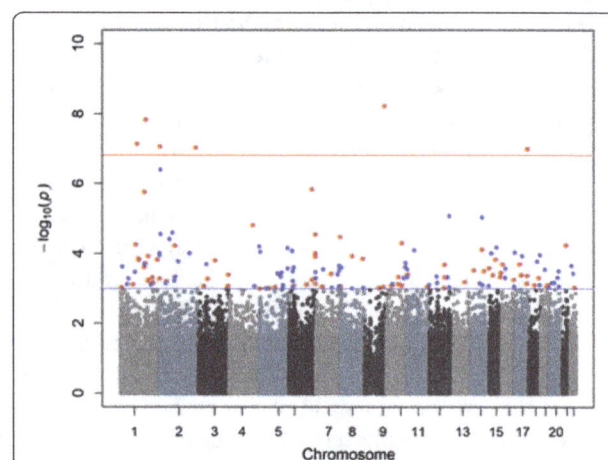

Fig. 1 Manhattan plot of the p values for the association for nicotine equivalents with DNA methylation. *Red line: Bonferroni corrected p value $p = 1.48 \times 10^{-7}$, blue line: $p = 1 \times 10^{-3}$. **Red dots indicate that the parameter estimate is in the positive direction, and blue dots indicate parameter estimates that are in the negative direction

Table 2 Association between NE and DNA methylation (p value $< 1.48 \times 10^{-7}$ from pan-ethnic and/or ethnic-specific analyses)*

Probe	Chr	Cytoband	Mapinfo	CGI region	Ref_Gene	Overall		Whites		Japanese Americans		Native Hawaiians	
						Estimate	P value	Estimate	P value	Estimate	P value	Estimate	P value
cg11413570	1	1p13.3	109260678	S_Shore	FNDC7	0.0056	7.15E−08	− 0.0010	0.3870	0.0012	0.2774	0.0142	2.84E−08
cg00812246	1	1p32.3	55464868		BSND	0.0071	5.35E−06	− 0.0017	0.4165	0.0012	0.6007	0.0186	2.78E−08
cg09168939	1	1q23.3	164652019		PBX1	0.0046	1.46E−08	− 0.0008	0.3237	0.0011	0.2119	0.0115	4.82E−09
cg01924952	2	2p25.1	8627933		–	− 0.0063	3.96E−07	− 0.0006	0.6050	0.0007	0.6307	− 0.0157	1.19E−07
cg11108534	2	2p25.2	5584457		–	0.0062	8.65E−08	0.0010	0.4293	0.0020	0.3853	0.0136	2.79E−09
cg15613292	2	2q37.1	232481541		–	0.0062	9.04E−08	− 0.0022	0.0736	0.0007	0.6079	0.0169	8.27E−10
cg13986536	9	9q34.2	133456512	S_Shore	FUBP3	0.0050	5.84E−09	0.0003	0.7671	0.0010	0.2783	0.0121	1.19E−08
cg21842914	17	17q25.3	80545869	S_Shore	FOXK2	0.0054	9.86E−08	− 0.0014	0.0514	0.0001	0.9237	0.0151	1.10E−08

*In order by chromosome

associations were detected ($p < 1.48 \times 10^{-7}$). In our data, NE and CPD were found to have a modest, but statistically significant correlation (Pearson's $r = 0.12$; $p < 0.001$).

We found that none of the 55 well-replicated probes (≥ 5 studies) linked with smoking status were associated with NE at a Bonferroni significance level. However, eight of the 55 were modestly associated with NE ($p < 0.05$) (Additional file 1: Tables S2 and S3). Six of these eight were among the 10 most frequently replicated probes (> 10 studies) with current smoker status; the other two probes, cg25949550 in contactin-associated protein-like 2 (*CNTNAP2*) and cg02657160 in coproporphyrinogen oxidase (*CPOX*), were previously found to be associated with smoking status and with cotinine in ever smokers [22]. The most statistically significant association being cg05575921 in *AHRR* (regression coefficient = − 0.0154; $p = 6 \times 10^{-5}$). Among current smokers, no significant associations between CPD and DNA methylation were detected in these 55 probes ($p > 1.48 \times 10^{-7}$). We found three of the 55 well-replicated probes were modestly

associated with CPD ($p < 0.05$): cg13193840 in 2q37.1, cg19859270 in GPR15, and cg24090911 in *AHRR* ($p = 0.018$, 0.035, and 0.047, respectively).

A gene list based on differentially methylated probes associated with NE ($p < 10^{-3}$) (Additional file 1: Tables S3 and S4) was used for pathway analysis. Based on Ingenuity Pathway Analysis (IPA) of the genes identified to have overall pan-ethnic or ethnic-specific association with NE, the vast majority of genes were identified as playing a role in cancer (86% of 117 genes for the pan-ethnic; 90% of the 278 genes for whites; 95% of the 108 genes for Japanese Americans; and 92% of the 206 genes for Native Hawaiians). Interestingly, we found that there was no overlap of genes or probes across all three ethnicities. Only four genes overlapped in whites and Japanese Americans, two overlapped in Japanese Americans and Native Hawaiians, and 10 in whites and Native Hawaiians (Additional file 2: Figure S1).

The IPA analysis from the ethnic-specific gene lists found that the top three canonical pathways in whites

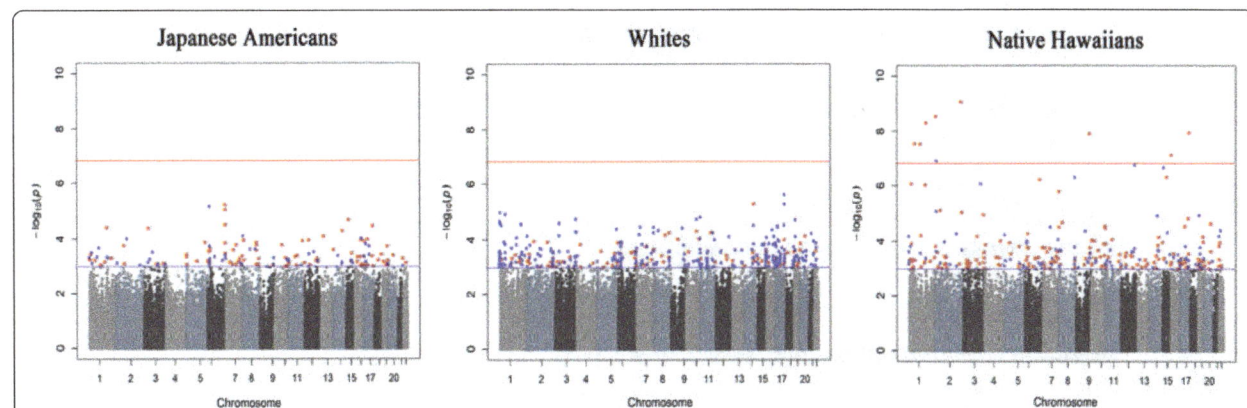

Fig. 2 Manhattan plots of the p values for the association for nicotine equivalents with DNA methylation, stratified by race/ethnicity. *Red line: Bonferroni corrected p value $p = 1.48 \times 10^{-7}$, blue line: $p = 1 \times 10^{-3}$. **Red dots indicate that the parameter estimate is in the positive direction and blue dots indicate parameter estimates that are in the negative direction

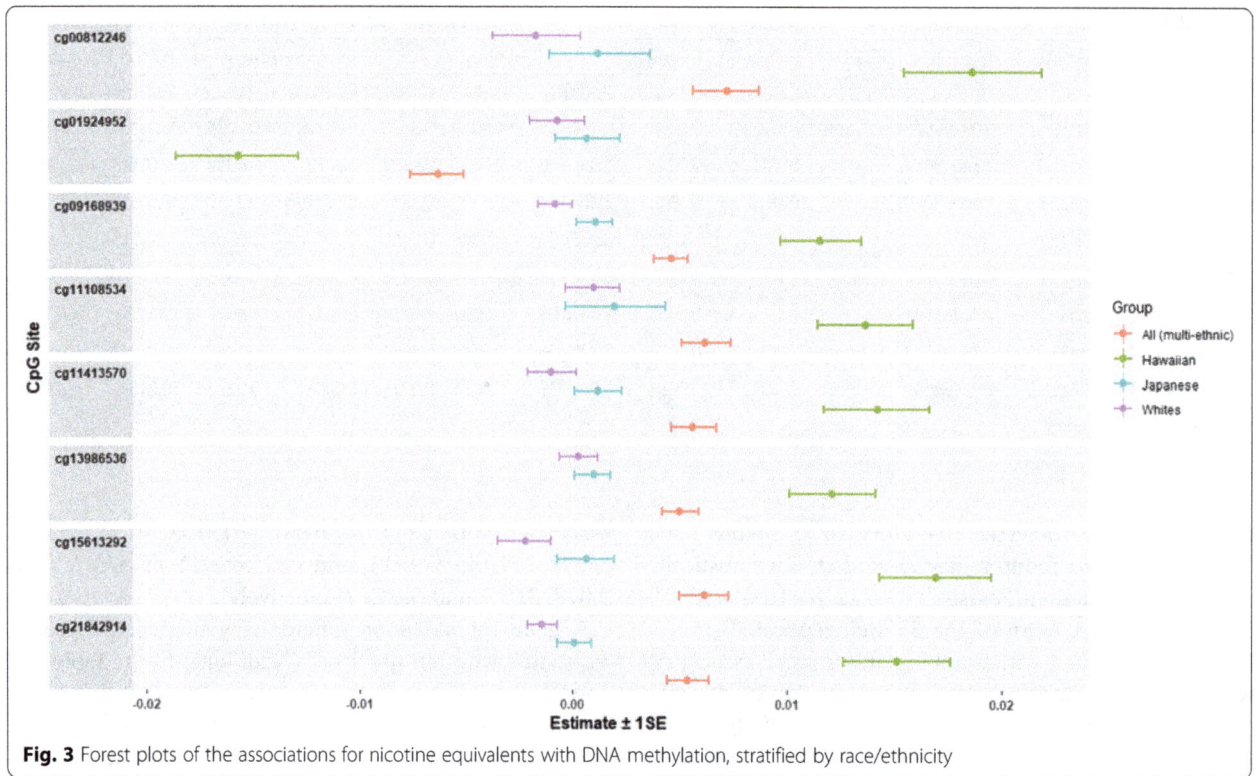

Fig. 3 Forest plots of the associations for nicotine equivalents with DNA methylation, stratified by race/ethnicity

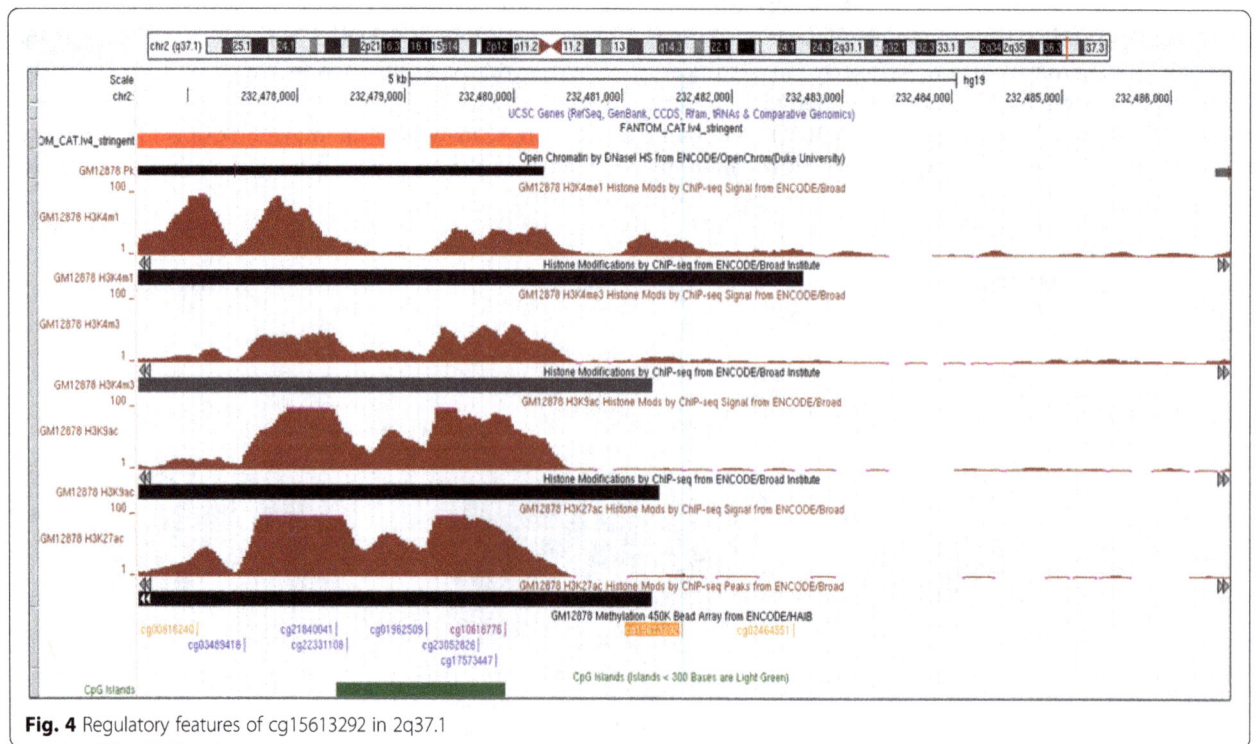

Fig. 4 Regulatory features of cg15613292 in 2q37.1

were reelin signaling in neurons ($p = 0.004$), thrombin signaling ($p = 0.01$), and tight junction signaling ($p = 0.01$) (Additional file 1: Table S5). In Native Hawaiians, the canonical pathways were dermatan sulfate degradation (Metazoa) ($p = 0.02$), netrin signaling ($p = 0.02$), and γ-glutamyl cycle ($p = 0.02$)). In Japanese Americans, the canonical pathways were ephrin B signaling ($p = 2.2 \times 10^{-5}$), IL-1 signaling ($p = 7.1 \times 10^{-5}$), and relaxin signaling ($p = 0.001$).

To gain insight into the possible functional role of the top eight significantly differentially methylated probes associated with NE from either our pan-ethnic or ethnic-specific analysis ($p < 1.48 \times 10^{-7}$), we utilized ENCODE publicly available epigenomic data [23] (Figs. 4 and 5 and Additional file 2: Figures S2–S7). None of the eight top probes are located within CpG islands. Three probes (cg15613292, cg21842914, and cg13986536) are located within a CpG shore, just downstream (< 2 Kb) of a CpG island (Fig. 4 and Additional file 2: Figures S2–S3). Three of the six top probes (cg15613292, cg01924952, and cg13986536) are in putative transcriptional regulatory domains in the GM12878 cell line (B-lymphocytes) (Figs. 4 and 5 and Additional file 2: Figure S2). Cg21842914 is in a putative transcriptional regulatory domain in CD20+ cells (B cells) and CD14+ cells (monocytes) (Additional file 2: Figure S3). Cg15613292 (2q37.1) is located in an intergenic region within 1 kb of a large enhancer and the closest gene (C2orf57) is located > 22 Kb away (Fig. 4). Cg13986536

(9q34.11) is located in intron 1 of the *FUBP3* gene near a region carrying DNAse hypersensitivity marks as well as histone promoter and enhancer marks (Additional file 2: Figure S2), possibly functioning to regulate expression of the *FUBP3* gene, or an adjacent uncharacterized long noncoding RNA (LOC100272217). Cg01924952 (2p25.1) is located in a putative enhancer in a large intergenic region, with the closest gene (> 150 Kb) encoding for a long non-coding RNA, *LINC00299* (Fig. 5).

Discussion

This is the first study to evaluate the association of a NE with DNA methylation in circulating leukocytes across multiple racial/ethnic populations with different smoking-related lung cancer risk. Overall, we found similar methylation patterns associated with smoking status as in other studies. Higher NE levels were statistically significantly associated with an increase in DNA methylation β values (Bonferroni correction $p < 1.48 \times 10^{-7}$) in Native Hawaiians, but not in whites or Japanese Americans. Our findings suggest that Native Hawaiians have greater differential DNA methylation patterns, compared to whites and Japanese Americans, in relation to internal smoking dose, as measured by NE.

DNA methylation in relation to smoking status has been one of the most frequently studied epigenetic modifiers. There are > 2000 probes that have been found associated with measures of smoking (e.g., status,

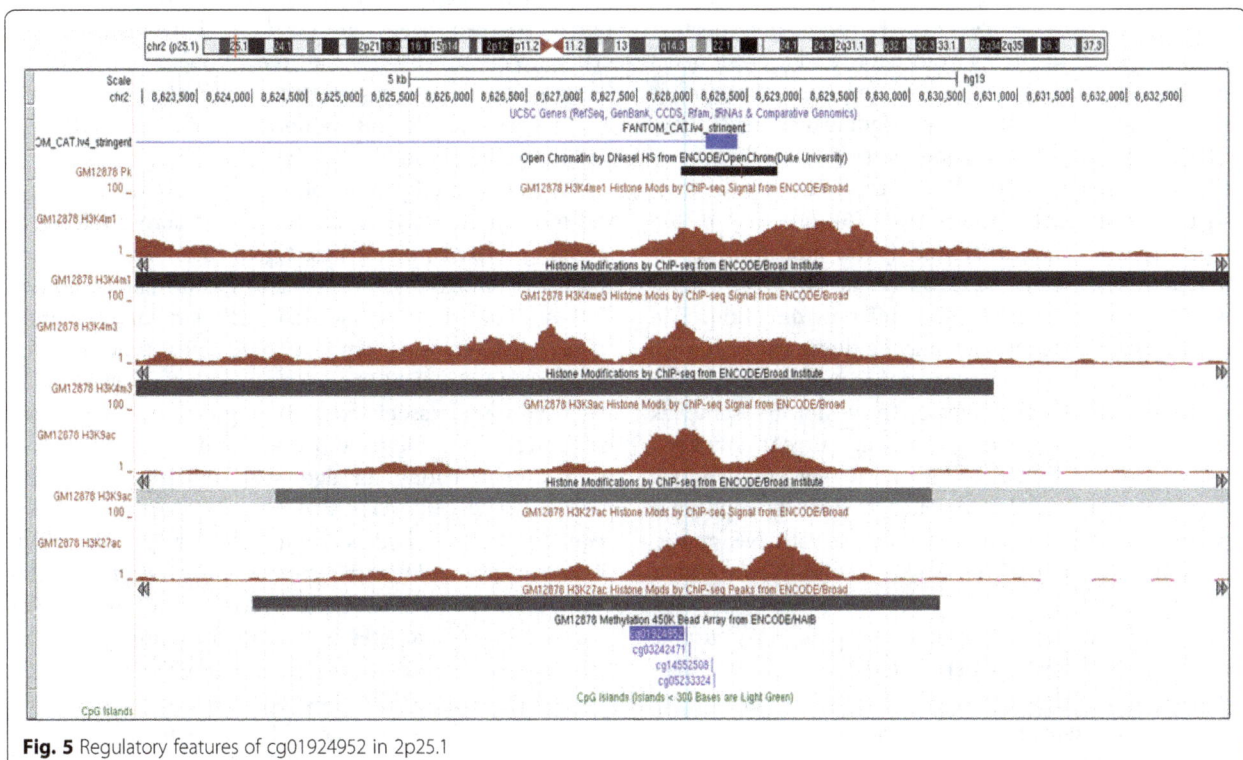

Fig. 5 Regulatory features of cg01924952 in 2p25.1

pack-years, time since quitting, dose) [18]. Among the four studies that have conducted EWAS of smoking dose [8, 10, 13, 22], all quantified dose by self-reported CPD and three of the four also conducted an EWAS of cotinine levels [10, 13, 22]. In addition, all four studies included both never and ever smokers in the discovery stage. In contrast, our study used NE, which is a better marker of smoking dose than CPD and cotinine, as it accounts for the variations of dose per cigarette from differences in smoking behavior (e.g., depth of inhalation) and/or nicotine metabolism present across multiethnic populations [5, 20]. Our study of NE was restricted to current smokers, as opposed to including both never and ever smokers. While the inclusion of never smokers improves the power to detect an association, such results also capture the associations with smoking status and not just with smoking dose.

In our EWAS of NE among current smokers, the top eight probes associated with NE were not among the probes most frequently associated with smoking status. We found that in seven of our top eight probes, higher NE was associated with an increase in methylation levels. These results are interesting, as previous epigenetic studies of smoking found that many markers associated with smoking status are found to be hypomethylated in current smokers compared to never or former smokers. However, importantly, smoking dose on the epigenome in only current smokers has not been systematically investigated. There has been only one other EWAS of smoking dose (self-reported CPD and cotinine) in current smokers [22]. Here, the investigators found that when including both never and ever smokers ($n = 1000$), 40 probes had a dose-response relationship with cotinine at a Bonferroni significance level ($p = 1.13 \times 10^{-7}$) [22]. All 40 probes were previously associated with smoking status [22]. When restricting the analysis to only current smokers ($n = 176$), only five of the 40 probes remained associated (p for non-linearity < 0.05) and one probe cg22132788 at $MYO1G$ had a dose-response relationship in a different direction. The loss of statistical significance may be the result of the reduction in sample size or suggest that methylated probes associated with smoking status may not be same as those affected by smoking dose in current smokers. Similarly, in our EWAS of NE in current smokers, we found that none of the 55 most frequently replicated smoking status probes were associated with NE at $p < 10^{-7}$ and only eight of these were modestly associated with NE ($p < 0.05$).

Moreover, in our multiethnic study of 612 current smokers (~ 200 samples per race/ethnicity), the epigenome of Native Hawaiians appeared to be differentially sensitive to the effects of internal smoking dose (Fig. 3), with eight probes mapping in or near six genes: $FNDC7$,

$BSND$, $PBX1$, $FUBP3$, $FOXK2$, and three in intergenic regions. These eight probes have not been previously identified as differentially methylated probes in relation to smoking dose (including never smokers). The majority of the previous EWAS of smoking dose were conducted in populations of European descent, whereas a small minority were conducted in populations of non-European descent (such as African or South Asian descent) [10, 11, 15, 17, 24], and no study included Native Hawaiians. No prior EWAS of smoking dose were conducted in populations of non-European descent. In the two multiethnic EWAS of smoking status, one study detected an interaction by race (South Asian and whites) with the DNA methylation beta values for cg05575921 (in $AHRR$) ($p = 2.0 \times 10^{-3}$) among 36 current smokers, where the median methylation beta values were higher in South Asian smokers than white smokers, even after adjusting for CPD [24]. The other study found that differential methylation of cg05575921 by smoking status was more significant in whites than in African Americans (p values = 1.45×10^{-62} vs. 4.61×10^{-16}) [17]. However, the authors stated that this difference was likely a result of the smaller sample size in African Americans and the p value for interaction was not shown [17]. In our current study, the sample size for each of the three ethnicities was similar ($n \sim 200$). Variations of cell type distribution across race/ethnicity may also have contributed the differential impact of NE on methylation across populations. A study of 20 smokers and 14 nonsmokers found that smoking may differentially affect the epigenome by cell type lineage [25]. For instance, for cg05575921 in $AHRR$, the reduction in methylation levels in smokers (compared to non-smokers) was greatest in granulocytes and monocytes, followed by B cells and not observed in T cells [25].

Differential methylation of probes in $AHRR$ is one of the most commonly replicated regions across EWAS of smoking-related phenotypes. Cg05575921 has served as marker of smoking status [26] and second-hand smoking [27] and has been associated with smoking quantity (pack-years) in ever smokers and quit time in past smokers [14, 28]. Differential methylation of cg05575921 has been found associated with lung cancer, where cases had lower DNA methylation beta values than controls, even after adjusting for age, sex, smoking status, and pack-years [29, 30]. AHRR serves as a negative feedback regulator of aryl hydrocarbon receptor (AHR), which plays a critical role in the metabolic activation of polycyclic aromatic hydrocarbons (PAHs), found in cigarette smoke. AHHR competes with AHR for binding with the aryl nuclear receptor translocator ($ARNT$). We recently showed that cg05575921 lies right adjacent to a tobacco smoke-inducible enhancer [31]. Hypomethylation of cg05575921, as well as the transcriptional activation of

AHRR, was replicated in vitro by treating A549 cells with cigarette smoke concentrate [31]. Thus, at least in some cases, changes in DNA methylation appear to be the result of changes in the activation of regulatory elements. The gain or loss of factors interacting with the DNA in response to environmental cues might alter the accessibility of CpGs to the maintenance DNA methyltransferase.

We found that three of the probes (cg13986536 in *FUBP3*, cg15613292 in 2q37.1, and cg21842914 in *FOXK2*) that were differentially methylated with smoking dose were located in CpG shores, just downstream (< 2 Kb) of CpG islands. All three are located in putative transcriptional regulatory domains based on their proximity to DNase hypersensitivity cluster and histone modification tracks in leukocytes. *FUBP3* is a member of a family of single-strand DNA binding proteins that bind to the far-upstream element (FUSE) of the *MYC* gene regulating its expression [32]. In a GWAS to study the stages of smoking progression, an intronic SNP (rs2304808) in *FUBP3* was associated with greater smoking tolerance (defined as "years from the age of daily smoking to the age when the heaviest smoking started"), independent of cigarette quantity [33]. The evaluation of methylation quantitative trait loci between this variant and cg13986536 is warranted. Cg15613292 is located in an intergenic region in 2q37.1, with the closest gene, *C2orf57* (also known as *TEX44*), more than 22 Kb away. However, two putative long non-coding RNA genes in the region (< 10 Kb away) were recently reported in the FANTOM5 project database [34]. Interestingly, the p interaction by race/ethnicity was most significant for cg15613292 ($p < 10^{-11}$) in Native Hawaiians; a log unit increase in NE was associated with a statistically significant increase in methylation beta-values. In contrast, in whites, the same log unit increase in NE was associated with a suggestive decrease in methylation beta-values. In addition, this probe is 4466 bp away from cg00816240, which was previously found to be inversely associated with current smoking status in an EWAS comprised of mostly European descent individuals [17]. Cg00816240 is also located in an exon of one of the putative long non-coding RNA identified in the FANTOM5 project.

Based on data from ENCODE, the differentially methylated probe, cg21842914 located in intron 8 of the *FOXK2* gene, is not located in a transcriptional regulatory region in GM12878 cells (B-lymphocytes) but is in a regulatory region for CD20+ and CD14+ cells based on histone modification levels. This genetic region has been found to be differentially methylated by smoking status in two other EWAS studies [17, 35]. In an EWAS of 31 current and 39 never Korean smokers to identify differential methylated regions (as opposed to only probes), the investigators found that probes within

80,545,020-80,545,869 bp of *FOXK2* were differentially methylated by current smoking status (cg21842914 is located at 80,545,869) [35]. Also, EWAS of current smoking status in primarily whites and some African Americans ($n = 15,907$) found that four probes in *FOXK2* (cg20412356, cg20173014, cg02094337, and cg16375265) were modestly associated with current smoking status ($p < 0.0015$) [17]. The most significant of the four probes, cg02094337 ($p = 2.3 \times 10^{-6}$), is 3751 bp away from cg21842914. We found that for cg21842914, a log unit increase in NE was associated with increasing methylated beta-values in Native Hawaiians and a modest decrease in methylated beta-values in whites. *FOXK2* is part of the family of forkhead transcription factors that control cell cycle and represses transcription of the cyclin-dependent kinase inhibitor gene p21 [36]. Thus, at least four of the top eight CpGs lie in or near regulatory regions that might be affected by environmental exposures such as smoking.

Based on the IPA analysis, the most significant of the implicated canonical pathways is ephrin B signaling, which has been shown to play an important role in lung cancer [37]. The ephrin type-B receptor 4 (EPHB4) tyrosine kinase has been shown to be overexpressed in lung tumors [38], and mutations in *EPHB4* identified in lung tumors can induce cellular proliferation and migration [38]. Ephrin type-B receptor 3 (EphB3) expression has been found to be higher in non-small cell lung cancer as well as associated with metastasis [39].

This study had some limitations worth noting. The generalizability of our findings is limited as we assessed methylation changes in leukocytes and not in the target tissue [40]. Also, we adjusted for predicted cell type measures with an algorithm that may not be valid for all racial/ethnic groups. In addition, we carried out IPA analysis using the genes nearest to the affected CpGs; however, it may not always be the nearest target gene whose expression is affected, in particular, if the CpG lies in or near the enhancer [31]. Lastly, a slightly more comprehensive measure of internal smoking dose, total nicotine equivalents (the sum of NE and nicotine N-oxide), was not measured in this study. However, on average, nicotine N-oxide only accounts for < 5% of the total nicotine equivalents. Strengths of this study include the multiethnic composition and relatively large sample size of current smokers, the use of a biomarker of internal smoking dose, and the ability to adjust for a range of potential confounders.

Conclusions

In conclusion, we identified eight differentially methylated probes in relation to internal smoking dose. These associations were primarily found in Native Hawaiians, suggesting that smoking may impact the epigenome differentially by race/ethnicity. Further investigation on how these methylation sites may influence transcriptional regulation and modify function within a biologic context is warranted. Our findings suggest that smoking dose may differentially impact the epigenome by ethnicity, which may provide insights into the mechanisms that contribute to the observed differences in lung cancer risk across these three populations.

Methods

Study population

The primary analysis was conducted in a study of only current smokers in Hawaii. The study has been described in detail previously [4, 41]. In brief, 612 smokers were randomly identified from either the Hawaii component of the Multiethnic Cohort study (MEC) (87%) or control groups of population-based case-control studies conducted in Hawaii (13%). The MEC is a prospective study of > 215,000 men and women of five racial/ethnic groups: African Americans, Japanese American, Native Hawaiian, Latinos, and whites, recruited from the state of Hawaii and from Southern California, primarily Los Angeles County, between 1993 and 1996 [42]. For the present study, eligible participants were identified among those who reported smoking at least 10 CPD on their respective study questionnaire, have had no previous history of cancer, and whose parents are both of Japanese or both of Caucasian ancestry or for whom one or both parents have any amount of Native Hawaiian ancestry. To confirm previously published associations between smoking status and DNA methylation, 35 randomly selected never smokers from the MEC (n = 12 Native Hawaiians, 11 Japanese Americans, and 12 whites) were included in the EWAS of smoking status. Never smoking status was identified by self-report at time of biospecimen collection.

Data collection

For this study, all interviews were conducted in the participants' home. Information was collected on lifetime tobacco and alcohol use and lung cancer-related occupational exposures. Participants were also instructed on how to keep a food record and a diary of all medications and dietary supplements for the 3 days preceding a 12-h overnight urine collection and a blood draw. Urine collection began between 5 and 9 pm for a period of 12 h which included all urine passed through the night and the first morning urine. The urine was kept on ice until processing, which occurred within 4 h of the last sample. Aliquots were subsequently stored in a − 80 °C freezer until analysis.

Laboratory analysis and quality control

Nicotine equivalents (NE) comprised of total cotinine (nmol/mL), total nicotine (nmol/mL), and total trans-3′-hydroxycotinine (3-HC, in nmol/mL) which includes their glucuronides. The methodology to measure these biomarkers was previously reported [4]. In brief, total urinary nicotine, cotinine, and 3-HC were measured by gas chromatography/mass spectrometry. For total nicotine (free + nicotine N-glucuronide) and total cotinine (free + cotinine N-glucuronide) concentration, the samples were treated with base to cleave the glucuronide conjugates, and the nicotine and cotinine were quantified by gas chromatography/mass spectrometry analysis [43]. For total 3-HC (3-HC + its glucuronide), the sample was first treated with h-glucuronidase and then analyzed 3-HC by gas chromatography/mass spectrometry, as described previously [44]. The sum of these metabolites accounts for over 75% of nicotine and its metabolites [45] and has been used to quantify the majority of nicotine uptake.

DNA methylation

DNA was extracted from buffy coat using the QIAamp DNA Blood Mini kit (Qiagen) and quantified using the Quant-iT Pico Green dsDNA Assay Kit (Invitrogen). DNA was normalized to 50 ng/ul and plated without regard to ethnicity. Five hundred nanograms of the extracted DNA was treated with bisulfite using EZ-96 DNA Methylation kit (Zymo Research, Orange, CA, USA), and 100–200 ng of bisulfite-converted DNA was hybridized onto the Infinium Human Methylation450 BeadChip (Illumina, San Diego, CA).

This array covers 485,512 loci, representing 96% of known CpG islands and 99% of RefSeq genes, with an average of 17 CpG sites per gene distributed across the upstream region of the transcription start sites (TSS) 1500, TSS200, 5′UTR, first exon, gene body, and 3′ UTR.

After hybridization, washing, and single nucleotide extension steps, the BeadChips were scanned on the Illumina iScan and the intensities of the images recorded in .IDAT files. The probe intensities were processed using the minfi package in Bioconductor [46, 47], with fluorescence intensities normalized utilizing various internal controls that are present on the Methylation450 BeadChip. Within-sample normalization consisted of background correction, dye-bias correction to normalize any imbalance due to intensities measured in two color channels, and type I and II probe intensity normalization to correct for differences in range of signal intensity due to two probe types [48, 49]. The DNA methylation score for each CpG site is represented by a β value between 0 (fully unmethylated) to 1 (fully methylated) calculated from the fluorescence intensity ratio between methylated and methylated + unmethylated probes for each tested CpG. β values can easily be interpreted as the proportion of methylated DNA at a given locus.

Each chip included a randomly selected mix of racial/ethnic groups, sex, and smoking levels to minimize the impact of any batch effects. To avoid gender- and genotype-associated biases [50], non-autosomal CpG loci and loci positioned at a single nucleotide polymorphism (SNP) (dbSNP build 137) were excluded. This resulted in 337,542 probes being retained for the analysis.

Cell-type calculations

Cell type proportions for CD4 T cells, CD8 T cells, B cells, natural killer cells, monocytes, and granulocytes were calculated using an online calculator [51, 52]. Adjusting for cell types was justified based on the known inflammation and immune response changes due to smoking [53].

Statistical methods

Pearson partial correlation coefficients, adjusting for age, sex, and race/ethnicity, were assessed between CPD and NE. Median and interquartile ranges were used to describe the cell type data distribution. ANOVA was used to evaluate cell type distribution differences across the three populations. NE was not normally distributed and thus log transformed. To evaluate the association of log NE with DNA methylation β values, linear regression models were used. We adjusted for age, sex, race/ethnicity (in pan-ethnic analyses, i.e., all races combined), and estimated cell-types distribution. Other variables such as BMI were considered. Findings did not change with the inclusion of BMI and thus were not presented. All tests for heterogeneity of effects by race/ethnicity were conducted by including an interaction term between log-NE and race/ethnicity. For the pan-ethnic analyses, we did not use random effects model as our study sample was a sample of convenience and not a random cluster sampling from an ideal super population. Thus, the variance from such a random effects model would not properly define the degree of heterogeneity in the super population. Moreover, our conclusions as to whether heterogeneity in the effects of methylation exists across these three populations would be the same whether we used a fixed or random effects model. An EWAS of smoking status ($n = 35$ never vs 612 current) was conducted to confirm previously identified DNA methylation findings. Also, after analyses were completed, the significant probes were evaluated for poor mapping quality [54]; those considered to be poor were excluded.

Bioinformatics analysis

Gene lists were generated based on proximity to the significant differentially methylated probes ($p < 10^{-3}$). The Ingenuity Pathway Analysis software (IPA; Ingenuity® Systems, www.ingenuity.com) was used to analyze our gene lists to identify an enrichment for genes functioning in specific signaling pathways and biological mechanisms associated with smoking dose.

We also used the Encyclopedia of DNA Elements (EN-CODE) Consortium data [23, 55] to determine if the significant probes were located in putative regulatory regions (e.g., DNase hypersensitivity and histone modification) in multiple cell types. We examined the regulatory features in human embryonic stem cells, an immortalized B-lymphocyte cell line (GM12878 cells within a 10 kb window of the eight CpGs), focusing on CpG islands, DNase hypersensitivity clusters and four histone modifications: histone 3 lysine 4 monomethylation (H3K4me1, a mark for poised or active enhancers), histone 3 lysine 4 trimethylation (H3K4me3, a promoter mark), histone 3 lysine 9 acetylation (H3K9ac, a mark found near transcription start sites), and histone 3 lysine 27 acetylation (H3K27ac, an active enhancer mark found at proximal and distal regions of transcription start sites). We also considered the regulatory features in CD20 and CD14 cell lines. The probes were considered as potential regulatory probes if they were in regions containing DNase hypersensitivity and/or histone modifications (H3K4me1, H3K4me3, H3K9ac, HeK27ac).

Abbreviations

AHRR: Aryl-hydrocarbon receptor repressor; *ALPPL2*: Alkaline phosphatase genes, placental-like; BMI: Body mass index; ENCODE: Encyclopedia of DNA Elements; EWAS: Epigenome-wide association study; *F2RL3*: Coagulation factor II (thrombin) receptor-like 3 gene; *GPR15*: G protein-coupled receptor; H3K27ac: Histone 3 lysine 27 acetylation; H3K4me1: Histone 3 lysine 4 monomethylation; H3K4me3: Histone 3 lysine 4 trimethylation; H3K9ac: Histone 3 lysine 9 acetylation; NE: Nicotine equivalents

Acknowledgements

We thank the staff and study participants for their time and important contributions.

Funding

This study was supported by the NIH grants R01CA85997 and P01CA138338, the Norris Comprehensive Cancer Center Core grant P30CA014089, the University of Southern California Provost Fellowship and Roy E. Thomas Foundation Award (DJM), and TRDRP grant 26IR-0019 (to IAO). The MEC study is supported by UM1CA164973.

Authors' contributions

SLP participated in the design of the study, data interpretation and drafted the manuscript. YMP performed the epigenome-wide association analyses. LWML carried out the IPA analyses and contributed to the data interpretation. DJM and IAO created the ENCODE figures and contributed to the data interpretation. AM contributed to the data interpretation. DOS and KS advised the statistical analyses. SEM performed the assays measuring nicotine equivalents in smokers. MT supervised the laboratory work for the methylation arrays and contributed to the data interpretation. LLM conceived of the study, participated in its design and coordination and contributed to the data interpretation. All authors helped draft the manuscript, participated in the manuscript editing, and read/approved the final manuscript.

Competing interests

The authors declare that they have no competing interests.

Author details

[1]Department of Preventive Medicine, Norris Comprehensive Cancer Center, Keck School of Medicine, University of Southern California, 1450 Biggy Street, NRT 1509G, Los Angeles, CA 90033, USA. [2]Epidemiology Program, University of Hawaii Cancer Center, 701 Ilalo Street, Honolulu, HI 96813, USA. [3]Department of Biochemistry and Molecular Biology, Keck School of Medicine, University of Southern California, Los Angeles, CA 90032, USA. [4]University of Hawaii John A. Burns School of Medicine, Honolulu, HI 96813, USA. [5]Masonic Cancer Center, University of Minnesota, Minneapolis, MN 55455, USA.

References

1. Hecht SS. Lung carcinogenesis by tobacco smoke. Int J Cancer. 2012;131:2724–32.
2. Haiman CA, Stram DO, Wilkens LR, Pike MC, Kolonel LN, Henderson BE, Le Marchand L. Ethnic and racial differences in the smoking-related risk of lung cancer. N Engl J Med. 2006;354:333–42.
3. Le Marchand L, Wilkens LR, Kolonel LN. Ethnic differences in the lung cancer risk associated with smoking. Cancer EpidemiolBiomarkers Prev. 1992;1:103–7.
4. Derby KS, Cuthrell K, Caberto C, Carmella SG, Franke AA, Hecht SS, Murphy SE, Le Marchand L. Nicotine metabolism in three ethnic/racial groups with different risks of lung cancer. Cancer Epidemiol Biomark Prev. 2008;17:3526–35.
5. Park SL, Tiirikainen MI, Patel YM, Wilkens LR, Stram DO, Le Marchand L, Murphy SE. Genetic determinants of CYP2A6 activity across racial/ethnic groups with different risks of lung cancer and effect on their smoking intensity. Carcinogenesis. 2016;37:269–79.
6. Laird PW. Principles and challenges of genome-wide DNA methylation analysis. Nat Rev Genet. 2010;11:191–203.
7. Breitling L, Yang R, Korn B, Burwinkel B, Brenner H. Tobacco-smoking-related differential DNA methylation: 27K discovery and replication. Am J Hum Genet. 2011;88:450–7.
8. Zeilinger S, Kühnel B, Klopp N, Baurecht H, Kleinschmidt A, Gieger C, Weidinger S, Lattka E, Adamski J, Peters A, et al. Tobacco smoking leads to extensive genome-wide changes in DNA methylation. PLoS One. 2013;8:e63812.
9. Monick MM, Beach SR, Plume J, Sears R, Gerrard M, Brody GH, Philibert RA. Coordinated changes in AHRR methylation in lymphoblasts and pulmonary macrophages from smokers. Am J Med Genet B Neuropsychiatr Genet. 2012;159B:141–51.
10. Philibert R, Beach SR, Lei M-K, Brody G. Changes in DNA methylation at the aryl hydrocarbon receptor repressor may be a new biomarker for smoking. Clin Epigenetics. 2013;5:19.
11. Dogan M, Shields B, Cutrona C, Gao L, Gibbons F, Simons R, Monick M, Brody G, Tan K, Beach S, Philibert R. The effect of smoking on DNA methylation of peripheral blood mononuclear cells from African American women. BMC Genomics. 2014;15:151.
12. Philibert RA, Beach SR, Brody GH. Demethylation of the aryl hydrocarbon receptor repressor as a biomarker for nascent smokers. Epigenetics. 2012;7:1331–8.
13. Shenker NS, Polidoro S, van Veldhoven K, Sacerdote C, Ricceri F, Birrell MA, Belvisi MG, Brown R, Vineis P, Flanagan JM. Epigenome-wide association study in the European Prospective Investigation into Cancer and Nutrition (EPIC-Turin) identifies novel genetic loci associated with smoking. Hum Mol Genet. 2013;22:843–51.
14. Shenker NS, Ueland PM, Polidoro S, van Veldhoven K, Ricceri F, Brown R, Flanagan JM, Vineis P. DNA methylation as a long-term biomarker of exposure to tobacco smoke. Epidemiology. 2013;24:712–6.
15. Sun Y, Smith A, Conneely K, Chang Q, Li W, Lazarus A, Smith J, Almli L, Binder E, Klengel T, et al. Epigenomic association analysis identifies smoking-related DNA methylation sites in African Americans. Hum Genet. 2013;132:1027–37.
16. Wan E, Qiu W, Baccarelli A, Carey V, Bacherman H, Rennard S, Agusti A, Anderson W, Lomas D, Demeo D. Cigarette smoking behaviors and time since quitting are associated with differential DNA methylation across the human genome. Hum Mol Genet. 2012;21:3073–82.
17. Joehanes R, Just AC, Marioni RE, Pilling LC, Reynolds LM, Mandaviya PR, 800 Guan W, Xu T, Elks CE, Aslibekyan S, et al. Epigenetic signatures of cigarette 801 smoking. Circ Cardiovasc Genet. 2016;9(5): 436–47.
18. Gao X, Jia M, Zhang Y, Breitling LP, Brenner H. DNA methylation changes of whole blood cells in response to active smoking exposure in adults: a systematic review of DNA methylation studies. Clin Epigenetics. 2015;7:113.
19. Lee K, Pausova Z. Cigarette smoking and DNA methylation. Front Genet. 2013;4:132.
20. Hukkanen J, Jacob P, Benowitz NL. Metabolism and disposition kinetics of nicotine. Pharmacol Rev. 2005;57:79–115.
21. Murphy SE, Park SL, Thompson EF, Wilkens LR, Patel Y, Stram DO, Le Marchand L. Nicotine N-glucuronidation relative to N-oxidation and C-oxidation and UGT2B10 genotype in five ethnic/racial groups. Carcinogenesis. 2014;35:2526–33.
22. Zhang Y, Florath I, Saum KU, Brenner H. Self-reported smoking, serum cotinine, and blood DNA methylation. Environ Res. 2016;146:395–403.
23. Sloan CA, Chan ET, Davidson JM, Malladi VS, Strattan JS, Hitz BC, Gabdank I, Narayanan AK, Ho M, Lee BT, et al. ENCODE data at the ENCODE portal. Nucleic Acids Res. 2016;44:D726–32.
24. Elliott H, Tillin T, McArdle W, Ho K, Duggirala A, Frayling T, Davey Smith G, Hughes A, Chaturvedi N, Relton C. Differences in smoking associated DNA methylation patterns in South Asians and Europeans. Clin Epigenetics. 2014;6:4.
25. Su D, Wang X, Campbell MR, Porter DK, Pittman GS, Bennett BD, Wan M, Englert NA, Crowl CL, Gimple RN, et al. Distinct epigenetic effects of tobacco smoking in whole blood and among leukocyte subtypes. PLoS One. 2016;11:e0166486.
26. Lee D-H, Hwang S-H, Lim MK, Oh J-K, Song DY, Yun EH, Park EY. Performance of urine cotinine and hypomethylation of AHRR and F2RL3 as biomarkers for smoking exposure in a population-based cohort. PLoS One. 2017;12:e0176783.
27. Reynolds LM, Magid HS, Chi GC, Lohman K, Barr RG, Kaufman JD, Hoeschele I, Blaha MJ, Navas-Acien A, Liu Y. Secondhand tobacco smoke exposure associations with DNA methylation of the aryl hydrocarbon receptor repressor. Nicotine Tob Res. 2017;19:442–51.
28. Guida F, Sandanger TM, Castagne R, Campanella G, Polidoro S, Palli D, Krogh V, Tumino R, Sacerdote C, Panico S, et al. Dynamics of smoking-induced genome-wide methylation changes with time since smoking cessation. Hum Mol Genet. 2015;24:2349–59.
29. Zhang Y, Elgizouli M, Schöttker B, Holleczek B, Nieters A, Brenner H. Smoking-associated DNA methylation markers predict lung cancer incidence. Clin Epigenetics. 2016;8:127.
30. Fasanelli F, Baglietto L, Ponzi E, Guida F, Campanella G, Johansson M, Grankvist K, Johansson M, Assumma MB, Naccarati A, et al. Hypomethylation of smoking-related genes is associated with future lung cancer in four prospective cohorts. Nat Commun. 2015;6:10192.
31. Stueve TR, Li W-Q, Shi J, Marconett CN, Zhang T, Yang C, Mullen D, Yan C, Wheeler W, Hua X, et al. Epigenome-wide analysis of DNA methylation in lung tissue shows concordance with blood studies and identifies tobacco smoke-inducible enhancers. Hum Mol Genet. 2017;26:3014–27.
32. Weber A, Kristiansen I, Johannsen M, Oelrich B, Scholmann K, Gunia S, May M, Meyer H-A, Behnke S, Moch H, Kristiansen G. The FUSE binding proteins FBP1 and FBP3 are potential c-myc regulators in renal, but not in prostate and bladder cancer. BMC Cancer. 2008;8:369.
33. He L, Pitkäniemi J, Heikkilä K, Chou Y-L, Madden PAF, Korhonen T, Sarin A-P, Ripatti S, Kaprio J, Loukola A. Genome-wide time-to-event analysis on smoking progression stages in a family-based study. Brain Behav. 2016;6: e00462-n/a.
34. Hon C-C, Ramilowski JA, Harshbarger J, Bertin N, Rackham OJL, Gough J, Denisenko E, Schmeier S, Poulsen TM, Severin J, et al. An atlas of human long non-coding RNAs with accurate 5′ ends. Nature. 2017;543:199–204.
35. Lee MK, Hong Y, Kim S-Y, London SJ, Kim WJ. DNA methylation and smoking in Korean adults: epigenome-wide association study. Clin Epigenetics. 2016;8:103.
36. Marais A, Ji Z, Child ES, Krause E, Mann DJ, Sharrocks AD. Cell cycle-dependent regulation of the forkhead transcription factor FOXK2 by CDK. cyclin complexes. J Biol Chem. 2010;285:35728–39.
37. Pasquale EB. Eph receptors and ephrins in cancer: bidirectional signaling and beyond. Nat Rev Cancer. 2010;10:165–80.
38. Ferguson BD, Liu R, Rolle CE, Tan YH, Krasnoperov V, Kanteti R, Tretiakova MS, Cervantes GM, Hasina R, Hseu RD, et al. The EphB4 receptor tyrosine kinase promotes lung cancer growth: a potential novel therapeutic target. PLoS One. 2013;8:e67668.
39. Ji X-D, Li G, Feng Y-X, Zhao J-S, Li J-J, Sun Z-J, Shi S, Deng Y-Z, Xu J-F, Zhu Y-Q, et al. EphB3 is overexpressed in non–small-cell lung cancer and promotes tumor metastasis by enhancing cell survival and migration. Cancer Res. 2011;71:1156–66.

40. Bergougnoux A, Claustres M, De Sario A. Nasal epithelial cells: a tool to study DNA methylation in airway diseases. Epigenomics. 2015;7:119–26.

41. Derby KS, Cuthrell K, Caberto C, Carmella S, Murphy SE, Hecht SS, Le Marchand L. Exposure to the carcinogen 4-(methylnitrosamino)-1-(3-pyridyl)-1-butanone (NNK) in smokers from 3 populations with different risks of lung cancer. Int J Cancer. 2009;125:2418–24.

42. Kolonel LN, Henderson BE, Hankin JH, Nomura AM, Wilkens LR, Pike MC, Stram DO, Monroe KR, Earle ME, Nagamine FS. A multiethnic cohort in Hawaii and Los Angeles: baseline characteristics. Am J Epidemiol. 2000;151:346–57.

43. Hecht SS, Carmella SG, Chen M, Koch JFD, Miller AT, Murphy SE, Jensen JA, Zimmerman CL, Hatsukami DK. Quantitation of urinary metabolites of a tobacco-specific lung carcinogen after smoking cessation. Cancer Res. 1999;59:590–6.

44. Hecht SS, Carmella SG, Murphy SE. Effects of watercress consumption on urinary metabolites of nicotine in smokers. Cancer Epidemiol Biomark Prev. 1999;8:907–13.

45. Tricker AR. Nicotine metabolism, human drug metabolism polymorphisms, and smoking behaviour. Toxicology. 2003;183:151–73.

46. Aryee MJ, Jaffe AE, Corrada-Bravo H, Ladd-Acosta C, Feinberg AP, Hansen KD, Irizarry RA. Minfi: a flexible and comprehensive Bioconductor package for the analysis of Infinium DNA methylation microarrays. Bioinformatics. 2014;30:1363–9.

47. Huber W, Carey VJ, Gentleman R, Anders S, Carlson M, Carvalho BS, Bravo HC, Davis S, Gatto L, Girke T, et al. Orchestrating high-throughput genomic analysis with Bioconductor. Nat Meth. 2015;12:115–21.

48. Maksimovic J, Gordon L, Oshlack A. SWAN: subset-quantile within array normalization for illumina infinium HumanMethylation450 BeadChips. Genome Biol. 2012;13:R44.

49. Triche JTJ, Weisenberger DJ, Van Den Berg D, Laird PW, Siegmund KD. Low-level processing of Illumina Infinium DNA Methylation BeadArrays. Nucleic Acids Res. 2013;41:e90.

50. Chen YA, Lemire M, Choufani S, Butcher DT, Grafodatskaya D, Zanke BW, Gallinger S, Hudson TJ, Weksberg R. Discovery of cross-reactive probes and polymorphic CpGs in the Illumina Infinium HumanMethylation450 microarray. Epigenetics. 2013;8:203–9.

51. Houseman E, Accomando W, Koestler D, Christensen B, Marsit C, Nelson H, Wiencke J, Kelsey K. DNA methylation arrays as surrogate measures of cell mixture distribution. BMC Bioinformatics. 2012;13:86.

52. Horvath S. DNA methylation age of human tissues and cell types. Genome Biol. 2013;14:R115.

53. Lee J, Taneja V, Vassallo R. Cigarette smoking and inflammation: cellular and molecular mechanisms. J Dent Res. 2012;91:142–9.

54. Zhou W, Laird PW, Shen H. Comprehensive characterization, annotation and innovative use of Infinium DNA methylation BeadChip probes. Nucleic Acids Res. 2017;45:e22.

55. ENCODE Project Consortium. An integrated encyclopedia of DNA elements in the human genome. Nature. 2012;489:57–74.

20

FADS1-FADS2 genetic polymorphisms are associated with fatty acid metabolism through changes in DNA methylation and gene expression

Zhen He[1,2], Rong Zhang[1], Feng Jiang[1], Hong Zhang[1], Aihua Zhao[3], Bo Xu[1], Li Jin[4], Tao Wang[1], Wei Jia[3], Weiping Jia[1] and Cheng Hu[1,2]*

Abstract

Background: Genome-wide association studies (GWASs) have shown that genetic variants are important determinants of free fatty acid levels. The mechanisms underlying the associations between genetic variants and free fatty acid levels are incompletely understood. Here, we aimed to identify genetic markers that could influence diverse fatty acid levels in a Chinese population and uncover the molecular mechanisms in terms of DNA methylation and gene expression.

Results: We identified strong associations between single-nucleotide polymorphisms (SNPs) in the fatty acid desaturase (*FADS*) region and multiple polyunsaturated fatty acids. Expression quantitative trait locus (eQTL) analysis of rs174570 on *FADS1* and *FADS2* mRNA levels proved that minor allele of rs174570 was associated with decreased *FADS1* and *FADS2* expression levels ($P < 0.05$). Methylation quantitative trait locus (mQTL) analysis of rs174570 on DNA methylation levels in three selected regions of *FADS* region showed that the methylation levels at four CpG sites in *FADS1*, one CpG site in intragenic region, and three CpG sites in *FADS2* were strongly associated with rs174570 ($P < 0.05$). Then, we demonstrated that methylation levels at three CpG sites in *FADS1* were negatively associated with *FADS1* and *FADS2* expression, while two CpG sites in *FADS2* were positively associated with *FADS1* and *FADS2* expression. Using mediation analysis, we further show that the observed effect of rs174570 on gene expression was tightly correlated with the effect predicted through association with methylation.

Conclusions: Our findings suggest that genetic variants in the *FADS* region are major genetic modifiers that can regulate fatty acid metabolism through epigenetic gene regulation.

Keywords: DNA methylation, Gene expression, Fatty acids, Genetic markers, Fatty acid desaturase

Background

In human physiology, fatty acids have multiple functions. Fatty acids serve as energy sources, substrates for multiple lipid mediators, constituents of cell membranes, and modulators of gene transcription. Fatty acids exist in various forms, including saturated fatty acids (SFAs), trans-fatty acids (TFAs), monounsaturated fatty acids (MUFAs), and polyunsaturated fatty acids (PUFAs) [1, 2]. Numerous prospective epidemiological studies and randomized controlled trials have been conducted to evaluate the involvement of diverse fatty acids in cardiovascular and metabolic diseases [3–5]. High-dose ω-3 fatty acid intake can reduce the risk of noninfarct myocardial fibrosis, while high TFA content in erythrocytes is associated with an elevated risk of coronary heart disease (CHD) [6, 7]. However, the association of ω-6-specific fatty acids with cardiovascular disease is still controversial [8]. Although some earlier experimental studies observed that

* Correspondence: alfredhc@sjtu.edu.cn
[1]Shanghai Diabetes Institute, Shanghai Key Laboratory of Diabetes Mellitus, Shanghai Clinical Center for Diabetes, Shanghai Jiao Tong University Affiliated Sixth People's Hospital, 600 Yishan Road, Shanghai 200233, China
[2]Institute for Metabolic Diseases, Fengxian Central Hospital, The Third School of Clinical Medicine, Southern Medical University, Shanghai, China
Full list of author information is available at the end of the article

ω-6-specific PUFA interventions tended to increase CHD risk, a recent meta-analysis based on 13 prospective cohort studies with a total of 310,602 individuals found that higher linoleic acid (LA) intake was associated with a lower risk of CHD events [9–11]. Considering the diverse roles of fatty acids in human diseases, an exploration of the determinants of fatty acid metabolism and concentrations in circulation is needed. Fatty acid levels vary widely according to the individual and to ethnicity, and such differences may be due to environmental factors, especially dietary and/or genetic differences. The mapping of genetic variants that affect serum fatty acid levels may help identify novel genetic markers, uncover disease pathogenesis, and provide pharmaceutical targets for cardiovascular and metabolic diseases.

Genome-wide association studies (GWASs) have identified multiple genetic loci that contribute to inter-individual variations in SFAs, TFAs, MUFAs, and PUFAs in whole plasma, plasma phospholipids, and erythrocyte membrane phospholipids in populations of European ancestry [12–14]. However, the vast majority of the identified loci are noncoding variants, and only a few of these loci have been linked to underlying mechanisms contributing to phenotypic outcome. A validated method for exploring noncoding variation and its influence on complex traits or diseases is linking genetic variants to gene expression or epigenetics in disease-associated tissues [15–17].

Epigenetics can be described as heritable changes that affect gene transcription regardless of the DNA sequence. DNA methylation is an important epigenetic mechanism through which a methyl group, most often a cytosine nucleotide preceding a guanine nucleotide, is added to the DNA sequence [18]. DNA methylation can be affected by both environmental and heritable factors, can affect chromatin structure, and can influence transcription [19].

In this study, we aim to identify genetic markers that could influence diverse fatty acid levels in a Chinese population. Then, by focusing on *FADS1* and *FADS2* (fatty acid desaturase1 and 2), we seek to explain the gene regulatory mechanisms including DNA methylation and gene transcription to help explain the relationships we observed between genomic variation and fatty acid levels.

Methods

Participants

The present study represents a subgroup analysis of participants from the Shanghai Obesity Study (SHOS). Detailed study methods have been published previously [20, 21]. Briefly, the SHOS is a community-based, prospective cohort study to investigate the occurrence and development of metabolic syndrome and its related diseases. Beginning in 2009, the SHOS recruited 5000

participants from four communities in Shanghai, China, which included a baseline study as well as 1.5-, 3-, and 5-year follow-up studies. Three hundred twelve adult participants (132 healthy subjects with normal BMI, 107 metabolically healthy participants with overweight or obese state, and 73 metabolically unhealthy participants with overweight or obese state) were recruited in a cross-sectional study for a project focusing on studying the association of serum free fatty acid with metabolic abnormalities. Of these participants, 304 subjects with genotype data available were further selected in our study (mean ± SD age of 48.4 ± 9.7 years and BMI 24.4 ± 3.8 kg/m^2). A participant flow chart is shown in Additional file 1: Figure S1. Blood samples were collected in the morning after a 12-h fast. EDTA-treated whole blood samples were used for DNA extraction and genotyping with the Infinium Exome BeadChip, and serum samples were used for measuring fatty acid levels.

Genome-wide genotyping, quality control

Genomic DNA was extracted from peripheral blood leucocytes in whole blood samples. The DNA samples were genotyped using the Infinium Exome-24 v1.0 BeadChip (Illumina, Inc., San Diego, CA, USA), which included a total of 247,870 SNPs. Quality control (QC) was assessed at the individual and SNP levels. First, individuals with high levels of missingness, excess autosomal heterozygosity, high relatedness, ambiguous gender, and ancestry outliers estimated by using ancestry principal component analysis (PCA) were excluded. Next, criteria such as call rate < 98%, significant departures from Hardy–Weinberg equilibrium ($P < 1 \times 10^{-6}$), significant differences in allele frequency between case and control ($P > 0.05$), not on chromosomes 1–22, and minor allele frequency (MAF) < 1% were applied for excluding SNPs in further analysis. Finally, 32,387 SNPs and 297 individuals were selected for subsequent analysis. The detailed QC results are shown in Additional file 1: Tables S1 and S2; Figures S2, S3, S4 and S5.

Measurement of serum free fatty acids

All serum samples were stored at − 80 °C until use. The sample preparation procedure for free fatty acid measurements has been described previously [20]. A panel of 42 free fatty acids (FFAs) including 17 SFAs, 12 MUFAs, and 13 PUFAs were subjected to ultra-performance liquid chromatography quadrupole-time-of-flight mass spectrometry (UPLC-QTOFMS) analysis (Waters Corporation, Milford, MA, USA). The ACQUITY-UPLC system was equipped with a binary solvent delivery system and an auto-sampler (Waters Corporation, Milford, USA), coupled to a tandem quadrupole-time-of-flight (Q-TOF) mass spectrometry (Waters Corporation, Milford, USA). A mixture of all the reference standards at an appropriate concentration was prepared and run after every ten serum samples for quality control. The raw data were processed with TargetLynx applications manager version 4.1 (Waters Corporation, Milford, MA, USA). After peak signal detection, standard curve confirmation was needed to calculate the absolute concentration of each FFA. Manual examination and correction were needed to ensure data quality. R version 3.2.1 and SIMCA 13.0.1 software (Umetrics, Sweden) were used for statistical computing and graphics. The relative concentrations of 42 individual fatty acids were expressed as the percentage of total serum fatty acids. Fatty acids with relative concentrations above 0.1% are listed in Table 1. The product-to-precursor ratios were used to estimate the activities of different desaturases as follows: δ-5 desaturase (D5D), arachidonic acid (AA)/dihomo-gamma--linolenic acid (DGLA), and δ-6 desaturase (D6D), gamma-linolenic acid (GLA)/linoleic acid (LA).

Table 1 Twenty-two free fatty acids with relative concentrations above 0.1% in 297 subjects

Characteristics	% of total fatty acids
14:0	3.89 ± 1.48
15:0	0.32 ± 0.07
16:0	22.95 ± 2.07
17:0	0.84 ± 0.19
18:0	22.41 ± 4.63
19:0	0.14 ± 0.03
20:0	0.51 ± 0.16
15:0 iso	0.26 ± 0.26
16:0 iso	0.17 ± 0.05
17:0 iso	0.65 ± 0.16
18:0 iso	1.61 ± 0.48
16:1n-7	1.01 ± 0.41
16:1n-9	0.17 ± 0.05
18:1n-9	13.59 ± 3.84
20:1n-9	0.14 ± 0.05
18:2n-6(LA)	20.04 ± 4.76
18:3n-6(GLA)	0.26 ± 0.07
20:2n-6(EDA)	0.32 ± 0.06
20:3n-6(DGLA)	0.36 ± 0.1
20:4n-6(AA)	2.94 ± 0.88
22:4n-6(ADA)	0.33 ± 0.07
22:5n-6	0.19 ± 0.05
18:3n-3(ALA)	0.70 ± 0.27
20:5n-3(EPA)	0.46 ± 0.19
22:5n-3(DPA)	0.58 ± 0.18
22:6n-3(DHA)	4.47 ± 2.00

Data are shown as the mean ± SD. *AA* arachidonic acid, *ADA* adrenic acid, *ALA* α-linolenic acid, *DGLA* dihomo-gamma-linolenic acid, *DHA* docosahexaenoic acid, *DPA* docosapentaenoic acid, *EDA* eicosadienoic acid, *EPA* eicosapentaenoic acid, *GLA* gamma-linolenic acid, *Iso* isomer, *LA* linoleic acid

Adipose tissue RNA isolation and quantitative PCR

Adipose tissues were previously collected from a metabolic surgery follow-up study [22]. Obese patients from the Department of Endocrinology and Metabolism were recruited in this study, and they received Roux-en-Y gastric bypass surgery. Visceral adipose tissue samples from 42 subjects (age, 43.04 ± 14.90 years; BMI, 34.34 ± 6.37 kg/m^2) were randomly selected and stored at − 80 ° C. RNA from the adipose tissues was extracted with the RNeasy Plus Universal Kit (QIAGEN, Valencia, CA, USA), and 1 µg of RNA was used to synthesize cDNA using the PrimeScript™ RT reagent kit with gDNA Eraser (Takara Bio, Japan). Template cDNAs were diluted 1:4, and the relative expression of *FADS1* and *FADS2* was quantified in triplicate 10-µl reactions by using ABI 7900 Applied Biosystems 7900HT Fast Real-Time PCR System (Applied Biosystems, Foster City, CA, USA) and normalized against the housekeeping gene RPLP0. An assay ID for each gene was assigned as follows: FADS1, Hs00203685_m1; FADS2, Hs00927433_m1; and RPLP0, Hs99999902_m1 (Assays on-demand; Applied Biosystems, Foster City, CA, USA). Each sample was run in triplicates, and the mean value was obtained. Relative quantitative method was used for quantification of mRNA levels.

Adipose tissue DNA isolation, DNA methylation analysis, and genotyping

Genomic DNA (500 ng) was extracted from the visceral adipose tissues according to the manufacturer's instructions with the QIAamp DNA Mini kit (Qiagen, Valencia, CA, USA). Bisulfite conversion was performed with the EpiTect Fast DNA Bisulfite kit (Qiagen, Valencia, CA, USA). Based on the CpG densities of the genes, two different methods were used to quantify the DNA methylation levels by matrix-assisted laser desorption ionization-TOF mass spectrometry with a MassARRAY Compact Analyzer (Agena Bioscience, San Diego, CA, USA) [23, 24]. The first method was used for the regions that had high densities of CpGs (CGI1 and CGI2). Specific primers for PCR amplicons covering the majority of the CpG-dense areas in the promoter and in the flanking regions of *FADS1* and *FADS2* were designed with the EpiDesigner tool (http://www.epidesigner.com). After in vitro RNA transcription and subsequent base-specific cleavage reactions, the products were processed in the MassARRAY system. All reactions were performed in duplicate. By comparing the differences in signal intensity between the mass signals derived from the methylated and nonmethylated template DNA, the relative amount of methylation was calculated with EpiTYPER software (Agena Bioscience, San Diego, CA, USA). The signal peaks with overlapping and duplicate units were eliminated in the calculations. The second method was used for the low-density CpG areas. Specific primers for PCR amplicons covering the CpG site were designed with MassARRAY Assay Design software (Agena Bioscience, San Diego, CA, USA). After multiplex amplification and extension of the bisulfite-treated DNA in a single reaction and processing in the MassARRAY system, the methylation data of the individual CpG sites were generated with the TyperAnalyzer software (Agena Bioscience, San Diego, CA, USA). Duplicate measurements with differences equal to or greater than 10% were discarded.

rs174570 was selected from the seven SNPs (rs102275, rs174546, rs174547, rs174550, rs174570, rs1535, and rs174583) that were significantly associated with FFA metabolism and genotyped in DNA samples from the visceral adipose tissues of 42 participants using 3500 Genetic Analyzer (Applied Biosystem, Foster City, CA, USA).

Statistical analysis

Data are presented as the mean ± SD or median (interquartile range). Variables with skewed distribution were appropriately transformed before analyses. The Hardy–Weinberg equilibrium was tested before the association analysis, and all seven SNPs were in accordance with the Hardy–Weinberg equilibrium (all $P > 0.05$). Linkage disequilibrium analysis was performed in Haploview 4.2, relying on all individuals in the population, and was assessed with D' and r^2 values. For each fatty acid, the distribution of P values was evaluated using a quantile–quantile plot. The Q–Q plots for the nine most studied PUFAs are shown in Additional file 1: Figure S5. To explore the possible molecular mechanism of DNA methylation and gene expression in gene–nutrition interaction, we further conducted a series of pre-specified analyses based on biological plausibility and the literature. Linear regression analysis was used to estimate the associations of genotypes with fatty acid levels and mRNA expression with adjustments for age, sex, and BMI with PLINK 1.07. The effects of rs174570 on the DNA methylation levels of the CpG sites were analyzed using the Kruskal–Wallis H test. Pearson's correlation analysis was applied to test the correlation between mRNA expression and the methylation level.

Mediation analysis was performed to explore the relationship between the predictor and outcome variables and was achieved with the PROCESS procedure implemented in SPSS20.0 [25]. Bootstrap analyses (with 5000 resamples) were performed to test the significance of the differences in the predictor–outcome associations after adding a mediator as a covariate. A mediation effect was considered significant if 0 was not included in the bootstrap confidence interval. In our study, we established models relating rs174570 as a predictor to FADS1 and FADS2 gene expression outcome including DNA methylation as a covariate. Analyses were adjusted for age, sex,

and BMI. The model assumes no unmeasured confounding or modification effect between the included variables.

Statistical analyses were carried out using SAS 9.3 (SAS Institute, Cary, NC, USA) unless specified otherwise. Statistical significance was defined as a two-tailed $P < 0.05$.

Results

Identification of SNPs involved in fatty acid metabolism

To explore the potential effects of genetic variants on fatty acid metabolism, we tested the association of 32,387 SNPs that passed the QC standards with 42 fatty acids in 297 subjects. A total of 317 linear mixed models of SNP–fatty acid combinations reached significant P values of less than 10^{-4}. A cluster of seven SNPs in tight linkage disequilibrium (rs174546, rs174547, rs174550, rs174570, rs1535, rs174583, and rs102275) in one locus that was on chromosome 11, containing FADS1, FADS2, and C11orf10, was significantly associated with multiple serum fatty acid levels. Characteristics of the seven SNPs analyzed in the C11orf10/FADS1/FADS2 gene cluster were listed (Additional file 1: Table S3). Based on the high linkage disequilibrium of these seven SNPs ($r^2 = 0.98–1$, Additional file 1: Figure S6), rs174570 was selected in the next analysis due to differences in the allele frequencies among different ethnicities from the International HapMap project. We showed that the minor allele (T) of rs174570 was associated with lower levels of GLA, AA, and adrenic acid (ADA) in the ω-6 pathway and with lower levels of docosapentaenoic acid (DPA) and eicosapentaenoic acid (EPA) in the ω-3 pathway (all $P < 0.05$). GLA was the product of the D6D-catalyzed reaction, while AA and ADA in the ω-6 pathway and DPA and EPA in the ω-3 pathway served as D5D products. However, no associations were evident between rs174570 and other fatty acids (Fig. 1 and Additional file 1: Table S4). The Manhattan plots in Fig. 2 show the genome-wide associations of AA, GLA, and ADA. Moreover, using ratios of ω-6 PUFAs as proxies of desaturase activities, we confirmed that the minor allele of rs174570 was associated with lower D5D and D6D activities (Fig. 1).

Expression quantitative trait locus (eQTL) analysis of rs174570 on gene expression

To better understand the potential functional roles of the significant genetic variant, we performed eQTL analysis with adjustments for age, sex, and BMI to test the association of rs174570 with the mRNA levels of FADS1 and FADS2 in the visceral adipose tissues of 42 participants. As shown in Fig. 3, the FADS1 and FADS2 mRNA levels were significantly reduced in the TT carriers compared with the CC and TT carriers ($P = 0.001$, $\beta \pm SE = -0.142 \pm 0.040$ for FADS1; $P = 0.016$, $\beta \pm SE = -0.094 \pm 0.037$ for FADS2). These data suggest that rs174570 is a strong eQTL and that the observed decrease in

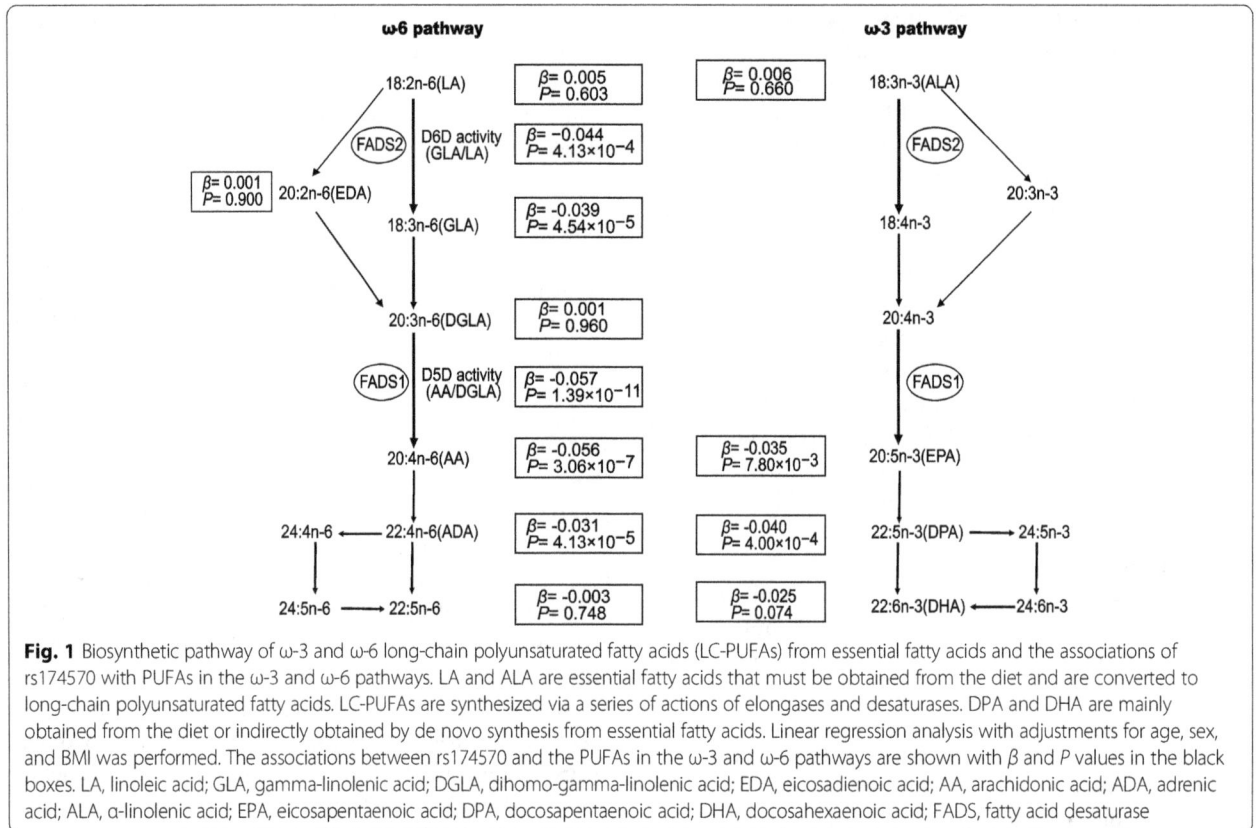

Fig. 1 Biosynthetic pathway of ω-3 and ω-6 long-chain polyunsaturated fatty acids (LC-PUFAs) from essential fatty acids and the associations of rs174570 with PUFAs in the ω-3 and ω-6 pathways. LA and ALA are essential fatty acids that must be obtained from the diet and are converted to long-chain polyunsaturated fatty acids. LC-PUFAs are synthesized via a series of actions of elongases and desaturases. DPA and DHA are mainly obtained from the diet or indirectly obtained by de novo synthesis from essential fatty acids. Linear regression analysis with adjustments for age, sex, and BMI was performed. The associations between rs174570 and the PUFAs in the ω-3 and ω-6 pathways are shown with β and P values in the black boxes. LA, linoleic acid; GLA, gamma-linolenic acid; DGLA, dihomo-gamma-linolenic acid; EDA, eicosadienoic acid; AA, arachidonic acid; ADA, adrenic acid; ALA, α-linolenic acid; EPA, eicosapentaenoic acid; DPA, docosapentaenoic acid; DHA, docosahexaenoic acid; FADS, fatty acid desaturase

desaturase activity is mediated by variant-dependent inhibition of *FADS1* and *FADS2* expression.

Methylation quantitative trait locus (mQTL) analysis of rs174570 on DNA methylation levels

To examine whether genetic variation was associated with DNA methylation levels in the human visceral fatty tissues, three regions (region1, region2, and region3) were selected for mQTL analysis. Region1 and region3 were selected due to the inclusion of two CpG islands (CGI1 and CGI2, respectively), each covering the first exons of *FADS1* and *FADS2*, respectively, with potential promoter activity (Fig. 4). Region2 with putative enhancer activity was selected to validate the results of previous studies conducted by Floyd H. Chilton et al. [26, 27]. These authors showed that the DNA methylation levels of multiple CpG sites in this region were associated with rs174537. A total of 27 CpG sites in region1 covering 4.2 kb, 8 CpG sites in region2 covering 1 kb, and 28 CpG sites in region3 covering 5.2 kb passed QC and were selected for further analysis. As shown in Fig. 4 (F, G), distinct patterns of the methylation levels were observed for CpG sites in the genome, with lower methylation levels for CpG sites in potential promoters than in other regions. Then, we compared the DNA methylation levels of the different groups according to the rs174570 genotype. The methylation levels of CpG sites CpG_9, CpG_10, CpG_11, and CpG_12 in region1 and

CpG_1 in region2 were significantly higher in the TT genotype group than in the CC and CT genotype groups ($P < 0.05$), while the CpG methylation levels of sites CpG_2, CpG_3, and CpG_4 in region3 were significantly lower in the TT group than in the CC and CT groups ($P < 0.05$). However, the methylation levels at the other sites, including four CpG sites (chr11:61587979, 61588092, 61588096, and 61588188 based on genome build GRCh37/hg19) that were found to be associated with rs174537 in another study, did not significantly differ ($P > 0.05$ for all). Consistent with the previous data suggesting that clusters of adjacent CpG sites are co-regulated, we showed that rs174570 had a directionally consistent effect on methylation levels at four CpG sites in *FADS1* and three CpG sites in *FADS2*. Table 2 provides an overview of the eight CpG sites, summarizing the location information and sequences around the CpG sites in the genome.

Correlation analysis of DNA methylation levels with gene expression

Then, we tested the correlations between gene expression and the DNA methylation levels of the eight CpG sites that were confirmed to be significantly associated with rs174570. We found that three CpG sites in region1 (CpG_9, CpG_10, and CpG_11) and two CpG sites (CpG_2 and CpG_3) in region3 were significantly associated with both *FADS1* and *FADS2* expression. However,

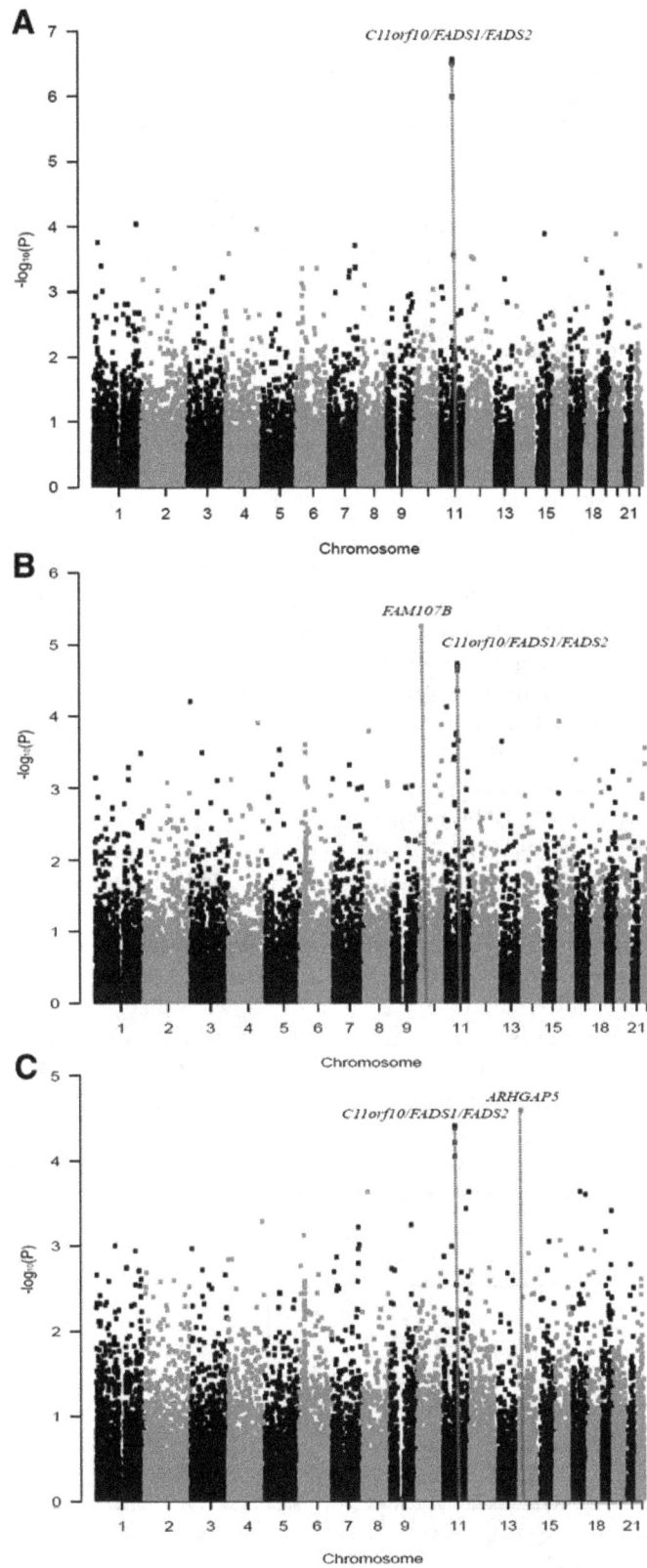

Fig. 2 (See legend on next page.)

(See figure on previous page.)
Fig. 2 Genome-wide Manhattan plot for arachidonic acid (**a**), gamma-linolenic acid (**b**), and adrenic acid (**c**). Plots of $-\log_{10}(P)$ values for associations tested by linear regression analysis with adjustments for age, sex, and BMI under an additive genetic model against fatty acid levels across the entire autosomal genome are shown. The red dots at each locus indicate the signals with $P < 10^{-4}$ detected in the genome-wide analysis. A total of 32,387 SNPs was used to generate the plots. FADS, fatty acid desaturase; ARHGAP5, P190-B RhoGAP; FAM107B, family with sequence similarity 107 member B

we did not observe a significant correlation between CpG_1 in region2 and gene expression. Notably, the *FADS1* and *FADS2* expression levels decreased with the increasing methylation levels of the three CpG sites in region1, while the *FADS1* and *FADS2* expression levels increased with the increasing methylation levels of the two CpG sites in region3 (Table 3).

Mediation analysis reveals that DNA methylation potentially mediates the genetic impact on mRNA expression

To investigate whether DNA methylation functioned as a mediator for the observed association between genotype and phenotype (gene expression), mediation analysis was conducted with the following two statistical criteria. First, the effect value of the original association was reduced with the addition of a potential mediator to the model. Second, the differences before and after the addition of the potential mediator were statistically significantly tested with a bootstrap analysis ($P < 0.05$). Bootstrap analysis was performed with DNA methylation levels at five CpG sites (CpG_9, CpG_10, and CpG_11 in region1 and CpG_2 and CpG_3 in region3) as the mediator, the genotyping of rs174570 as the independent variable, and the FADS1 or FADS2 expression levels as the dependent variable. Based on the two statistical criteria, we found that the differences before and after the addition of DNA methylation levels at CpG_9, CpG_10, CpG_2, or CpG_3 were significant for *FADS1* gene expression. However, only the difference in the regression coefficient with and without the addition of the CpG_2 methylation level was significant for *FADS2* gene expression (Table 4). These data demonstrate that the

DNA methylation levels of four CpG sites mediated the effect of rs174570 on *FADS1* gene expression, while only DNA methylation of one CpG site mediated the effect of rs174570 on *FADS2* gene expression.

Discussion

In this exome-wide association study of fatty acid levels in a Chinese population, we identified several strong signals on the *FADS* region and confirmed the associations of polymorphisms in FADS gene cluster with decreased GLA, AA, ADA, EPA, and DPA, but the strongest associations were with D5D activity in the ω-6 pathway. Long-chain ω-3 and ω-6 PUFAs, including AA, EPA, and DPA, are products of the ω-3 and ω-6 pathways that are converted from essential fatty acids (LA and ALA) by fatty acid desaturases and elongases (Fig. 1). AA is a precursor of multiple pro-inflammatory factors, including prostaglandin E2 and thromboxane A2 which have a harmful impact on the development of cardiovascular disease, while EPA improves biomarkers of inflammation and has a protective effect [28–30]. Thus, major allele (C) carriers with greater desaturase activity should have both pro-inflammatory and anti-inflammatory outcomes. Due to competition between ω-3 and ω-6 PUFAs for the same desaturases and due to the higher levels of LA intake than ALA intake in the modern Western diet, individuals with the CC genotype may be vulnerable to inflammatory disorders when consuming a diet that is rich in ω-6 fatty acids. Thus, CC carriers should consume a diet that is rich in ALA, which may reduce the synthesis of ω-6 PUFAs, or adopt a diet containing more EPA and docosahexaenoic acid (DHA), which directly balance AA.

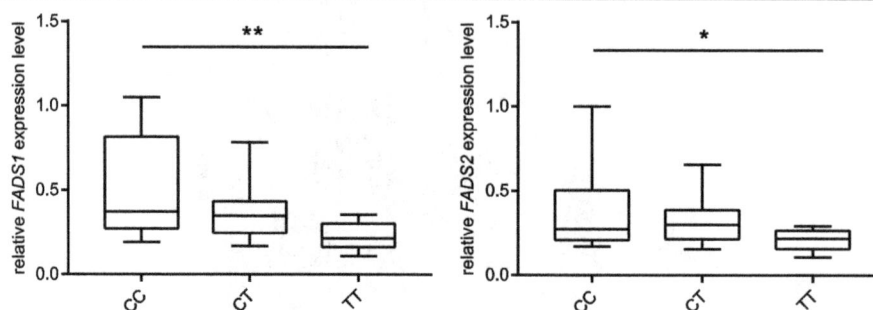

Fig. 3 The relative *FADS1* and *FADS2* mRNA levels of the CC ($n = 13$), CT ($n = 17$), and TT ($n = 12$) carriers at rs174570 were quantified by qPCR with *RPLP0* as the reference gene. For each box, the median is indicated by the band inside the box. The first and third quartiles are shown at the bottom and top of the box, respectively. **$P < 0.01$, *$P < 0.05$ tested by linear regression analysis with adjustments for age, sex, and BMI. FADS, fatty acid desaturase; RPLP0, ribosomal protein lateral stalk subunit P0

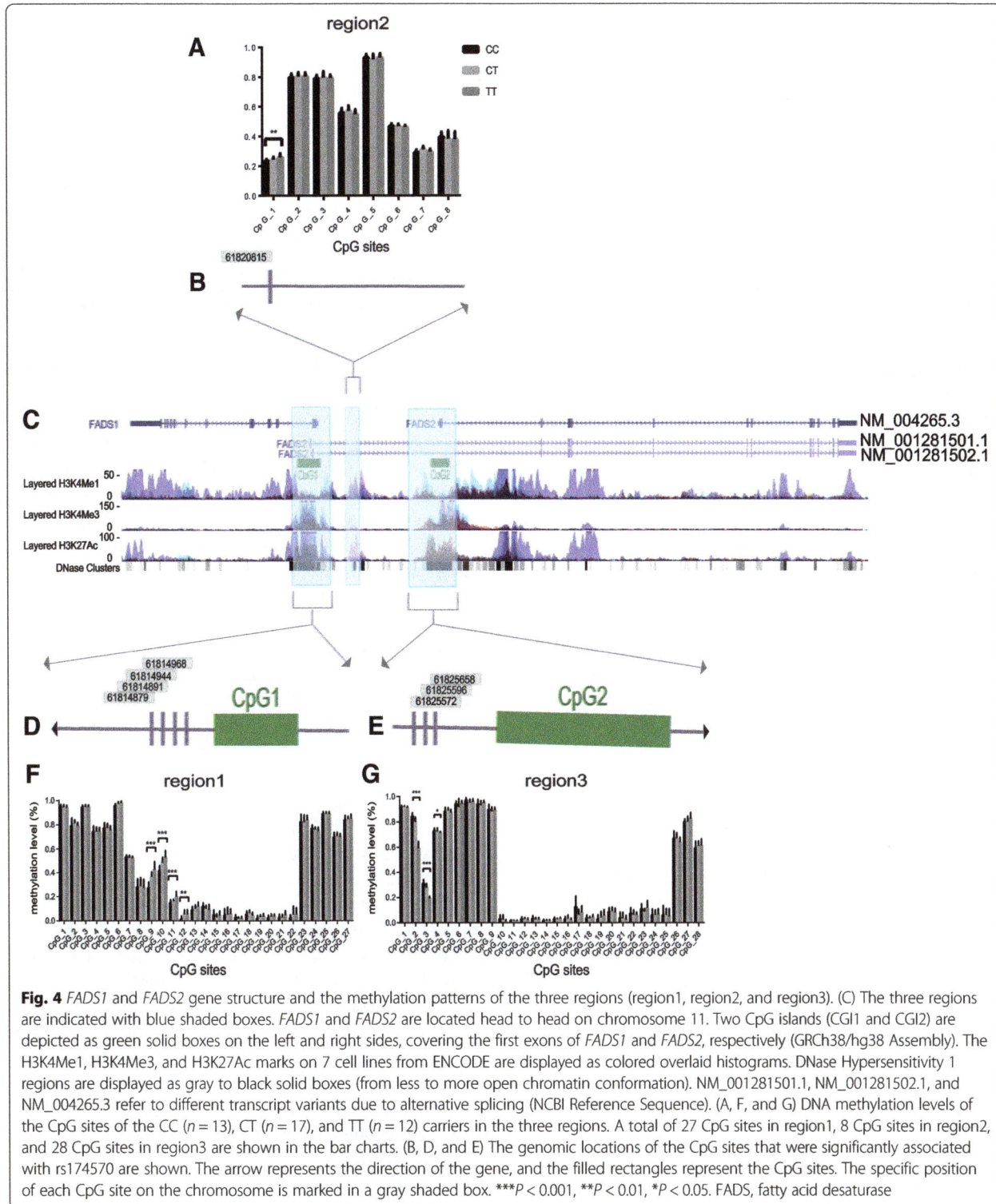

Fig. 4 *FADS1* and *FADS2* gene structure and the methylation patterns of the three regions (region1, region2, and region3). (C) The three regions are indicated with blue shaded boxes. *FADS1* and *FADS2* are located head to head on chromosome 11. Two CpG islands (CGI1 and CGI2) are depicted as green solid boxes on the left and right sides, covering the first exons of *FADS1* and *FADS2*, respectively (GRCh38/hg38 Assembly). The H3K4Me1, H3K4Me3, and H3K27Ac marks on 7 cell lines from ENCODE are displayed as colored overlaid histograms. DNase Hypersensitivity 1 regions are displayed as gray to black solid boxes (from less to more open chromatin conformation). NM_001281501.1, NM_001281502.1, and NM_004265.3 refer to different transcript variants due to alternative splicing (NCBI Reference Sequence). (A, F, and G) DNA methylation levels of the CpG sites of the CC ($n = 13$), CT ($n = 17$), and TT ($n = 12$) carriers in the three regions. A total of 27 CpG sites in region1, 8 CpG sites in region2, and 28 CpG sites in region3 are shown in the bar charts. (B, D, and E) The genomic locations of the CpG sites that were significantly associated with rs174570 are shown. The arrow represents the direction of the gene, and the filled rectangles represent the CpG sites. The specific position of each CpG site on the chromosome is marked in a gray shaded box. ***$P < 0.001$, **$P < 0.01$, *$P < 0.05$. FADS, fatty acid desaturase

Although numerous studies have focused on how polymorphisms in *FADS1* and *FADS2* alter fatty acid profiles or desaturase activity, few have investigated whether these polymorphisms regulate fatty acid metabolism by altering gene expression and epigenetic modifications in human tissues. By performing the eQTL and mQTL analyses in this study, we showed that rs174570 was associated with gene expression and methylation levels at multiple local CpG sites in the visceral adipose tissue. These results suggest that both

Table 2 Specific genomic information of CpG sites shown to be associated with the rs174570

Region	CpG site	Location	Sequence
Region1	CpG_9	Chr11: 61814879	GAAAGACCCGCAAGAAGGGA [CG]GAAGTCTCATAGCCCTGAGA
	CpG_10	Chr11: 61814891	AAGGGACTTATTGAAAGACC [CG]CAAGAAGGGACGGAAGTCTC
	CpG_11	Chr11: 61814944	CGTAGGGAAGTCTTCCTCTT [CG]TGGTTTTTGGAGAACCCTAG
	CpG_12	Chr11: 61814968	AACGCAGAAGTGCCCCAGTT [CG]GACGTAGGGAAGTCTTCCTC
Region2	CpG_1	Chr11: 61820815	CTTTGCCTCCTGGGTTCAAG [CG]ATTCTCCTGCCTCACCCCCA
Region3	CpG_2	Chr11: 61825572	AGGTTGCAGTGAGCTGAGAT [CG]CACCACTGCACTCCAGCCTG
	CpG_3	Chr11: 61825596	CCACTGCACTCCAGCCTGGG [CG]ACAGAGTGAGACCCTGTCTC
	CpG_4	Chr11: 61825658	GAAAAAGCCCTTTGGGAGGC [CG]AGGCAGGTGGATCACGAGGT

Region1, region2, and region3 indicate the selected regions used for DNA methylation analysis; sequence indicates 20 bp upstream and downstream of the CpG site in the genome (GRCh38/hg38 Assembly). *Chr* chromosome

DNA methylation and gene transcription may account for the association between genetic variants in the *FADS* region and different PUFA levels.

DNA methylation has long been considered an important regulator of gene expression, and DNA methylation levels of CpG sites in different regions may have different effects on gene expression [31, 32]. In our study, we observed a negative correlation between DNA methylation and gene expression in region1 with putative promoter activity. This is consistent with a previous concept that DNA methylation in promoter regions may suppress gene expression by affecting the physical access of transcription factors. However, the underlying mechanism has not been clarified. We used publicly available UCSC annotations (GRCh38/hg38 Assembly) to evaluate histone modification and transcription factor binding sites. The results from UCSC show that region1 is an active promoter site, as indicated by the tri-methylation of lysine 4 of the H3 histone protein. There are several transcription factor binding sites near our highlighted CpGs in region1, one of which, namely, SP1, has been shown to be involved in the regulation of *FADS1* expression by Pan et al. [33]. This study demonstrated that the

minor allele of rs174557, which was approximately 1 kb away from our highlighted CpGs, was associated with the activating complex of SP1 and sterol regulatory element-binding protein (SREBP1c), together decreasing *FADS1* expression level. SREBP1c is an important transcription factor that regulates *FADS* expression and has been investigated intensively [34, 35]. Thus, future studies are needed to determine whether SREBP1c or other factors play roles in the effect of DNA methylation on *FADS* expression. In contrast to methylation in promoter regions, gene-body methylation is not necessarily associated with repression. One major explanation may link DNA methylation to alternative splicing, and another possible mechanism may be that DNA methylation promotes more efficient transcriptional elongation of upstream promoters while simultaneously repressing spurious transcription from intragenic promoters [36–39]. Our data suggested a positive correlation of methylation levels at CpG sites in region3 with *FADS1* and *FADS2* expression. These data are consistent with a previous genome-wide study showing that 35.4% of the associations between gene expression and DNA methylation levels at intragenic CpGs in human pancreatic islets are positive. Notably, three transcript variants of *FADS2*, including NM_004265.3, NM_001281501.1, and NM_001281502.1, exist. The first transcript is the traditional isoform and is located downstream of the last two transcripts (Fig. 4). Thus, *FADS2* may have at least two TSSs, and the downstream start sites are within the "bodies" of the transcriptional units of the upstream promoters, providing a foundation for what we observed in our study.

In addition, we note that other studies conducted by Floyd H. Chilton et al. [26, 27] have focused on exploring the effects of genetic variation on DNA methylation and found a significant association between rs174537 and the methylation statuses of multiple CpG sites between *FADS1* and *FADS*. In our study, eight CpG sites in this region were selected for DNA methylation analysis and the methylation level of only one CpG site

Table 3 Correlations of DNA methylation levels with *FADS1* and *FADS2* gene expression

Region	CpG site	*FADS1* mRNA levels		*FADS2* mRNA levels	
		r	P^1	r	P^2
Region1	CpG_9	− 0.501	< 0.001	− 0.363	0.020
	CpG_10	− 0.527	< 0.001	− 0.420	0.006
	CpG_11	− 0.428	0.005	− 0.419	0.006
	CpG_12	− 0.157	0.328	− 0.085	0.600
Region2	CpG_1	− 0.134	0.397	− 0.118	0.456
Region3	CpG_2	0.548	< 0.001	0.478	0.001
	CpG_3	0.565	< 0.001	0.459	0.003
	CpG_4	0.200	0.2062	0.235	0.135

P^1 and P^2 separately indicate the correlation of DNA methylation of CpG site with *FADS1* or *FADS2* gene expression tested by Pearson's correlation analysis. *FADS* fatty acid desaturase

Table 4 Mediation effects of DNA methylation levels on the association between rs174570 and gene expression

Outcome	Total effect		Model	Direct effect		Bootstrap analysis	
	$\beta \pm SE$	P^1		$\beta \pm SE$	P^2	Boot LLCI	Boot ULCI
FADS1 mRNA level	-0.142 ± 0.040	0.001	Adjusted for CpG_9	-0.019 ± 0.068	0.782	*-0.264*	*-0.023*
			Adjusted for CpG_10	-0.066 ± 0.055	0.235	*-0.173*	*-0.014*
			Adjusted for CpG_11	-0.115 ± 0.054	0.042	-0.090	0.068
			Adjusted for CpG_2	0.002 ± 0.080	0.976	*-0.284*	*-0.005*
			Adjusted for CpG_3	0.043 ± 0.075	0.572	*-0.295*	*-0.047*
FADS2 mRNA level	-0.094 ± 0.037	0.016	Adjusted for CpG_9	0.002 ± 0.063	0.977	-0.217	0.004
			Adjusted for CpG_10	-0.038 ± 0.519	0.472	-0.162	0.004
			Adjusted for CpG_11	-0.055 ± 0.050	0.275	-0.103	0.032
			Adjusted for CpG_2	0.042 ± 0.074	0.571	*-0.265*	*-0.008*
			Adjusted for CpG_3	0.066 ± 0.070	0.350	-0.243	0.005

P^1 represents the total effect of rs174570 on *FADS1* or *FADS2* gene expression without adjustment for DNA methylation; P^2 represents the effect of rs174570 on *FADS1* or *FADS2* gene expression controlling for DNA methylation. A mediation effect was considered significant when 0 was not included in the bootstrap confidence interval. The characters shown in italics refer to a significant mediation effect. *Boot LLCI*, Boot low limit confidence interval; *Boot ULCI*, Boot upper limit confidence interval; *FADS*, fatty acid desaturase

(CpG_1 in region2) was associated with rs174570. However, Floyd H. Chilton et al. [26, 27] did not find an association between rs174537 and the methylation level of CpG_1. The reason for the lack of association between rs174570 and the methylation levels at the CpG sites identified in the other study may have been that the different SNPs from different races were used in the two studies (rs174537 from European Americans and African Americans in the other study versus rs174570 from a Chinese population in our study). Furthermore, the authors in the other study did not identify the CpG sites that were shown to be statistically significant in our study. Indeed, the Illumina HumanMethylation450 array covers less than 2% of the estimated 30 million CpG sites in the human genome [40]. Among the 63 CpG sites analyzed in our study, only one CpG site (CpG_16 in region3) was assessed with the 450K array. These results suggest that studies focusing on methylation levels of CpG sites in potential regulatory elements are potent complement for global DNA methylation studies to identify novel CpG sites that are associated with related phenotypes. In addition, we did not observe a correlation between the DNA methylation level of CpG_1 in region2 and gene expression in our study, which was not shown in studies conducted by Floyd H. Chilton et al. [26, 27]. Thus, further studies in different populations are needed to elucidate whether the DNA methylation levels of CpG sites in this region contribute to variations in gene expression.

We performed mediation analysis to investigate the potential mediator effect of methylation on the relationship between rs174570 and gene expression. Mediation analysis has been used in several studies to evaluate the mediation effect of DNA methylation levels on interactions between predictor and outcome variables [41, 42].

In this study, we identified DNA methylation levels at several CpG sites as mediators by applying this approach. However, not all significant CpG sites that were associated with both rs174570 and gene expression mediated the genetic effect on expression. These results suggest that DNA methylation is not the only pathway explaining the association between rs174570 and gene expression.

In addition to the observation that genetic variants of *FADS* cluster exerted an effect on gene expression by changing DNA methylation levels, substantial evidence suggests that dietary supplementation can modulate DNA methylation status of *FADS* gene cluster that affect gene transcription [43, 44]. These findings suggest that epigenetics may serve as a common pathway mediating both the genetic and environmental effect on gene function and as an underlying mechanism for gene–environment interaction, which are now recognized as an important implication for complex phenotypes [45, 46]. It is possible that genetically controlled methylation sites are sensitive to environmental changes and can serve as mediators of disease susceptibility [47]. Thus, understanding the impact of polymorphisms on the epigenetics provides instruction on early dietary interventions to modify long-term disease risk. However, it is still not clear whether DNA methylation status of *FADS* gene cluster conveys the information from gene–environment interactions to specific disease disorders. Clinical trials on investigating the effect of nutrition intake on DNA methylation with the consideration of genotypes are urgently needed.

The limitation of our study was that we did not consider the effect of dietary fatty acids on DNA methylation. There is growing evidence that complex interactions among food components and genetic factors lead to a dynamic modification of DNA methylation that controls the phenotype [48, 49]. However, we did not have the relevant data for dietary fatty acid intake in this study, and thus, we could not evaluate the effects of dietary fatty acids on DNA methylation.

Conclusions

Overall, our results support that DNA methylation and gene regulation have important implications for the interpretation of the effects of noncoding sequence variations on phenotypic outcomes. Further studies are needed to investigate how rs174570 in the intronic region of *FADS2* influences DNA methylation and to uncover the mechanisms underlying the specific effects of DNA methylation on *FADS1* and *FADS2* expression.

Abbreviations

AA: Arachidonic acid; ADA: Adrenic acid; D5D: δ-5 Desaturase; D6D: δ-6 Desaturase; DGLA: Dihomo-gamma-linolenic acid; DPA: Docosapentaenoic acid; eQTL: Expression quantitative trait locus; FADS: Fatty acid desaturase; GLA: Gamma-linolenic acid; GWASs: Genome-wide association studies; LA: Linoleic acid; mQTL: Methylation quantitative trait locus; MUFAs: Monounsaturated fatty acids; QC: Quality control; SHOS: Shanghai Obesity Study; SNPs: Single-nucleotide polymorphisms; SREBP1c: Sterol regulatory element-binding protein; TFAs: Trans-fatty acids

Acknowledgements

We would like to thank our participants and staff in this study for the valuable contributions.

Funding

This work was supported by grants from the National Key Research and Development Project of China [2016YFA0502003], National Natural Science Foundation of China grants [81570713, 91649112], Outstanding Academic Leaders of Shanghai Health System [2017BR008], National Program for Support of Top-notch Young Professionals, Yangtze River Scholar, and Shanghai Municipal Education Commission-Gaofeng Clinical Medicine Grant Support [20152527].

Authors' contributions

CH and Weiping J designed the research; ZH, BX, TW, FJ, and RZ conducted the research; AZ and Wei J collected and interpreted the data. ZH, LJ, and HZ analyzed the data; ZH was a major contributor in writing the manuscript. CH had primary responsibility for the final content. All authors read and approved the final manuscript.

Author details

[1]Shanghai Diabetes Institute, Shanghai Key Laboratory of Diabetes Mellitus, Shanghai Clinical Center for Diabetes, Shanghai Jiao Tong University Affiliated Sixth People's Hospital, 600 Yishan Road, Shanghai 200233, China. [2]Institute for Metabolic Diseases, Fengxian Central Hospital, The Third School of Clinical Medicine, Southern Medical University, Shanghai, China. [3]Shanghai Key Laboratory of Diabetes Mellitus and Center for Translational Medicine, Shanghai Jiao Tong University Affiliated Sixth People's Hospital, Shanghai, China. [4]National Clinical Research Center of Kidney Diseases, Jinling Hospital, Nanjing University School of Medicine, Nanjing, China.

References

1. Tvrzicka E, Kremmyda LS, Stankova B, Zak A. Fatty acids as biocompounds: their role in human metabolism, health and disease--a review. Part 1: classification, dietary sources and biological functions. Biomed Pap Med Fac Univ Palacky Olomouc Czech Repub. 2011;155:117–30.
2. Kremmyda LS, Tvrzicka E, Stankova B, Zak A. Fatty acids as biocompounds: their role in human metabolism, health and disease: a review. Part 2: fatty acid physiological roles and applications in human health and disease. Biomed Pap Med Fac Univ Palacky Olomouc Czech Repub. 2011;155:195–218.
3. Saglimbene VM, Wong G, Ruospo M, Palmer SC, Campbell K, Larsen VG, et al. Dietary n-3 polyunsaturated fatty acid intake and all-cause and cardiovascular mortality in adults on hemodialysis: the DIET-HD multinational cohort study. Clin Nutr. 2017; https://doi.org/10.1016/j.clnu.2017.11.020.
4. Alfaddagh A, Elajami TK, Ashfaque H, Saleh M, Bistrian BR, Welty FK. Effect of eicosapentaenoic and docosahexaenoic acids added to statin therapy on coronary artery plaque in patients with coronary artery disease: a randomized clinical trial. J Am Heart Assoc. 2017;6:12.
5. Ma W, Wu JH, Wang Q, Lemaitre RN, Mukamal KJ, Djousse L, et al. Prospective association of fatty acids in the de novo lipogenesis pathway with risk of type 2 diabetes: the cardiovascular health study. Am J Clin Nutr. 2015;101:153–63.
6. Heydari B, Abdullah S, Pottala JV, Shah R, Abbasi S, Mandry D, et al. Effect of omega-3 acid ethyl esters on left ventricular remodeling after acute myocardial infarction: the OMEGA-REMODEL randomized clinical trial. Circulation. 2016;134:378–91.
7. Sun Q, Ma J, Campos H, Hankinson SE, Manson JE, Stampfer MJ, et al. A prospective study of trans fatty acids in erythrocytes and risk of coronary heart disease. Circulation. 2007;115:1858–65.
8. Harris WS, Shearer GC. Omega-6 fatty acids and cardiovascular disease: friend, not foe? Circulation. 2014;130:1562–4.
9. Ramsden CE, Hibbeln JR, Majchrzak SF, Davis JM. n-6 fatty acid-specific and mixed polyunsaturate dietary interventions have different effects on CHD risk: a meta-analysis of randomised controlled trials. Br J Nutr. 2010;104: 1586–600.
10. Ramsden CE, Zamora D, Leelarthaepin B, Majchrzak-Hong SF, Faurot KR, Suchindran CM, et al. Use of dietary linoleic acid for secondary prevention of coronary heart disease and death: evaluation of recovered data from the Sydney Diet Heart Study and updated meta-analysis. BMJ. 2013;346:e8707.
11. Farvid MS, Ding M, Pan A, Sun Q, Chiuve SE, Steffen LM, et al. Dietary linoleic acid and risk of coronary heart disease: a systematic review and meta-analysis of prospective cohort studies. Circulation. 2014;130:1568–78.
12. Wu JH, Lemaitre RN, Manichaikul A, Guan W, Tanaka T, Foy M, et al. Genome-wide association study identifies novel loci associated with concentrations of four plasma phospholipid fatty acids in the de novo lipogenesis pathway: results from the cohorts for heart and aging research in genomic epidemiology (CHARGE) consortium. Circ Cardiovasc Genet. 2013;6:171–83.
13. Tintle NL, Pottala JV, Lacey S, Ramachandran V, Westra J, Rogers A, et al. A genome-wide association study of saturated, mono- and polyunsaturated red blood cell fatty acids in the Framingham Heart Offspring Study. Prostaglandins Leukot Essent Fatty Acids. 2015;94:65–72.
14. Mozaffarian D, Kabagambe EK, Johnson CO, Lemaitre RN, Manichaikul A, Sun Q, et al. Genetic loci associated with circulating phospholipid trans fatty acids: a meta-analysis of genome-wide association studies from the CHARGE consortium. Am J Clin Nutr. 2015;101:398–406.
15. Volkov P, Olsson AH, Gillberg L, Jorgensen SW, Brons C, Eriksson KF, et al. A genome-wide mQTL analysis in human adipose tissue identifies genetic variants associated with DNA methylation, gene expression and metabolic traits. PLoS One. 2016;11:e0157776.
16. Olsson AH, Volkov P, Bacos K, Dayeh T, Hall E, Nilsson EA, et al. Genome-wide associations between genetic and epigenetic variation influence mRNA expression and insulin secretion in human pancreatic islets. PLoS Genet. 2014;10:e1004735.
17. Gibbs JR, van der Brug MP, Hernandez DG, Traynor BJ, Nalls MA, Lai SL, et al. Abundant quantitative trait loci exist for DNA methylation and gene expression in human brain. PLoS Genet. 2010;6:e1000952.
18. Robertson KD. DNA methylation and human disease. Nat Rev Genet. 2005;6: 597–610.

19. Fraga MF, Ballestar E, Paz MF, Ropero S, Setien F, Ballestar ML, et al. Epigenetic differences arise during the lifetime of monozygotic twins. Proc Natl Acad Sci U S A. 2005;102:10604–9.

20. Zhao L, Ni Y, Ma X, Zhao A, Bao Y, Liu J, et al. A panel of free fatty acid ratios to predict the development of metabolic abnormalities in healthy obese individuals. Sci Rep. 2016;6:28418.

21. Bao Y, Ma X, Yang R, Wang F, Hao Y, Dou J, et al. Inverse relationship between serum osteocalcin levels and visceral fat area in Chinese men. J Clin Endocrinol Metab. 2013;98:345–51.

22. Liu F, Di J, Yu H, Han J, Bao Y, Jia W. Effect of Roux-en-Y gastric bypass on thyroid function in euthyroid patients with obesity and type 2 diabetes. Surg Obes Relat Dis. 2017;13:1701–7.

23. D'Avola A, Drennan S, Tracy I, Henderson I, Chiecchio L, Larrayoz M, et al. Surface IgM expression and function are associated with clinical behavior, genetic abnormalities, and DNA methylation in CLL. Blood. 2016;128:816–26.

24. Huang JY, Gavin AR, Richardson TS, Rowhani-Rahbar A, Siscovick DS, Hochner H, et al. Accounting for life-course exposures in epigenetic biomarker association studies: early life socioeconomic position, candidate gene DNA methylation, and adult cardiometabolic risk. Am J Epidemiol. 2016;184:520–31.

25. Preacher KJ, Hayes AF. Asymptotic and resampling strategies for assessing and comparing indirect effects in multiple mediator models. Behav Res Methods. 2008;40:879–91.

26. Rahbar E, Ainsworth HC, Howard TD, Hawkins GA, Ruczinski I, Mathias R, et al. Uncovering the DNA methylation landscape in key regulatory regions within the FADS cluster. PLoS One. 2017;12:e0180903.

27. Howard TD, Mathias RA, Seeds MC, Herrington DM, Hixson JE, Shimmin LC, et al. DNA methylation in an enhancer region of the FADS cluster is associated with FADS activity in human liver. PLoS One. 2014;9:e97510.

28. Skulas-Ray AC, Flock MR, Richter CK, Harris WS, West SG, Kris-Etherton PM. Red blood cell docosapentaenoic acid (DPA n-3) is inversely associated with triglycerides and C-reactive protein (CRP) in healthy adults and dose-dependently increases following n-3 fatty acid supplementation. Nutrients. 2015;7:6390–404.

29. Del Gobbo LC, Imamura F, Aslibekyan S, Marklund M, Virtanen JK, Wennberg M, et al. Omega-3 polyunsaturated fatty acid biomarkers and coronary heart disease: pooling project of 19 cohort studies. JAMA Intern Med. 2016;176:1155–66.

30. Nasrallah R, Hassouneh R, Hebert RL. PGE2, kidney disease, and cardiovascular risk: beyond hypertension and diabetes. J Am Soc Nephrol. 2016;27:666–76.

31. Jones PA. Functions of DNA methylation: islands, start sites, gene bodies and beyond. Nat Rev Genet. 2012;13:484–92.

32. Ehrlich M, Lacey M. DNA methylation and differentiation: silencing, upregulation and modulation of gene expression. Epigenomics. 2013;5:553–68.

33. Pan G, Ameur A, Enroth S, Bysani M, Nord H, Cavalli M, et al. PATZ1 down-regulates FADS1 by binding to rs174557 and is opposed by SP1/SREBP1c. Nucleic Acids Res. 2017;45:2408–22.

34. Nakamura MT, Nara TY. Gene regulation of mammalian desaturases. Biochem Soc Trans. 2002;30:1076–9.

35. Nakamura MT, Nara TY. Essential fatty acid synthesis and its regulation in mammals. Prostaglandins Leukot Essent Fatty Acids. 2003;68:145–50.

36. Shukla S, Kavak E, Gregory M, Imashimizu M, Shutinoski B, Kashlev M, et al. CTCF-promoted RNA polymerase II pausing links DNA methylation to splicing. Nature. 2011;479:74–9.

37. Maunakea AK, Nagarajan RP, Bilenky M, Ballinger TJ, D'Souza C, Fouse SD, et al. Conserved role of intragenic DNA methylation in regulating alternative promoters. Nature. 2010;466:253–7.

38. Lee SM, Choi WY, Lee J, Kim YJ. The regulatory mechanisms of intragenic DNA methylation. Epigenomics. 2015;7:527–31.

39. Lev Maor G, Yearim A, Ast G. The alternative role of DNA methylation in splicing regulation. Trends Genet. 2015;31:274–80.

40. Kato N, Loh M, Takeuchi F, Verweij N, Wang X, Zhang W, et al. Trans-ancestry genome-wide association study identifies 12 genetic loci influencing blood pressure and implicates a role for DNA methylation. Nat Genet. 2015;47:1282–93.

41. Cao-Lei L, Veru F, Elgbeili G, Szyf M, Laplante DP, King S. DNA methylation mediates the effect of exposure to prenatal maternal stress on cytokine production in children at age 13(1/2) years: Project Ice Storm. Clin Epigenetics. 2016;8:54.

42. Ma Y, Follis JL, Smith CE, Tanaka T, Manichaikul AW, Chu AY, et al. Interaction of methylation-related genetic variants with circulating fatty acids on plasma lipids: a meta-analysis of 7 studies and methylation analysis of 3 studies in the cohorts for heart and aging research in genomic epidemiology consortium. Am J Clin Nutr. 2016;103:567–78.

43. Hoile SP, Clarke-Harris R, Huang RC, Calder PC, Mori TA, Beilin LJ, et al. Supplementation with N-3 long-chain polyunsaturated fatty acids or olive oil in men and women with renal disease induces differential changes in the DNA methylation of FADS2 and ELOVL5 in peripheral blood mononuclear cells. PLoS One. 2014;9:e109896.

44. Karimi M, Vedin I, Freund Levi Y, Basun H, Faxen Irving G, Eriksdotter M, et al. DHA-rich n-3 fatty acid supplementation decreases DNA methylation in blood leukocytes: the OmegAD study. Am J Clin Nutr. 2017;106:1157–65.

45. Lu Y, Feskens EJ, Dolle ME, Imholz S, Verschuren WM, Muller M, et al. Dietary n-3 and n-6 polyunsaturated fatty acid intake interacts with FADS1 genetic variation to affect total and HDL-cholesterol concentrations in the Doetinchem Cohort Study. Am J Clin Nutr. 2010;92:258–65.

46. Park JY, Paik JK, Kim OY, Chae JS, Jang Y, Lee JH. Interactions between the APOA5-1131T>C and the FEN1 10154G>T polymorphisms on omega6 polyunsaturated fatty acids in serum phospholipids and coronary artery disease. J Lipid Res. 2010;51:3281–8.

47. Meaburn EL, Schalkwyk LC, Mill J. Allele-specific methylation in the human genome: implications for genetic studies of complex disease. Epigenetics. 2010;5:578–82.

48. Lai CQ, Smith CE, Parnell LD, Lee YC, Corella D, Hopkins P, et al. Epigenomics and metabolomics reveal the mechanism of the APOA2-saturated fat intake interaction affecting obesity. Am J Clin Nutr. 2018;108:188–200.

49. Sun D, Heianza Y, Li X, Shang X, Smith SR, Bray GA, et al. Genetic, epigenetic and transcriptional variations at NFATC2IP locus with weight loss in response to diet interventions: the POUNDS Lost Trial. Diabetes Obes Metab. 2018;20:2298–303.

21

Epigenetic regulation of MAGE family in human cancer progression-DNA methylation, histone modification, and non-coding RNAs

Yishui Lian[1†], Lingjiao Meng[1,2†], Pingan Ding[1] and Meixiang Sang[1,2*] (iD)

Abstract

The melanoma antigen gene (MAGE) proteins are a group of highly conserved family members that contain a common MAGE homology domain. Type I MAGEs are relevant cancer-testis antigens (CTAs), and originally considered as attractive targets for cancer immunotherapy due to their typically high expression in tumor tissues but restricted expression in normal adult tissues. Here, we reviewed the recent discoveries and ideas that illustrate the biological functions of MAGE family in cancer progression. Furthermore, we also highlighted the current understanding of the epigenetic mechanism of MAGE family expression in human cancers.

Keywords: MAGE, Epigenetics, Transcription regulator, E3 RING ubiquitin ligases

Background

The first member of the melanoma antigen gene (MAGE) was discovered in 1991, when Van der Bruggen et al. performed experiments to identify tumor antigens from melanoma cells [1]. The human MAGE family was divided into two categories in the light of their chromosomal location and expression pattern [2–4]. Nowadays, MAGE family was well known as tumor-associated antigens and comprises more than 60 genes, which share a conserved MAGE homology domain (MHD) [5]. Type I MAGEs are relevant cancer-testis antigens (CTAs) which contain MAGE-A, -B and -C subfamily members [6], and therefore are rarely expressed in normal adult tissues, but highly expressed in various cancers, including melanoma, breast cancer, prostate cancer, lung adenocarcinoma, esophageal squamous cell carcinoma, gastric cancer, bladder cancer, ovarian cancer, hepatocellular carcinoma, and brain cancer [7–16]. Type II MAGEs contain the MAGE-D, -E, -F, -G, -H, -L, and necdin genes, which are not limited to the X chromosome and are expressed in various tissues, such as brain, embryonic, and adult tissues [2–4].

MAGE family has specific functions in normal development and tumor progression. Type I MAGEs express normally only in testis or placenta, and their restricted expression suggests that they may function in germ cell development. Many studies have consistently showed that MAGE-A family may play an important role in spermatogenesis and embryonic development [4]. MAGE-B4 was found to be expressed during premeiotic germ cell differentiation, indicating that MAGE proteins may also play a role in developing oocytes [17]. MAGE-A proteins were detected by immunohistochemistry in the early development of the central nervous system (CNS) and the spinal cord and brainstem of peripheral nerves, revealing that MAGE-A protein was also involved in neuronal development [18]. Type II MAGEs are highly expressed in the brain and participate in various neural processes. These MAGE proteins might perform important functions in differentiation and neurodevelopment, thus their loss of function leads to a range of cognitive, behavioral, and developmental defects [4]. However, the biological functions and underlying regulatory mechanism of MAGE family expression in cancer is still not fully understood. The

* Correspondence: mxsang@hotmail.com
†Yishui Lian and Lingjiao Meng contributed equally to this work.
[1]Research Center, the Fourth Affiliated Hospital of Hebei Medical University, Shijiazhuang 050017, Hebei, People's Republic of China
[2]Tumor Research Institute, the Fourth Affiliated Hospital of Hebei Medical University, Shijiazhuang 050017, Hebei, People's Republic of China

known tumor-related functions of MAGE family were summarized in Table 1.

In this review, we summarized these exciting advances and discoveries concerning the biological functions of MAGE family in cancer progression. We also take a comprehensive look at the current understanding of the epigenetic mechanism of MAGE family expression in human cancers. This provides an outlook on cancer therapeutic approaches that target MAGE family.

Biological functions of MAGEs in cancer progression

MAGEs function as regulators of E3 RING ubiquitin ligases

Some studies have explored the function of MAGE proteins in cancer cells, and they were observed to promote cancer cell survival, tumor formation, and metastasis [19, 20]. Members of all type I MAGE protein families promoted tumor cell viability and inhibited cell apoptosis, therefore providing a growth advantage to melanoma and other malignancies [21]. MAGE-A3 and A6 were critical for cancer cell survival, and MAGE-A3/6-TRIM28 E3 ubiquitin ligase complex was found to degrade AMPKα1 resulting in downregulating AMPK signaling during tumorigenesis [22].

Recently, multiple MAGE proteins were found to form complexes with RING domain proteins, such as MAGE-A2/C2-TRIM28, MAGE-B18-LNX, MAGE-G1-NSE1 complexes, etc. [23, 24]. RING domain is a cysteine-rich domain that normally forms a cross-brace structure that typically coordinates two zinc ions [25]. RING domain proteins are proved to be a big E3 ubiquitin ligase family, which bind to and localize E2 ubiquitin-conjugating enzymes to substrates for ubiquitylation [26, 27]. MAGE proteins bind directly to RING domain proteins and act as scaffold of RING domain proteins to their substrates, thus regulating the ubiquitin ligase activity of RING domain proteins (Fig. 1). In particular, MAGE-A2, -A3, -A6, and -C2 were found to bind TRIM28, also known as KAP1, TIF-1beta or Krip125, therefore inducing the degradation of tumor suppressor p53 [23]. Recently, Potts and their colleagues reported MAGE-A3/6-TRIM28 complex ubiquitinates and degrades the tumor suppressor AMPKα1, thus leading to the inhibition of autophagy and activation of mTOR signaling [22, 28]. MAGE I binding to KAP1 induced the poly-ubiquitination and degradation of the substrate ZNF382 [29]. ZNF382 is one of KRAB domain zinc finger transcription factors (KZNFs) family member, which is involved in cell apoptosis and tumor suppression [30]. KZNFs bind the KAP1 protein and direct KAP1 to specific DNA sequences where it suppresses gene expression by inducing localized herterochromatin characterized by histone 3 lysine 9 trimethylation (H3K9me3). The binding of MAGE to KAP1 induces the degradation of ZNF382 leading to the decreased KAP1 binding to ID1 and the increased expression of

oncogene ID1 [29]. Thus, it appears that cancer-specific up-regulation of MAGE family triggers ubiquitination and degradation of multiple tumor suppressors, such as p53, AMPKα1, and ZNF382 through binding to RING domain protein KAP1, promoting tumorigenesis and aggressive growth. Therefore, identification of novel small molecules that inhibit protein–protein interactions between MAGE and KAP1 may be a potential therapeutic strategy for cancer-bearing MAGE expression [31].

RING-box protein 1 (Rbx1), another RING domain containing protein, is a RING component of the largest E3 ligases SCF complex [32]. SCF complex consists of Rbx1, Cullin1, Skp1, and F-box protein family, and degradation of SCF-dependent proteolysis can cause a variety of diseases including cancer [32–34]. MAGE-C2 binds directly to Rbx1 and inhibits ubiquitin-dependent degradation of cyclin E, and promotes melanoma cell cycle progression at G1-S transition [35]. In addition, MAGE-A2 was reported to associate with MDM2, a RING finger-type E3 ligase that mediates ubiquitylation of more than 20 substrates including mainly p53, MDM2 itself, and MDM4. And the interaction of MAGE-A2 with MDM2 inhibits the E3 ubiquitin ligase activity of MDM2, thus increasing the level of MDM4. However, it does not affect p53 turnover mediated by MDM2 [36]. MAGE-A11 interacts with Skp2, the substrate recognition protein of the Skp1-Cullin1-F-box E3 ubiquitin ligase, and increases Skp2-mediated degradation of cyclin A and p130, but decreases Skp2-mediated degradation of E2F1 and Skp2 self-ubiquitination by sequestering and inactivating Skp2 via forming an E2F1-MAGE-A11-Skp2 complex [37].

MAGEs function as transcriptional regulators

The binding of MAGE-C2 to KAP1 increases the interaction between KAP1 and ATM, and increased KAP1-Ser824 phosphorylation. Therefore, MAGE-C2 may promote tumor growth by phosphorylation of KAP1-Ser824 and the enhancement of DNA damage repair [38]. KAP1 seems to function as a molecular scaffold that coordinates at least four activities necessary for gene-specific silencing, including (a) targeting of specific promoters through the KRAB protein zinc finger motifs; (b) promotion of histone deacetylation via the NuRD/histone deacetylase complex; (c) histone H3-K9 methylation via SETDB1; and (d) recruitment of HP1 protein [39]. KAP1 also regulates DNA repair through the phosphorylation of KAP1-Serine 824 (Ser824) by ataxia telangicctasia-mutated (ATM) kinase [40] (Fig. 2-1). As a scaffolding protein, KAP1 interacts with p53 and acts as a co-repressor of p53 expression and function. MAGE suppression decreases KAP1 complexing with p53, increases acetylation of p53, and activates p53 responsive reporter genes. Class I MAGE protein may promote tumor

Table 1 The known tumor-related functions of MAGE family

Type	Subtype	Gene name	Highly expressed tumor type	Biological functions
MAGE-I	MAGE-A	MAGE-A1	Melanoma; gastric cancer; endometrial cancer; esophageal squamous cell carcinoma; head and neck cancer	Activating p-C-JUN directly or through ERK-MAPK pathways; Repressing transcription by binding to SKIP and recruiting HDAC1
		MAGE-A2	Glioma; breast cancer	Degradation of P53, MDM2, MDM4; Increasing ER-dependent signaling
		MAGE-A3	Non-small-cell lung cancer; hepatocellular carcinoma	Degradation of P53, AMPKα1; Enhancing TRIM28-dependent degradation of FBP1
		MAGE-A4	Hepatocellular carcinoma; lung cancer	Inactivate the oncoprotein gankyrin
		MAGE-A5	Head and neck cancer; non-small-cell lung cancer	Not well characterized
		MAGE-A6	Breast, colon, and lung cancer	Degradation of P53, AMPKα1
		MAGE-A7	Non-small-cell lung cancer	Not well characterized
		MAGE-A8	Bladder cancer	Not well characterized
		MAGE-A9	Head and neck cancer; hepatocellular carcinoma; esophageal squamous cell carcinoma; breast, colorectal, lung, bladder cancer	Not well characterized
		MAGE-A10	Breast cancer; stomach cancer; melanoma; esophageal and head and neck squamous carcinoma; bladder, lung, hepatocellular carcinoma	Not well characterized
		MAGE-A11	Breast cancer; esophageal squamous cell carcinoma; head and neck cancer; non-small cell lung cancer; prostate cancer	Increasing Skp2-mediated degradation of cyclin A and p130; Decreasing Skp2-mediated degradation of E2F1 and Skp2 self-ubiquitination; Increasing the AR transcriptional activity
		MAGE-A12	Prostatic carcinoma and colorectal cancer; melanoma, bladder, lung, esophageal carcinoma; head and neck cancer	Promoting the ubiquitination of p21
	MAGE-B	MAGE-B1	Hepatocellular carcinoma	Not well characterized
		MAGE-B2	Hepatocellular carcinoma	Not well characterized
		MAGE-B3	Colorectal cancer	Not well characterized
		MAGE-B4–18	Not well characterized	Not well characterized
	MAGE-C	MAGE-C1	Cutaneous melanoma; breast, lung cancer	Not well characterized
		MAGE-C2	Hepatocellular carcinoma; breast, lung cancer; melanoma; gastrointestinal stromal tumors	Enhancing TRIM28-dependent degradation of FBP1; Inhibiting degradation of cyclinE; Increasing KAP1-Ser824 phosphorylation
		MAGE-C3–7	Not well characterized	Not well characterized
MAGE-II	MAGE-D	MAGE-D1	Breast cancer	Not well characterized
		MAGE-D2	Melanoma; gastric, colorectal cancer; hepatocellular carcinoma	Suppressing TRAIL-induced apoptosis
		MAGE-D3	Not well characterized	Not well characterized
		MAGE-D4	Glioma; hepatocellular carcinoma Colorectal, esophageal, lung cancer	Not well characterized
	MAGE-E	MAGE-E1	Glioma	Not well characterized
		MAGE-E2–3	Not well characterized	Not well characterized
	MAGE-F	MAGE-F1	Colorectal, ovarian, breast, cervical cancer; melanoma and leukemia	Not well characterized
	MAGE-G	MAGE-G1	Not well characterized	Not well characterized
	MAGE-H	MAGE-H1	Breast cancer; colorectal cancer	Upregulating mir-200a/b expression via association with p73
	MAGE-L2	MAGE-L2	Not well characterized	Not well characterized
	NECDIN	NECDIN	Melanoma, prostate and breast cancer; leukemia; urothelial carcinoma	Repression in a STAT3-dependent manner

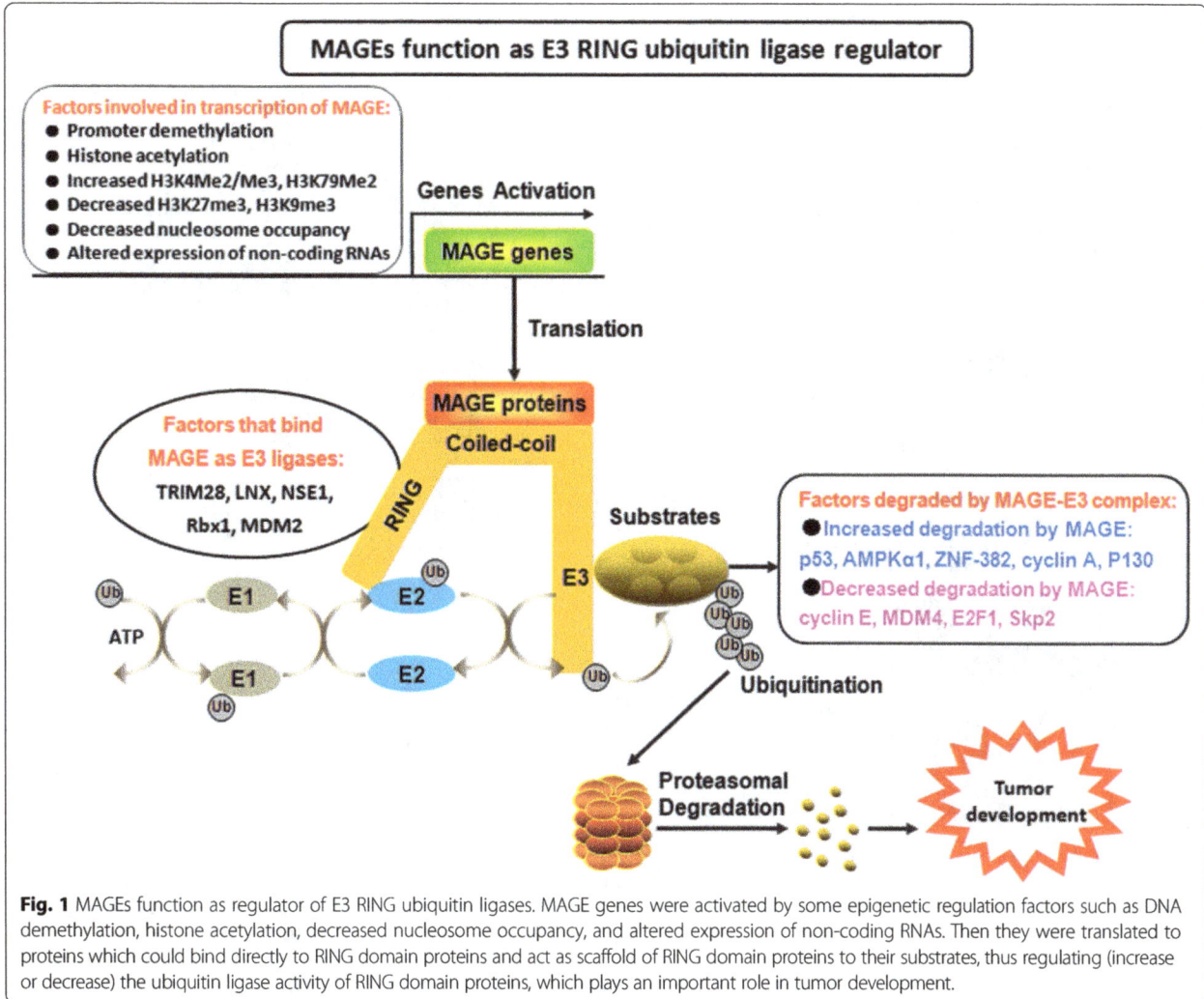

Fig. 1 MAGEs function as regulator of E3 RING ubiquitin ligases. MAGE genes were activated by some epigenetic regulation factors such as DNA demethylation, histone acetylation, decreased nucleosome occupancy, and altered expression of non-coding RNAs. Then they were translated to proteins which could bind directly to RING domain proteins and act as scaffold of RING domain proteins to their substrates, thus regulating (increase or decrease) the ubiquitin ligase activity of RING domain proteins, which plays an important role in tumor development.

development at least in part through inhibiting p53 activation [21]. In addition, MAGE-A proteins can directly interact with p53. This direct interaction may occlude the binding of p53 to p53-responsive promoters, lead to the decreased p53-dependent transcription, cell cycle arrest, and apoptosis [41]. In multiple myeloma, the interaction of MAGE-A proteins with p53 was shown to inhibit apoptosis through repression of bax and stabilization of survivin [42]. MAGE-A proteins also inhibit p53 transcription functions, at least in part by recruiting HDAC3 to the binding sites of p53 promoter, leading to resistance to anti-tumor agents [43]. MAGE-A1 was reported to repress transcription through binding to ski interacting protein (SKIP), a transcription regulator, and recruiting HDAC1 [44]. Through forming complex with p53 and estrogen receptor α (ERα), MAGE-A2 represses p53 pathway and increases ER-dependent signaling, therefore contributing to tamoxifen-resistance of ER-positive breast cancer [45] (Fig. 2-2).

MAGE-A11 was found to play a crucial role in the androgen receptor (AR) signaling network in prostate cancer. MAGE-A11 forms a complex with AR by binding NH2-terminal FXXLF motif of AR and increases the AR transcriptional activity by modulating AR interdomain interaction [46, 47]. The increased expression of MAGE-11 facilitates prostate cancer progression by enhancing AR-dependent tumor growth [48]. Epidermalgrowth factor (EGF) stabilizes the AR-MAGE-A11 complex and increases androgen-dependent AR transcription activity through the site-specific phosphorylation of Thr-360, and subsequent ubiquitinylation of Lys-240 and Lys-245 within MAGE homology domain [49]. Further studies showed that the interaction between AR and MAGE-A11 is mediated by AR NH2-terminal FXXLF motif binding to a highly conserved MAGE-A11 F-box (residues 329-369) in the MAGE homology domain, and that the interaction is modulated by serum stimulation of mitogen-activated protein kinase phosphorylation of MAGE-A11 Ser-174 [50] (Fig. 2-3). In

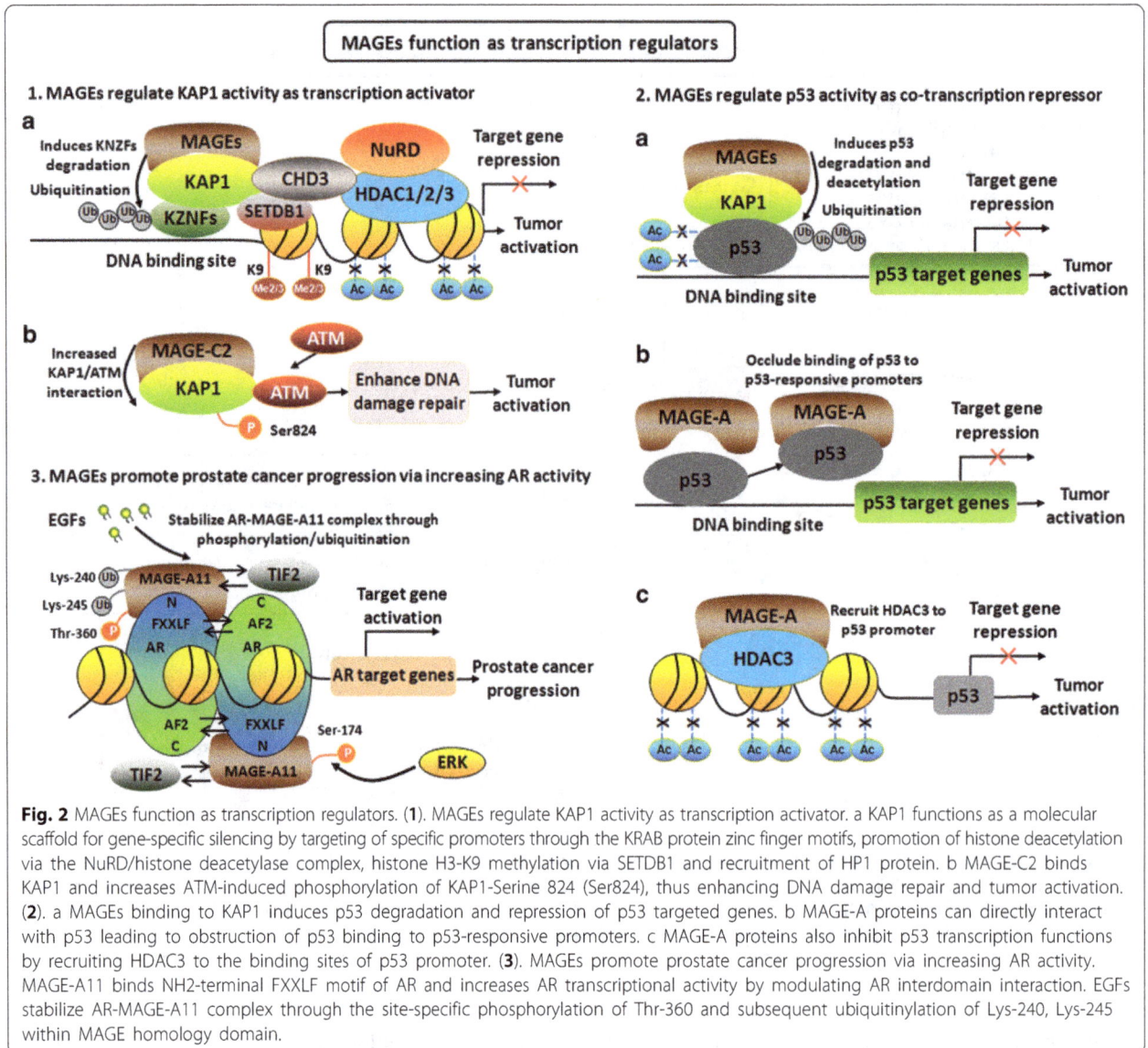

Fig. 2 MAGEs function as transcription regulators. (**1**). MAGEs regulate KAP1 activity as transcription activator. a KAP1 functions as a molecular scaffold for gene-specific silencing by targeting of specific promoters through the KRAB protein zinc finger motifs, promotion of histone deacetylation via the NuRD/histone deacetylase complex, histone H3-K9 methylation via SETDB1 and recruitment of HP1 protein. b MAGE-C2 binds KAP1 and increases ATM-induced phosphorylation of KAP1-Serine 824 (Ser824), thus enhancing DNA damage repair and tumor activation. (**2**). a MAGEs binding to KAP1 induces p53 degradation and repression of p53 targeted genes. b MAGE-A proteins can directly interact with p53 leading to obstruction of p53 binding to p53-responsive promoters. c MAGE-A proteins also inhibit p53 transcription functions by recruiting HDAC3 to the binding sites of p53 promoter. (**3**). MAGEs promote prostate cancer progression via increasing AR activity. MAGE-A11 binds NH2-terminal FXXLF motif of AR and increases AR transcriptional activity by modulating AR interdomain interaction. EGFs stabilize AR-MAGE-A11 complex through the site-specific phosphorylation of Thr-360 and subsequent ubiquitinylation of Lys-240, Lys-245 within MAGE homology domain.

addition, MAGE-A11 also functions as a transcriptional coregulator through interacting with progesterone receptor (PR), steroid receptor-associated p300 and p160 coactivators, and contributes to cell cycle progression through interacting with p107 and E2F1 transcription factors which are important for cell cycle progression and induction of apoptosis [51, 52].

Epigenetic regulation of MAGE family in cancer

As a CTA subfamily, type I MAGE-A gene expression is restricted to cancer cells and testis. However, the precise regulatory mechanisms of MAGE family expression are still not fully understood. Epigenetic regulation seems to play an important role in MAGE expression.

DNA methylation plays critical role in the regulation of MAGEs expression

Contrary to the high homology of MAGE genes, their promoters are less homologous. These promoter regions contain some binding sites for the transcription factors. The hypermethylation of these sites may be involved in the silence of MAGE genes. For example, the promoter of MAGE-A1 gene contains binding sites for the transcription factors Ets and Sp1, whereby the Ets proteins are responsible for the high transcriptional activation. The hypermethylation of CpG dinucleotides on the MAGE-A promoters may prevent the binding of these activators to their motif, and consequently inhibiting the promoter activity [53, 54]. MAGE-A1 promoter was reported to be highly methylated in somatic tissues. In contrast, it is largely unmethylated in male germ cells and in tumor cells that express this gene [55]. Moreover, the expression of MAGE-A1 can be induced by the demethylating agents in cells that do not express this gene. These observations suggested that DNA methylation is an essential component of MAGE-A1 repression in somatic cells. MAGE-A11 expression is increased during prostate cancer progression and castration-recurrent growth of prostate cancer, which is resulted from the hypomethylation of CpG sites directly proximal to the MAGE-A11 transcription start site (TSS) [54]. MAGE-A11 expression is also correlated with DNA hypomethylation at its TSS in epithelial ovarian cancer, which is associated with the global DNA hypomethylation [54]. The demethylating agent decitabine was able to reduce MAGE-A11 promoter methylation levels. Its promoter activity is partially dependent on the transcription factor Sp1. Sp1 inhibitor mithramycin A (MitA) could cause a dose-dependent reduction in MAGE-A11 promoter activity and endogenous MAGE-A11 expression. In addition, DNA demethylating agent-mediated MAGE-A11 induction could be inhibited by MitA treatment [56]. Taken together, DNA methylation plays a primary role in MAGE-A11 gene silencing.

In mammalian, DNA methylation is regulated by two DNA methyltransferases (DNMTs) families: the so-called "de novo" methyltransferase of DNMT3 family and the "maintenance" methyltransferase DNMT1 [57]. In colon cancer cells, genetic knockout of DNMT1 caused moderate activation of X-link cancer/germline (CG-X) genes including MAGE-A1, NY-ESO-1, and XAGE-1, and DNMT3b knockout had a negligible effect on CG-X gene activation. However, double knockout of DNMT1 and DNMT3b caused dramatic hypomethylation of promoters and robust induction of these CG-X genes [58]. Similarly, in MZ2-MEL cells, down-regulation of DNMT1, but not DNMT3A and DNMT3B, induced the activation of MAGE-A1 gene, suggesting that DNMT1 has a predominant role for methylation maintenance of MAGE-A1 [59]. Therefore, both DNMT1 and DNMT3 family, participate in, and are necessary for, effective CpG island hypermethylation of MAGE genes.

Some methyl-CpG-binding domain (MBD) proteins, which are able to bind methylated DNA, have been reported to contribute to the silencing of MAGE-A genes as modulator [60]. Most hypermethylated promoters are occupied by MBD proteins, whereas unmethylated promoters generally lack MBDs. Treatment of demethylating agents causes hypomethylation of CpG islands, MBD release, and gene re-activation, reinforcing the notion that the association of MBDs with methylated promoters is methylation-dependent [61]. In all MBD-containing proteins, MBD1 differs from other members due to its unique structure and specific function in gene regulation. Except for the

conserved MBD domain at its N-terminal, it also has a transcriptional repression domain (TRD) at its C-terminal [62]. These two domains are related to the interaction between MBD1 and other proteins. However, the MBD domain mediates the binding of MBD1 to the methylated DNA, but the TRD domain regulates the transcriptional repression of target genes. In addition, MBD1 has two or three specific CXXC domains distinct from other MBD-containing proteins. The number of CXXC motifs varies among different MBD1 isoforms and depends on whether MBD1 binds to the unmethylated DNA. The first two CXXC domains (CXXC1 and CXXC2) allow MBD1 to bind to the methylated DNA, but the presence of the third CXXC domain (CXXC3) enables MBD1 to bind to DNA irrespective of its methylation status [63]. MBD1 binds to methylated as well as unmethylated MAGE-A gene promoters, and leads to the repression of the promoters. Repression of unmethylated genes depends on the third CXXC domain, and repression of methylated genes requires the MBD domain. MBD1mut, which lacks the MBD domain and harbors a non-functional TRD, showed no effect on MAGE-A gene expression [60]. The isoform MBD1v1 which contains the additional third CXXC domain could repress MAGE-A gene promoters regardless of their methylation status. However, although MBD1v3 lacks the third CXXC domain, it also has a weak repression on the unmethylated MAGE-A gene promoters, suggesting that the two other CXXC domains may also contribute to the repression of unmethylated MAGE-A promoters, however, with a weaker affinity [60]. These two kinds of binding to both methylated and unmethylated DNA enable MBD1 to act in different epigenetic regulations for MAGE-A genes. Another methyl-CpG binding protein, MeCP2, was also found to regulate MAGE-A11 expression in ESCC progression [64].

MAGE-A gene promoters contain Ets motifs, and the transcription factor Ets has been shown to be responsible for the high transcriptional activation of MAGE-A1 [65]. Ets-1 over-expression could result in the activation of MAGE-A promoters. However, the trans-activator Ets-1 could not abrogate the MBD-1 mediated suppression, suggesting that binding of MBD1 to the unmethylated MAGE-A gene promoter lead to gene repression which could not be abrogated by Ets-1 [60]. MAGE-A11 was also reported to be stimulated via DNA demethylation, histone acetylation and histone methylation, resulting in strengthened ESCC proliferation [64]. These data revealed why promoter demethylation results in the activation of MAGE-A genes. In general, DNA methylation is dominant over other epigenetic mechanisms for CTA (including MAGE) gene repression [66].

Post-translational modifications of histone play accessory roles in the regulation of MAGE expression

DNA methylation is intertwined with the post translational modification of histone [67]. Although hypermethylation of CpG-rich MAGE-A promoters plays a crucial role in the silencing of MAGE-A genes, several studies have shown that up-regulation of MAGE-A genes could not be always observed, although tumor cells were treated by the DNA methylase inhibitor DAC. Histone deacetylases inhibitor trichostatin A (TSA) was able to significantly up-regulate DAC-induced MAGE-A gene transcription, although treatment of several tumor cells with TSA alone had only small influence on MAGE-A gene expression, suggesting that histone deacetylation, which leads to a compact and transcriptionally inactive chromatin structure, also contributes to the repression of MAGE genes [58, 68]. The increased abundance of Ac-H3K9 at MAGE-A gene promoters correlates with increased MAGE-A gene expression. In addition, dual DNMT1/DNMT3b knockout resulted in large increases of AC-H3K9 level at MAGE-A promoters, which correlated with increased MAGE-A expression in cells [58]. Fibroblast growth factor receptor 2-IIIb (FGFR2-IIIb) could suppress MAGE-A3/A6 gene expression through increasing histone deacetylation and histone methylation in thyroid cancer [69]. These studies suggested that not only DNA hypermethylation but also histone deacetylation is responsible for the mechanism underlying MAGE-A gene silencing. Histone deacetylation could lead to a compact and transcriptional inactive chromatin structure, which is involved in the partial repression of MAGE-A genes in tumor cells and may impede their activation. However, in the DNA hypermethylated cells, MAGE-A genes could not be induced by TSA, suggesting that DNA methylation plays a primary role in MAGE-A gene repression, and histone deacetylation plays an accessory role in cells with hypermethylated MAGE-A genes (Fig. 3).

Histone lysine methylation also affects MAGE genes expression in cancer cells [70]. The increased level of H3K9me2 at MAGE-A promoters correlates with a lack of gene expression, whereas an increased abundance of H3K4me2 at these promoters correlates with increased MAGE-A gene expression [59]. MAGE-A high-expressed tumor cells exhibited increased occupancy of RNA polymerase II, enrichment of euchromatin/activation marks such as H3K4Me2, H3K4Me3, H3K79Me2, total H3Ac, H3K9Ac, toal H4Ac, and H4K16Ac, with decreased occupancy of SirT1 as well as polycomb repressor complex (PRC-2) components (KMT6, EED, and SUZ12), and associated PRC-2 mediated repression mark, H3K27me3 [64]. Knockdown of LSD-1 (KDM1) and JARID1B (KDM5B) that mediate demethylation of mono-, di-, and trimethylated H3K4, or the histone lysine methytransferase KMT6

that mediateds trimethylation of H3K27 significantly enhanced DAC-mediated activation of MAGE-A genes in lung cancer cells [70]. DZNep, as an EZH2 inhibitor, could decrease KMT6 and H3K27me3 levels within MAGE-A promoters, and significantly enhanced DAC-mediated induction of MAGE-A genes (Fig. 3).

Nucleosome occupancy in the regulation of MAGE expression

Nucleosomes are the basic structural units of eukaryotic chromatin [71]. Increasing evidences revealed that nucleosomes and their position, in concert with other epigenetic mechanisms, such as DNA methylation, histone modifications, changes in histone variants, as well as small noncoding regulatory RNAs, play essential roles in the control of gene expression [72]. Most importantly, nucleosomes are depleted at promoter, enhancer, and terminator regions, which allow the access of transcription factors and other regulatory proteins [73, 74]. Nucleosome occupancy and positioning are dynamic processes during development as well as in response to different environmental conditions. Therefore, nucleosome positioning and occupancy are determined by combined action of DNA sequence features, transcription factors, chromatin remodelers, and histone modifications [75]. Nucleosome positioning can direct DNA methylation patterns, whereas DNA methylation also can dictate nucleosome occupancy at numerous genomic loci in human cancer cells [76]. For the epigenetic regulation of MAGE-A11, DNA methylation regulates nucleosome occupancy specifically at the − 1 positioned nucleosome of MAGEA11. Methylation of a single Ets site near the transcriptional start site correlated with − 1 nucleosome occupancy and, by itself, strongly repressed MAGEA11 promoter activity. Thus, DNA methylation regulates nucleosome occupancy at MAGEA11, and this appears to function cooperatively with sequence-specific transcription factors to regulate *MAGE-A11* gene expression [56].

Crosstalk between DNA methylation, histone modifications, and nucleosome occupancy

In addition to performing their individual roles, DNA methylation, histone modifications, and nucleosome occupancy work together at multiple levels to determine gene expression status [77]. The crosstalk between DNA methylation and histone modifications can occur in two ways. Firstly, DNA methylation established can lead to the recruitment of MBPs and other transcription regulatory proteins. These proteins can recruit the "writers" of histone modifications followed by the recruitment of "readers" and/ or "erasers". Secondly, histone modifications can directly or indirectly recruit the methyl writers (such as DNMTs) to establish DNA methylation. Furthermore, DNA methylation and nucleosome positioning appear to be linked with

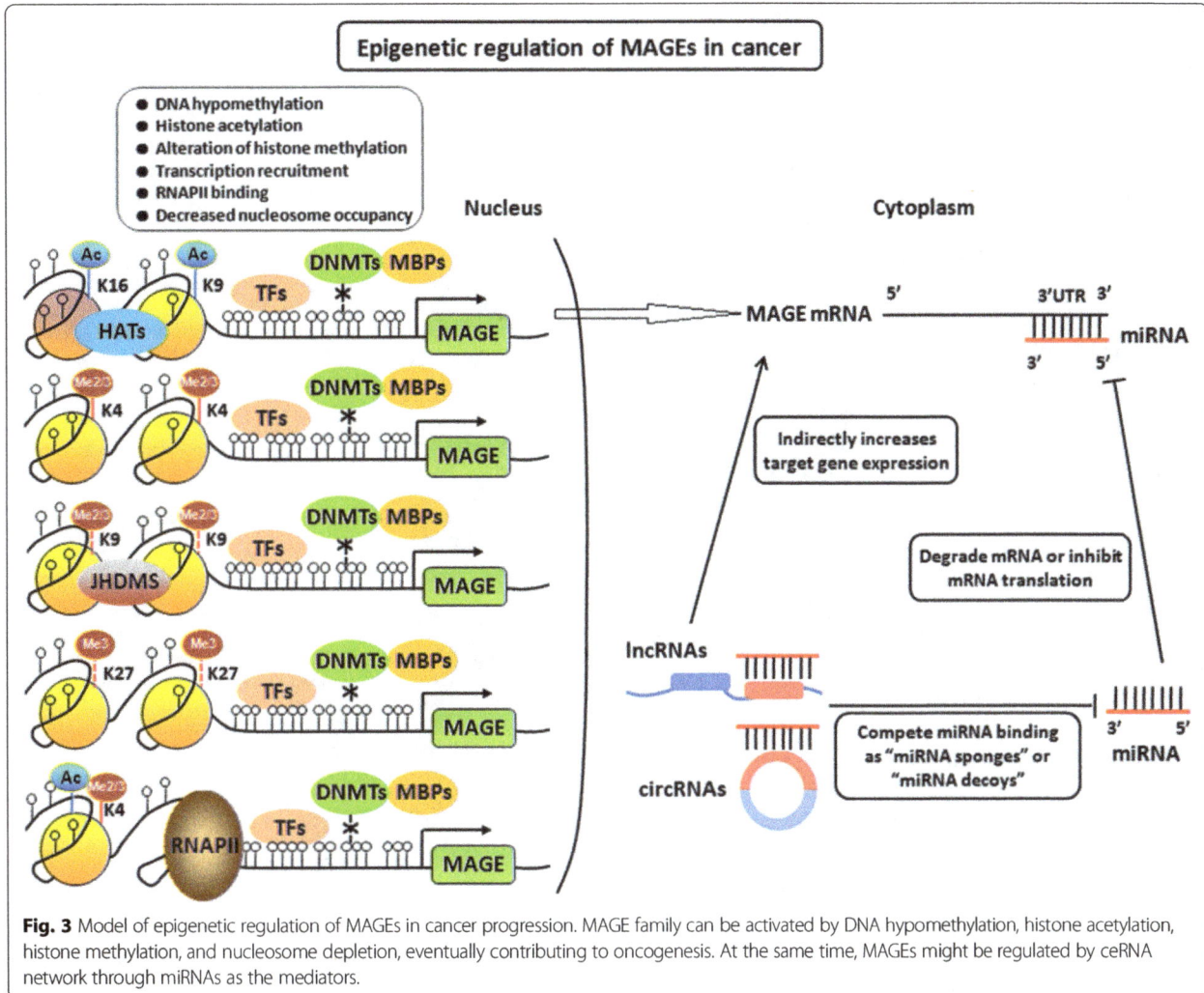

Fig. 3 Model of epigenetic regulation of MAGEs in cancer progression. MAGE family can be activated by DNA hypomethylation, histone acetylation, histone methylation, and nucleosome depletion, eventually contributing to oncogenesis. At the same time, MAGEs might be regulated by ceRNA network through miRNAs as the mediators.

transcription factor binding and gene expression in a complex manner [78, 79]. The crosstalk between DNA methylation, histone modifications, and nucleosome occupancy further enhance the complexity of epigenetic regulation of MAGE gene expression, which determines and maintains their function in cancer cells (Fig. 3).

Non-coding RNAs including microRNAs (miRNAs) and competing endogenous RNA (ceRNA) regulate MAGEs expression in cancer progression

It has been demonstrated that approximately 5–10% of the sequence is transcribed in human genome. Among transcripts, about 10–20% are the protein-coding RNAs, and the rest 80–90% are non-protein-coding RNAs (ncRNAs). MAGE family was also regulated by ncRNAs. MiRNAs, a novel class of gene regulator, are a class of small non-coding RNAs of ~ 22 nucleotides in length that regulate gene expression through post-transcriptional silencing of target genes [80]. Sequence-specific base pairing of miRNAs with 3′ untranslated region (3′UTR) of target

mRNA within the RNA-induced silencing complex results in the degradation or translational inhibition of target mRNAs [81]. There also exist a lot of miRNAs-binding sites at the 3′UTR of MAGE gene mRNAs. MiR-34a was reported to directly bind the 3′UTR of several MAGE-A mRNAs including MAGE-A2, -A3, -A6, and -A12, and thus inhibiting the expression of MAGE-A members [82]. In addition, miR-874 could directly bind the 3′UTR of MAGE-C2 and at least in part negatively regulate the expression of MAGE-C2 in cancer cells [83]. In addition, miRNAs can also modulate epigenetic regulatory mechanisms in cells by targeting enzymes responsible for DNA methylation or histone modifications, which potentially could indirectly influence MAGE expressions [84, 85].

For many years, it is believed that miRNAs regulate gene expression in a simple "miRNA→mRNA→protein" pattern. However, in recent years, it has been found that some RNAs contain the same conservative miRNA binding sites and reduce miRNA availability for its mRNA targets by competing for miRNA binding as "miRNA sponges" or "miRNA decoys" [86, 87]. Based on these finding, the competing endogenous RNA hypothesis was proposed [88]. According to the ceRNA hypothesis, the role of miRNAs in regulating gene expression has thus been amended from that of an "initiator" to a "mediator," and the regulation pattern has been amended from "miR-NA→mRNA" to network-based "ceRNAs→miRNAs→mR-NAs" [89]. Long non-coding RNAs (lncRNAs), circular RNAs (circRNAs), mRNAs and pseudogene transcripts are all revealed to act as ceRNAs and regulate the target genes by competing for the same miRNAs in the available miRNA pools [90–93]. In our recent study, MAGE-A family was found to be regulated by the circRNA-miRNA-mRNA axis in ESCC progression [94]. Taken together, MAGE family might be regulated by ceRNA network through miRNAs as the mediators (Fig. 3).

Conclusion

MAGEs are expressed in a variety of human cancers, and drive tumor progression through various mechanisms, which eventually results in the tumor growth, metastasis, and recurrence. Although recent studies have made great progress towards elucidating the epigenetic regulation of MAGE family, the transcriptional programs controlling their aberrant expression are still not fully understood and much yet is to be discovered. More mechanism studies concerning MAGE function and regulation will provide some new alternative strategies targeting MAGEs in multiple types of cancers.

Abbreviations

3'UTR: 3' Untranslated region; AR: Androgen receptor; ATM: Ataxia-telangiectasia-mutated; CG-X: X-link cancer/germline; CNS: Central nervous system; CTAs: Cancer-testis antigens; DNMTs: DNA methyltransferases; EGF: Epidermalgrowth factor; ERα: Estrogen receptor α; FGFR2-IIIb: Fibroblast growth factor receptor 2-IIIb; H3K9me3: Histone 3 lysine 9 trimethylation; KZNFs: KRAB domain zinc finger transcription factors; lncRNAs: Long non-coding RNAs; MAGE: Melanoma Antigens Genes; MBD: Methyl-CpG binding domain; MitA: Mithramycin A; ncRNAs: Non-protein-coding RNAs; PR: Progesterone receptor; PRC-2: Polycomb repressor complex; Rbx1: RING Box protein-1; SKIP: Ski interacting protein; TRD: Transcriptional repression domain; TSA: Histone deacetylases inhibitor trichostatin A; TSS: Transcription start site

Acknowledgements

The authors would like to greatly appreciate Dr. Qianglin Duan, a skilled English proofreader from Tongji University for paper revision. We also apologize to many authors whose work could not be cited due to space limitations. We recognize that our conclusions are based on the efforts of many.

Funding

This work was supported by Nature Science Foundation of Hebei Province (no. 2016206410).

Authors' contributions

YL, LM, and PD acquired the materials and wrote the manuscript draft. SM designed the draft, and reviewed and edited the manuscript. All authors read and approved the final manuscript.

References

1. Van d BP, Traversari C, Chomez P, Lurquin C, De Plaen E, Van den Eynde B, et al. A gene encoding an antigen recognized by cytolytic T lymphocytes on a human melanoma. Science. 1991;254:1643–7.
2. Chomez P, De BO, Bertrand M, De PE, Boon T, Lucas S. An overview of the MAGE gene family with the identification of all human members of the family. Cancer Res. 2001;61:5544–51.
3. Barker PA, Salehi A. The MAGE proteins: emerging roles in cell cycle progression, apoptosis, and neurogenetic disease. J Neurosci Res. 2002;67:705–12.
4. Anna KL , Patrick RP. A comprehensive guide to the MAGE family of ubiquitin ligases. J Mol Biol 2017; 429:1114–1142.
5. Sang M, Wang L, Ding C, Zhou X, Wang B, Wang L, et al. Melanoma-associated antigen genes - an update. Cancer Lett. 2011;302:85–90.
6. Simpson AJ, Caballero OL, Jungbluth A, Chen YT, Old LJ. Cancer/testis antigens, gametogenesis and cancer. Nat Rev Cancer. 2005;5:615–25.
7. Wang D, Wang J, Ding N, Li Y, Yang Y, Fang X, et al. MAGE-A1 promotes melanoma proliferation and migration through C-JUN activation. Biochem Biophys Res Commun. 2016;473:959–65.
8. Lian Y, Sang M, Ding C, Zhou X, Fan X, Xu Y, et al. Expressions of MAGE-A10 and MAGE-A11 in breast cancers and their prognostic significance: a retrospective clinical study. J Cancer Res Clin Oncol. 2012;138:519–27.
9. Heninger E, Krueger TE, Thiede SM, Sperger JM, Byers BL, Kircher MR, et al. Inducible expression of cancer-testis antigens in human prostate cancer. Oncotarget. 2016;7:84359–74.
10. Sang M, Gu L, Yin D, Liu F, Lian Y, Zhang X, et al. MAGE-A family expression is correlated with poor survival of patients with lung adenocarcinoma: a retrospective clinical study based on tissue microarray. J Clin Pathol. 2017; 70:533–40.
11. Sang M, Gu L, Liu F, Lian Y, Yin D, Fan X, et al. Prognostic significance of MAGE-A11 in esophageal squamous cell carcinoma and identification of related genes based on DNA microarray. Arch Med Res. 2016;47:151–61.
12. Ogata K, Aihara R, Mochiki E, Ogawa A, Yanai M, Toyomasu Y, et al. Clinical significance of melanoma antigen-encoding gene-1 (MAGE-1) expression and its correlation with poor prognosis in differentiated advanced gastric cancer. Ann Surg Oncol. 2011;18:1195–203.
13. Mengus C, Schultz-Thater E, Coulot J, Kastelan Z, Goluza E, Coric M, et al. MAGE-A10 cancer/testis antigen is highly expressed in high-grade non-muscle-invasive bladder carcinomas. Int J Cancer. 2013;132:2459–63.
14. Sang M, Wu X, Fan X, Sang M, Zhou X, Zhou N. Multiple MAGE-A genes as surveillance marker for the detection of circulating tumor cells in patients with ovarian cancer. Biomarkers. 2014;19:34–42.
15. Gu X, Fu M, Ge Z, Zhan F, Ding Y, Ni H, et al. High expression of MAGE-A9 correlates with unfavorable survival in hepatocellular carcinoma. Sci Rep. 2014;4:6625.
16. Scarcella DL, Chow CW, Gonzales MF, Economou C, Brasseur F, Ashley DM. Expression of MAGE and GAGE in high-grade brain tumors: a potential target for specific immunotherapy and diagnostic markers. Clin Cancer Res. 1999;5:335–41.
17. Osterlund C, Tohonen V, Forslund KO, Nordqvist K. Mage-b4, a novel melanoma antigen (MAGE) gene specifically expressed during germ cell differentiation. Cancer Res. 2000;60:1054–61.
18. Gjerstorff MF, Harkness L, Kassem M, Frandsen U, Nielsen O, Lutterodt M, et al. Distinct GAGE and MAGE-A expression during early human development indicate specific roles in lineage differentiation. Hum Reprod. 2008;23:2194–201.
19. Yang B, O'Herrin S, Wu J, Reagan-Shaw S, Ma Y, Nihal M, et al. Select cancer testes antigens of the MAGE-A, -B, and -C families are expressed in mast cell lines and promote cell viability in vitro and in vivo. J Invest Dermatol. 2007; 127:267–75.
20. Liu W, Cheng S, Asa SL, Ezzat S. The melanoma-associated antigen A3 mediates fibronectin-controlled cancer progression and metastasis. Cancer Res. 2008;68:8104–12.
21. Yang B, O'Herrin SM, Wu J, Reagan-Shaw S, Ma Y, Bhat KM, et al. MAGE-A, mMage-b, and MAGE-C proteins form complexes with KAP1 and suppress p53-dependent apoptosis in MAGE-positive cell lines. Cancer Res. 2007;67: 9954–62.
22. Pineda CT, Ramanathan S, Fon TK, Weon JL, Potts MB, Ou YH, et al. Degradation of AMPK by a cancer-specific ubiquitin ligase. Cell. 2015;160:715–28.
23. Doyle JM, Gao J, Wang J, Yang M, Potts PR. MAGE-RING protein complexes comprise a family of E3 ubiquitin ligases. Mol Cell. 2010;39:963–74.

24. Feng Y, Gao J, Yang M. When MAGE meets RING: insights into biological functions of MAGE proteins. Protein Cell. 2011;2:7–12.

25. Borden KL. RING domains: master builders of molecular scaffolds? J Mol Biol. 2000;295:103–1112.

26. Lorick KL, Jensen JP, Fang S, Ong AM, Hatakeyama S, Weissman AM. RING fingers mediate ubiquitin-conjugating enzyme (E2)-dependent ubiquitination. Proc Natl Acad Sci U S A. 1999;6:364–11369.

27. Jackson PK, Eldridge AG, Freed E, Furstenthal L, Hsu JY, Kaiser BK, et al. The lore of the RINGs: substrate recognition and catalysis by ubiquitin ligases. Trends Cell Biol. 2000;10:429–39.

28. Pineda CT, Potts PR. Oncogenic MAGEA-TRIM28 ubiquitin ligase downregulates autophagy by ubiquitinating and degrading AMPK in cancer. Autophagy. 2015;112:844–6.

29. Xiao TZ, Bhatia N, Urrutia R, Lomberk GA, Simpson A, Longley BJ. MAGE I transcription factors regulate KAP1 and KRAB domain zinc finger transcription factor mediated gene repression. PLoS One. 2011;6:e23747.

30. Angelo L, Elena C, Giorgia M, Diana Z, Paola L, Paola C. KRAB-zinc finger proteins: a repressor family displaying multiple biological functions. Curr Genomics. 2013;14:268–78.

31. Bhatia N, Yang B, Xiao TZ, Peters N, Hoffmann MF, Longley BJ. Identification of novel small molecules that inhibit protein-protein interactions between MAGE and KAP-1. Arch Biochem Biophys. 2011;508:217–21.

32. Zheng N, Schulman BA, Song L, Mille JJ, Jeffrey PD, Wang P, et al. Structure of the Cul1-Rbx1-Skp1-F boxSkp2 SCF ubiquitin ligase complex. Nature. 2002;416:703–9.

33. Nakayama KI, Nakayama K. Ubiquitin ligases: cell-cycle control and cancer. Nat Rev Cancer. 2006;6:369–81.

34. Petroski MD, Deshaies RJ. Function and regulation of cullin-RING ubiquitin ligases. Nat Rev Mol Cell Biol. 2005;6:9–20.

35. Hao J, Song X, Wang J, Guo C, Li Y, Li B, et al. Cancer-testis antigen MAGE-C2 binds Rbx1 and inhibits ubiquitin ligase-mediated turnover of cyclin E. Oncotarget. 2015;6:42028–39.

36. Marcar L, Ihrig B, Hourihan J, Bray SE, Quinlan PR, Jordan LB, et al. MAGE-A cancer/testis antigens inhibit MDM2 ubiquitylation function and promote increased levels of MDM4. PLoS One. 2015;10:e0127713.

37. Su S, Chen X, Geng J, Bray SE, Quinlan PR, Jordan LB, et al. Melanoma antigen-A11 regulates substrate-specificity of Skp2-mediated protein degradation. Mol Cell Endocrinol. 2017;439:1–9.

38. Bhatia N, Xiao TZ, Rosenthal KA, Siddiqui IA, Thiyagarajan S, Smart B, et al. MAGE-C2 promotes growth and tumorigenicity of melanoma cells, phosphorylation of KAP1, and DNA damage repair. J Invest Dermatol. 2013; 133:759–67.

39. Schultz DC, Ayyanathan K, Negorev D, Maul GG, Rauscher FJ 3rd. SETDB1: a novel KAP-1-associated histone H3, lysine 9-specific methyltransferase that contributes to HP1-mediated silencing of euchromatic genes by KRAB zinc-finger proteins. Genes Dev. 2002;16:919–32.

40. Li X, Lee YK, Jeng JC, Yen Y, Schultz DC, Shih HM, et al. Role for KAP1 serine 824 phosphorylation and sumoylation/desumoylation switch in regulating KAP1-mediated transcriptional repression. J Biol Chem. 2007;282:36177–89.

41. Marcar L, Maclaine NJ, Hupp TR, Meek DW. Mage-A cancer/testis antigens inhibit p53 function by blocking its interaction with chromatin. Cancer Res. 2010;70:10362–70.

42. Nardiello T, Jungbluth AA, Mei A, Diliberto M, Huang X, Dabrowski A, et al. MAGE-A inhibits apoptosis in proliferating myeloma cells through repression of bax and maintenance of survivin. Clin Cancer Res. 2011; 17:4309–19.

43. Monte M, Simonatto M, Peche LY, Bublik DR, Gobessi S, Pierotti MA, et al. MAGE-A tumor antigens target p53 transactivation function through histone deacetylase recruitment and confer resistance to chemotherapeutic agents. Proc Natl Acad Sci U S A. 2006;103:11160–5.

44. Laduron S, Deplus R, Zhou S, Kholmanskikh O, Godelaine D, De Smet C, et al. MAGE-A1 interacts with adaptor SKIP and the deacetylase HDAC1 to repress transcription. Nucleic Acids Res. 2004;32:4340–50.

45. Wong PP, Yeoh CC, Ahmad AS, Chelala C, Gillett C, Speirs V, et al. Identification of MAGEA antigens as causal players in the development of tamoxifen-resistant breast cancer. Oncogene. 2014;33:4579–88.

46. Bai S, Grossman G, Yuan L, Lessey BA, French FS, Young SL, et al. Hormone control and expression of androgen receptor coregulator MAGE-11 in human endometrium during the window of receptivity to embryo implantation. Mol Human Reprod. 2008;14:107–16.

47. Bai S, Wilson EM. Epidermal-growth-factor-dependent phosphorylation and ubiquitinylation of MAGE-11 regulates its interaction with the androgen receptor. Mol Cell Biol. 2008;28:1947–63.

48. Wilson EM. Androgen receptor molecular biology and potential targets in prostate cancer. Ther Adv Urol. 2010;2:105–17.

49. Bai S, He B, Wilson EM. Melanoma antigen gene protein MAGE-11 regulates androgen receptor function by modulating the interdomain interaction. Mol Cell Biol. 2005;25:1238–57.

50. Askew EB, Bai S, Hnat AT, Minges JT, Wilson EM. Melanoma antigen gene protein-A11 (MAGE-11) F-box links the androgen receptor NH2-terminal transactivation domain to p160 coactivators. J Biol Chem. 2009;284:34793–808.

51. Su S, Blackwelder AJ, Grossman G, Minges JT, Yuan L, Young SL, et al. Primate-specific melanoma antigen-A11 regulates isoform-specific human progesterone receptor-B transactivation. J Biol Chem. 2012;287:34809–24.

52. Su S, Minges JT, Grossman G, Blackwelder AJ, Mohler JL, Wilson EM. Proto-oncogene activity of melanoma antigen-A11 (MAGE-A11) regulates retinoblastoma-related p107 and E2F1 proteins. J Biol Chem. 2013;288:24809–24.

53. De Smet C, Lurquin C, Lethé B, Martelange V, Boon T. DNA methylation is the primary silencing mechanism for a set of germ line- and tumor-specific genes with a CpG-rich promoter. Mol Cell Biol. 1999;19:7327–35.

54. Karpf AR, Bai S, James SR, Mohler JL, Wilson EM. Increased expression of androgen receptor coregulator MAGE-11 in prostate cancer by DNA hypomethylation and cyclic AMP. Mol Cancer Res. 2009;7:523–35.

55. De Smet C, Loriot A, Boon T. Promoter-dependent mechanism leading to selective hypomethylation within the 5' region of gene MAGE-A1 in tumor cells. Mol Cell Biol. 2004;24:4781–90.

56. Smitha RJ, Carlos DC, Ashok S, Wa Z, James LM, Kunle O, et al. DNA methylation and nucleosome occupancy regulate the cancer germline antigen gene MAGEA11. Epigenetics. 2013;8:849–63.

57. Elliott EN, Sheaffer KL, Kaestner KH. The 'de novo' DNA methyltransferase Dnmt3b compensates the Dnmt1-deficient intestinal epithelium. Elife. 2016;5.

58. James SR, Link PA, Karpf AR. Epigenetic regulation of X-linked cancer/germline antigen genes by DNMT1 and DNMT3b. Oncogene. 2006;25: 6975–85.

59. Loriot A, De PE, Boon T, De Smet C. Transient down-regulation of DNMT1 methyltransferase leads to activation and stable hypomethylation of MAGE-A1 in melanoma cells. J Biol Chem. 2006;281:10118–26.

60. Wischnewski F, Friese O, Pantel K, Schwarzenbach H. Methyl-CpG binding domain proteins and their involvement in the regulation of the MAGE-A1, MAGE-A2, MAGE-A3, and MAGE-A12 gene promoters. Mol Cancer Res. 2007; 5:749–59.

61. Lopez-Serra L, Ballestar E, Fraga MF, Alaminos M, Setien F, Esteller M. A profile of methyl-CpG binding domain protein occupancy of hypermethylated promoter CpG islands of tumor suppressor genes in human cancer. Cancer Res. 2006;66:8342–6.

62. Ng HH, Jeppesen P, Bird A. Active repression of methylated genes by the chromosomal protein MBD1. Mol Cell Biol. 2000;20:1394–406.

63. Jorgensen HF, Ben-Porath I, Bird AP. MBD1 is recruited to both methylated and nonmethylated CpGs via distinct DNA binding domains. Mol Cell Biol. 2004;24:3387–95.

64. Liu S, Liu F, Huang W, Gu L, Meng L, Ju Y, et al. MAGE-A11 is activated through TFCP2/ZEB1 binding sites demethylation as well as histone modification and facilitates ESCC tumor growth. Oncotarget. 2017;9:3365–78.

65. De Smet C, Courtois SJ, Faraoni I, Lurquin C, Szikora JP, De Backer O, et al. Involvement of two Ets binding sites in the transcriptional activation of the MAGE1 gene. Immunogenetics. 1995;42:282–90.

66. Akers SN, Odunsi K, Karpf AR. Regulation of cancer germline antigen gene expression: implication for cancer immunotherapy. Future Oncol. 2010;6:717–32.

67. Bartke T, Vermeulen M, Xhemalce B, Robson SC, Mann M, Kouzarides T. Nucleosome-interacting proteins regulated by DNA and histone methylation. Cell. 2010;143:470–84.

68. Wischnewski F, Pantel K, Schwarzenbach H. Promoter demethylation and histone acetylation mediate gene expression of MAGE-A1, -A2, -A3, and -A12 in human cancer cells. Mol Cancer Res. 2006;4:339–49.

69. Kondo T, Zhu X, Asa SL, Ezzat S. The cancer/testis antigen melanoma-associated antigen-A3/A6 is a novel target of fibroblast growth factor receptor 2-IIIb through histone H3 modifications in thyroid cancer. Clin Cancer Res. 2007;13:4713–20.

70. Rao M, Chinnasamy N, Hong JA, Zhang Y, Zhang M, Xi S, et al. Inhibition of histone lysine methylation enhances cancer-testis antigen expression in lung cancer cells: implications for adoptive immunotherapy of cancer. Cancer Res. 2011;71:4192–204.

71. Richmond TJ, Davey CA. The structure of DNA in the nucleosome core. Nature. 2003;423:145–50.

72. Andreu-Vieyra CV, Liang G. Nucleosome occupancy and gene regulation during tumorigenesis. Adv Exp Med Biol. 2013;754:109–34.

73. Bell O, Tiwari VK, Thomä NH, Schübeler D. Determinants and dynamics of genome accessibility. Nat Rev Genet. 2011;12:554–64.

74. Henikoff S. Nucleosomes at active promoters: unforgettable loss. Cancer Cell. 2007;12:407–9.

75. Lorch Y, Kornberg RD. Chromatin-remodeling and the initiation of transcription. Q Rev Biophys. 2015;48:465–70.

76. Chodavarapu RK, Feng S, Bernatavichute YV, Chen PY, Stroud H, Yu Y, et al. Relationship between nucleosome positioning and DNA methylation. Nature. 2010;466:388–92.

77. Teif VB, Beshnova DA, Vainshtein Y, Marth C, Mallm JP, Höfer T, et al. Nucleosome repositioning links DNA (de)methylation and differential CTCF binding during stem cell development. Genome Res. 2014;24:1285–95.

78. Cedar H, Bergman Y. Linking DNA methylation and histone modification: patterns and paradigms. Nat Rev Genet. 2009;10:295–304.

79. Collings CK, Anderson JN. Links between DNA methylation and nucleosome occupancy in the human genome. Epigenetics Chromatin. 2017;10:18.

80. He L, Hannon GJ. MicroRNAs: small RNAs with a big role in gene regulation. Nat Rev Genet. 2004;5:522–31.

81. Filipowicz W, Bhattacharyya SN, Sonenberg N. Mechanisms of post-transcriptional regulation by microRNAs: are the answers in sight? Nat Rev Genet. 2008;9:102–14.

82. Weeraratne SD, Amani V, Neiss A, Teider N, Scott DK, Pomeroy SL, et al. miR-34a confers chemosensitivity through modulation of MAGE-A and p53 in medulloblastoma. Neuro-Oncology. 2011;13:165–75.

83. Song X, Song W, Wang Y, Wang J, Li Y, Qian X, et al. MicroRNA-874 functions as a tumor suppressor by targeting cancer/testis antigen HCA587/MAGE-C2. J Cancer. 2016;7:656–63.

84. Fabbri M, Garzon R, Cimmino A, Liu Z, Zanesi N, Callegari E, et al. MicroRNA-29 family reverts aberrant methylation in lung cancer by targeting DNA methyltransferases 3A and 3B. Proc Natl Acad Sci U S A. 2007;104:15805–10.

85. Friedman JM, Liang G, Liu CC, Wolff EM, Tsai YC, Ye W, et al. The putative tumor suppressor microRNA-101 modulates the cancer epigenome by repressing the polycomb group protein EZH2. Cancer Res. 2009;69:2623–9.

86. Ebert MS, Neilson JR, Sharp PA. MicroRNA sponges: competitive inhibitors of small RNAs in mammalian cells. Nat Methods. 2007;4:721–6.

87. Poliseno L, Salmena L, Zhang J, Carver B, Haveman WJ, Pandolfi PP. A coding-independent function of gene and pseudogene mRNAs regulates tumour biology. Nature. 2010;465:1033–8.

88. Salmena L, Poliseno L, Tay Y, Kats L, Pandolfi PP. A ceRNA hypothesis: the Rosetta stone of a hidden RNA language? Cell. 2011;146:353–8.

89. Yang C, Wu D, Gao L, Liu X, Jin Y, Wang D, et al. Competing endogenous RNA networks in human cancer: hypothesis, validation, and perspectives. Oncotarget. 2016;7:13479–90.

90. Huang M, Zhong Z, Lv M, Shu J, Tian Q, Chen J. Comprehensive analysis of differentially expressed profiles of lncRNAs and circRNAs with associated co-expression and ceRNA networks in bladder carcinoma. Oncotarget. 2016;7:47186–200.

91. Wang W, Zhuang Q, Ji K, Wen B, Lin P, Zhao Y, et al. Identification of miRNA, lncRNA and mRNA-associated ceRNA networks and potential biomarker for MELAS with mitochondrial DNA A3243G mutation. Sci Rep. 2017;7:41639.

92. Hansen TB, Jensen TI, Clausen BH, Bramsen JB, Finsen B, Damgaard CK, et al. Natural RNA circles function as efficient microRNA sponges. Nature. 2013;495:384–8.

93. An Y, Furber KL, Ji S. Pseudogenes regulate parental gene expression via ceRNA network. J Cell Mol Med. 2017;21:185–92.

94. Sang M, Meng L, Sang Y, Liu S, Ding P, Ju Y, et al. Cicular RNA ciRS-7 accelerates ESCC progression through acting as a miR-876-5p sponge to enhance MAGE-A family expression. Cancer Lett. 2018;426:37–46.

22

DNA methylation and repressive histones in the promoters of PD-1, CTLA-4, TIM-3, LAG-3, TIGIT, PD-L1, and galectin-9 genes in human colorectal cancer

Varun Sasidharan Nair[1], Salman M. Toor[1], Rowaida Z. Taha[1], Hibah Shaath[1] and Eyad Elkord[1,2]*

Abstract

Background: Colorectal cancer (CRC) is the third most commonly diagnosed human malignancy worldwide. Upregulation of inhibitory immune checkpoints by tumor-infiltrating immune cells (TIICs) or their ligands by tumor cells leads to tumor evasion from host immunosurveillance. Changes in DNA methylation pattern and enrichment of methylated histone marks in the promoter regions could be major contributors to the upregulation of immune checkpoints (ICs) in the tumor microenvironment (TME).

Methods: Relative expressions of various immune checkpoints and ligands in colon normal tissues (NT) and colorectal tumor tissues (TT) were assessed by qRT-PCR. The epigenetic modifications behind this upregulation were determined by investigating the CpG methylation status of their promoter regions using bisulfite sequencing. Distributions of histone 3 lysine 9 trimethylation (H3K9me3) and histone 3 lysine 27 trimethylation (H3K27me3) in promoter regions of these genes were assessed by chromatin immunoprecipitation (ChIP) assay.

Results: We found that the expression levels of PD-1, CTLA-4, TIM-3, TIGIT, PD-L1, and galectin-9 were significantly higher in colorectal tumor tissues, compared with colon normal tissues. To study the role of DNA methylation, we checked the promoter CpG methylation of ICs and ligands and found that only CTLA-4 and TIGIT, among other genes, were significantly hypomethylated in TT compared with NT. Next, we checked the abundance of repressive histones (H3K9me3 and H3K27me3) in the promoter regions of ICs/ligands. We found that bindings of H3K9me3 in PD-1 and TIGIT promoters and H3K27me3 in CTLA-4 promotor were significantly lower in TT compared with NT. Additionally, bindings of both H3K9me3 and H3K27me3 in the TIM-3 promoter were significantly lower in TT compared with NT.

Conclusion: This study shows that both DNA hypomethylation and H3K9me3 and H3K27me3 repressive histones are involved in upregulation of CTLA-4 and TIGIT genes. However, repressive histones, but not DNA hypomethylation, are involved in upregulation of PD-1 and TIM-3 genes in CRC tumor tissue. These epigenetic modifications could be utilized as diagnostic biomarkers for CRC.

Keywords: Colorectal cancer, Immune checkpoints, PD-L1, Galectin-9, DNA methylation, Histone trimethylation

* Correspondence: eelkord@hbku.edu.qa; eyad.elkord@manchester.ac.uk
[1]Cancer Research Center, Qatar Biomedical Research Institute, College of Science and Engineering, Hamad Bin Khalifa University, Qatar Foundation, Doha, Qatar
[2]Institute of Cancer Sciences, University of Manchester, Manchester, UK

Background

Colorectal cancer (CRC) is the third most common cancer worldwide [1]. Approximately 20% of CRC patients show distinct metastases at diagnosis, and the death rate is estimated to be 26% in both genders [1, 2]. The relationship between immune cells and cancer cells within the tumor microenvironment (TME) attains a great interest among researchers. Immune cell-mediated tumor evasion is one of the key mechanisms for the progression and survival of malignant cells [3]. T cells are the chief cytotoxic effector cells that recognize and eliminate tumor cells. Immune response against tumor is initiated by recognition of tumor-antigenic peptides by T cell receptors (TCR) along with co-stimulatory signals, which are required for an effective and prolonged immune response against tumor antigens for successful elimination of malignant cell. In addition to co-stimulatory signals, co-inhibitory signals (immune checkpoints; ICs) are indispensable for maintaining peripheral tolerance and in preventing autoimmunity. The balance between co-stimulatory and co-inhibitory signals determines the amplitude of T cell response [4, 5]. The expression of these ICs is utilized by tumor cells to escape from host immunosurveillance [6, 7].

It has been reported that epigenetic regulation is one of the key mechanisms behind ICs expression in the TME [8]. Three important epigenetic modifications are reported in the colorectal TME; DNA methylation, post-translational modifications in chromatin-protein interactions, and expression of non-coding RNAs [9, 10]. In particular, hypermethylation of the CpG islands (CGIs) enriched in the promoter regions of tumor suppressor genes, induce silencing of these genes [11]. Active demethylation of DNA occurs by the oxidation of 5-methyl cytosine (5-mc) to 5-hydroxymethyl cytosine (5-hmc) and finally to 5-cytosine (5-c) by enzymes belonging to the ten-eleven translocation (TET) family [12]. Mammalian TET family consists of three members; TET1, TET2, and TET3 [12]. It has been reported that promoter demethylation and distribution of repressive histones work together for the upregulation of many genes in cancers [13]. A report showed that the enrichment of repressive histones, histone 3 lysine 9 trimethylation (H3K9me3) and histone 3 lysine 27 trimethylation (H3K27me3) in the promoter regions along with CpG hypermethylation, were the common epigenetic modifications in the colorectal TME [14]. The epigenetic modifications of ICs in colorectal tumor are still not elucidated.

In this study, we investigated expression levels of different immune checkpoints/their ligands, and the epigenetic modifications that could be involved in their upregulation in the colorectal TME. PD-1, CTLA-4, TIM-3, LAG-3, TIGIT immune checkpoints and PD-L1, and galactin-9 ligands were selected due to their important role in tumor immune evasion and their potential as therapeutic targets for immune-mediated therapies. Interestingly, we found that ICs including PD-1, CTLA-4, TIM-3 and TIGIT, and IC ligands including PD-L1 and galactin-9 were significantly upregulated in colorectal tumor tissues (TT), compared with colon normal tissues (NT). Additionally, we found that both DNA hypomethylation and repressive histone binding in the promoter regions are involved in the transcriptional upregulation of CTLA-4 and TIGIT. However, distribution of repressive histones, but not DNA hypomethylation, seems to be involved in the upregulation of PD-1 and TIM-3 in colorectal tumor tissue.

Results

Multiple immune checkpoints/ligands are upregulated in colorectal tumor tissue

Reports showed that tumors attain various mechanisms to circumvent host immunosurveillance [15, 16]. One such mechanism is the upregulation of ICs by TIICs and their ligands by tumor cells in the TME. To investigate the transcriptional expression of ICs/ligands in the colorectal TME, we performed real time PCR to determine mRNA levels of ICs/ligands in NT and TT. We found that ICs including PD-1, CTLA-4, TIM-3 and TIGIT, (Fig. 1a) and IC ligands including PD-L1 and galactin-9 (Fig. 1b) were significantly upregulated in TT compared with NT. However, there was no significant change in LAG-3 expression in TT compared to NT (Fig. 1a). These data show that in the colorectal TME, multiple ICs and ligands are upregulated, which may assist tumor cells to evade host immunosurveillance.

DNA demethylation enzymes are overexpressed in colorectal tumor microenvironment

DNA methylation has a predominant role in the silencing of tumor suppressor genes in the TME, and any imbalance in DNA methylation/demethylation genes could result in disease onset and progression [17]. It has been reported that TET1, TET2, and TET3 exhibit both overlapping and discrete functions [18]. In CRC, somatic mutations have been reported in all three TET proteins [19]. These reports prompted us to check the expression of TET1, TET2, and TET3 and methylation enzymes including DNMT3a and DNMT3b in NT and TT. Interestingly, we found all three TETs were significantly increased and DNMTs were significantly decreased in TT compared with NT (Fig. 1c). Out of all TETs, TET2 was more significantly upregulated in TT compared with NT, indicating that TET2 might play a pivotal role in demethylation than TET1 and TET3 in the colorectal TME (Fig. 1c). The reciprocal expressions of TETs and DNMTs are in line with previous findings that the methylation status of the gene is dynamically regulated by TETs and DNMTs [20, 21].

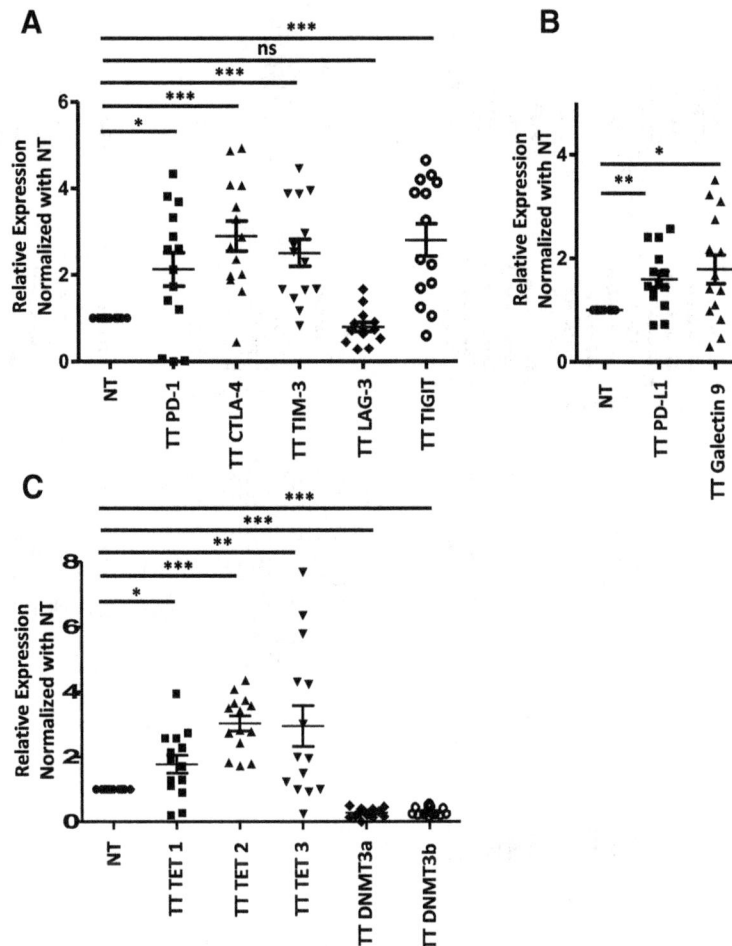

Fig. 1 Expression of immune checkpoints/ligands and methylation/demethylation genes in colorectal tumor and normal colon tissues. RNA isolated from tissues from 14 patients was reverse transcribed to cDNA. Quantitative RT-PCR was performed to assess the expression level of immune checkpoints PD-1, CTLA-4, TIM-3, LAG-3, and TIGIT (**a**); immune checkpoint ligands PD-L1 and galectin-9 (**b**); demethylation/methylation enzymes TET1, TET2, TET3, DNMT3a, and DNMT3b (**c**) from both NT and TT. The relative expression of each gene was normalized to β-actin

Analyses of DNA methylation in the promoter regions of immune checkpoints/ligands in the colorectal tumor microenvironment

Hypermethylation of CpG islands (CpGIs) located in the promoter regions have a major role in gene inactivation in the TME and has been defined in almost all malignancies [22]. In order to check the promoter methylation profile of ICs/ligands, we selected CpGIs in the promotors of PD-1, CTLA-4, TIM-3, LAG-3, TIGIT, and PD-L1 as described previously [23]. In addition to this, we also selected 12 CpGIs in the promoter region of galectin-9. We found that the average demethylation percentages of CTLA-4 and TIGIT in TT were significantly higher compared with NT (Figs. 2b, e and 3a). Additionally, the average demethylation percentages of PD-1 and TIM-3 were higher in TT compared to NT, but not significant (Figs. 2a, c and 3a). In contrast, the demethylation of LAG-3 was reduced in TT compared

to NT (Figs. 2d and 3a). These results are in accordance with real-time data that LAG-3 was the only gene, which has lower expression in TT compared to NT (Fig. 1a). Additionally, there were no differences in the demethylation percentages for IC ligands, PD-L1 and galectin-9, in TT compared to NT (Figs. 2f, g and 3a). Interestingly, PD-L1 was completely demethylated in both NT and TT (Fig. 2f). This is similar to our findings in breast tumor tissues [23]. These data show that all genes do not follow similar mechanisms for their transcriptional upregulation in the TME. The transcriptional upregulation of CTLA-4 and TIGIT might be under the control of DNA hypomethylation. We also checked the corrected demethylation percentage by subtracting the demethylation percentage of NT from corresponding TT and found that the percentages of CTLA-4 and TIGIT were higher than other genes, and there were no significant differences between them (Fig. 3b). In addition, we checked

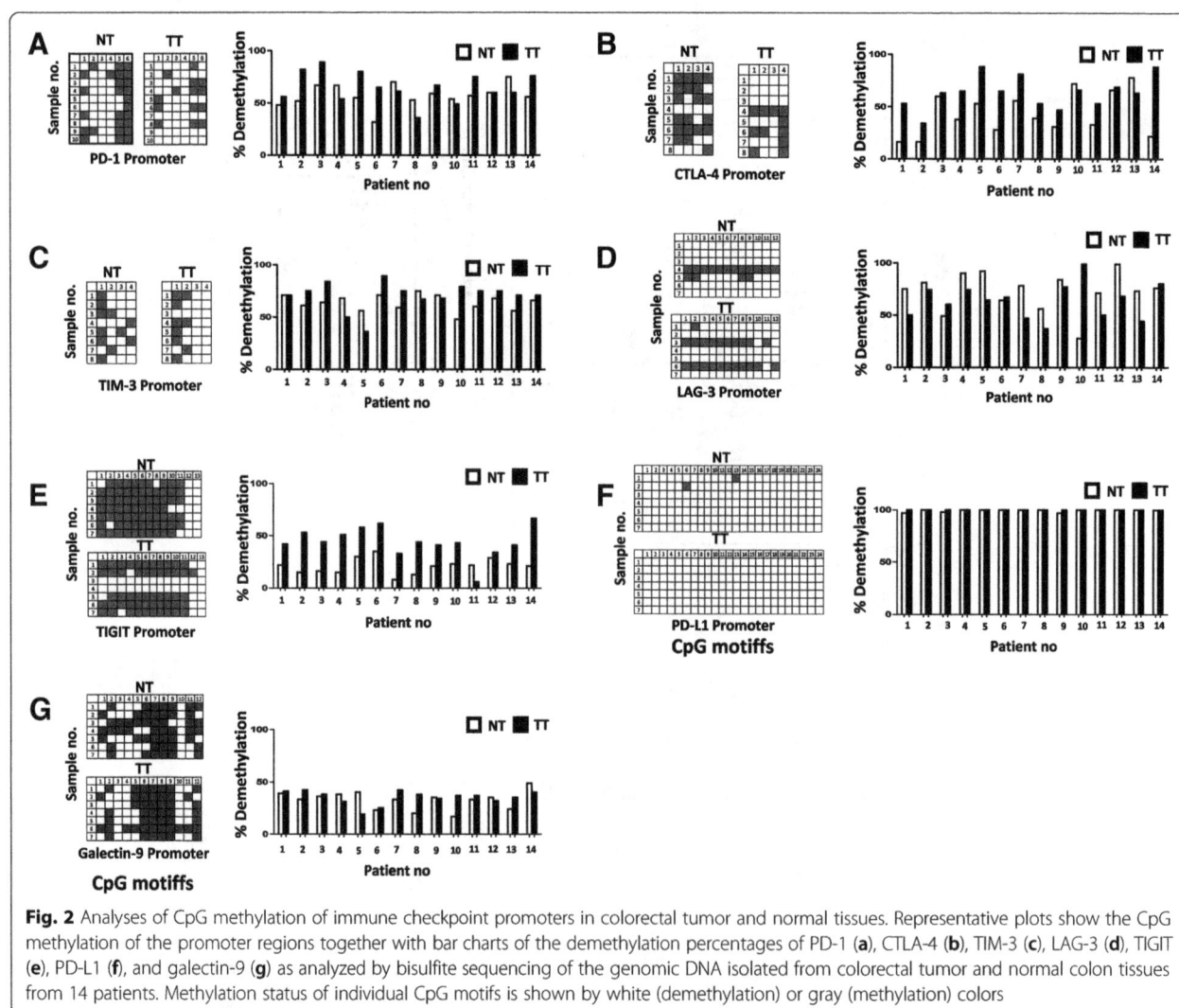

Fig. 2 Analyses of CpG methylation of immune checkpoint promoters in colorectal tumor and normal tissues. Representative plots show the CpG methylation of the promoter regions together with bar charts of the demethylation percentages of PD-1 (**a**), CTLA-4 (**b**), TIM-3 (**c**), LAG-3 (**d**), TIGIT (**e**), PD-L1 (**f**), and galectin-9 (**g**) as analyzed by bisulfite sequencing of the genomic DNA isolated from colorectal tumor and normal colon tissues from 14 patients. Methylation status of individual CpG motifs is shown by white (demethylation) or gray (methylation) colors

the corrected demethylation percentages of all genes in individual patients and found that the percentages of CTLA-4 and TIGIT were higher in most of patients compared with other genes (Fig. 3 c, d). These data show that demethylation in promotors might play an important role in the expression of ICs in the TME.

Analyses of the abundance of repressive histones in the promoter regions of immune checkpoints/ligands in the colorectal tumor microenvironment

Our DNA methylation data show that the transcriptional upregulation of ICs/ligands are not completely dependent on the hypomethylation of promoter regions. These results prompted us to check the presence of repressive H3K9me3 and H3K27me3 in the promoter regions of PD-1, CTLA-4, TIM-3, LAG-3, TIGIT, PD-L1, and galectin-9 in the colorectal TME by chromatin immunoprecipitation assays. As controls, we precipitated

chromatin from both NT and TT with anti-H3 antibody and confirmed that there is no difference in the distribution of H3 in the promoter regions of all ICs/ligands between NT and TT (Fig. 4). We also used rabbit-IgG as an isotype negative control to confirm that there were no non-specific enrichments (Fig. 4). Interestingly, the abundance of H3K9me3 was significantly lower in TT compared with NT in the promoter regions of PD-1 (Fig. 4a) and TIGIT (Fig. 4e), while H3K27me3 was lower in CTLA-4 promotor (Fig. 4b). Moreover, both H3K9me3 and H3K27me3 were significantly lower in TT in TIM-3 promoter (Fig. 4c). Of note, there was no difference in the distribution of either H3K9me3 or H3K27m3e in the promoter regions of LAG-3, PD-L1, and galectin-9 (Fig. 4d, f, g). These data show that in the colorectal TME, abundance of repressive histones in TT was significantly lower in the promoter regions of PD-1, CTLA-4, TIM-3, and TIGIT, which may in turn lead to their transcriptional upregulation in TT compared with NT.

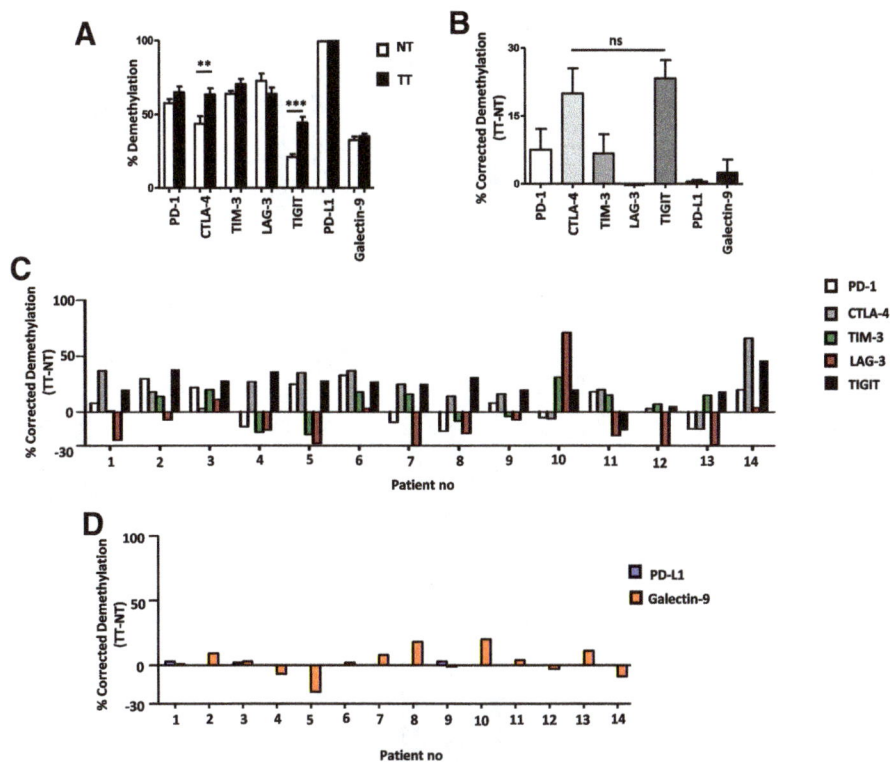

Fig. 3 Corrected demethylation percentage of immune checkpoint promoters in tumor tissues. CpG methylation status of the promoter regions of PD-1, CTLA-4, TIM-3, LAG-3, PD-L1, TIGIT, and galectin-9 was analyzed by bisulfite sequencing of the genomic DNA isolated from colorectal tumor and normal colon tissues from 14 patients. A bar diagram shows the average demethylation percentage from the 14 NT and TT samples of each gene (**a**). A bar diagram shows the corrected demethylation percentage of immune checkpoints by subtracting average demethylation percentage of NT from TT (**b**). A bar diagram shows the corrected demethylation percentage of immune checkpoints (**c**) and their ligands (**d**) in 14 individual patients

Discussion

Evidence shows that immune system actively participates in tumor development by promoting the uncontrolled growth of tumor cells [24]. Cancer cells bind to co-inhibitory molecules on T cell surface such as CTLA-4, PD-1, TIM-3, and LAG-3 which in turn secrete immune-suppressive mediators such as IDO (indoleamine 2,3-dioxygenase) to create an immune subversive environment in the TME [25, 26]. We have recently reported that in the breast TME, ICs including PD-1, CTLA-4, TIM-3, and LAG-3 were transcriptionally upregulated in TT compared with NT and both DNA and histone modifications in the TME might be actively involved in this upregulation [23]. Additionally, it has been reported by us and other groups that ICs show elevated expression in the colorectal tumor tissues compared with colon normal tissues [5, 27, 28]. However, the epigenetic modifications behind this upregulation are still not disclosed.

In this study, we found that expression of ICs including PD-1, CTLA-4, TIM-3, TIGIT, and IC ligands including PD-L1 and galectin-9 was significantly higher in colorectal tumor tissues compared with normal tissues (Fig. 1a, b). These findings are in line with our pervious report that

the expression of multiple ICs was elevated in the breast TME [23]. In contrast to CRC TME, we did not find IC ligands, PD-L1 and galectin-9 upregulation in the breast TME [23]. These data show that the expressions of ICs/ligands are different in each cancer type, and precise characterization of the ICs and ligands in each cancer type could have prognostic significance. Moreover, we have previously shown that there were more T cell infiltrates in the colorectal TT compared with NT [28]. In this study, we used tissue samples from the same patients that we had used in our previous study [28].

In order to check DNA epigenetic modifications behind the upregulation of ICs/ligands, we checked the expression of demethylation enzymes (TETs) and methylation enzymes (DNMTs) in the tumor and normal tissues and found that the expressions of demethylation enzymes were significantly higher and methylation enzymes were lower in TT (Fig. 1c). It has been reported that the TET protein level was upregulated in solid tumors [29]. These data prompted us to check the CpG methylation profile of the promoter regions of ICs/ligands. We found that the promoter regions of CTLA-4 and TIGIT were significantly hypomethylated in TT compared with NT. These data

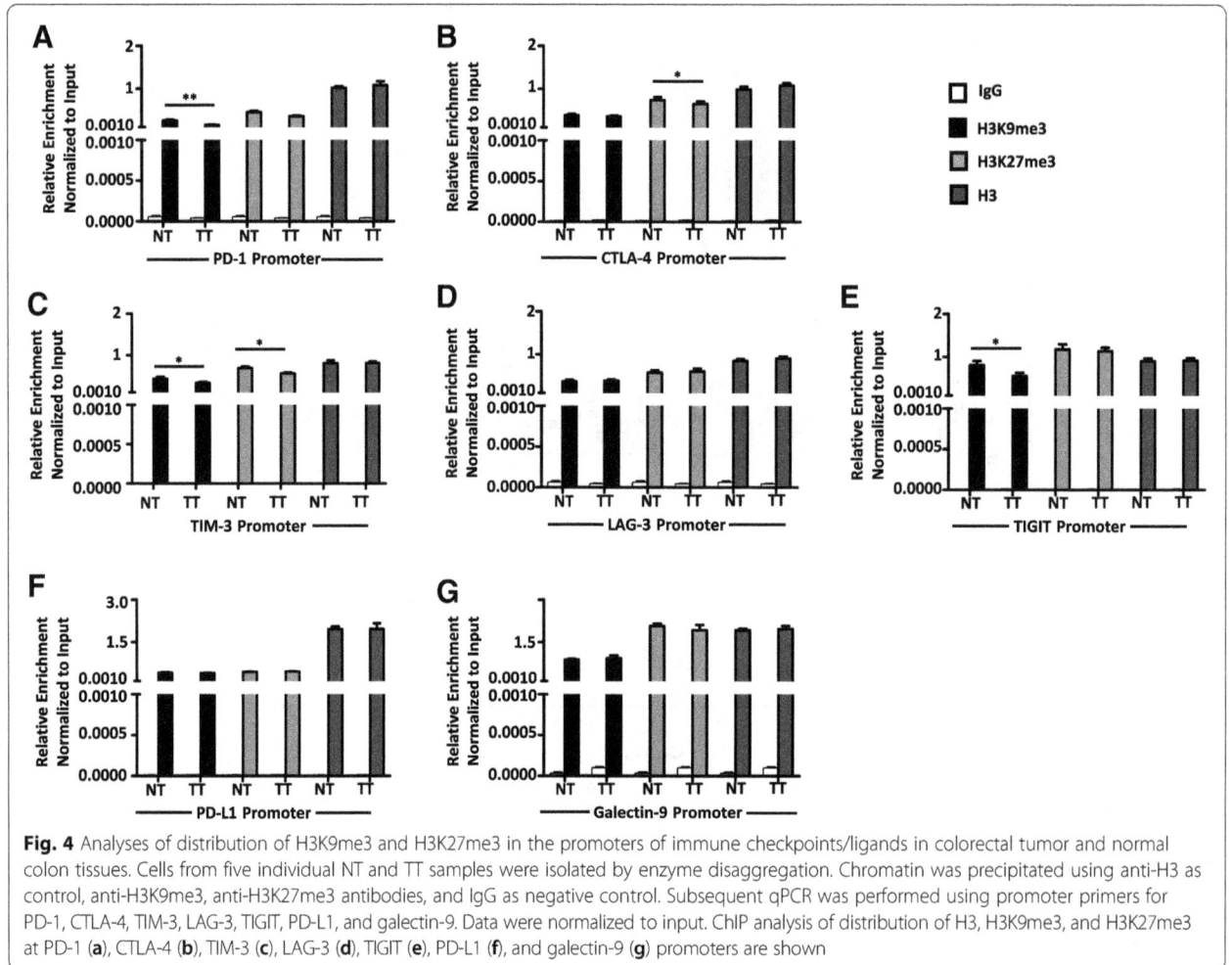

Fig. 4 Analyses of distribution of H3K9me3 and H3K27me3 in the promoters of immune checkpoints/ligands in colorectal tumor and normal colon tissues. Cells from five individual NT and TT samples were isolated by enzyme disaggregation. Chromatin was precipitated using anti-H3 as control, anti-H3K9me3, anti-H3K27me3 antibodies, and IgG as negative control. Subsequent qPCR was performed using promoter primers for PD-1, CTLA-4, TIM-3, LAG-3, TIGIT, PD-L1, and galectin-9. Data were normalized to input. ChIP analysis of distribution of H3, H3K9me3, and H3K27me3 at PD-1 (**a**), CTLA-4 (**b**), TIM-3 (**c**), LAG-3 (**d**), TIGIT (**e**), PD-L1 (**f**), and galectin-9 (**g**) promoters are shown

suggest that not all ICs are following similar epigenetic modifications to upregulate their expression in the TME. Additionally, there was no significant difference in the demethylation percentage in LAG-3 promoter between NT and TT (Fig. 3a). These results are similar to our previous findings in the breast TME that the promoter regions of PD-1, CTLA-4, and TIM-3 were significantly hypomethylated in TT compared with NT and no change in LAG-3 [23]. Compared to our previous study [23], we found that in both NT and TT of colorectal and breast tumors, the CpGs in the promoter region of PD-L1 have been totally demethylated (Fig. 2f), but the relative expression of PD-L1 was significantly higher only in the colorectal TT compared with NT (Fig. 1b). Taken together, our data suggest that the transcriptional upregulation of ICs/ligands does not solely depend on promoter CpG hypomethylation but also on malignant type.

In addition to CpG methylation, we also investigated whether the histone modifications also participate in the upregulation of ICs/ligands in the colorectal TME. It has been reported that promoter region hypermethylation is often associated with H3K9me3 and H3K27me3 for transcriptional silencing [30]. Herein, we checked H3K9me3 and H3K27me3 markings in the promoter regions of PD-1, CTLA-4, TIM-3, LAG-3, TIGIT, PD-L1, and galectin-9 (Fig. 4). In accordance with our previous findings in breast tumors [23], the distribution of H3K9me3 was lower in colorectal TT of PD-1 (Fig. 4a) and H3K27me3 was lower in TT of the CTLA-4 (Fig. 4b) and TIM-3 (Fig. 4c) promoter regions compared with NT. Moreover, there was no change in distribution of either H3K9me3 or H3K27me3 in the promoter regions of LAG-3, PD-L1 and galectin-9 in colorectal TT compared to NT (Fig. 4d, f, g). We have reported that in the breast TME, the relative expression of LAG-3 was higher in TT compared with NT, and also the distribution of both H3K9me3 and H3K27me3 was lower in TT compared with NT [23]. Of note, in CRC tumor tissue, there was no upregulation in the expression of LAG-3 and also no difference in the distribution of either H3K9me3 or H3K27me3 in TT compared to NT (Figs. 1a and 4d). Taken together, these data show that the expression of ICs and the epigenetic modifications in the TME differ in different malignancy types.

Conclusions

This study advances our knowledge in both molecular and epigenetic modifications behind the upregulation of ICs/ligands in the colorectal TME. We showed that multiple ICs/ligands including PD-1, CTLA-4, TIM-3, TIGIT, PD-L1, and galectin-9 are upregulated in the colorectal TME. The epigenetic modifications, including DNA hypomethylation and less abundance of H3K9me3/H3K27me3 in the promoter regions, could be responsible for their upregulation. Moreover, the transcriptional upregulation of CTLA-4 in tumor tissue might be under the control of both DNA hypomethylation and lower H3K27me3 enrichment, while DNA hypomethylation and lower H3K9me3 enrichment regulate TIGIT expression. Additionally, lower enrichment of H3K9me3 or both H3K9me3 and H3K27me3 markings could be behind the upregulation of PD-1 and TIM-3 expressions in the CRC TME, respectively. These examinations of promoter DNA methylation and distribution of repressive histones in different ICs/ligands could be further utilized as a diagnostic tool for colorectal cancer.

Methods

Sample collection

Tumor tissues (TT) and adjacent non-cancerous normal tissues (NT) were obtained from 14 colorectal cancer patients who underwent surgery. All patients provided written informed consent prior to sample collection and none of the patients included in this study received any treatment prior to surgery. Table 1 shows the clinical and pathological characteristics of all patients. The study was executed under ethical approval by the Qatar Biomedical Research Institute, Doha, Qatar (Protocol no. 2017–006).

Table 1 Characteristic features of study population

S no.	Patient ID	Age	Sex	Histological grade	TNM stage
1	CRC 09	56	F	Poorly differentiated	I
2	CRC 12	39	F	Moderately differentiated	IIA
3	CRC 14	41	F	Poorly differentiated	IIIC
4	CRC 15	46	M	Moderately differentiated	IIC
5	CRC 16	67	M	Moderately differentiated	I
6	CRC 18	52	M	Moderately differentiated	IIIB
7	CRC 21	62	M	Poorly differentiated	IIIC
8	CRC 22	41	F	Poorly differentiated	IIIB
9	CRC 26	60	M	Moderately differentiated	IIA
10	CRC 28	39	F	Poorly differentiated	IVB
11	CRC 29	41	F	Moderately differentiated	IIA
12	CRC 30	40	M	Well differentiated	IIIB
13	CRC 32	39	F	Moderately differentiated	IIIB
14	CRC 33	36	M	Moderately differentiated	IIIC

All experiments were performed in accordance with relevant guidelines and regulations.

RNA and DNA isolation

RNA and DNA were isolated using RNA/DNA/Protein Purification Plus Kit (Norgen Biotek Corp, Ontario, Canada) as per manufacturer's instructions, from 14 fresh-frozen TT and their corresponding NT. Briefly, frozen tissues were grinded thoroughly using mortar and pestle with adequate amount of liquid nitrogen. Tissue fragments were then resuspended with lysis buffer and incubated at 55 °C for 10 min. DNA extraction was then performed using the DNA extraction column. The flow-through from DNA extraction was used for RNA purification using RNA extraction column. The flow-through from RNA extraction was then used for protein extraction using the same column. RNA and DNA concentrations were measured using Nanodrop 2000c (Thermo Scientific, MA, USA), and aliquots were stored at − 80 °C.

Quantitative real-time PCR (RT-qPCR)

One microgram of RNA from each sample was reverse transcribed into cDNA using QuantiTect Reverse Transcription Kit (Qiagen, Hilden, Germany). RT-qPCR was performed on QuantStudio 7 Flex qPCR (Applied Biosystems, CA, USA) using PowerUP SYBER Green Master Mix, and all data were normalized to β-actin. Non-specific amplifications were checked by using melting curve and agarose gel electrophoresis. The relative changes in target gene expression were determined using comparative threshold cycle (CT) method $2^{-\Delta\Delta CT}$ between NT and TT. The primers were designed using Primer3 (http://www.ncbi.nlm.nih.gov/tools/primer-blast/) and Harvard Primer Bank (http://pga.mgh.harvard.edu/primerbank/). Primer sequences are provided in Additional file 1: Table S1a.

CpG methylation analysis by bisulfite sequencing

CpG methylation analyses were performed through bisulfite sequencing as previously described [23]. Briefly, genomic DNA was extracted from NT and TT, and bisulfite treatment was performed using the EZ DNA Methylation Kit (Zymo Research, Irvine, CA, USA). PCR was then performed on the bisulfite-treated DNA for amplification of the promoter regions of PD-1, CTLA-4, TIM-3, LAG-3, TIGIT, PD-L1, and galectin-9 using hot start TaKaRa Taq DNA polymerase (TaKaRa Bio, Shiga, Japan). PCR primers were designed using MethPrimer software (http://www.urogene.org/methprimer/index1.html). Primer details are provided in Additional file 1: Table S1b. PCR products were cloned into the pGemT-easy vector (Promega, Madison, USA) using DNA Ligation Kit, Mighty Mix (TaKaRa Bio). Ten individual clones from each sample were purified using Wizard® Plus SV Minipreps DNA Purification System (Promega) and sequenced using M13-reverse/forward primers (Additional file 1: Table S1c). The promoter regions amplified for CpG methylation profile in this study were as previously described [23].

Enzyme disaggregation of tumor and normal tissues for cell isolation

Cell suspensions for ChIP experiments were obtained from frozen NT and TT of five CRC patients by enzyme disaggregation (ED), as previously described [23]. Briefly, thawed tissues were first washed with phosphate-buffered saline (PBS) and mechanically cut into small fragments (2–4 mm) using a surgical scalpel. Tissues were then suspended into RPMI-1640 with 1% penicillin/streptomycin and enzyme cocktail consisting of 1 mg/ml collagenase and 100 µg/ml hyluronidase type V (all from Sigma-Aldrich, UK) and incubated at 37 °C under slow rotation for 60 min. The resulting cell suspension was then passed through a 100 µm BD Falcon cell strainer (BD Biosciences, Oxford, UK), washed with serum free RPMI-1640, and resuspended in RPMI-1640 enriched with 10% FCS and 1% penicillin/streptomycin for further analyses.

Chromatin immunoprecipitation assay (ChIP)

ChIP analysis was performed using Magna ChIP A/G chromatin immunoprecipitation kit (Merck Millipore, MA, USA) as per manufacturer's protocol on cells isolated from NT and TT by ED. Briefly, nuclear lysate was prepared as per manufacturer's protocol and sonicated using Covaris S2 system (Covaris, MA, USA) to make small DNA fragments (100–200 base pairs) and then incubated with ChIP grade anti-Histone H3 rabbit mAb (Active Motif, CA, USA), anti-Histone H3 (tri methyl K9) rabbit mAb (Abcam Cambridge, UK), and anti-Histone H3 (tri methyl K27) rabbit mAb (Abcam). Isotype-matched control antibodies were used as negative controls. Immune complexes containing DNA fragments were precipitated using Magna A/G beads (supplied with the kit). Relative enrichment of target regions in the precipitated DNA fragments was analyzed by qPCR using PowerUP SYBER Green Master Mix (Applied Biosystems) on QuantStudio 7 Flex platform (Applied Biosystems). Sequences of primers are listed in Additional file 1: Table S1d. All data were normalized to input controls. Non-specific amplification was checked by using melting curve and agarose gel electrophoresis.

Sanger sequencing

Purified plasmid DNA samples were subjected to sequencing using 3130X Genetic Analyzer (Applied Biosystems). Cycle sequencing reactions of samples were performed using M-13 forward/reverse primers and Big-Dye Treminator V3.1 (Applied Biosystems), using thermal conditions: 95 °C for 5 min, 35 cycles of 95 °C for 30 s, and 60 °C for 4 min. DNA was precipitated after PCR reaction using 125 mm EDTA and 95% ethanol and incubated at – 20 °C for 30 min. DNA was then washed twice with 70% ethanol followed by denaturation using formaldehyde. Denatured DNA was then loaded into analyzer for sequencing. Sequencing data were analyzed using Bisulfite Sequencing DNA Methylation Analysis (BISMA) software (Jacobs University, Germany).

Statistical analyses

Statistical analyses were performed using GraphPad Prism 5 software (GraphPad Software, USA). Paired t test was carried out on samples within groups that passed the Shapiro–Wilk normality test. Nonparametric/Wilcoxon matched-pairs signed-rank tests were performed on samples that did not pass normality test. A P value of < 0.05 was considered statistically significant. The P values are represented as ***$P < 0.001$, **$P < 0.01$, *$P < 0.05$. The data are presented as mean + standard error of the mean (SEM).

Abbreviations

ChIP: Chromatin immunoprecipitation; CpGI: CpG islands; CTLA-4: Cytotoxic T lymphocyte-associated protein 4; DNMT: DNA methyltransferase; DNMTi: DNA methyltransferase inhibitor; ED: Enzyme disaggregation; H3K27me3: Histone 27 lysine 9 trimethylation; H3K9me3: Histone 3 lysine 9 trimethylation; LAG-3: Lymphocyte-activation gene 3; NT: Normal tissue; PBS: Phosphate-buffered saline; PD-1: Programmed cell death protein-1; PD-L1: Programmed death-ligand 1; RT-qPCR: Quantitative real-time PCR; SEM: Standard error of the mean; TET: Ten-eleven translocation dioxygenase; TIGIT: T cell immunoreceptor with Ig and ITIM domains; TIM-3 : T cell immunoglobulin and mucin-domain containing-3; TT: Tumor tissue

Acknowledgements

We are grateful to all patients for donating their samples. We are also grateful to Dr Haytham El Salhat, Oncology Department, Al Noor Hospital, Abu Dhabi, UAE, for collecting patient samples. We also would like to thank the genomics core facility at Qatar Biomedical Research Institute for Sanger sequencing.

Funding

This work was supported by a start-up grant [VR04] for Dr. Eyad Elkord from Qatar Biomedical Research Institute, Qatar Foundation.

Authors' contributions

VSN performed experimental work, data analysis, and wrote the manuscript. SMT performed the experimental work and contributed to the sample collection, figures preparation, and to manuscript preparation. RZT and HS helped in experimental work. EE conceived the idea, designed the study, obtained funds, supervised the project, analyzed and interpreted data, and wrote and revised the manuscript. All authors were involved in the final approval of the manuscript.

References

1. Siegel RL, Miller KD, Jemal A. Cancer statistics, 2017. CA Cancer J Clin. 2017;67:7–30.
2. van der Geest LG, Lam-Boer J, Koopman M, Verhoef C, Elferink MA, de Wilt JH. Nationwide trends in incidence, treatment and survival of colorectal cancer patients with synchronous metastases. Clin Exp Metastasis. 2015;32:457–65.
3. Hanahan D, Weinberg RA. Hallmarks of cancer: the next generation. Cell. 2011;144:646–74.

4. Emambux S, Tachon G, Junca A, Tougeron D. Results and challenges of immune checkpoint inhibitors in colorectal cancer. Expert Opin Biol Ther. 2018;18:561–73.

5. Passardi A, Canale M, Valgiusti M, Ulivi P. Immune checkpoints as a target for colorectal cancer treatment. Int J Mol Sci. 2017;18:1324.

6. Chaudhary B, Elkord E. Regulatory T cells in the tumor microenvironment and cancer progression: role and therapeutic targeting. Vaccines (Basel). 2016;4:28.

7. Sasidharan Nair V, Elkord E. Immune checkpoint inhibitors in cancer therapy: a focus on T-regulatory cells. Immunol Cell Biol. 2018;96:21–33.

8. Heninger E, Krueger TE, Lang JM. Augmenting antitumor immune responses with epigenetic modifying agents. Front Immunol. 2015;6:29.

9. Jia Y, Guo M. Epigenetic changes in colorectal cancer. Chin J Cancer. 2013; 32:21–30.

10. Lao VV, Grady WM. Epigenetics and colorectal cancer. Nat Rev Gastroenterol Hepatol. 2011;8:686–700.

11. Issa JP. CpG island methylator phenotype in cancer. Nat Rev Cancer. 2004;4: 988–93.

12. Tahiliani M, Koh KP, Shen Y, Pastor WA, Bandukwala H, Brudno Y, et al. Conversion of 5-methylcytosine to 5-hydroxymethylcytosine in mammalian DNA by MLL partner TET1. Science. 2009;324:930–5.

13. Schlesinger Y, Straussman R, Keshet I, Farkash S, Hecht M, Zimmerman J, et al. Polycomb-mediated methylation on Lys27 of histone H3 pre-marks genes for de novo methylation in cancer. Nat Genet. 2007;39:232–6.

14. Derks S, Bosch LJ, Niessen HE, Moerkerk PT, van den Bosch SM, Carvalho B, et al. Promoter CpG island hypermethylation- and H3K9me3 and H3K27me3-mediated epigenetic silencing targets the deleted in colon cancer (DCC) gene in colorectal carcinogenesis without affecting neighboring genes on chromosomal region 18q21. Carcinogenesis. 2009;30:1041–8.

15. Khong HT, Restifo NP. Natural selection of tumor variants in the generation of "tumor escape" phenotypes. Nat Immunol. 2002;3:999–1005.

16. Kim R, Emi M, Tanabe K. Cancer immunoediting from immune surveillance to immune escape. Immunology. 2007;121:1–14.

17. Huang Y, Rao A. Connections between TET proteins and aberrant DNA modification in cancer. Trends Genet. 2014;30:464–74.

18. Pastor WA, Aravind L, Rao A. TETonic shift: biological roles of TET proteins in DNA demethylation and transcription. Nat Rev Mol Cell Biol. 2013;14:341–56.

19. Seshagiri S, Stawiski EW, Durinck S, Modrusan Z, Storm EE, Conboy CB, et al. Recurrent R-spondin fusions in colon cancer. Nature. 2012;488:660–4.

20. An J, Rao A, Ko M. TET family dioxygenases and DNA demethylation in stem cells and cancers. Exp Mol Med. 2017;49:e323.

21. Nair VS, Song MH, Ko M, Oh KI. DNA demethylation of the Foxp3 enhancer is maintained through modulation of ten-eleven-translocation and DNA methyltransferases. Mol Cell. 2016;39:888–97.

22. Esteller M. CpG island hypermethylation and tumor suppressor genes: a booming present, a brighter future. Oncogene. 2002;21:5427–40.

23. Sasidharan Nair V, El Salhat H, Taha RZ, John A, Ali BR, Elkord E. DNA methylation and repressive H3K9 and H3K27 trimethylation in the promoter regions of PD-1, CTLA-4, TIM-3, LAG-3, TIGIT, and PD-L1 genes in human primary breast cancer. Clin Epigenetics. 2018;10:78.

24. Gubin MM, Zhang X, Schuster H, Caron E, Ward JP, Noguchi T, et al. Checkpoint blockade cancer immunotherapy targets tumour-specific mutant antigens. Nature. 2014;515:577–81.

25. Mahoney KM, Rennert PD, Freeman GJ. Combination cancer immunotherapy and new immunomodulatory targets. Nat Rev Drug Discov. 2015;14:561–84.

26. Postow MA, Callahan MK, Wolchok JD. Immune checkpoint blockade in cancer therapy. J Clin Oncol. 2015;33:1974–82.

27. Rosenbaum MW, Bledsoe JR, Morales-Oyarvide V, Huynh TG, Mino-Kenudson M. PD-L1 expression in colorectal cancer is associated with microsatellite instability, BRAF mutation, medullary morphology and cytotoxic tumor-infiltrating lymphocytes. Mod Pathol. 2016;29:1104–12.

28. Syed Khaja AS, Toor SM, El Salhat H, Ali BR, Elkord E. Intratumoral FoxP3(+)Helios(+) regulatory T cells upregulating immunosuppressive molecules are expanded in human colorectal cancer. Front Immunol. 2017;8:619.

29. Ficz G, Gribben JG. Loss of 5-hydroxymethylcytosine in cancer: cause or consequence? Genomics. 2014;104:352–7.

30. Ohm JE, McGarvey KM, Yu X, Cheng L, Schuebel KE, Cope L, et al. A stem cell-like chromatin pattern may predispose tumor suppressor genes to DNA hypermethylation and heritable silencing. Nat Genet. 2007;39:237–42.

23

The polyphenol quercetin induces cell death in leukemia by targeting epigenetic regulators of pro-apoptotic genes

Marisa Claudia Alvarez, Victor Maso, Cristiane Okuda Torello, Karla Priscilla Ferro and Sara Teresinha Olalla Saad[*]

Abstract

Background: In the present study, we investigated the molecular mechanisms underlying the pro-apoptotic effects of quercetin (Qu) by evaluating the effect of Qu treatment on DNA methylation and posttranslational histone modifications of genes related to the apoptosis pathway. This study was performed in vivo in two human xenograft acute myeloid leukemia (AML) models and in vitro using HL60 and U937 cell lines.

Results: Qu treatment almost eliminates DNMT1 and DNMT3a expression, and this regulation was in part STAT-3 dependent. The treatment also downregulated class I HDACs. Furthermore, treatment of the cell lines with the proteasome inhibitor, MG132, together with Qu prevented degradation of class I HDACs compared to cells treated with Qu alone, indicating increased proteasome degradation of class I HDACS by Qu. Qu induced demethylation of the pro-apoptotic BCL2L11, *DAPK1* genes, in a dose- and time-dependent manner. Moreover, Qu (50 µmol/L) treatment of cell lines for 48 h caused accumulation of acetylated histone 3 and histone 4, resulting in three- to ten fold increases in the promoter region of *DAPK1*, *BCL2L11*, *BAX*, *APAF1*, *BNIP3*, and *BNIP3L*. In addition, Qu treatment significantly increased the mRNA levels of all these genes, when compared to cells treated with vehicle only (control cells) (*$p < 0.05$*).

Conclusions: In summary, our results showed that enhanced apoptosis, induced by Qu, might be caused in part by its DNA demethylating activity, by HDAC inhibition, and by the enrichment of H3ac and H4ac in the promoter regions of genes involved in the apoptosis pathway, leading to their transcription activation.

Keywords: Quercetin, HDACs, DNMTs, Epigenetics, Leukemia

Background

The myelodysplastic syndromes (MDSs) are a group of diverse and heterogeneous disorders characterized by clonal proliferation, bone marrow failure, and an increased risk of the development of acute myelogenous leukemia (AML) [1]. Leukemia has traditionally been considered to be the consequence of genetic alterations; however, in recent years, a body of evidence has demonstrated that the neoplastic phenotypes, including leukemia, may also be mediated by epigenetic alterations [2–4]. Epigenetics, broadly, refers to stimuli-triggered changes in gene expression due to processes that arise independentless of changes in the underlying DNA sequence. Some of these

processes include DNA methylation [5], histone modifications and chromatin-remodeling proteins [6], and DNA silencing by noncoding RNAs (ncRNA) [7]. The reversability of epigenetics makes this mechanism a potential target for novel therapeutic approaches.

Quercetin (Qu) is an important dietary flavonoid, present in different vegetables, fruits, nuts, tea, red wine, and propolis [8–10]. Its study as potential therapeutic agent is assuming importance considering its involvement in the suppression of many tumor-related processes including oxidative stress, apoptosis, proliferation, and metastasis. Qu has also received attention as a pro-apoptotic flavonoid with a specific and almost exclusive effect on tumor cell lines rather than normal, non-transformed cells [11].

A previous study from our group showed that Qu caused pronounced apoptosis in leukemia cells, in vivo and in vitro (xenograft model), followed by *BCL-2*,

---
* Correspondence: sara@unicamp.br
Hematology and Transfusion Medicine Center-University of Campinas/
Hemocentro-UNICAMP, Instituto Nacional de Ciencia e Tecnologia do
Sangue, Rua Carlos Chagas, 480, CEP, Campinas, SP 13083-878, Brazil

BCL-XL, MCL-1 downregulation, BAX upregulation, and mitochondrial translocation, triggering cytochrome c release and caspase activation [12]. In the present study, we investigated the molecular mechanisms underlying the pro-apoptotic effects of Qu by evaluating the effect of Qu treatment on DNA methylation and posttranslational histone modifications of genes related to the apoptosis pathway. Qu treatment of the myeloid leukemia cells, in vitro or in a human tumor xenograft, induced apoptosis, in part, through the reversal of epigenetic alterations.

Results

Gene-specific promoter methylation of apoptosis-related genes

We examined the DNA methylation status at the promoter CpG islands of 24 apoptosis-related genes in the HL60 cell line. Of the 24 genes assayed in the cell line,

the extent of promoter methylation in five genes (BCL2L11, DAPK1, HRK, TNFRSF21, TNFRSF25) exceeded 90% (Fig. 1a). In order to determine whether quercetin affected CpG methylation, we further validated the promoter methylation of BCL2L11 and DAPK1 by MSP-PCR in samples treated with 50 and 75 μmol/L of Qu for 48 and 72 h. After 72 h of Qu treatment, there was partial demethylation of BCL2L11 and DAPK1 gene promoters in HL60 cells (Fig. 1b, c). The partial demethylation of DAPK1 promoter was confirmed by bisulfite sequencing (Fig. 1d-f). Concentrations of 1 and 2 μM concentration of 5-aza-dC were chosen as positive control. The U937 cell line was also treated with Qu (same concentrations and period of time as for HL60 cells). This cell line was unmethylated in the promoter region of DAPK1 and hemimethylated in the promoter region of BCL2L11. No demethylation was observed after Qu treatment (Fig. 1c).

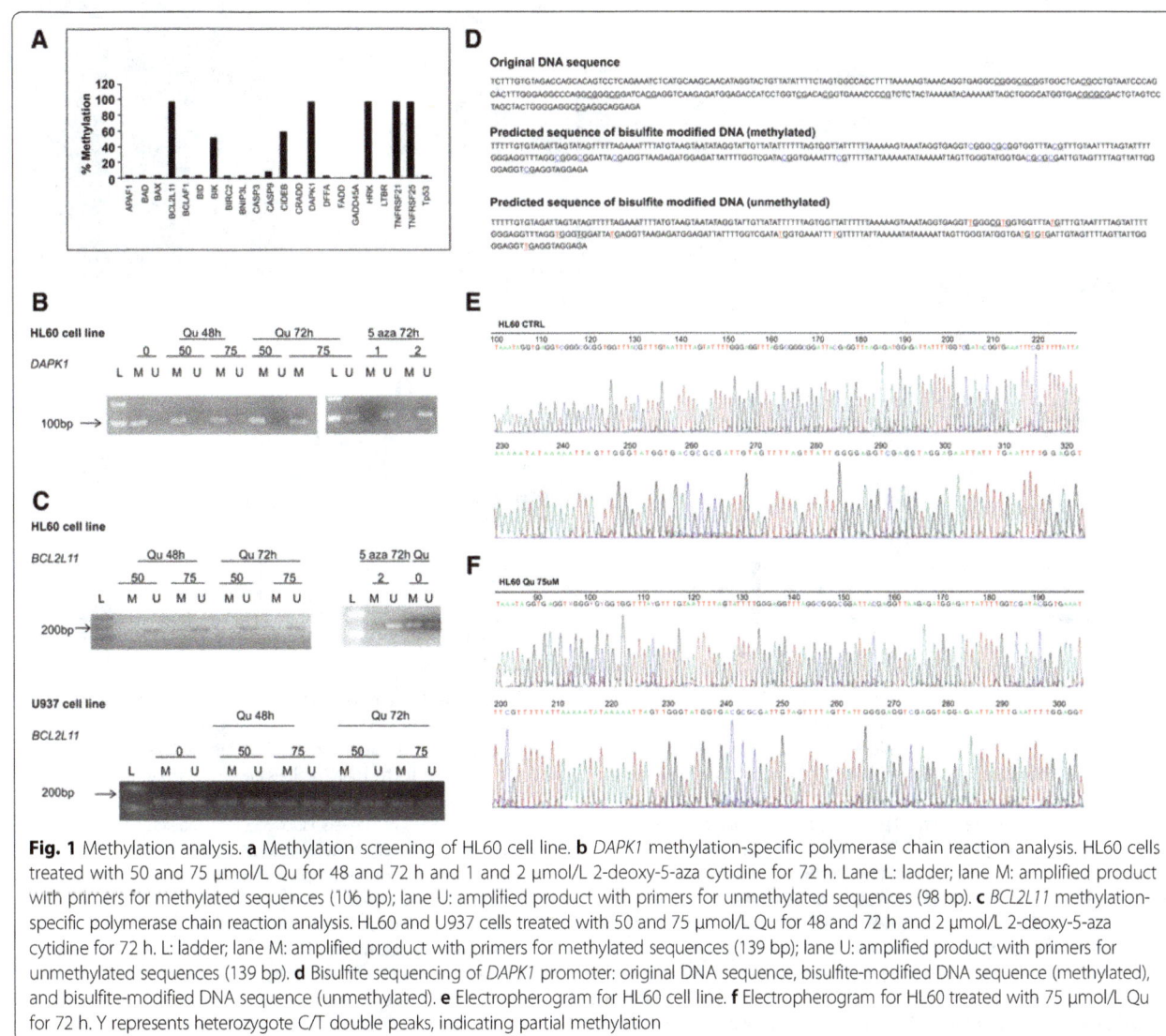

Fig. 1 Methylation analysis. a Methylation screening of HL60 cell line. b DAPK1 methylation-specific polymerase chain reaction analysis. HL60 cells treated with 50 and 75 μmol/L Qu for 48 and 72 h and 1 and 2 μmol/L 2-deoxy-5-aza cytidine for 72 h. Lane L: ladder; lane M: amplified product with primers for methylated sequences (106 bp); lane U: amplified product with primers for unmethylated sequences (98 bp). c BCL2L11 methylation-specific polymerase chain reaction analysis. HL60 and U937 cells treated with 50 and 75 μmol/L Qu for 48 and 72 h and 2 μmol/L 2-deoxy-5-aza cytidine for 72 h. L: ladder; lane M: amplified product with primers for methylated sequences (139 bp); lane U: amplified product with primers for unmethylated sequences (139 bp). d Bisulfite sequencing of DAPK1 promoter: original DNA sequence, bisulfite-modified DNA sequence (methylated), and bisulfite-modified DNA sequence (unmethylated). e Electropherogram for HL60 cell line. f Electropherogram for HL60 treated with 75 μmol/L Qu for 72 h. Y represents heterozygote C/T double peaks, indicating partial methylation

Quercetin downregulates DNMTs and STAT3

Since Qu induced partial demethylation in the promoter regions of highly methylated genes, Western blot analyses using anti-DNMT1 (DNA methyltransferase 1) and anti-DNMT3a (DNA methyltransferase 3a) antibodies were performed. Qu treatment decreased the levels of both proteins. Next, since the STAT3 pathway direct regulates DNMTs [13], we investigated whether Qu treatment modulates these proteins. Western blot analysis, RT-PCR, and confocal microscopy showed that Qu treatment downregulated STAT3 expression and phosphorylation ($*p < 0.05$). These data provide evidence that Qu downregulates DNMTs through STAT3 pathway (Fig. 2a–c).

Quercetin induces H3 and H4 global acetylation

Like DNA methylation, the acetylation or methylation of histone proteins comprise major epigenetic processes on the chromatin structure, altering nucleosomal architecture and leading to gene activation or repression. In order to determine whether Qu also affects histones, we determined the effect of Qu treatment on global acetylation of histones 3 and 4. For this purpose, Western blotting of the acid extracted proteins of the HL60 cell line were exposed to 50 μmol/L Qu for 48 h and western blotting was performed. After Qu treatment, a global increase in H3ac and H4ac was observed compared to cells treated with vehicle only (Fig. 2d).

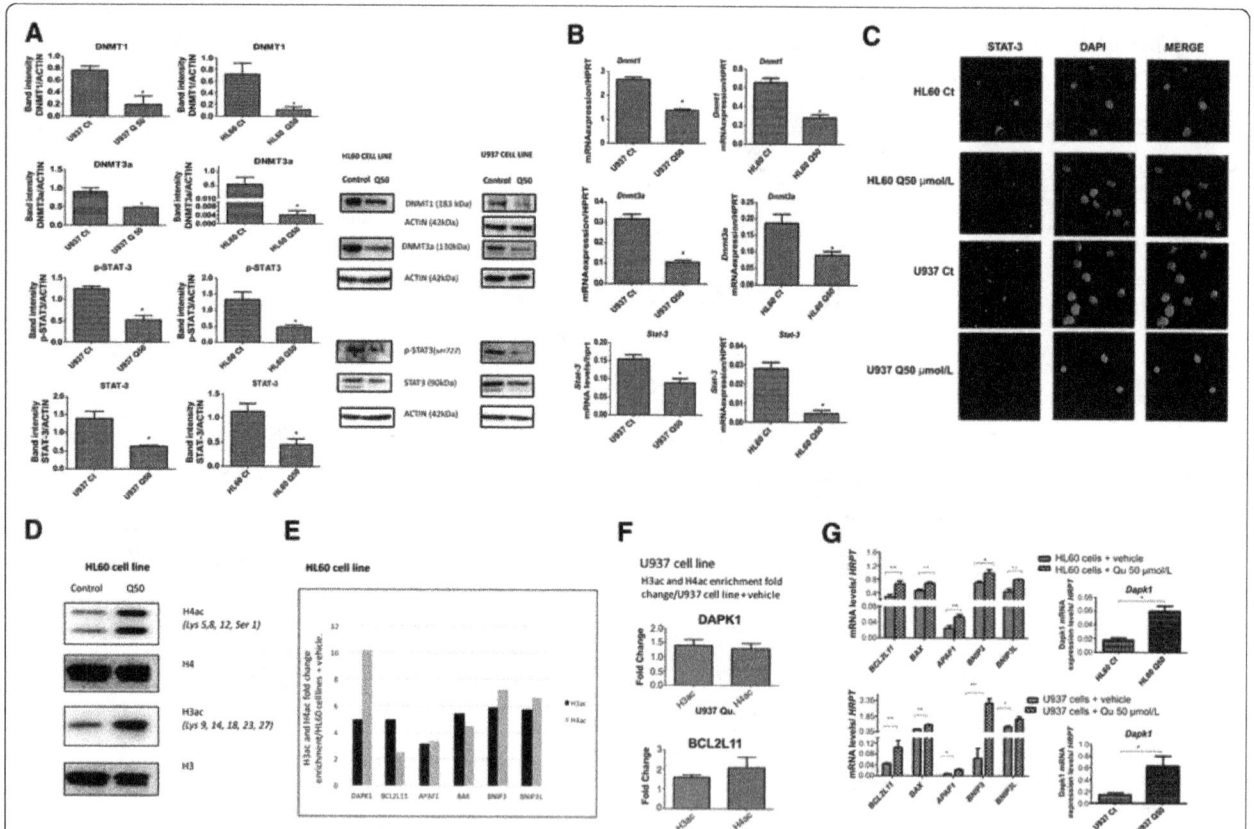

Fig. 2 Quercetin treatment decreases DNMTs, in STAT3-dependent manner, increases global acetylation of H3 and H4, and increases the enrichment of acetylated histone H3 and H4 to the promoters of genes related to the apoptosis pathway. **a** HL60 and U937 cell lines were treated with 50 μmol/L Qu for 48 h. Western blotting was performed for DNMT1, DNMT3a, p-STAT3, and STAT3 proteins. Values are means ± SD of three independent assays. $*p < 0.05$ when compared to cell lines treated with vehicle only. One experiment in three is shown. **b** The mRNA values are expressed as mean ± SD of three independent experiments. $*p < 0.05$; $** p < 0.005$ when compared to HL60 or U937 cells treated with vehicle only. **c** Confocal microscopy view of HL60 and U937 cells treated with 50 μmol/L Qu for 48 h, incubated with STAT3 antibody and probed with Alexa Fluor 555 (red)-labeled secondary antibody showing a decreased STAT3 expression after treatment. DAPI was used to stain nuclei. **d** Western blotting analysis of acid extracted proteins of HL60 cell line exposed to 50 μmol/l Qu for 48 h. Qu treatment increases acetylated levels of H3 and H4. One representative experiment in three is shown. **e** Treatment of HL60 cells with 50 μmol/L Qu for 48 h. *Apoptosis ChIP human PCR array* for association of acetylated histone H3 and H4 with the promoters of *DAPK1*, *BCL2L11*, *APAF1*, *BAX*, *BNIP3*, and *BNIP3L* was performed; details are provided in the "Methods" section. **f** Chromatin immunoprecipitation assay was performed for association of acetylated H3 and H4 histones with the promoters of *DAPK1* and *BCL2L11* in U937 cells treated with 50 μmol/L Qu for 48 h. Qu treatment caused increased association of acetylated histones H3 and H4 to the promoters of *DAPK1* and *BCL2L11*. **g** *BCL2L11*, *BAX*, *APAF1*, *BNIP3*, and *BNIP3L* mRNA expression levels of HL60 and U937 cells treated with 50 μmol/L Qu for 48 h. The mRNA values are expressed as mean ± SD of three independent experiments. $*p < 0.05$, $**p < 0.005$, when compared to HL60 or U937 cells + vehicle

Quercetin enriched H3ac and H4ac in the promoter region of the apoptosis pathway genes and increased their transcription levels

We then wondered whether this increase in acetylation of H3 and H4 also occurred at promoter regions of genes involved in the apoptosis pathway. To verify this, an *Apoptosis ChIP human PCR array* (SAbiosciences, Qiagen) was performed. HL60 cells treated with 50 µmol/L Qu, for 48 h induced a three- to ten fold enrichment of H3ac and H4ac in the promoter regions of *APAF1*, *BAX*, *BCL2L11*, *BNIP3 BNIP3*, and *DAPK1* (Fig. 2e). We further analyzed the mRNA expression levels of these genes in HL60 and U937 samples treated with 50 µmol/L Qu for 48 h. Qu treatment significantly increased the mRNA levels of all these genes in both cell lines, when compared to control cells (**$p < 0.005$; *$p < 0.05$) (Fig. 2g). As the *DAPK1* gene promoter is unmethylated and Qu treatment did not induce demethylation of promoter region of *BCL2L11* in the U937 cell line, furthermore, Qu treatment upregulated mRNA expression levels of *DAPK1* and *BCL2L11*, we proceeded to investigate whether Qu treatment also induced an enrichment of H3 and H4 acetylation in the promoter regions of *DAPK1* and *BCL2L11* in U937 cell line.

Using anti acetylated histone H3 and H4 antibodies, followed by RT-PCR with specific primers for *DAPK1* and *BCL2L11* promoters, a chromatin immunoprecipitation assay was performed. As shown in Fig. 2f, Qu treatment resulted in an increase in the amount of acetylated H3 and H4 associated with both *DAPK1* and *BCL2L11* promoters.

To confirm that Qu effect on apoptosis was via *DAPK1* and *BCL2L11*, we proceeded to stably inhibit these genes in the cell lines. Further, the transduced cell lines were treated with 50 µmol/L of Qu for 48 h, and apoptosis was detected by flow cytometry. It was observed that in both *BCL2L11* shRNA-transduced cell lines, Qu induced apoptosis at a lesser extend when compared to control shRNA-transduced cell lines (*$p < 0.05$; **$p < 0.001$) (Fig. 3a–c). It was not possible to accomplish *DAPK1* inhibition. For both cell lines, the shRNA lentiviral particle caused too much damage and cells did not recover from transduction.

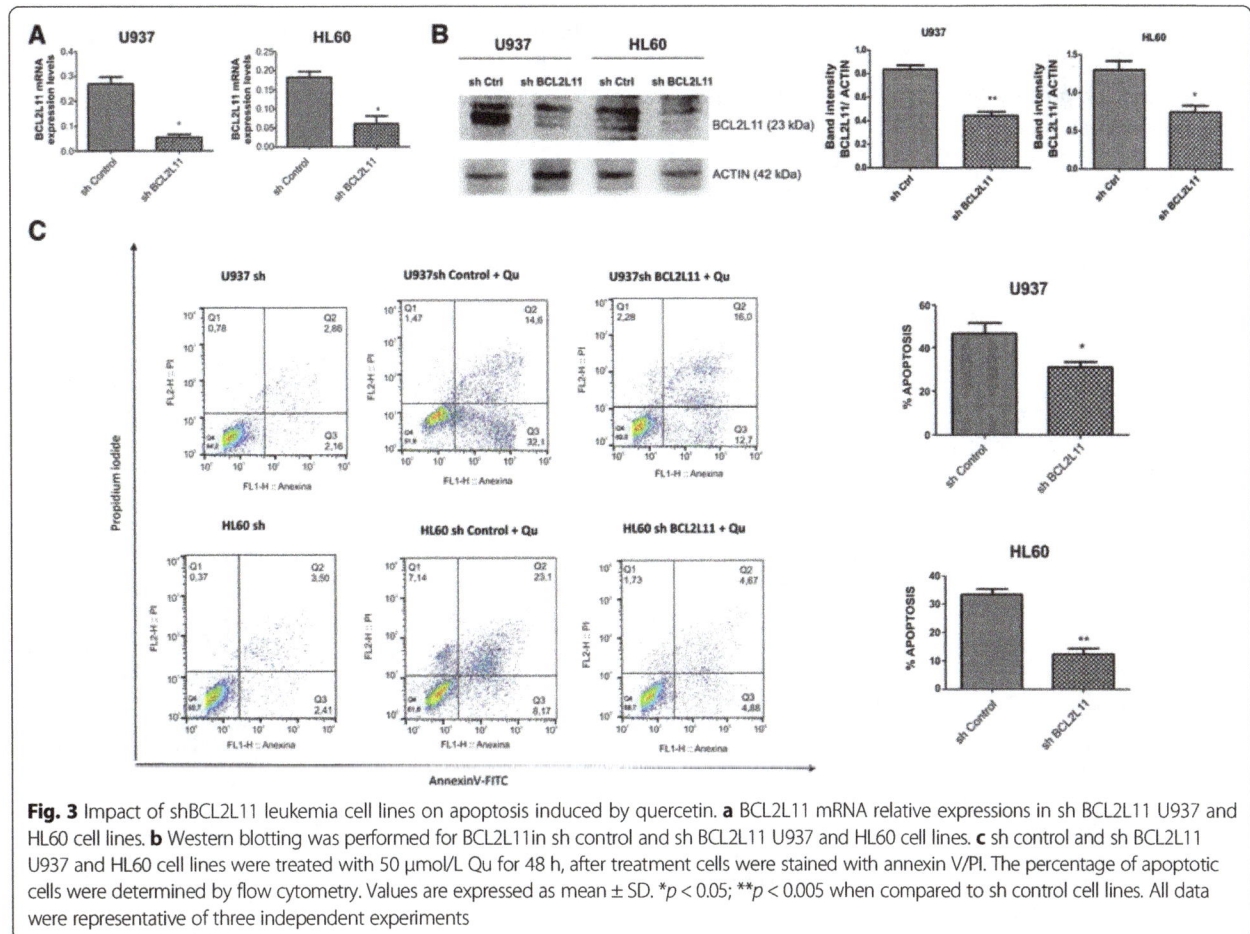

Fig. 3 Impact of shBCL2L11 leukemia cell lines on apoptosis induced by quercetin. **a** BCL2L11 mRNA relative expressions in sh BCL2L11 U937 and HL60 cell lines. **b** Western blotting was performed for BCL2L11in sh control and sh BCL2L11 U937 and HL60 cell lines. **c** sh control and sh BCL2L11 U937 and HL60 cell lines were treated with 50 µmol/L Qu for 48 h, after treatment cells were stained with annexin V/PI. The percentage of apoptotic cells were determined by flow cytometry. Values are expressed as mean ± SD. *$p < 0.05$; **$p < 0.005$ when compared to sh control cell lines. All data were representative of three independent experiments

Quercetin decreases the protein expression of class I histone deacetylases (HDACs) in leukemia cells

Given the data described herein and the fact that HADCs are found in corepressor complexes, we investigated whether the global increment of the acetylation of H3 and H4 affected the expression levels of HADCs. To establish whether Qu treatment alters the protein expression of class I HADCs, we performed Western blot analysis on total cell lysates of HL60 and U937 cells treated with 50 μmol/L Qu for 48 h. Exposure of cells to Qu caused a decrease in the levels of HADCs 1 and 2 (*$p < 0.05$) (Fig. 4) but not of HDAC 3 and 8 in both cell lines (data not shown).

Quercetin caused proteasome-mediated protein degradation of HADCs in leukemia cells

Furthermore, we determined whether proteasome-mediated degradation was involved in the downregulation of HADCs in cells exposed to Qu. HL60 and U937 cell lines were exposed to 50 μmol/L Qu for 40 h in duplicate, followed by the addition of 10 μmol/L MG132 (an inhibitor of proteasome) to one group and incubated for an additional 8 h. Compared to cells treated only with Qu, MG132 caused a significant increase in HADC expression in both cell lines, demonstrating that Qu treatment downregulates these proteins through proteasome degradation (Fig. 4).

Quercetin downregulates DNMTs and HADCs at the protein levels, in xenograft models

Our in vitro results encouraged us to proceed with an in vivo model; mice were subcutaneously engraftment with

HL60 and/or U937 cells, as described in the "Methods" section. Accordingly, Qu treatment almost eliminated DNMT protein levels, and this occurred in part through the downregulation of STAT3 and p-STAT3 at the protein and message levels (*$p < 0.05$; **$p < 0.005$) (Fig. 5a). mRNA expression levels of *DAPK1*, *BCL2L11*, *BAX*, *BNIP3*, *BNIP3L*, and *APAF1* were significantly upregulated compared to those of the control mice (*$p < 0.05$; **$p < 0.005$) (Fig. 5b). Moreover, in treated animals, decreased protein levels of HDAC 1 and 2 were also observed (*$p < 0.05$; **$p < 0.005$) (Fig. 5c).

Discussion

Epigenetic mechanisms involving modifications in the DNA (methylation) and histones (acetylation, methylation, among others) and their corresponding effects on gene regulation have gained considerable interest. The pattern of modifications on histones and DNA constitutes an epigenetic program that is unique for the cell type and is replicated during successive cell divisions. Alterations of these patterns, particularly in the promoter region of genes, can have profound effects on gene expression. Studies from various cancers have revealed that these alterations affect genes involved in different cellular pathways including apoptosis. Cancer cells have the ability to avoid apoptosis, and this is considered to be one of the prime factors that aid the evolution of cancer [14].

Previously, we have shown that Qu upregulated the expression of pro-apoptotic proteins [12]. Then, in this study, we first performed a screening of the promoter methylation status of 24 apoptosis-related genes in human

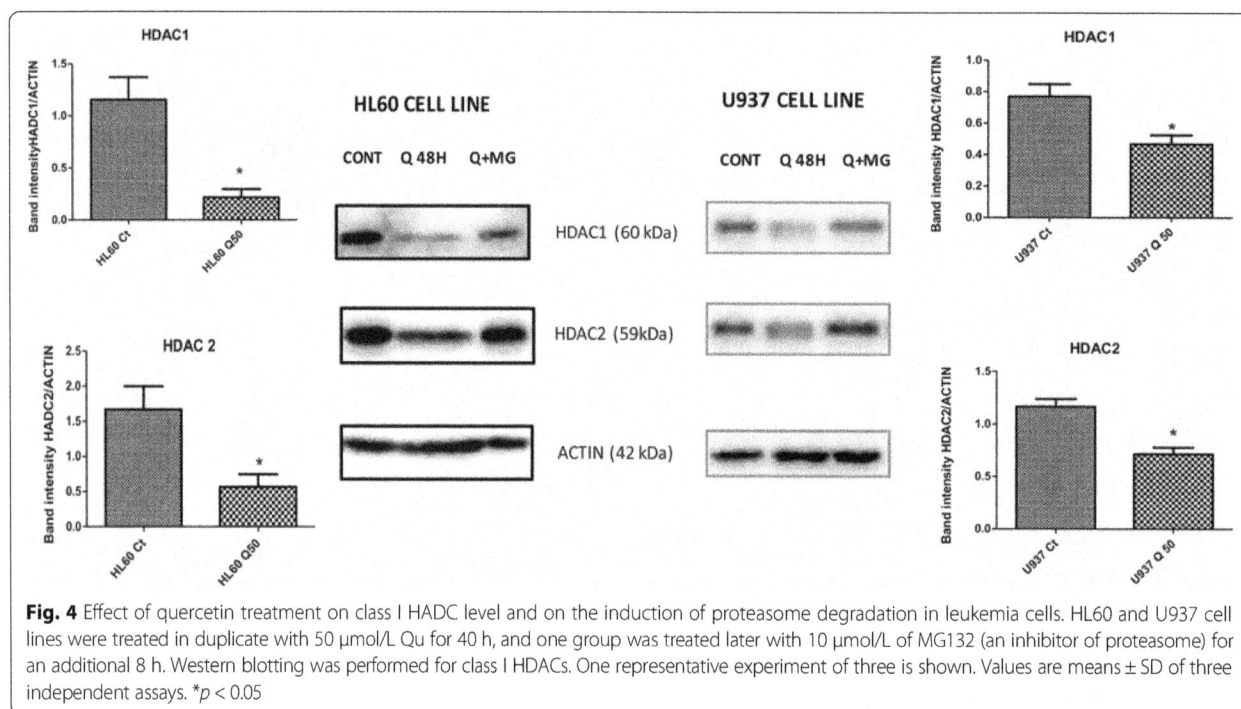

Fig. 4 Effect of quercetin treatment on class I HADC level and on the induction of proteasome degradation in leukemia cells. HL60 and U937 cell lines were treated in duplicate with 50 μmol/L Qu for 40 h, and one group was treated later with 10 μmol/L of MG132 (an inhibitor of proteasome) for an additional 8 h. Western blotting was performed for class I HDACs. One representative experiment of three is shown. Values are means ± SD of three independent assays. *$p < 0.05$

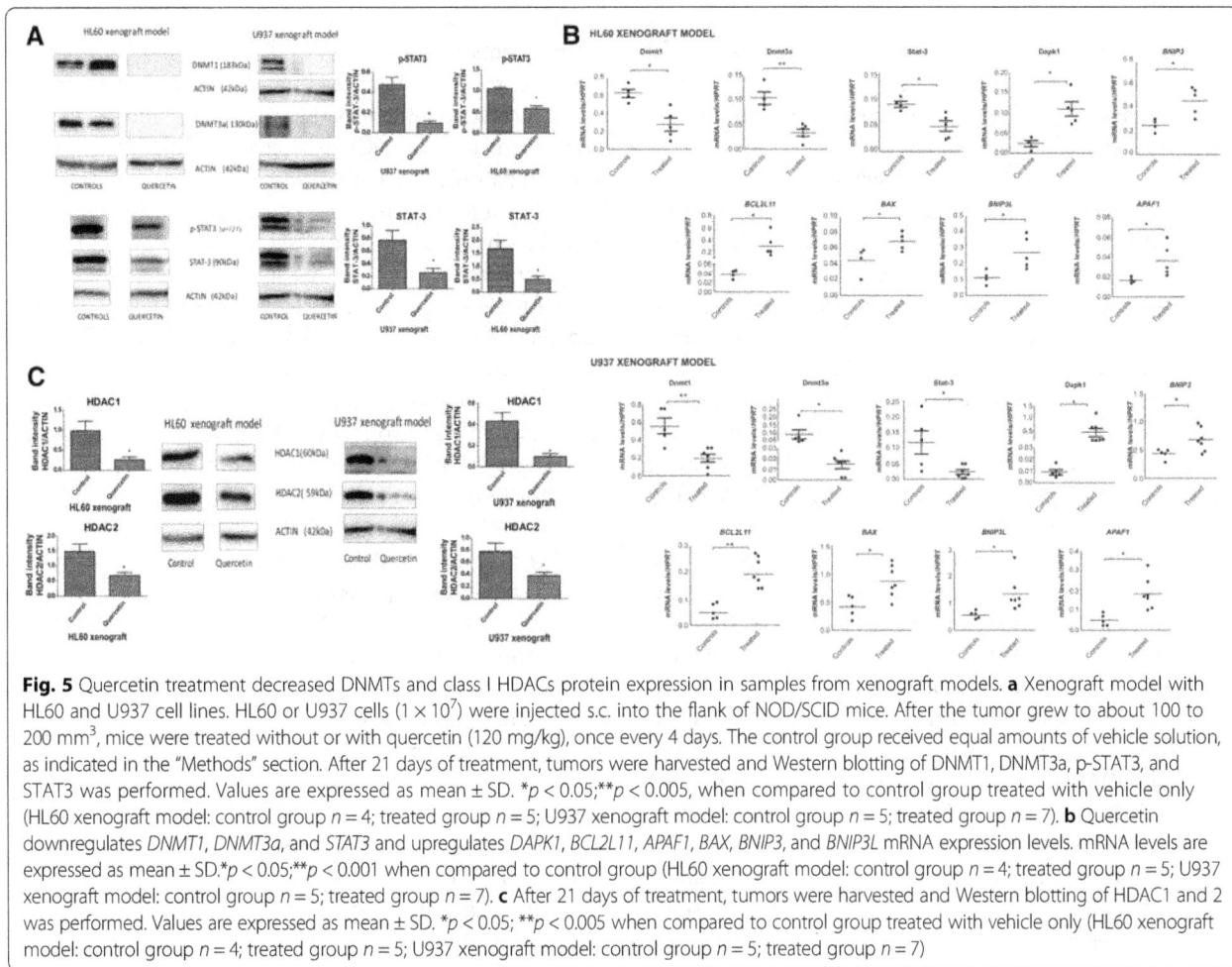

Fig. 5 Quercetin treatment decreased DNMTs and class I HDACs protein expression in samples from xenograft models. **a** Xenograft model with HL60 and U937 cell lines. HL60 or U937 cells (1×10^7) were injected s.c. into the flank of NOD/SCID mice. After the tumor grew to about 100 to 200 mm^3, mice were treated without or with quercetin (120 mg/kg), once every 4 days. The control group received equal amounts of vehicle solution, as indicated in the "Methods" section. After 21 days of treatment, tumors were harvested and Western blotting of DNMT1, DNMT3a, p-STAT3, and STAT3 was performed. Values are expressed as mean ± SD. *$p < 0.05$;**$p < 0.005$, when compared to control group treated with vehicle only (HL60 xenograft model: control group $n = 4$; treated group $n = 5$; U937 xenograft model: control group $n = 5$; treated group $n = 7$). **b** Quercetin downregulates *DNMT1*, *DNMT3a*, and *STAT3* and upregulates *DAPK1*, *BCL2L11*, *APAF1*, *BAX*, *BNIP3*, and *BNIP3L* mRNA expression levels. mRNA levels are expressed as mean ± SD.*$p < 0.05$;**$p < 0.001$ when compared to control group (HL60 xenograft model: control group $n = 4$; treated group $n = 5$; U937 xenograft model: control group $n = 5$; treated group $n = 7$). **c** After 21 days of treatment, tumors were harvested and Western blotting of HDAC1 and 2 was performed. Values are expressed as mean ± SD. *$p < 0.05$; **$p < 0.005$ when compared to control group treated with vehicle only (HL60 xenograft model: control group $n = 4$; treated group $n = 5$; U937 xenograft model: control group $n = 5$; treated group $n = 7$)

HL60 cells. The analysis revealed that five of these genes were highly methylated, including *BCL2L11*, *DAPK1*, *HRK*, *TNFRSF21*, and *TNFRSF25*. Furthermore, we validated the methylation pattern of *BCL2L11* and *DAPK1* using MSP-PCR in samples treated with Qu and observed that the treatment with Qu totally and partially demethylated *BCL2L11* and *DAPK1*, respectively. This demethylation was both dose and time dependent.

DAPK1 (death-associated protein kinase 1) is a pro-apoptotic gene that induces cellular apoptosis in response to internal and external apoptotic stimulants [15]. Therefore, silencing of *DAPK1* may result in uncontrolled cell proliferation, indicating that this gene may have a role in tumor suppression. Several studies have demonstrated promoter methylation of *DAPK1* in different types of cancer such as renal [15] and cervical cancer [16], B cell lymphoma [17], myelodysplastic syndrome, acute myeloblastic leukemia [18], and chronic myeloid leukemia [19–21]. Our data show that Qu partially demethylates the promoter region of this gene in both a dose- and time-dependent manner, and this may contribute to the increased apoptosis observed in a previous

study realized by our group [12]. Consistent with the demethylating effect of Qu, a previous study reported that different concentrations of Qu partially reverted *P16INK4a* promoter methylation and increased its expression in RKO cells after 5 days of treatment [22].

DNA methylation at the cytosine 5 nucleotide is catalyzed by DNA methyltransferases (DNMTs). This family of proteins is vitally important in epigenetic regulation to modulate gene expression [23]. In our study, Qu treatment almost eliminated DNMT1 and DNMT3a at the protein and message levels, in vitro and in human xenograft models. A previous study, in a gastric cancer cell line, showed that quercetin and isoliquiritigenin decreased DNMT1 and DNMT3a protein levels, causing slight demethylation of the promoter region of the BCL7A gene [24]. We further investigated the expression levels of p-STAT3 and STAT3. STAT3 is a member of a family of transcription factors that regulates proliferation, apoptosis, differentiation, and oncogenesis, and it also regulates DNMT transcription [13]. We found that Qu decreased STAT3 at the protein and at the message level and p-STAT3 at the protein level. The decrease in STAT3 was also confirmed by confocal microscopy. Unlike this previous study [24], we observed that Qu decreased DNMTs in a STAT3-dependent manner, demonstrating that the mode of action of specific natural compounds depends on their cellular origin.

BCL2L11 (BCL2-interacting mediator, (BIM)) is a member of the BH3-only death activator family and a key determinant of cell fate upon cytokine withdrawal. Its expression is regulated by transcriptional and post-transcriptional mechanisms [25]. BCL2L11 downregulation has a central role in the survival of clonal progenitors of chronic myeloid leukemia (CML), and this low expression was ascribed to DNA hypermethylation at the gene promoter [26–28]. Moreover, BCL2L11 re-expression has a key role in BCR-ABL1-expressing cell apoptosis in response to imatinib (IM) [29]. We also observed an upregulation of mRNA levels of this gene in vitro and in vivo (xenograft models), induced by Qu treatment. However, in xenograft models, this upregulation was independent of the demethylation of the promoter region of the gene. This upregulation may be the consequence of the augmentation in H3ac and H4ac observed in the promoter region. Moreover, a study in NPM/ALK+ anaplastic large cell lymphoma (ALCL) cell lines and NPM/ALK+ ALCL lymph node biopsies showed that BCL2L11 is epigenetically silenced and that treatment with the deacetylase inhibitor trichostatin A restores histone acetylation, strongly upregulates BCL2L11 expression, and induces cell death [30]. In addition, a study realized by Lee et al. [31] showed that Qu induced apoptosis in leukemia HL60 cells by enhancing the expression of Fas-L, in part through the promotion of H3 acetylation.

We observed in vitro that 50 µmol/L Qu increased the enrichment of H3ac and H4ac by three- to ten fold, after 48 h, in the promoter region of DAPK1, BCL2L11, BAX, BNIP3, BNIP3L, and APAF1, compared to control cells. Further, we analyzed mRNA levels of these genes in vitro and in vivo (in samples from xenograft models) and observed that all of them were upregulated, compared to control samples. It is known that histone acetylation mainly occurs at the promoter regions of genes in the process of transcription, whereas histone deacetylation cooperates with gene silencing. Histone deacetylases (HDACs) deacetylate lysine residues of histone tails leading to condensation and closed chromatin formation and transcriptional repression [32].

In the present study, we showed that Qu treatment decreased HDAC1 and HDAC2 protein levels in vitro and in vivo, in the xenograft models, and induced its proteasomal degradation. Many important molecular cell processes are performed by large multisubunit protein complexes, and HDACs do it in the same way. HDAC1 and 2 exist together in at least three distinct multiprotein CoREST complexes [33], and these corepressor complexes are recruited by specific DNA sequences to promoter regions, resulting in transcriptional repression [34].

A potential mechanism to induce apoptosis through histone deacetylase inhibitors (HDACi) is the upregulation of apoptotic genes. HADCi can activate components of the intrinsic pathway, including BAX and APAF1. APAF1 has been shown to be upregulated by HDACi including suberoylanilide hydroxamic acid SAHA [35, 36]. APAF1 binds to cytochrome C, forming the apoptosome and initiating the caspase cascade. BAX is a cytosolic protein that undergoes conformational change during apoptosis and migrates to the mitochondria, while APAF1 cooperates with the release of cytochrome c. In addition, a recent study showed that two HDACi, kendine 92 and SAHA, induced apoptosis in CLL cells by increasing BAD, BNIP3, BNIP3L, BIM, PUMA, and AIF mRNA expression levels and decreasing expression of BCL-W, BCL-2, BFL-1, XIAP, and FLIP. Thus, this study indicates global changes in the apoptosis mRNA expression profile, consistent with the apoptotic outcome [37]. Moreover, Qu has also been shown to inhibit cell cycle and induce apoptosis through inhibition of HDAC and DNMT1, thus suppressing tumor growth and angiogenesis in an induced model of hamster buccal pouch carcinoma [38].

Conclusions

In summary, our results showed that enhanced apoptosis, induced by Qu, might be caused in part by its DNA demethylating activity, by HDAC inhibition, and by the enrichment of H3ac and H4ac in the promoter regions of genes involved in the apoptosis pathway, leading to their transcription activation. Our results provide the first evidence that Qu acts as an inhibitor of the expression of class I HDAC in leukemia cells. We have also demonstrated that this inhibitory effect of class I HDACs by Qu is due to increased proteasomal degradation. The decrease in HDAC expression coincides with increased global as well as local acetylation of H3 and H4 on the DAPK1 and BCL2L11 promoters in both cell lines. Further studies on the effect of Qu on histone acetyltransferases (HATs) and HDAC activity as well as other affected molecular pathways in leukemia cells are encouraged.

Methods

Reagents and antibodies

Quercetin (> 98% pure) was obtained from Sigma Chemical Co. Antibodies used were as follows: DNMT1, STAT3, HDAC1, HDAC2, acetylated H4 (Ser 1/Lys5/Lys 8/Lys12) actin, DAPK1, BCL2L11, and control shRNA (h) lentiviral particles from Santa Cruz Biotechnology. DNMT3a and p-STAT3 were from Cell Signalling Technology. Acetylated H3 (Lys 9/Lys 18/Lys 23/Lys 27), H3, and H4 were from Abcam Inc. Anti-rabbit, anti-mouse, and anti-goat per-oxidase-conjugated antibodies were from KPL, Inc.

DAPI, Alexa Fluor 555, and Alexa Fluor 488 molecular probes were from Invitrogen. The FITC–Annexin V Apoptosis Detection Kit I was from BD Pharmingen.

Cell lines and treatment

HL60 and U937 cell lines were purchased from the American Type Culture Collection (ATCC, Philadelphia, PA) and were cytogenetically tested and authenticated before being frozen. HL60 and U937 cells were cultured in RPMI-1640 medium containing 10%n FBS, in a 37 °C humidified atmosphere containing CO_2. Qu (> 98% pure, Sigma Chemical Co) was dissolved in (DMSO) at a final concentration of 0.1% (*v*/*v*) in RPMI. The cells were treated with Qu at 50 and 75 μmol/L for 48 or 72 h. Control cells were treated with vehicle alone.

shRNA lentivirus particle transduction

HL60 and U937 cells were infected with DAPK1 or BCL2L11 or control shRNA lentivirus particles in the presence of 5 μg/mL Polybrene (Sigma). Infected cells were selected for 14 days in the presence of 2 μg/mL puromycin (Sigma). Expression of DAPK1 and BCL2L11 in infected cells were verified by real-time PCR (RT-PCR) and western blot analysis.

Detection of apoptosis by flow cytometry

HL60 and U937 cells transduced with shRNA-targeted *BCL2L11* were seeded on 12-well plates and treated with 50 μmol/L Qu. After 48 h, the cells were washed twice with ice-cold PBS and resuspended in a binding buffer containing 1 mg/mL propidium iodide (PI) and 1 mg/mL FITC-labeled annexin V. All specimens were analyzed on FACSCalibur after incubation for 15 min at room temperature in a light-protected area. Ten thousand events were acquired for each sample.

Confocal microscopy

Control and treated cells were fixed with 4% PFA (paraformaldehyde) at room temperature for 15 min. Fixed cells were permeabilized with perm buffer (0.2% saponin and 0.1% BSA), blocked with 5% BSA, and incubated overnight in anti-Stat3 antibody at 4 °C. Cells were washed and incubated again with Alexa Fluor 455-conjugated secondary antibody for 2 h at room temperature along with nuclear stain DAPI (4′,6-diamidino-2-phenylindole). Confocal imaging was performed with a Zeiss LSM 710 NLO laser scan confocal microscope using a × 63 objective magnification.

Methylation analyses
Epitec Methyl II PCR Array Human Apoptosis

For the initial screening of the methylation profile of HL60 cell line, the *Epitec Methyl II PCR Array Human Apoptosis* was used. Briefly, input genomic DNA was aliquoted into four equal portions and subjected to mock

(Mo), methylation sensitive (Ms), methylation dependent (Md), and double (Msd) restriction endonuclease digestion. After digestion, the enzyme reactions were mixed directly with qPCR master mix and aliquoted into a PCR array plate containing pre-dispensed primer mixes. The plate was run then in real-time PCR using specified cycling conditions. The relative fractions of methylated and unmethylated DNA were subsequently determined by comparing the amount in each digest with that of a mock (no enzymes added) digest using the ΔCt method.

Bisulfite treatment and methylation-specific PCR (MSP-PCR)

Bisulfite treatment was performed on 1 μg of DNA previously extracted from cells treated with Qu and from frozen samples from xenograft models using the EpiTect Bisulfite kit (Qiagen, Valencia, CA, USA). Methylation-specific PCR (MSP) [39] was performed for the promoter region of *DAPK* and *BCL2L11* with primers that were specific for the methylated or unmethylated sequences (M or U sets, respectively; Table 1). The reaction products were separated by electrophoresis on 2% agarose gels.

Bisulfite sequencing

Bisulfite sequence assay was performed to demonstrate the methylation status of DAPK1 promoters in the cell line. Genomic DNA from cell lines was isolated with DNeasy kit (Qiagen, Valencia, CA, USA). Genomic DNA was subjected to bisulfite conversion with Epitect Bisulfite kit (Qiagen, Valencia, CA, USA) according to the manufacturer's instructions. The BSP primers for DAPK1 promoter region were 5′- GAGGTTTTTAGTGGATATG GGATT-3′ (sense) and 5′-TCCACCTCCAAAATTCAAA TAATT-3′ (antisense), designed by Methyl Primer Express v1.0. Amplified PCR products were purified and sequenced on an ABI Prism 3500 Genetic Analyzer.

Extraction and expression of acetylated histone proteins

Leukemia cells HL60 and U937 were treated with 50 μmol/L Qu for 48 h and were harvested and washed twice with ice-cold phosphate-buffered saline (PBS) supplemented with 5 mM sodium butyrate. After washing, cells were resuspended in Triton extraction buffer [PBS containing 0.5% Triton X-100 (vol/vol), 2 mM phenylmethylsulfonyl fluoride, 0.02%(wt/vol) NAN3] and lysed on ice for 10 min with gentle stirring, centrifuged at 2000 r.p.m. for 10 min at 4 °C. The pellet was washed in Triton extraction buffer and then resuspended in 0.2 N HCl. Histones were acid extracted overnight at 4 °C and centrifuged at 2000 r.p.m. for 10 min at 4 °C. Samples were processed for the analysis of histones using immunoblotting.

Table 1 Primers used for MSP-PCR and real-time PCR

Genes		Primer sense (5′–3′)	Primer antisense (5′–3′)
BCL2L11	M	AGTATTTTCGGTAAATAATGGGGT	GAATAAATCAAAAACTCCCAACG
	U	GTATTTTTGGTAAATAATGGGGTTG	CAAATAAATCAAAAACTCCCAACA
DAPK1	M	GGATAGTCGGATCGAGTTAACGTC	CCCTCCCAAACGCCGA
	U	GGAGGATAGTTGGATTGAGTTAATGTT	CAAATCCCTCCCAAACACCAA
APAF1		CCCAGAGGCTTCCACTTAATATTG	CAAACATCATCCAAGATCAAGAGAGA
BAX		TGAGTACTTCACCAAGATTGCCA	AGTCAGGCCATGCTGGTAGAC
BCL2L11		TGTCTGACTCTCTCCGGACTG	TGACCACATCGAGCTTTAGCCAGTCA
BNIP3		CCAGAACATCATCCCTGCAT	TTCCAGTAGGGTCTCGACTTG
BNIP3L		CTCAGGATCCACAGCAAACA	CCAGACTGGACTCTGCCTTC
DNMT1		CCATCAGGCATTCTACCA	CGTTCTCCTTGTCTTCTCT
DNMT3a		TATTCATGAGCGCACAAGAGAGC	GGGTGTTCCAGGGTAACATTGAG
STAT3		CACCTTGGATTGAGAGTCAAGAC	AGGAATCGGCTATATTGCTGGT

M methylated, U unmethylated

Western blot analysis

Total cell protein was extracted in RIPA buffer. Protein concentrations were quantified by the Bio-Rad Protein Assay Kit. Equal protein amounts were loaded on 8 to 15% SDS polyacrylamide gels and electrophoretically transferred to nitrocellulose membrane. Nonspecific binding sites were blocked by incubation with a buffer containing Tris (10 mmol/L, pH 7.4), NaCl (150 mmol/L), Tween 20 (0.1%), and fat-free dry milk (5%). Membranes were incubated overnight with a specific primary antibody, at 4 °C, followed by horseradish peroxidase-conjugated secondary antibody, at room temperature for 1 h. Immunoreactivities were visualized by ECL Western Blot Analysis System (Amersham Pharmacia Biotech).

Posttranscriptional histone modifications
Chromatin immunoprecipitation (ChIP)

Apoptosis ChIP human PCR array (SAbiosciences, Qiagen) was used to evaluate whether Qu treatment induces an enrichment of modified histones such as acetylated histone 3 and histone 4 (H3ac, H4ac) in the promoter regions of genes associated to apoptosis pathway. After cross-linking cells with formaldehyde, chromatin containing covalent complexes of genomic DNA and nuclear factors were isolated and sheared by sonication into fragments of between 500 and 1500 bp. The DNA sequences and the posttranslational histone modifications were then immunoprecipitated with specifically antibodies for anti H3ac and H4ac. Next, cross-linking was reversed followed by nucleic acid purification to detect DNA by real-time PCR.

RNA extraction and real-time PCR

The cells treated with Qu and the samples from the xenotransplants were collected, snap frozen, and stored at − 80 °C in RNAlater® (Qiagen, Valencia, CA, USA).

Total RNA was isolated using the miRNeasy mini kit® (Qiagen). Single-stranded cDNA was synthesized from the RNA using the high capacity cDNA archive kit® (Applied Biosystems, Foster City, CA, USA) following the manufacturer's protocol.

Quantitative PCR (Sybr Green®) was performed on a 7500 real-time PCR system (Applied Biosystems) using threshold cycle numbers as determined by the RQ Study software (Applied Biosystems). The reactions were run in triplicate, and the threshold cycle numbers were averaged.

DNMT1, DNMT3a, STAT3, DAPK1, BCL2L11, BAX, BNIP3, BNIP3L, and *APAF1* expressions were measured and normalized using *HPRT* as an endogenous control. The relative expression was calculated according to the formula $2^{(-\Delta\Delta Ct)}$ [40], and the results were expressed as average gene expression ± SD.

Human tumor xenograft model

Female (NOD.CB17-Prkdc^{scid}/J lineage) 8–11-week-old animals, from the Jackson Laboratory, bred at the Animal Facility Centre at The University of Campinas, under specific pathogen-free conditions, were matched for body-weight before use. Animal experiments were performed following institutional protocols and guidelines of the Institutional Animal Care and Use Committee. Mice were inoculated, s.c, in the dorsal region, on day 0 with 0.1 mL of HL60 or U937 cell suspension (1×10^7 cells/mice). Every 7 days, tumor volumes were evaluated according to the formula: tumor volume (mm^3) = (length × width^2)/2. Qu treatment (HL60 xenograft model, treated group *n* = 5; U937 xenograft model, treated group *n* = 7) was initiated after tumors reached 100 to 200 mm^3 and was administered once every 4 days by i.p injection at 120 mg/kg body weight. The control group (HL60 xenograft model *n* = 4; U937 xenograft model *n* = 5) received equal amounts of vehicle solution, as previously described [41].

Mice were sacrificed after 21 days. Tumors were then removed, minced, snap frozen, and stored at – 80 °C in RNAlater® (Qiagen, Valencia, CA, USA).

Statistical analysis

The results of the real-time PCR were expressed as means ± SD. All the experiments were realized in triplicate. Student's *t* test was used to determine the statistical difference between treated and control group. The data were considered significant if $p < 0.05$.

Abbreviations

AML: Acute myelogenous leukemia; BCL2L11: BCL2-interacting mediator, (*BIM*); CML: Chronic myeloid leukemia; ChIP: Chromatin immunoprecipitation; DAPK1: Death-associated protein kinase 1; DNMTs: DNA methyltransferases; DNMT1: DNA methyltransferase 1; DNMT3a: DNA methyltransferase 3a; HATs: Histone acetyltransferases; H3ac: Acetylated histone 3; H4ac: Acetylated histone 4; HDACs: Histone deacetylases; HDACi: Histone deacetylase inhibitors; IM: Imatinib; MDSs: Myelodysplastic syndromes; MSP-PCR: Methylation-specific PCR; ncRNA: Noncoding RNAs; Qu: Quercetin; SAHA: Suberoylanilide hydroxamic acid

Acknowledgements

The authors would like to thank Nicola Conran and Raquel S Foglio for the English revision and Irene Santos and Tereza Salles for their valuable technical assistance.

Funding

This work was supported by grants from the Fundaçao de Amparo a Pesquisa do Estado de Sao Paulo (FAPESP), grant number 2015/21164-7, and Conselho Nacional de Desenvolvimento Científico e Tecnológico (Cnpq), grant number 150171\2014-5.

Authors' contributions

MCA and STOS contributed to the conception and design and analysis and interpretation of data. MCA contributed to the development of methodology and acquisition of data. VM, COT, and KPF contributed in the manipulation of animals. MCA and STO contributed to the writing, review, and revision of the manuscript. All authors read and approved the final manuscript.

References

1. Steensma DP. Myelodysplastic syndromes: diagnosis and treatment. Mayo Clin Proc. 2015;90(7):969–83.
2. Hatziapostolou M, et al. Epigenetic aberrations during oncogenesis. Cell Mol Life Sci. 2011;68(10):1681–702.
3. Galm O, et al. The fundamental role of epigenetics in hematopoietic malignancies. Blood Rev. 2006;20(1):1–13.
4. Chen J, et al. Leukemogenesis: more than mutant genes. Nat Rev Cancer. 2010;10(1):23–36.
5. Suzuki M, et al. DNA methylation landscapes: provocative insights from epigenomics. Nature Reviews Genet. 2008;9:465–76.
6. Bannister AJ, et al. Regulation of chromatin by histone modifications. Cell Res. 2011;21(3):381–95.
7. Storz G. An expanding universe of noncoding RNAs. Sci. 2002;296(5571):1260–3.
8. Beecher GR, et al. Analysis of tea polyphenols. Proc Soc Exp Biol Med. 1999; 220(4):267–70.
9. Formica JV, et al. Review of the biology of quercetin and related bioflavonoids. Food Chem Toxicol. 1995;33(12):1061–80.
10. Hollman PC, et al. Dietary flavonoids: intake, health effects and bioavailability. Food Chem Toxicol. 1999;37(9-10):937–42.
11. Lugli E, et al. Quercetin inhibits lymphocyte activation and proliferation without inducing apoptosis in peripheral mononuclear cells. Leuk Res. 2009; 33(1):140–50.
12. Maso V, et al. Multitarget effects of quercetin in leukemia. Cancer Prev Res (Phila). 2014;7(12):1240–50.
13. Herman JG, et al. Methylation-specific PCR: a novel PCR assay for methylation status of CpG islands. Proc Natl Acad Sci U S A. 1996;93(18):9821–6.
14. Livak KJ, et al. Analysis of relative gene expression data using real-time quantitative PCR and the 2 (−Delta Delta (CT)) method. Methods. 2001;25:402–8.
15. Wang K, et al. Quercetin induces protective autophagy in gastric cancer cells: involvement of Akt-mTOR- and hypoxia-induced factor 1α-mediated signaling. Autophagy. 2011;7(9):966–78.
16. Hino R, et al. Activation of DNA methyltransferase 1 by EBV latent membrane protein 2A leads to promoter hypermethylation of PTEN gene in gastric carcinoma. Cancer Res. 2009;69:2766–74.
17. Hanahanh D, et al. Hallmarks of cancer: the next generation. Cell. 2011; 144(5):646–74.
18. Ahmad S, et al. Methylation of the APAF-1 and DAPK-1 promoter region correlates with progression of renal cell carcinoma in North Indian population. Tumor Biol. 2012;33:395–402.
19. Tanaka K et al. (2014) Gynecological Cancer Registry of Niigata: Promoter methylation of DAPK1, FHIT, MGMT, and CDKN2A genes in cervical carcinoma. Int J Clin Oncol;19: 127–132.
20. Kristensen LS, et al. Investigation of MGMT and DAPK1 methylation patterns in diffuse large B-cell lymphoma using allelic MSP-pyrosequencing. Sci Rep. 2013;3:2789.
21. Claus N, et al. Quantitative analyses of DAPK1 methylation in AML and MDS. Int J Cancer. 2012;131:E138–42.
22. Katzenellenbogen R, et al. Hypermethylation of the DAP-kinase CpG island is a common alteration in B-cell malignancies. Blood. 1999;93:4347–53.
23. Imtiyaz A, et al. Epigenetic silencing of DAPK1 gene is associated with faster disease progression in India populations with chronic myeloid leukemia. J Cancer Sci Ther. 2013;5:144–9 2013.
24. Qian J, et al. Aberrant methylation of the death-associated protein kinase 1 (DAPK1) CpG island in CpG island in chronic myeloid leukemia. Eur J Haematol. 2009;82:119–23 2009. CpG island in chronic myeloid leukemia. Eur J Haematol; 82: 119–123.
25. Tan S, et al. Quercetin is able to demethylate the p16INK4a gene promoter. Chemotherapy. 2009;55(1):6–10.
26. Klose RJ, et al. Genomic DNA methylation: the mark and its mediators. Trends Biochem Sci. 2006;31:89–97.
27. Minjung L, et al. Quercetin-induced apoptosis prevents EBV infection. Oncotarget. 2015;6(14):12603–24.
28. Youle RJ, et al. The BCL-2 protein family: opposing activities that mediate cell death. Nat Rev Mol Cell Biol. 2008;9(1):47–59.
29. Kuribara R, et al. Roles of Bim in apoptosis of normal and Bcr-Abl-expressing hematopoietic progenitors. Mol Cell Biol. 2004;24(14):6172–83.
30. Aichberger KJ, et al. Low-level expression of proapoptotic Bcl-2-interacting mediator in leukemic cells in patients with chronic myeloid leukemia: role of BCR/ABL, characterization of underlying signaling pathways, and reexpression by novel pharmacologic compounds. Cancer Res. 2005;65(20):9436–44.
31. San José-Eneriz E, et al. Epigenetic down-regulation of BIM expression is associated with reduced optimal responses to imatinib treatment in chronic myeloid leukaemia. Eur J Cancer. 2009;45(10):1877–89.
32. Kuroda J, et al. Bim and Bad mediate imatinib-induced killing of Bcr/Abl+ leukemic cells, and resistance due to their loss is overcome by a BH3 mimetic. Proc Natl Acad Sci U S A. 2006;103(40):14907–12.
33. Piazza M, et al. Epigenetic silencing of the proapoptotic gene BIM in anaplastic large cell lymphoma through an MeCP2/SIN3a deacetylating complex. Neoplasia. 2013;15(5):511–22.
34. Lee WJ, et al. Quercetin induces FasL-related apoptosis, in part, through promotion of histone H3 acetylation in human leukemia HL-60 cells. Oncol Rep. 2011;25(2):583–91.
35. Forsberg EC, et al. Histone acetylation beyond promoters: long-range acetylation patterns in the chromatin world. Bioessays. 2001;23(9):820–30.
36. Ayer DE. Histone deacetylases: transcriptional repression with SINers and NuRDs. Trends Cell Biol. 1999;9:193–8.
37. Yang XJ, et al. Collaborative spirit of histone deacetylases in regulating chromatin structure and gene expression. Curr Opin Genet Dev. 2003;13:143–53.
38. Peart MJ, et al. Identification and functional significance of genes regulated by structurally different histone deacetylase inhibitors. Proc Natl Acad Sci U S A. 2005;102(10):3697–702.
39. Wang S, et al. Activation of mitochondrial pathway is crucial for tumor selective induction of apoptosis by LAQ824. Cell Cycle. 2006;5(15):1662–8.
40. Pérez-Perarnau A, et al. Analysis of apoptosis regulatory genes altered by histone deacetylase inhibitors in chronic lymphocytic leukemia cells. Epigenetics. 2011;6(10):1228–35.
41. Priyadarsini RV, et al. The flavonoid quercetin modulates the hallmark capabilities of hamster buccal pouch tumors. Nutr Cancer. 2011;63(2):218–26.

Permissions

List of Contributors

Aditi Chandra and Raghunath Chatterjee
Human Genetics Unit, Indian Statistical Institute, 203 B. T. Road, Kolkata, West Bengal 700108, India

Swapan Senapati
Uttarpara, Hooghly, West Bengal 712258, India

Sudipta Roy
MDDC, Lansdowne Place, Kolkata, West Bengal, India

Gobinda Chatterjee
Department of Dermatology, IPGMER/SSKM Hospital, Kolkata, West Bengal, India

Lexie Prokopuk and Patrick S. Western
Centre for Reproductive Health, Hudson Institute of Medical Research and Department of Molecular and Translational Science, Monash University, Clayton, Victoria 3168, Australia

Jessica M. Stringer
Centre for Reproductive Health, Hudson Institute of Medical Research and Department of Molecular and Translational Science, Monash University, Clayton, Victoria 3168, Australia
Monash Biomedicine Discovery Institute, Monash University, Clayton, Victoria 3800, Australia

Craig R. White
Centre for Geometric Biology, School of Biological Sciences, Monash University, Clayton, Victoria 3800, Australia

Rolf H. A. M. Vossen and Stefan J. White
Leiden Genome Technology Centre, Department of Human Genetics, Leiden University Medical Center, Leiden, the Netherlands

Ana S. A. Cohen and William T. Gibson
Department of Medical Genetics, University of British Columbia and British Columbia Children's Hospital Research Institute, Vancouver, BC, Canada

Hao Wang and Zelian Qin
Medical Research Center, Peking University Third Hospital, Beijing, China

Ran Peng and Junjie Wang
Department of Radiation Oncology, Peking University Third Hospital, Beijing, China

Lixiang Xue
Medical Research Center, Peking University Third Hospital, Beijing, China
Department of Radiation Oncology, Peking University Third Hospital, Beijing, China

Maher Jedi, Susan E. Byrne, Dawn Bastin and Graeme P. Young
Flinders Centre for Innovation in Cancer, College of Medicine and Public Health, Flinders University of South Australia, Bedford Park, South Australia 5042, Australia

Erin L. Symonds
Flinders Centre for Innovation in Cancer, College of Medicine and Public Health, Flinders University of South Australia, Bedford Park, South Australia 5042, Australia
Bowel Health Service, Flinders Medical Centre, Bedford Park, South Australia, Australia

Susanne K. Pedersen, Rohan T. Baker and David H. Murray
Clinical Genomics Pty Ltd, North Ryde, New South Wales, Australia

Philippa Rabbitt
Colorectal Surgery, Division of Surgery and Perioperative Medicine, Flinders Medical Centre, Bedford Park, South Australia, Australia

A. M. Di Blasio
Istituto Auxologico Italiano IRCCS, 20095 Cusano Milanino, Italy

D. Gentilini
Istituto Auxologico Italiano IRCCS, 20095 Cusano Milanino, Italy
Department of Brain and Behavioral Sciences, University of Pavia, 27100 Pavia, Italy

E. Somigliana
Infertility Unit, Fondazione Ca' Granda, Ospedale Maggiore Policlinico, 20122 Milan, Italy

L. Pagliardini, E. Papaleo, and P. Viganò and E. Rabellotti
Reproductive Sciences Laboratory, Division of Genetics and Cell Biology, IRCCS Ospedale San Raffaele, Via Olgettina 58, 20132 Milan, Italy

P. Garagnani
Department of Experimental, Diagnostic and Specialty Medicine, University of Bologna, 40138 Bologna, Italy

L. Bernardinelli
Department of Brain and Behavioral Sciences, University of Pavia, 27100 Pavia, Italy

M. Candiani
Obstetrics and Gynaecology Unit, IRCCS Ospedale San Raffaele, 20132 Milan, Italy

María Gallardo-Gómez, María Páez de la Cadena, Vicenta Soledad Martínez-Zorzano, Francisco Javier Rodríguez-Berrocal and Loretta De Chiara
Department of Biochemistry, Genetics and Immunology, Centro Singular de Investigación de Galicia (CINBIO), University of Vigo, Campus As Lagoas-Marcosende s/n, 36310 Vigo, Spain

Sebastian Moran and Manel Esteller
Cancer Epigenetics and Biology Program (PEBC), Bellvitge Biomedical Research Institute (IDIBELL), Barcelona, Spain

Mar Rodríguez-Girondo
Department of Medical Statistics and Bioinformatics, Leiden University Medical Centre, Leiden, The Netherlands
SiDOR Research Group and Centro de Investigaciones Biomédicas (CINBIO), Faculty of Economics and Business Administration, University of Vigo, Vigo, Spain

Joaquín Cubiella
Department of Gastroenterology, Complexo Hospitalario Universitario de Ourense, Instituto de Investigación Biomédica Galicia Sur, Centro de Investigación Biomédica en Red de Enfermedades Hepáticas y Digestivas (CIBERehd), Ourense, Spain

Luis Bujanda
Department of Gastroenterology, Instituto Biodonostia, Centro de Investigación Biomédica en Red de Enfermedades Hepáticas y Digestivas (CIBERehd), Universidad del País Vasco (UPV/EHU), San Sebastián, Spain

Antoni Castells and Francesc Balaguer
Gastroenterology Department, Hospital Clínic, IDIBAPS, CIBERehd, University of Barcelona, Barcelona, Spain

Rodrigo Jover
Department of Gastroenterology, Hospital General Universitario de Alicante, Alicante, Spain

Nisreen Al-Moghrabi, Nujoud Al-Yousef, Bedri Karakas and Hannah Almubarak
Head of Cancer Epigenetic Section, Molecular Oncology Department, King Faisal Specialist Hospital and Research Centre, PO BOX 3354, Riyadh 11211, Kingdom of Saudi Arabia

Maram Al-Showimi and Bushra Al-Shahrani
Cancer Epigenetic section, Department of Molecular Oncology, King Faisal Specialist Hospital and Research Centre, PO BOX 3354, Riyadh 11211, Kingdom of Saudi Arabia

Lamyaa Alghofaili
Al Faisal University College of Medicine, PO BOX 50927, Riyadh 11533, Kingdom of Saudi Arabia

Safia Madkhali
King Saud bin Abdulaziz University for Health Sciences, PO BOX 22490, Riyadh 3130, Kingdom of Saudi Arabia

Hind Al Humaidan
Department of pathology and Laboratory Medicine, King Faisal Specialist Hospital and Research Centre, PO BOX 3354, Riyadh 11211, Kingdom of Saudi Arabia

A. T. Lely and A. Franx
Department of Obstetrics, Wilhelmina Children's Hospital Birth Center, University Medical Center Utrecht, Utrecht, the Netherlands

J. A. Joles
Department of Nephrology and Hypertension, University Medical Center Utrecht, Utrecht, the Netherlands

P. G. Nikkels
Department of Pathology, University Medical Center Utrecht, Utrecht, the Netherlands

M. Mokry
Division of Pediatrics, University Medical Center Utrecht, Utrecht, the Netherlands

N. D. Paauw
Department of Obstetrics, Wilhelmina Children's Hospital Birth Center, University Medical Center Utrecht, Utrecht, the Netherlands
Division Woman and Baby, University Medical Center Utrecht, Postbus 85090, 3508 AB Utrecht, the Netherlands

B. B. van Rijn
Department of Obstetrics, Wilhelmina Children's Hospital Birth Center, University Medical Center Utrecht, Utrecht, the Netherlands

Academic Unit of Human Development and Health, University of Southampton, Southampton, UK
Division Woman and Baby, University Medical Center Utrecht, Postbus 85090, 3508 AB Utrecht, the Netherlands

Aline Kaletsch, Maria Pinkerneil, Michèle J. Hoffmann, Ananda A. Jaguva Vasudevan, Wolfgang A. Schulz and Günter Niegisch
Department of Urology, Medical Faculty, Heinrich Heine University, Moorenstr. 5, 40225 Duesseldorf, Germany

Chenyin Wang, Finn K. Hansen, Christoph Gertzen, Holger Gohlke, Matthias U. Kassack and Thomas Kurz
Institute for Pharmaceutical and Medical Chemistry, Heinrich Heine University, Duesseldorf, Germany

Constanze Wiek and Helmut Hanenberg
Department of Otorhinolaryngology and Head and Neck Surgery, Medical Faculty, Heinrich Heine University, Duesseldorf, Germany

Wan Li, Xiangjin Zheng, Weiqi Fu, Liwen Ren, Jinhua Wang and Guanhua Du
The State Key Laboratory of Bioactive Substance and Function of Natural Medicines, Beijing, China
Key Laboratory of Drug Target Research and Drug Screen, Institute of Materia Medica, Chinese Academy of Medical Science and Peking Union Medical College, Beijing 100050, China

Li Li
Key Laboratory of Drug Target Research and Drug Screen, Institute of Materia Medica, Chinese Academy of Medical Science and Peking Union Medical College, Beijing 100050, China

Jie Yi
Department of Clinical Laboratory, Peking Union Medical College Hospital, Beijing 100730, China

Shiwei Liu
Department of Endocrinology, Shanxi DAYI Hospital, Shanxi Medical University, Taiyuan 030002, Shanxi, China

Dave S. B. Hoon
Department of Translational Molecular Medicine, John Wayne Cancer Institute (JWCI) at Providence Saint John's Health Center, Santa Monica, CA 90404, USA

Kristin M. Junge, Beate Leppert, Stefan Röder, Mario Bauer and Saskia Trump
Department of Environmental Immunology, Helmholtz Centre for Environmental Research (UFZ), Leipzig, Germany

Susanne Jahreis and Tobias Polte
Department of Environmental Immunology, Helmholtz Centre for Environmental Research (UFZ), Leipzig, Germany
Department of Dermatology, Venerology and Allergology, Leipzig University Medical Center, Leipzig, Germany

Ralph Feltens
Department Molecular Systems Biology, Helmholtz Centre for Environmental Research (UFZ), Leipzig, Germany

Dirk K. Wissenbach
Department Molecular Systems Biology, Helmholtz Centre for Environmental Research (UFZ), Leipzig, Germany
Institute of Forensic Medicine, University Hospital Jena, Jena, Germany

Melanie Bewerunge-Hudler
German Cancer Research Center (DKFZ), 69120 Heidelberg, Germany

Konrad Grützmann
Department of Environmental Immunology, Helmholtz Centre for Environmental Research (UFZ), Leipzig, Germany
Core Unit for Molecular Tumor Diagnostics (CMTD), National Center for Tumor Diseases (NCT) Dresden, 01307 Dresden, Germany
German Cancer Consortium (DKTK), Dresden, Germany
German Cancer Research Center (DKFZ), 69120 Heidelberg, Germany

Tobias Bauer
German Cancer Research Center (DKFZ), Division of Theoretical Bioinformatics, Heidelberg, Germany

Matthias Schick
German Cancer Research Center (DKFZ), Genomics and Proteomics Core Facility, Heidelberg, Germany

Angela Schulz
Medical Faculty, Rudolf-Schönheimer-Institute of Biochemistry, University of Leipzig, Leipzig, Germany

Michael Borte
Children's Hospital, Municipal Hospital "St. Georg", Leipzig, Germany

Antje Körner, Wieland Kiess and Kathrin Landgraf
LIFE-Leipzig Research Centre for Civilization Diseases, University of Leipzig, Leipzig, Germany
Hospital for Children and Adolescents-Centre for Pediatric Research, University of Leipzig, Leipzig, Germany

Martin von Bergen
Department Molecular Systems Biology, Helmholtz Centre for Environmental Research (UFZ), Leipzig, Germany
Faculty of Biosciences, Pharmacy and Psychology, Institute of Biochemistry, University of Leipzig, Leipzig, Germany

Naveed Ishaque
German Cancer Research Center (DKFZ), Division of Theoretical Bioinformatics, Heidelberg, Germany
Institute of Agriculture and Nutritional Sciences, Martin Luther University Halle-Wittenberg, Halle (Saale), Germany

Gabriele I. Stangl
Institute of Agriculture and Nutritional Sciences, Martin Luther University Halle-Wittenberg, Halle (Saale), Germany
Competence Cluster for Nutrition and Cardiovascular Health (nutriCARD), Halle-Jena Leipzig, Germany

Loreen Thürmann
Department of Environmental Immunology, Helmholtz Centre for Environmental Research (UFZ), Leipzig, Germany
Berlin Institute of Health and Charité-Universitätsmedizin Berlin, Center for Digital Health, Berlin, Germany

Roland Eils
German Cancer Research Center (DKFZ), Heidelberg Center for Personalized Oncology, DKFZ-HIPO, Heidelberg, Germany
Berlin Institute of Health and Charité-Universitätsmedizin Berlin, Center for Digital Health, Berlin, Germany
Health Data Science Unit, Heidelberg University Hospital, Heidelberg, Germany

Irina Lehmann
Department of Environmental Immunology, Helmholtz Centre for Environmental Research (UFZ), Leipzig, Germany
Unit for Molecular Epidemiology, Berlin Institute of Health (BIH) and Charitè - Universitätsmedizin Berlin, Berlin, Germany

Lu Gao, Xiaochen Liu, Joshua Millstein, Kimberly D. Siegmund, Louis Dubeau and Carrie V. Breton
Department of Preventive Medicine, USC Keck School of Medicine, 2001 N. Soto Street, Los Angeles, CA 90032, USA

Rachel L. Maguire and Cathrine Hoyo
Department of Biological Sciences, Center for Human Health and the Environment, North Carolina State University, Raleigh, NC 27695, USA

Junfeng (Jim) Zhang
Nicholas School of the Environment and Duke Global Health Institute, Duke University, Durham, NC 27701, USA

Bernard F. Fuemmeler
Department of Health Behavior and Policy, Massey Cancer Center, Virginia Commonwealth University, Richmond, VA 23219, USA

Scott H. Kollins
Department of Psychiatry and Behavioral Sciences, Duke University Medical Center, Durham, NC 27705, USA

Susan K. Murphy
Division of Reproductive Sciences, Department of Obstetrics and Gynecology, Duke University School of Medicine, Durham, NC 27708, USA

Masato Kantake, Natsuki Ohkawa, Naho Ikeda, Atsuko Awaji and Nobutomo Saito
Neonatal Medical Center, Juntendo University Shizuoka Hospital, 1192 Nagaoka, Izunokuni, Shizuoka 410-2295, Japan

Tomohiro Iwasaki, Hiromichi Shoji and Toshiaki Shimizu
Division of Pediatrics, Juntendo University School of Medicine, 3-1-3, Hongo, Bunkyo 113-8421, Japan

Cheng Peng, Augusto A. Litonjua and Dawn L. DeMeo
Channing Division of Network Medicine and the Division of Pulmonary and Critical Care Medicine, Department of Medicine, Brigham and Women's Hospital, Harvard Medical School, 181 Longwood Avenue, 4th Floor, Boston, MA 02115, USA

Andres Cardenas, Sheryl L. Rifas-Shiman and Emily Oken
Division of Chronic Disease Research Across the Lifecourse, Department of Population Medicine, Harvard Medical School and Harvard Pilgrim Health Care Institute, Boston, MA, USA

Marie-France Hivert
Division of Chronic Disease Research Across the Lifecourse, Department of Population Medicine, Harvard Medical School and Harvard Pilgrim Health Care Institute, Boston, MA, USA

Diabetes Unit, Massachusetts General Hospital, Boston, MA, USA

Diane R. Gold
Channing Division of Network Medicine and the Division of Pulmonary and Critical Care Medicine, Department of Medicine, Brigham and Women's Hospital, Harvard Medical School, 181 Longwood Avenue, 4th Floor, Boston, MA 02115, USA
Department of Environmental Health, Harvard T. H. Chan School of Public Health, Boston, MA, USA

Thomas A. Platts-Mills
Division of Allergy and Clinical Immunology, University of Virginia School of Medicine, Charlottesville, VA, USA

Xihong Lin
Department of Biostatistics, Harvard T. H. Chan School of Public Health, Boston, MA, USA

Andrea A. Baccarelli
Department of Environmental Health Sciences, Columbia University Mailman School of Public Health, New York, NY, USA

Jing-dong Zhou, Ting-juan Zhang, Xi-xi Li, Yu Gu, Wei Zhang and Jun Qian
Department of Hematology, Affiliated People's Hospital of Jiangsu University, 8 Dianli Rd, 212002 Zhenjiang, People's Republic of China
The Key Lab of Precision Diagnosis and Treatment of Zhenjiang City, Zhenjiang, Jiangsu, People's Republic of China

Yu-xin Wang
Department of Nephrology and Endocrinology, Traditional Chinese Medicine Hospital of Kunshan City, Kunshan, Jiangsu, People's Republic of China

Ji-chun Ma and Jiang Lin
The Key Lab of Precision Diagnosis and Treatment of Zhenjiang City, Zhenjiang, Jiangsu, People's Republic of China
Laboratory Center, Affiliated People's Hospital of Jiangsu University, 8 Dianli Rd., 212002 Zhenjiang, People's Republic of China

Jiaying You and Pingzhao Hu
Department of Biochemistry and Medical Genetics and Department of Electrical and Computer Engineering, University of Manitoba, Winnipeg, Canada

Yan Cheng
Department of Biochemistry and Medical Genetics and Department of Electrical and Computer Engineering, University of Manitoba, Winnipeg, Canada

Experimental Center, Northwest University for Nationalities, Lanzhou, People's Republic of China

Cátia Monteiro
Molecular Oncology Group, Portuguese Institute of Oncology, Porto, Portugal
Research Department, Portuguese League Against Cancer–North, Porto, Portugal

Andreia Matos
Laboratory of Genetics and Environmental Health Institute, Faculty of Medicine, University of Lisboa, Lisbon, Portugal
Tumor and Microenvironment Interactions, i3S/INEB, Institute for Research and Innovation in Health, and Institute of Biomedical Engineering, University of Porto, Porto, Portugal

Avelino Fraga
Tumor and Microenvironment Interactions, i3S/INEB, Institute for Research and Innovation in Health, and Institute of Biomedical Engineering, University of Porto, Porto, Portugal
Department of Urology, Centro Hospitalar Universitário do Porto, Porto, Portugal

Carina Pereira
Molecular Oncology Group, Portuguese Institute of Oncology, Porto, Portugal
CINTESIS, Center for Health Technology and Services Research, Faculty of Medicine, e, University of Porto, Porto, Portugal

Victoria Catalán, Amaia Rodríguez and Javier Gómez-Ambrosi
Metabolic Research Laboratory, Universidad de Navarra, Pamplona, Spain
CIBER Fisiopatología de la Obesidad y Nutricion, Instituto de Salud Carlos III, Madrid, Spain

Gema Frühbeck
Metabolic Research Laboratory, Universidad de Navarra, Pamplona, Spain
CIBER Fisiopatología de la Obesidad y Nutricion, Instituto de Salud Carlos III, Madrid, Spain
Department of Endocrinology, Clínica Universidad de Navarra, Pamplona, Spain

Ricardo Ribeiro
Molecular Oncology Group, Portuguese Institute of Oncology, Porto, Portugal
Laboratory of Genetics and Environmental Health Institute, Faculty of Medicine, University of Lisboa, Lisbon, Portugal
Tumor and Microenvironment Interactions, i3S/INEB, Institute for Research and Innovation in Health, and Institute of Biomedical Engineering, University of Porto, Porto, Portugal

Department of Clinical Pathology, Centro Hospitalar e Universitário de Coimbra, Coimbra, Portugal
i3S/INEB, Instituto de Investigação e Inovação em Saúde/Instituto Nacional de Engenharia Biomédica, Universidade do Porto, Tumor and Microenvironment Interactions, Rua Alfredo Allen, 208 4200-135 Porto, Portugal

Liang-Shun Wang
Division of Thoracic Surgery, Department of Surgery, Shuang Ho Hospital, Taipei Medical University, New Taipei City, Taiwan

Kuang-Tai Kuo
Division of Thoracic Surgery, Department of Surgery, Shuang Ho Hospital, Taipei Medical University, New Taipei City, Taiwan
Division of Thoracic Surgery, Department of Surgery, School of Medicine, College of Medicine, Taipei Medical University, Taipei, Taiwan

Wen-Chien Huang
Division of Thoracic Surgery, Department of Surgery, MacKay Memorial Hospital, Taipei, Taiwan
MacKay Medical College, Taipei, Taiwan

Oluwaseun Adebayo Bamodu and Chi-Tai Yeh
Department of Medical Research and Education, Shuang Ho Hospital, Taipei Medical University, New Taipei City, Taiwan
Division of Hematology/Oncology, Department of Medicine, Shuang Ho Hospital, Taipei Medical University, New Taipei City, Taiwan

Wei-Hwa Lee
Department of Pathology, Shuang Ho Hospital, Taipei Medical University, New Taipei City, Taiwan

Chun-Hua Wang
Department of Dermatology, Taipei Tzu Chi Hospital, Buddhist Tzu Chi Medical Foundation, New Taipei City, Taiwan
School of Medicine, Buddhist Tzu Chi University, Hualien, Taiwan

M. Hsiao
Genomics Research Center, Academia Sinica, Taipei, Taiwan

Biyu He, Zhongqi Li, Huan Song and Peiyi Shi
Department of Epidemiology, School of Public Health, Nanjing Medical University, 101 Longmian Ave, Nanjing 211166, People's Republic of China

Min Wang
Department of Epidemiology, School of Public Health, Nanjing Medical University, 101 Longmian Ave, Nanjing 211166, People's Republic of China

Department of Preventive Health Care, People's Hospital of Suzhou High-tech Zone, Suzhou, People's Republic of China

Weimin Kong
Department of Nursing, The First People's Hospital of Yancheng City, Yancheng, People's
Republic of China

Jianming Wang
Department of Epidemiology, School of Public Health, Nanjing Medical University, 101 Longmian Ave, Nanjing 211166, People's Republic of China
Key Laboratory of Infectious Diseases, School of Public Health, Nanjing Medical University, Nanjing, People's Republic of China

Sungshim L. Park, Yesha M. Patel, Daniel O. Stram and Kimberly Siegmund
Department of Preventive Medicine, Norris Comprehensive Cancer Center, Keck School of Medicine, University of Southern California, 1450 Biggy Street, NRT 1509G, Los Angeles, CA 90033, USA

Lenora W. M. Loo, Maarit Tiirikainen and Loïc Le Marchand
Epidemiology Program, University of Hawaii Cancer Center, 701 Ilalo Street, Honolulu, HI 96813, USA

Daniel J. Mullen and Ite A. Offringa
Department of Biochemistry and Molecular Biology, Keck School of Medicine, University of Southern California, Los Angeles, CA 90032, USA

Alika Maunakea
University of Hawaii John A. Burns School of Medicine, Honolulu, HI 96813, USA

Sharon E. Murphy
Masonic Cancer Center, University of Minnesota, Minneapolis, MN 55455, USA

Rong Zhang, Feng Jiang, Hong Zhang, Bo Xu, Tao Wang and Weiping Jia
Shanghai Diabetes Institute, Shanghai Key Laboratory of Diabetes Mellitus, Shanghai Clinical Center for Diabetes, Shanghai Jiao Tong University Affiliated Sixth People's Hospital, 600 Yishan Road, Shanghai 200233, China

Zhen He and Cheng Hu
Shanghai Diabetes Institute, Shanghai Key Laboratory of Diabetes Mellitus, Shanghai Clinical Center for Diabetes, Shanghai Jiao Tong University Affiliated Sixth People's Hospital, 600 Yishan Road, Shanghai 200233, China
Institute for Metabolic Diseases, Fengxian Central Hospital, The Third School of Clinical Medicine, Southern Medical University, Shanghai, China

Aihua Zhao and Wei Jia
Shanghai Key Laboratory of Diabetes Mellitus and Center for Translational Medicine, Shanghai Jiao Tong University Affiliated Sixth People's Hospital, Shanghai, China

Li Jin
National Clinical Research Center of Kidney Diseases, Jinling Hospital, Nanjing University School of Medicine, Nanjing, China

Yishui Lian and Pingan Ding
Research Center, the Fourth Affiliated Hospital of Hebei Medical University, Shijiazhuang 050017, Hebei, People's Republic of China

Lingjiao Meng and Meixiang Sang
Research Center, the Fourth Affiliated Hospital of Hebei Medical University, Shijiazhuang 050017, Hebei, People's Republic of China
Tumor Research Institute, the Fourth Affiliated Hospital of Hebei Medical University, Shijiazhuang 050017, Hebei, People's Republic of China

Varun Sasidharan Nair, Salman M. Toor, Rowaida Z. Taha and Hibah Shaath
Cancer Research Center, Qatar Biomedical Research Institute, College of Science and Engineering, Hamad Bin Khalifa University, Qatar Foundation, Doha, Qatar

Eyad Elkord
Cancer Research Center, Qatar Biomedical Research Institute, College of Science and Engineering, Hamad Bin Khalifa University, Qatar Foundation, Doha, Qatar
Institute of Cancer Sciences, University of Manchester, Manchester, UK

Marisa Claudia Alvarez, Victor Maso, Cristiane Okuda Torello, Karla Priscilla Ferro and Sara Teresinha Olalla Saad
Hematology and Transfusion Medicine Center-University of Campinas/ Hemocentro-UNICAMP, Instituto Nacional de Ciencia e Tecnologia do Sangue, Rua Carlos Chagas, 480, CEP, Campinas, SP 13083-878, Brazil

Index

www.ingramcontent.com/pod-product-compliance
Lightning Source LLC
Chambersburg PA
CBHW061330190326
41458CB00011B/3954